Master Techniques in Orthopaedic Surgery®

Soft Tissue Surgery

SECOND EDITION

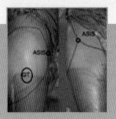 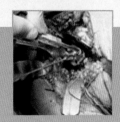 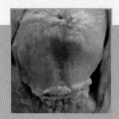 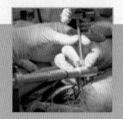 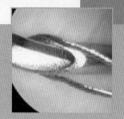
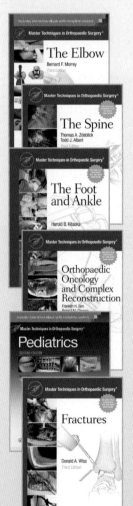
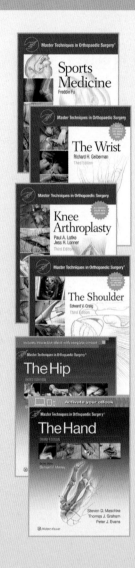
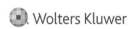

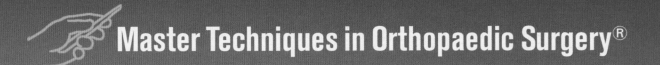

Master Techniques in Orthopaedic Surgery®

Soft Tissue Surgery

SECOND EDITION

Steven L. Moran, MD
Professor and Chair of Plastic Surgery
Professor of Orthopedic Surgery
Mayo Clinic
Rochester, Minnesota

S. Andrew Sems, MD
Assistant Professor of Orthopedics
Department of Orthopedic Surgery
Mayo Clinic
Rochester, Minnesota

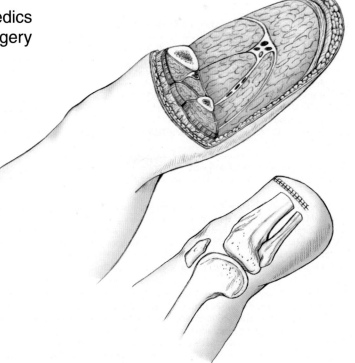

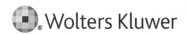
Wolters Kluwer

Philadelphia • Baltimore • New York • London
Buenos Aires • Hong Kong • Sydney • Tokyo

Acquisitions Editor: Brian Brown
Product Development Editor: Dave Murphy
Marketing Manager: Daniel Dressler
Production Project Manager: David Saltzberg
Design Coordinator: Stephen Druding
Manufacturing Coordinator: Beth Welsh
Prepress Vendor: SPi Global

2nd edition

Library of Congress Cataloging-in-Publication Data
Names: Moran, Steven L., editor. | Sems, S. Andrew (Stephen Andrew), editor.
Title: Soft tissue surgery / [edited by] Steven L. Moran, Dr. S. Andrew Sems.
Other titles: Soft tissue surgery (Moran) | Master techniques in orthopaedic surgery.
Description: Second edition. | Philadelphia : Wolters Kluwer, [2017] | Series: Master techniques in orthopaedic surgery | Includes bibliographical references and index.
Identifiers: LCCN 2016028693 | ISBN 9781496329004
Subjects: | MESH: Soft Tissue Injuries—surgery | Extremities—surgery | Skin Transplantation | Surgical Flaps | Wound Healing
Classification: LCC RD93 | NLM WO 700 | DDC 617.4/7—dc23 LC record available at https://lccn.loc.gov/2016028693

Contributors

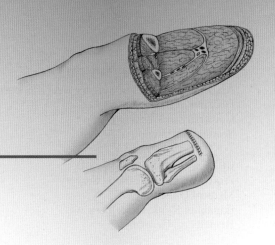

Julie E. Adams, MD
Associate Professor of Orthopedic Surgery
Mayo Clinic
Rochester, Minnesota

Annika Arsalan-Werner, MD
Department of Plastic, Hand, and Reconstructive
    Surgery
BG Trauma Center
Frankfurt, Germany

Morad Askari, MD
Assistant Professor of Surgery
Division of Plastic and Reconstructive Surgery,
    Department of Surgery
Assistant Professor of Orthopedics
Division of Hand and Upper Extremity Surgery,
    Department of Orthopedics
University of Miami Miller School of Medicine
Miami, Florida

Karim Bakri, MBBS
Assistant Professor of Plastic Surgery
Department of Plastic Surgery
Mayo Clinic
Rochester, Minnesota

Emily A. Borsting, MD
Department of Plastic Surgery
University of California, Irvine
Irvine, California

Sean R. Cantwell, BS
Mayo Medical School
Mayo Clinic
Rochester, Minnesota

Brian T. Carlsen, MD
Associate Professor
Departments of Orthopedic Surgery
    and Plastic Surgery
Mayo Clinic
Rochester, Minnesota

Harvey Chim, MD
Assistant Professor of Clinical Surgery
Division of Plastic Surgery
University of Miami Miller School of Medicine
Miami, Florida

Jimmy H. Chim, MD
Resident Fellow
Division of Plastic and Reconstructive Surgery
Department of Surgery
University of Miami
Jackson Memorial Hospital
Miami, Florida

Randall R. DeMartino, MD, MS
Assistant Professor of Surgery
Division of Vascular and Endovascular Surgery
Mayo Clinic
Rochester, Minnesota

Seth D. Dodds, MD
Associate Professor, Hand and Upper Extremity Surgery
Department of Orthopaedic Surgery and Rehabilitation
University of Miami
Millier School of Medicine
Bascom Palmer Institute
Miami, Florida

Bassem T. Elhassan, MD
Department of Orthopedic Surgery
Mayo Clinic
Rochester, Minnesota

David Elliot, MA (Oxon), BM, BCh
Consultant Hand and Plastic Surgeon
St. Andrew's Centre for Plastic Surgery
Broomfield Hospital
Chelmsford, England, United Kingdom

Ida K. Fox, MD
Assistant Professor of Plastic and Reconstructive Surgery
Department of Surgery
Washington University School of Medicine in St Louis
Saint Louis, Missouri

Jeffrey B. Friedrich, MD, FACS
Associate Professor of Surgery and Orthopaedics
Division of Plastic Surgery
University of Washington
Seattle, Washington

Günter Germann, MD, PhD
Professor of Plastic-Hand Surgery
Medical Director
Ethianum Klinic Heidelberg
Heidelberg, Germany

Oren Goltzer, MD
Resident
Department of Orthopaedic Surgery
Banner University Medical Center
Phoenix, Arizona

Kanu Goyal, MD
Assistant Professor
Division of Hand Surgery
Department of Orthopedic Surgery
The Ohio State University Wexner Medical Center
Columbus, Ohio

Douglas P. Hanel, MD
Professor of Orthopedic Surgery
University of Washington
Harborview Medical Center
Seattle, Washington

Christin A. Harless, MD
Resident Physician
Division of Plastic and Reconstructive Surgery
Department of Surgery
Mayo Clinic
Rochester, Minnesota

Mark Henry, MD
Hand and Wrist Center of Houston
Houston, Texas

James P. Higgins, MD
Chief of Hand Surgery
The Curtis National Health Center
MedStar Union Memorial Hospital
Baltimore, Maryland

Thomas F. Higgins, MD
Professor of Orthopaedic Surgery
Chief of Orthopaedic Trauma
University of Utah
Salt Lake City, Utah

John B. Hijjawi, MD
Assistant Professor of Plastic and Reconstructive
   Surgery
Medical College of Wisconsin
Milwaukee, Wisconsin

Matt T. Houdek, MD
Department of Orthopedic Surgery
Mayo Clinic
Rochester, Minnesota

Lance Jacobson, MD
Department of Orthopaedics
University of Utah School of Medicine
Salt Lake City, Utah

David J. Jacofsky, MD
Chairman and CEO
The CORE Institute
Phoenix, Arizona

Kathleen M. Kollitz, MD
Department of Orthopedic Surgery
Mayo Clinic
Rochester, Minnesota

Salvatore C. Lettieri, MD
Division of Plastic Surgery
Mayo Clinic
Rochester, Minnesota

L. Scott Levin, MD, FACS
Paul B. Magnuson Professor of Bone and Joint Surgery
Chairman, Department of Orthopaedic Surgery
Professor of Surgery (Plastic Surgery)
Perelman School of Medicine
University of Pennsylvania
Philadelphia, Pennsylvania

Laura W. Lewallen, MD
Department of Orthopedic Surgery
Mayo Clinic
Rochester, Minnesota

Chih-Hung Lin, MD
Vice-President
Head Professor of Plastic Surgery
Plastic Surgery Laboratory Director
Chang-Gung Memorial Hospital and Chang-Gung University
Taoyuan County, Taiwan

M. Claire Manske, MD
Fellow
Hand and Microvascular Surgery
Department of Orthopedic Surgery
University of Washington
Harborview Medical Center
Seattle, Washington

Samir Mardini, MD
Professor of Surgery
Mayo Clinic College of Medicine
Program Director
Division of Plastic Surgery
Department of Surgery
Mayo Clinic
Rochester, Minnesota

Hassan R. Mir, MD, MBA, FACS
Associate Professor and Director of Orthopaedic Residency
  Program
Department of Orthopaedic Surgery
University of South Florida
Director of Orthopaedic Trauma Research
Florida Orthopaedic Institute
Tampa, Florida

Anita T. Mohan, MRCS, MBBS, BSc
Division of Plastic Surgery
Mayo Clinic
Rochester, Minnesota

Amy M. Moore, MD
Assistant Professor of Plastic and Reconstructive Surgery
Washington University School of Medicine in St. Louis
St. Louis, Missouri

Steven L. Moran, MD
Professor and Chair of Plastic Surgery
Professor of Orthopedic Surgery
Mayo Clinic
Rochester, Minnesota

Emily N. Morgan, MD
Hand Fellow
Walter Reed National Military Medical Center
Bethesda, Maryland

Mohamed Morsy, MBBCh, MSc
Division of Plastic Surgery
Department of Surgery
Mayo Clinic
Rochester, Minnesota
Assistant Lecturer
Department of Orthopedic Surgery
Assiut University Hospital
Assiut University
Assiut, Egypt

George Nanos III, MD
Commander, Medical Corps, United States Navy
Navy Orthopaedic Specialty Leader and Associate
  Professor in Surgery
Walter Reed National Military Medical Center and the
  Uniformed Services University of the Health Sciences
Bethesda, Maryland

Jason Nascone, MD
Associate Professor of Orthopaedics
University of Maryland Medical Center
Baltimore, Maryland

Michael W. Neumeister, MD, FRCS(C), FACS
Professor and Chair
Department of Surgery
Southern Illinois University School of Medicine
Springfield, Illinois

Gustavo S. Oderich, MD
Professor of Surgery
Division of Vascular and Endovascular Surgery
Mayo Clinic
Rochester, Minnesota

William C. Pederson, MD, FACS
Professor of Surgery, Orthopaedics, and Pediatrics
Baylor College of Medicine
Head of Hand and Microsurgery
Texas Children's Hospital
Houston, Texas

Nicholas Pulos, MD
Fellow
Division of Hand and Microvascular Surgery
Department of Orthopaedic Surgery
Mayo Clinic
Rochester, Minnesota

Marco Rizzo, MD
Chair, Division of Hand Surgery
Professor of Orthopedic Surgery
Mayo Clinic
Rochester, Minnesota

Handel R. Robinson, MD, FACS
Assistant Professor of Surgery
University of Miami Miller School of Medicine
Miami, Florida

Peter S. Rose, MD
Associate Professor
Department of Orthopedic Surgery
Mayo Clinic
Rochester, Minnesota

S. Raja Sabapathy, MS, MCh, DNB, FRCS Ed, MAMS
Chairman
Department of Plastic Surgery, Hand and Reconstructive
  Microsurgery and Burns
Ganga Hospital
Coimbatore, Tamil Nadu, India

Michel Saint-Cyr, MD, FRCS
Director
Division of Plastic Surgery
Wigley Professorship in Plastic Surgery
Baylor Scott and White
Temple, Texas

Christopher J. Salgado, MD
Professor of Surgery
Division of Plastic Surgery
Section Chief
University of Miami Hospital
Miami, Florida

Roy W. Sanders, MD
Professor and Chairman
University of South Florida Department of Orthopaedic
  Surgery
President
Florida Orthopaedic Institute
Tampa, Florida

Michael Sauerbier, MD, PhD
Professor and Chair
Department for Plastic, Hand and Reconstructive Surgery
BG Trauma Center
Frankfurt, Germany

Ryan W. Schmucker, MD
Institute for Plastic Surgery
Southern Illinois University School of Medicine
Springfield, Illinois

S. Andrew Sems, MD
Assistant Professor of Orthopedics
Department of Orthopedic Surgery
Mayo Clinic
Rochester, Minnesota

Frances Sharpe, MD
Assistant Clinical Professor of Orthopedic Surgery
Department of Orthopedic Surgery
University of Southern California, Keck School of Medicine
Los Angeles, California
Attending Orthopedic Surgeon
Department of Orthopedic Surgery
Southern California Permanente Medical Group
Fontana, California

Alexander Y. Shin, MD
Professor and Consultant
Division of Hand and Microvascular Surgery
Department of Orthopedic Surgery
Mayo Clinic
Rochester, Minnesota

Thomas C. Shives, MD
Consultant
Department of Orthopedic Surgery
Mayo Clinic
Rochester, Minnesota

Adam Sierakowski, RCS (Plast), BSc(Hons), MBBS
Consultant Hand and Plastic Surgeon
St. Andrew's Centre for Plastic Surgery
Broomfield Hospital
Chelmsford, England, United Kingdom

Franklin H. Sim, MD
Department of Orthopedic Surgery
Mayo Clinic
Rochester, Minnesota

Scott P. Steinmann, MD
Professor of Orthopedics
Mayo Clinic
Rochester, Minnesota

Milan Stevanovic, MD, PhD
Professor of Orthopedics and Surgery
Director, Joseph H. Boyes Hand Fellowship
Department of Orthopedic Surgery
University of Southern California, Keck School of Medicine
Los Angeles, California

Yoo Joon Sur, MD, PhD
Associate Professor
Department of Orthopedic Surgery
Uijeongbu St. Mary's Hospital
College of Medicine
The Catholic University of Korea
Uijeongbu, Gyeonggi-do, South Korea

Shian Chao Tay, MBBS, FRCS, FAMS, MSc
Adjunct Associate Professor, Duke-NUS Medical School
Senior Consultant, Department of Hand Surgery, Singapore General Hospital
Director, Biomechanics Laboratory, Singapore General Hospital
Singapore

Lam Chuan Teoh, MD
Clinical Associate Professor
Hand Section
Orthopaedic Surgery
Tan Tock Seng Hospital
Singapore

Ryan P. Ter Louw, MD
Department of Plastic Surgery
Georgetown University Hospital
Washington, District of Columbia

Laura K. Tom, MD
Division of Plastic and Reconstructive Surgery
University of Washington
Seattle, Washington

Norman S. Turner, MD
Consultant
Department of Orthopedic Surgery
Mayo Clinic
Rochester, Minnesota

Ian L. Valerio, MD, MS, MBA, FACS
Associate Professor
Division Chief of Burn, Wound, and Trauma in Plastic Surgery
Department of Plastic Surgery
The Ohio State University Wexner Medical Center
Columbus, Ohio

Hari Venkatramani, MS, MCh, EDHS
Senior Consultant
Department of Plastic, Hand and Reconstructive Microsurgery
Ganga Hospital
Coimbatore, Tamil Nadu, India

Sang-Hyun Woo, MD, PhD
W Institute for Hand and Reconstructive Microsurgery
W Hospital
Daegu, South Korea

Eduardo A. Zancolli, MD
Orthopaedics and Traumatology
National Academy of Medicine
Buenos Aires, Argentina

Yasmina Zoghbi, MS
MD Candidate
University of Miami School of Medicine
Miami, Florida

Preface

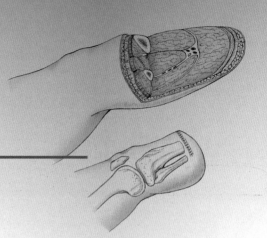

We are honored that the interest in the first edition of *Master Techniques in Orthopaedic Surgery: Soft Tissue Surgery* has created the demand for a second edition. The key educational goal of the text is to demonstrate how to avoid wound problems in the realm of orthopedic surgery and how to cover them if they occur. While the principles of surgical exposure and surgical debridement have not changed, a great deal has advanced our ability to manipulate the wound environment in preparation for wound closure. We have provided needed updates on the use of negative pressure wound therapy and newer wound dressings, which can prepare the wound for skin grafting and closure. Additional chapters have been devoted to coverage of difficult areas such as the elbow, back, and knee, and newer concepts of soft tissue coverage including the keystone flaps, perforator flaps, and free flaps have been added to increase the surgeon's armamentarium for managing soft tissue loss. We have again drawn on the vast experience of our military colleagues to discuss the topics of debridement and early wound management as these are the cornerstones of a successful outcome.

The book's format continues to emphasize the pertinent anatomy, indications, and surgical approach to allow the reader to quickly incorporate these techniques into his or her practice. We have expanded the content with video techniques for some of our newer chapters. As with the first edition, the reader may not feel comfortable performing every procedure described, but at least, you will know what to expect or request during specialist consultation. Finally, the book has continued to emphasize the importance of a team approach to the management of these difficult issues. Over the past decade, we have utilized this team approach at the Mayo Clinic to provide our patients with a broad perspective for the management of bone and soft tissue injury, allowing for improved limb salvage and successful outcomes.

Stephen L. Moran, MD
S. Andrew Sems, MD

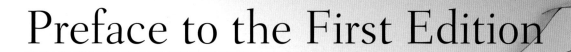

Preface to the First Edition

Over the past 30 years, options for the soft tissue management of traumatic defects have increased with an improved understanding of pedicled flaps, the advent of microsurgery, and the development of negative pressure sponge therapy. Wound complications have decreased due to advances in antibiotic therapy and better debridement techniques. Improved knowledge of surgical anatomy has helped to develop surgical incisions, which provide better exposure while preserving regional blood supply. Despite these advances, there is still a need for every surgeon to know the techniques of debridement, soft tissue management, and proper incision placement—for these are the foundation of successful surgery.

The educational goal of this text is to demonstrate how to avoid wound problems and how to cover wound problems if they should occur. Chapters illustrate pertinent anatomy, indications and contraindications for specific incisions, and methods for flap coverage in cases of soft tissue loss. Step-by-step accounts of the technical details are provided to carry out these exposures and procedures so that readers will feel they are watching over the shoulder of the contributing author in the operating room. Contributors are experienced in both soft tissue and bony management. Though all surgeons may not feel comfortable with performing all procedures presented in this book, they will at least know what they can expect or request during specialist consultation. This volume of the *Master Techniques in Orthopaedic Surgery* series focuses on the management of the soft tissues as they relate to orthopedic trauma but is a text designed for all traumatologists, orthopedic surgeons, plastic surgeons, and anyone who has had the pleasure (or displeasure) of taking care of a difficult wound.

Steven L. Moran, MD
William P. Cooney III, MD

Series Preface

Since its inception in 1994, the *Master Techniques in Orthopaedic Surgery* series has become the gold standard for both physicians in training and experienced surgeons. Its exceptional success may be traced to the leadership of the original series editor, Roby Thompson, whose clarity of thought and focused vision sought "to provide direct, detailed access to techniques preferred by orthopedic surgeons who are recognized by their colleagues as 'masters' in their specialty," as he stated in his series preface. It is personally very rewarding to hear testimonials from both residents and practicing orthopedic surgeons on the value of these volumes to their training and practice.

A key element of the success of the series is its format. The effectiveness of the format is reflected by the fact that it is now being replicated by others. An essential feature is the standardized presentation of information replete with tips and pearls shared by experts with years of experience. Abundant color photographs and drawings guide the reader through the procedures step by step.

The second key to the success of the *Master Techniques* series rests in the reputation and experience of our volume editors. The editors are truly dedicated "masters" with a commitment to share their rich experience through these texts. We feel a great debt of gratitude to them and a real responsibility to maintain and enhance the reputation of the *Master Techniques* series that has developed over the years. We are proud of the progress made in formulating the third edition volumes and are particularly pleased with the expanded content of this series. Six new volumes will soon be available covering topics that are exciting and relevant to a broad cross section of our profession. While we are in the process of carefully expanding *Master Techniques* topics and editors, we are committed to the now-classic format.

The first of the new volumes is—Relevant Surgical Exposures—which I have had the honor of editing. The second new volume is Pediatrics. Subsequent new topics to be introduced are Soft Tissue Reconstruction, Management of Peripheral Nerve Dysfunction, Advanced Reconstructive Techniques in the Joint, and finally Essential Procedures in Sports Medicine. The full library thus will consist of 16 useful and relevant titles. I am pleased to have accepted the position of series editor, feeling so strongly about the value of this series to educate the orthopedic surgeon in the full array of expert surgical procedures. The true worth of this endeavor will continue to be measured by the ever-increasing success and critical acceptance of the series. I remain indebted to Dr. Thompson for his inaugural vision and leadership, as well as to the *Master Techniques* volume editors and numerous contributors who have been true to the series style and vision. As I indicated in the preface to the second edition of The Hip volume, the words of William Mayo are especially relevant to characterize the ultimate goal of this endeavor: "The best interest of the patient is the only interest to be considered." We are confident that the information in the expanded *Master Techniques* offers the surgeon an opportunity to realize the patient-centric view of our surgical practice.

Bernard F. Morrey, MD

The creation of this text was the result of a tremendous effort of many people. Wolters Kluwer has provided us with incredible resources and a dedicated knowledgeable staff. We are deeply indebted to the team of Brian Brown, Executive Editor; Grace Caputo, Developmental Editor; and David Murphy, Editorial Coordinator. We are also deeply indebted to our medical illustrator Bernie Kida, who has provided the countless hours of work bringing the surgeons' sketches to life. We would also like to thank Dr. Bernard Morrey for giving us the opportunity to produce this second edition. Finally, we are deeply indebted to our countless who have provided insightful, organized, and beautifully illustrated chapters explaining the techniques involved in these reconstructive procedures. It is through their hard work that we are able to provide you with this text.

Steven L. Moran and S. Andrew Sems

Contents

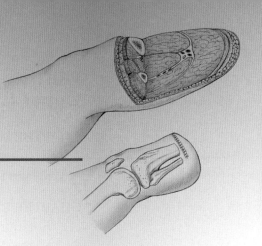

PART I Overview and Foundation 1

PART II   Management of Soft Tissues Within the Upper Extremity   90

PART III   Management of Soft Tissues Within the Hand and Wrist   196

Video List

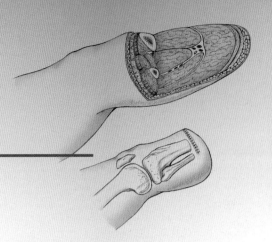

Chapter 4 Integra Bilayer Wound Matrix in Combination with Negative Pressure Wound Therapy for Treatment of Extremity Wounds

Case 1. Eleven videos illustrating details of the surgical technique and the Integra BWM application in 41-year-old woman with a history of common variable immune deficiency and multiple prior cutaneous bacterial infections who suffered a necrotizing soft tissue infection of her left dorsal forearm.

Video 4-1 Case 1 Dorsal Forearm Part 1
Video 4-1 Case 1 Dorsal Forearm Part 2
Video 4-1 Case 1 Dorsal Forearm Part 3
Video 4-1 Case 1 Dorsal Forearm Part 4
Video 4-1 Case 1 Dorsal Forearm Part 5
Video 4-1 Case 1 Dorsal Forearm Part 6
Video 4-1 Case 1 Dorsal Forearm Part 7
Video 4-1 Case 1 Dorsal Forearm Part 8
Video 4-1 Case 1 Dorsal Forearm Part 9
Video 4-1 Case 1 Dorsal Forearm Part 10
Video 4-1 Case 1 Dorsal Forearm Part 11

Case 2. Four videos illustrating details of surgical technique in a 40-year-old man who sustained an open distal tibial shaft fracture with an open medial leg wound that necessitated soft tissue coverage.

Video 4-2 Case 2 Medial Leg Part 1
Video 4-2 Case 2 Medial Leg Part 2
Video 4-2 Case 2 Medial Leg Part 3
Video 4-2 Case 2 Medial Leg Part 4

Case 3. One video illustrating ankle motion after healed soft tissue reconstruction with Integra DRT and skin graft in a 33-year-old man who sustained multiple gunshot wounds.

Video 4-3 Case 2 Achilles Tendon

Chapter 33 Propeller Flaps and Keystone Flaps in the Lower Extremity

Video 33-1 Propeller Flap: Planning, design, and harvest of a peroneal perforator flap for a lower leg traumatic defect with bony exposure.
Video 33-2 Keystone Flap: Planning and harvest of a keystone flap for an anterior thigh defect following sarcoma resection.

Chapter 34 Fasciotomies of the Lower Extremity

Video 34-1 From Maryland Shock Trauma shows the fascial compartment release of the lower extremity for compartment syndrome. (Provided by Dr. Jason Nascone.)

Chapter 42 Replantation of Digits

Video 42-1 Replantation of Digits

PART I
OVERVIEW AND FOUNDATION

1 Why Wounds Fail to Heal

Christin A. Harless and Steven L. Moran

Surgical wound complications can be a significant problem resulting in prolonged hospital stay, reoperations, and significant morbidity for our patients. Often, the surgeon can predict preoperatively which patients will have problems healing wounds or will need additional soft tissue coverage. Surgical planning should include not only the surgical approach but also an assessment of the patient's healing risks. It is our hope that preoperative risk reduction may avoid wound healing complications.

Prevention of wound healing complications starts with an understanding of the healing process. Risk factors can be recognized and modified. Techniques and practices that are proven to prevent wound infections must be employed. This chapter focuses on understanding wound healing and identifying patients at risk for wound complications; we also attempt to offer the surgeon a means to minimize risk factors for complications through surgical technique and preoperative planning.

PHASES OF WOUND HEALING

Surgically induced wounds heal in several stages. The wound passes through phases of coagulation, inflammation, matrix synthesis and deposition, angiogenesis, fibroplasia, epithelialization, contraction, and remodeling. These processes have been grouped into the three main stages of wound healing: inflammation, fibroplasia, and maturation. Interruption in any one of these stages can lead to wound healing complications.

The inflammatory phase of wound healing involves cellular responses to clear the wound of debris and devitalized tissue. Increased capillary permeability and leukocyte infiltration occur secondary to inflammatory mediators and vasoactive substances. Polymorphonuclear cells (PMNs) are the first cell population in the wound followed by mononuclear leukocytes, which mature into wound macrophages. Inflammatory cells clean the wound of harmful bacteria and devitalized tissue. Adequate tissue oxygen tension is necessary for the release of oxygen free radicals by neutrophils. Following the initial introduction of PMNs into the wound, lymphocytes enter the wound in great number, clearing the wound of old neutrophils and secreting important cytokines and chemoattractants for fibroblasts. Fibronectin and hyaluronate deposition from fibroblasts in the first 24 to 48 hours provides scaffolding for further fibroblast migration.

The fibroblast proliferation phase starts within the initial 2 to 3 days as large populations of fibroblasts migrate to the wound. Fibroblasts secrete a variety of substances necessary for wound healing, including large quantities of glycosaminoglycans and collagen. Ground substance formed from the four main glycosaminoglycans (hyaluronic acid, chondroitin 4 sulfate, dermatan sulfate, and heparin sulfate) acts as an amorphous gel that is necessary for collagen aggregation. Collagen levels rise for approximately 3 weeks, corresponding to increasing tensile strength within the wound. After 3 weeks, the rate of degradation equals the rate of deposition. Angiogenesis is an important aspect of the fibroblast proliferation phase as it helps to support new cells in the healing wound.

The maturation phase starts around 3 weeks and lasts up to 2 years. It is characterized by collagen remodeling and wound strengthening. Collagen is the principal building block of connective tissue and has at least 13 different types. Types I to IV are the most common in the human body. Each has a distinct feature and is found in different levels in many tissues. For example, type III collagen is high in hydroxyproline and low in hydroxylysine. It is commonly found in skin, arteries, bowel wall, and healing wounds. Type I collagen is found in the skin, tendon, and bone, is low in hydroxylysine content, and is the most common collagen type, accounting for more than 90% of body collagen. Early wounds are composed of a majority of type III collagen. As the wound matures, type III collagen is replaced by type I collagen. Collagen cross-linking improves tensile strength. There is a rapid increase in strength of the wound by 6 weeks as the wound reaches 70% of the strength of normal tissue. The wound then gradually plateaus to 80% of normal strength but never returns to preinjury levels.

Wound re-epithelialization occurs as adjacent cells migrate through a sequence of mobilization, migration, mitosis, and cellular differentiation of epithelial cells. Wound contraction starts at about 1 week. It is facilitated by the transformation of certain fibroblasts into myofibroblasts containing α-smooth muscle actin. These cells adhere to the wound margins as well as each other and effect contraction of the wound. These stages are imperative for proper wound healing as interruption of these processes results in chronic wound complications.

RISK FACTORS

The identification of patients at risk for aberrant wound healing allows the surgeon to make appropriate plans for skin closure technique, flap utilization, and postoperative wound management. This will ideally result in modification of risk factors prior to surgery. In cases of chronic diseases or nonmodifiable risk factors, patients must be informed of the increased risk of wound healing complications. The following discussion focuses on commonly encountered risk factors with recommendations to ameliorate their effects.

Diabetes

Patients with diabetes are both more likely to undergo surgery and develop perioperative complications than nondiabetic patients. This leads to longer hospital stay with higher health care costs and increased perioperative mortality. Diabetic patients have increased rates of hypertension, cardiac disease, and renal failure. These factors lead to much higher wound healing complications. Diabetes inhibits wound healing through many mechanisms. It affects small vessels, which are critical in supplying nutrients to the healing wound. Elevated glucose levels also affect a myriad of inflammatory systems. Neutrophil adherence, chemotaxis, phagocytosis, and intracellular bactericidal activity are all impaired. Pseudohypoxia develops as a result of altered redox reactions and vascular permeability secondary to hyperglycemia. Furthermore, glucose is a proinflammatory mediator stimulating cytokine production and inhibiting endothelial nitric oxide levels. This translates clinically into higher infectious complications. *Tight control of glucose in the perioperative period mitigates the postoperative complications seen in the diabetic patient.* This has been found in both the intensive care setting as well as routine operative cases.

Management of patients with diabetes starts in the preoperative period. There is good evidence to suggest that a preoperative hemoglobin A1C of less than 7% drastically decreases postoperative infectious complications. Physicians should aggressively improve glucose management using diet, oral hypoglycemic agents, and insulin as needed. Perioperative management should include sliding scale insulin or continuous insulin infusion to maintain glucose levels below 150 mg/dL. Evidence suggests that improved outcomes are possible with tighter control of glucose levels between 80 and 110 mg/dL in critically ill patients. After dismissal from the hospital, the patient should continue their preoperative diabetic regiment.

Obesity

Obese patients have a higher rate of wound infections, dehiscence, hematomas, seromas, and pressure ulcers. This is thought to be due to multiple factors including difficulty with the operation, altered immune response, increased tension with closure, increased dead space, decreased microperfusion, and decreased mobility postoperatively. Patients should be encouraged to lose weight prior to elective operations. Increased levels of physical activity preoperatively translate to an improved post-operative rehabilitation process. Successful weight loss is difficult to achieve in most patients. This has prompted some surgeons to recommend gastric bypass surgery prior to certain operations such as joint replacement. This has been associated with improved outcomes in hip replacement patients with morbid obesity.

Smoking

Numerous studies have consistently found that smokers have significantly higher rates of wound healing complications than nonsmokers. This is related to several causes including the vasoactive effect of cigarette smoke through the sympathetic alpha receptors, increased levels of carboxy-hemoglobin with a reduction in oxygen-carrying capacity, increased platelet activation leading to microangiopathic thrombosis, increased levels of fibrinogen with decreased fibrinolytic activity, endothelial injury, and increased hemoglobin levels leading to increased blood viscosity. Regardless of the mechanism, the effect is significant. Complication rates of 2.5% to 6% in nonsmokers versus 7.5% to 49% in smokers are reported in the literature.

The increased risk of wound complications in smokers is most pronounced in cases where a large area of tissue is undermined. This is most likely related to failure of the dermal and subdermal plexus supplying the resultant skin flap (Fig. 1-1). Poor outcome in smokers prompts many clinicians to postpone elective procedures until the patient has quit smoking for at least 3 to 4 weeks, particularly if the procedure involves large areas of undermining. Aggressive use of smoking cessation programs should be implemented. Still, other surgeons feel that this would restrict too many patients from receiving necessary surgery. We prefer to delay surgery for 4 weeks prior to elective surgical procedures where soft tissue coverage may be an issue and advocate early referral to a nicotine dependence unit. If smoking cessation is not possible, the patient is informed of the likelihood of additional flap coverage for wound closure and a higher likelihood of postoperative wound complications.

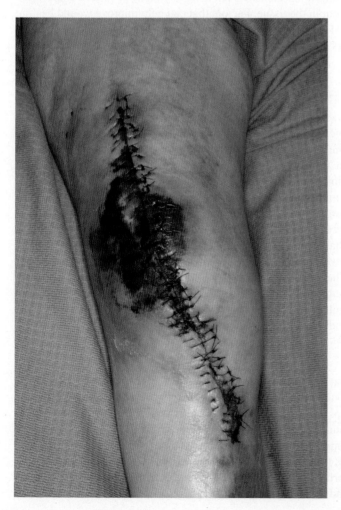

FIGURE 1-1

Following total knee arthroplasty, this 76-year-old diabetic smoker developed wound complications necessitating wound debridement and flap coverage.

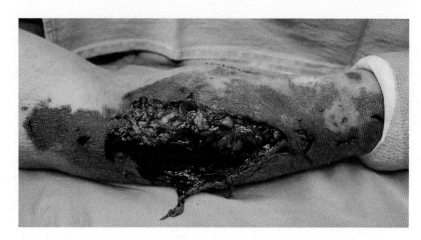

Chronic steroid use leads to increased skin and vessel fragility. This skin avulsion injury occurred in this 76-year-old steroid-dependent man following a fall from a chair.

Immunosuppressive Medications

Patients with intrinsic or acquired immunodeficiencies are at increased risks for wound healing complications. Patients with MHC class II deficiency have impaired wound healing because of altered T-cell immune function. Patient populations at risk for wound healing problems due to altered immune function include patients with hereditary, infectious, and iatrogenic immunodeficiencies.

Corticosteroids inhibit wound healing by their anti-inflammatory effect. Decreased numbers of inflammatory cells are noted at the wound site; delays in collagen synthesis, fibroblast proliferation, angiogenesis, wound contracture rates, and epithelial migration are also observed (Fig. 1-2). Vitamin A has been shown to counteract the effects of steroids on wound healing in all areas except wound contraction and infection. The exact mechanism is not known but may be related to the TGF-beta, IGF-I, and hydroxyproline content in the tissue. Factors that can help improve wound healing in immunocompromised states include prevention of malnutrition, hypoxia, endocrine disorders, anemia, and other metabolic disorders. Dead tissue, foreign bodies, tissue ischemia, and hematoma should be minimized.

Radiation and Chemotherapy

Radiation and chemotherapy are known to cause delays in wound healing. Operations in irradiated fields are particularly problematic due to dense fibrosis and decreased perfusion caused by small-vessel injury (Fig. 1-3). Irradiated fields are more susceptible to infection and delayed healing. Postoperative radiation initiated after the initial 3 to 4 weeks of primary wound healing does not seem to have marked an effect on wound healing but can lead to contracture, wound breakdown, and flap necrosis. Neoadjuvant chemotherapy can alter wound healing, especially in cases where chemotherapy has led to neutropenia. Surgery would be ideally delayed until full recovery of platelets and leukocytes. Healing seems to proceed normally in patients who receive their chemotherapy 3 to 4 weeks after surgery, as the wound has been allowed to proceed through the first stages of healing. Certain chemotherapeutic agents, however, can have a negative effect on wound healing far longer than 4 weeks; for example, Avastin (bevacizumab), which inhibits vascular endothelial growth factor, has an extremely long half-life ranging from days 11 to 50 and has been shown to inhibit wound healing when given in the neoadjuvant setting. Surgeons should have a good understanding of specific complications associated with individual chemotherapeutic regimens.

Malnutrition

It has been known for many years that malnutrition has deleterious effects on wound healing. Loss of nutrients alters host immunity through decreased T-cell function, phagocytosis, complement, and antibody levels. Certain patient groups are at particular risk of malnutrition. Severe catabolic states can be induced after multisystem trauma, sepsis, and burns. Significant increases in metabolic rate can also follow uncomplicated abdominal surgery (increase by 10%), uncomplicated injuries such as femoral fracture (20%), peritonitis (40%), and fever (10% for every 18C above normothermia). This is particularly alarming considering the high portion of trauma patients who are unable to eat for extended periods leading up to and following surgery.

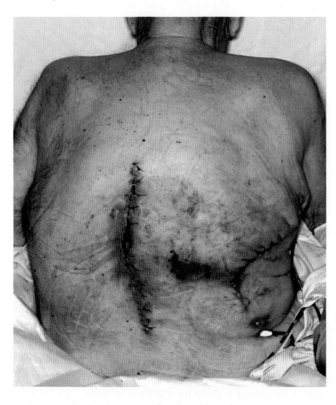

FIGURE 1-3

Signs of trouble in this 80-year-old man who had undergone preoperative radiation with subsequent resection of a spinal tumor and coverage with a latissimus flap. Spinal tumor resection and flap harvest were performed through separate and parallel incisions. The parallel incision in conjunction with the radiation damage led to ischemia within the center portion of skin bridge, which shows signs of early ischemia with epidermolysis and ulceration.

Assessment of nutritional status becomes an important task for the surgeon. Patients at risk include those with moderate weight loss (10% to 20%), severe weight loss (over 20%), and serum albumin below 3.2 to 2.5 g/dL. Other groups include patients with trauma, burns, gastrointestinal (GI) dysfunction, cancer, and fever and those on chemotherapy. Consideration for preoperative total parenteral nutrition (TPN) should be given to patients who are severely malnourished; however, this must be weighted against the risks associated with line infection and liver failure. Prealbumin is a laboratory value that can be followed as a surrogate of albumin due to its shorter half-life.

Postoperatively, patients should be started on a diet as soon as possible. Rapid diet advancement has been shown to decrease postoperative complications and decrease hospital stay. In patients who are unable to restart a diet but have a functioning GI tract, tube feeds should be administered. TPN should be started early on patients who are expected to not tolerate GI feeds. The benefit-risk ratio of TPN is equal for patients with normal metabolic demands after 1 week of fasting or inability to take oral intake. Patients with hypermetabolic states can benefit from earlier initiation of TPN.

Peripheral Vascular Disease

Peripheral artery disease is present in an estimated 0.9% of patients aged 40 to 49 compared with 15% to 29% of patients over the age of 70. Risk factors for the development of PVD include diabetes mellitus, hyperlipidemia, cigarette smoking, and hypertension. Patients at risk for PVD should be screened with blood pressure measurements of the arm and ankle to determine the patient's ankle brachial index; a normal value should produce a ratio above 0.9. Symptoms of PVD include claudication, rest pain, atypical leg pain, and ischemic tissue loss. Aggressive lifestyle and risk factor modification is indicated to prevent progression of disease and death from cardiovascular or cerebrovascular events. These patients should undergo cardiac risk evaluation as perioperative myocardial infarction and stroke are very common.

Wounds in the setting of peripheral vascular disease heal very slowly and can be difficult to manage. Patients with nonhealing wounds in spite of maximal medical management should undergo evaluation for revascularization or flap coverage if vital structures are exposed. Amputation may be considered in the absence of target vessels for revascularization. Transcutaneous oxygen measurements in peripheral occlusive disease can be helpful to determine healing potential. $TcPO_2$ levels greater than 30 mm Hg correlate with a high likelihood of healing, whereas levels less than 15 mm Hg rarely heal. CT angiograms can be used to evaluate the status of blood vessels within the zone of injury for evidence of occlusive disease. Prior to performing any type of flap closure for wounds in the patients with peripheral vascular disease, we routinely get CT angiograms (Fig. 1-4).

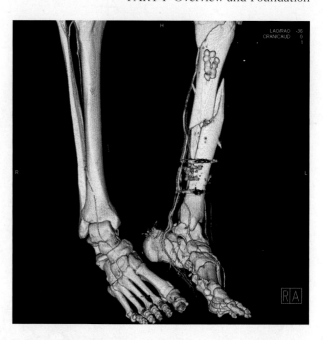

FIGURE 1-4

CT angiogram with three-dimensional reconstruction in a patient following comminuted tibial fracture. Image shows patency of posterior tibial vessels but shows occlusion of anterior tibial vessel, most likely due to trauma. CT angiograms are helpful in identifying vessel occlusion due to trauma or peripheral vascular disease.

Infection

Surgical site infections are a major impediment to wound healing and contribute to substantial morbidity and mortality. Postoperative infections increase the hospital length of stay by 7 to 10 days and increase charges by $2,000 to $5,000. Rates of surgical infections vary by type of procedure, health of the patient, and skill of the surgeon. Wound classification corresponds with expected rates of infection as follows: clean (1.3% to 2.9%), clean contaminated (2.4% to 7.7%), contaminated (6.4% to 15.2%), and dirty (5.1% to 40%). Other risk factors for the development of postoperative infections include diabetes, obesity, smoking, steroids, malnutrition, colonization with *S. aureus*, preoperative hospitalization, and patient health.

The most important factors that can be used to prevent surgical site infections are timely use of preoperative antibiotics and operative technique. Other practices that are helpful include preoperative showering with antimicrobial soap, scrubbing and draping the patient with sterile drapes, handwashing, gloving, and the use of sterile gowns, masks, and hats by surgical personnel. These practices are aimed at reducing the amount of skin-associated bacteria. Pathogens are not eliminated because approximately 20% of bacteria reside in the hair follicles and sweat glands where antiseptics do not reach. Although numerous studies have been aimed at identifying the best skin antiseptic, a systematic review failed to show superiority of one antiseptic over another.

Preoperative antibiotics administered within 2 hours of incision correlate strongly with the lowest rate of infections. Choices of antibiotics along with common pathogens are listed in Table 1-1.

TABLE 1-1	Antimicrobial Prophylaxis for Surgery		
Nature of Operation	**Common Pathogens**	**Recommended Antimicrobials**	**Adult Dosage before Surgery[a]**
Cardiac	*Staphylococcus aureus*	Cefazolin *or*	1–2 g IV[c]
	S. epidermis	Cefuroxime *or*	1.5 g IV[c]
		Vancomycin[b]	1 g IV
Gastrointestinal			
Esophageal, gastroduodenal	Enteric gram-negative bacilli, gram-positive cocci	*High risk[d] only:* cefazolin[e]	1–2 g IV
Biliary tract	Enteric gram-negative bacilli, enterococci, clostridia	*High risk[f] only:* cefazolin[e]	1–2 g IV
Colorectal	Enteric gram-negative bacilli, anaerobes, enterococci	*Oral:* neomycin + erythromycin base[g] *or* metronidazole[g]	
		Parenteral: cefoxitin[e] *or* cefazolin	1–2 g IV
		plus metronidazole[e] *or* ampicillin/	1–2 g IV
		sulbactam	0.5 g IV
			3 g IV

TABLE 1-1   Antimicrobial Prophylaxis for Surgery (Continued)

Nature of Operation	Common Pathogens	Recommended Antimicrobials	Adult Dosage before Surgery[a]
Appendectomy, nonperforated[h]	Enteric gram-negative bacilli, anaerobes, enterococci	Cefoxitin[e] or cefazolin *plus* metronidazole[e] or ampicillin/sulbactam[e]	1–2 g IV 1–2 g IV 0.5 g IV 3 g IV
Genitourinary	Enteric gram-negative bacilli, enterococci	*High risk only*[i]: ciprofloxacin	500 mg PO or 400 mg IV
Gynecologic and obstetric			
Vaginal, abdominal, or laparoscopic hysterectomy	Enteric gram-negative bacilli, anaerobes, group B strep, enterococci	Cefoxitin[e] or cefazolin[e] or ampicillin/sulbactam[e]	1–2 g IV 1–2 g IV 3 g IV
Cesarean section	Same as for hysterectomy	Cefazolin[e]	1–2 g IV after cord clamping
Abortion	Same as for hysterectomy	*First trimester, high risk*[j]: aqueous penicillin G or doxycycline *Second trimester*: cefazolin[e]	2 mill units IV 300 mg PO[k] 1–2 g IV
Head and neck			
Incisions through oral or pharyngeal mucosa	Anaerobes, enteric gram-negative bacilli, S. aureus	Clindamycin *plus* Gentamicin or Cefazolin	600–900 mg IV 1.5 mg/kg IV 1–2 g IV
Neurosurgery	S. aureus, S. epidermis	Cefazolin or Vancomycin[b]	1–2 g IV 1 g IV
Ophthalmic	S. epidermis, S. aureus, streptococci, enteric gram-negative bacilli, Pseudomonas spp.	Cefazolin or Gentamicin or tobramycin or ciprofloxacin or gatifloxacin or Levofloxacin or Moxifloxacin or Ofloxacin or Neomycin-gramicidin-polymyxin B	100 mg subconjunctivally multiple drops Topically over 2–24 h
Orthopedic	S. aureus, S. epidermis	Cefazolin[l] or Cefuroxime[l] or Vancomycin[b,l]	1–2 g IV 1.5 g IV 1 g IV
Thoracic (noncardiac)	S. aureus, S. epidermis, streptococci, enteric gram-negative bacilli	Cefazolin or Cefuroxime or Vancomycin[b]	1–2 g IV 1.5 g IV 1 g IV
Vascular			
Arterial surgery involving a prosthesis, the abdominal aorta, or a groin incision	S. aureus, S. epidermis, enteric gram-negative bacilli	Cefazolin or Vancomycin[b]	1–2 g IV 1 g IV
Lower extremity amputation for ischemia	S. aureus, S. epidermis, enteric gram-negative bacilli, clostridia	Cefazolin or Vancomycin[b]	1–2 g IV 1 g IV

[a]Parenteral prophylactic antimicrobials can be given as a single IV dose begun 60 min or less before the operation. For prolonged operations (>4 h), or those with major blood loss, additional intraoperative doses should be given at intervals 1 times the half-life of the drug for the duration of the procedure in patients with normal renal function. If vancomycin or a fluoroquinolone is used, the infusion should be started 60 to 120 min before the initial incision in order to minimize the possibility of an infusion reaction close to the time of induction of anesthesia and to have adequate tissue levels at the time of incision.

[b]Vancomycin is used in hospitals in which methicillin-resistant S. aureus and S. epidermis are a frequent cause of postoperative wound infection, for patients previously colonized with MRSA or for those who are allergic to penicillins or cephalosporins. Rapid IV administration may cause hypotension, which could be especially dangerous during induction of anesthesia. Even when the drug is given over 60 min, hypotension may occur; treatment with diphenhydramine (Benadryl and others) and further slowing of the infusion rate may be helpful. Some experts would give 15 mg/kg of vancomycin to patients weighing more than 75 kg, up to a maximum of 1.5 g, with a slower infusion rate (90 min for 1.5 g). To provide coverage against gram-negative bacteria, most Medical Letter consultants would also include cefazolin or cefuroxime in the prophylaxis regimen for patients not allergic to cephalosporins; ciprofloxacin, levofloxacin, gentamicin, or aztreonam, each one in combination with vancomycin, can be used in patients who cannot tolerate a cephalosporin.

[c]Some consultants recommend an additional dose when patients are removed from bypass during open-heart surgery.

[d]Morbid obesity, esophageal obstruction, decreased gastric acidity, or gastrointestinal motility.

[e]For patients allergic to penicillins and cephalosporins, clindamycin with gentamicin, ciprofloxacin, levofloxacin, or aztreonam is a reasonable alternative.

[f]Age >70 years, acute cholecystitis, nonfunctioning gall bladder, obstructive jaundice, or common duct stones.

[g]After appropriate diet and catharsis, 1 g of neomycin plus 1 g of erythromycin at 1 PM, 2 PM, and 11 PM or 2 g of neomycin plus 2 g of metronidazole at 7 PM and 11 PM the day before an 8 AM operation.

[h]For a ruptured viscus, therapy is often continued for about 5 days. Ruptured viscus in postoperative setting (dehiscence) requires antibacterials to include coverage of nosocomial pathogens.

[i]Urine culture positive or unavailable, preoperative catheter, transrectal prostatic biopsy, and placement of prosthetic material.

[j]Patients with previous pelvic inflammatory disease, previous gonorrhea, or multiple sex partners.

[k]Divided into 100 mg 1 h before the abortion and 200 mg one and half hour later.

[l]If a tourniquet is to be used in the procedure, the entire dose of antibiotic must be infused prior to its inflation.

Reproduced from Antimicrobial prophylaxis for surgery. *Treat Guide Med Lett*. 2006;4(52):83–88, with permission.

Endocarditis prophylaxis may need to be added in susceptible patients. In spite of clear benefits with the use of preoperative antibiotics, compliance is not perfect. Institutional policies should be constructed to promoting 100% compliance.

Hair removal is commonly performed prior to surgical procedures; however, most studies have shown that this is not necessary and is associated with an increased risk of surgical site infections. If hair removal is preferred, clippers or depilatory creams are safer than shaving and should be used just prior to skin incision. Razors are associated with microtrauma to the skin and should not be used secondary to increased infection rates.

Hypothermia has benefits of decreasing tissue oxygen consumption and is tissue protective in cardiac bypass and organ transplant. However, hypothermia may predispose to infection through cutaneous vasoconstriction. It has been shown that perioperative normothermia is associated with reduced rates of surgical site infections.

Several health care improvement initiative studies have shown that surgical site infection surveillance is effective in reducing the infection rates. The mechanism is unknown, but many researchers postulate that surveillance is associated with a greater awareness of sterile technique. Operative teams more rapidly recognize problems and find solutions. Surgeons should seek a program at their institution for health care improvement and operative safety. The Institute for Healthcare Improvement (IHI) is a nonprofit organization that leads health care improvement initiatives. They organized the 100,000 Lives Campaign to implement changes in US hospitals, which focused on increased compliance to four areas: appropriate use of antibiotics, removing razors from operative rooms, maintaining glucose control, and ensuring perioperative normothermia. Hospitals in compliance with these changes reported a 27% reduction in surgical site infections.

SURGICAL TECHNIQUE

Numerous studies aimed at discovering risk factors for complications have identified surgeons as independent risk factors. This could be due to numerous factors including clinical judgment, baseline characteristics of patient populations, procedure type, and surgical technique. There is no doubt that meticulous surgical technique can improve outcomes. This is particularly important when dealing with a patient at risk for complications. Excess intraoperative blood loss has been associated with surgical site infections and poor wound healing. Blood loss leading to hypotension with subsequent vasoconstriction and tissue hypoxia is one explanation for increased wound healing complications. Techniques aimed at improving sterility, minimizing tissue destruction, maintaining meticulous hemostasis, improving speed and accuracy, minimizing foreign body placement, and attention to closure are expected to reduce complications.

The choice of suture and method of suture placement can also have an impact on wound healing. There is a wide array of suture types. In general, sutures can be divided by life expectancy (permanent, absorbable, fast absorbable) and consistency (braided vs. monofilament). Permanent suture is indicated in situations where suture absorption is not desired (e.g., vasculature anastomosis). Drawbacks include development of suture abscesses and chronic infection. Stitch abscesses are less problematic with absorbable sutures but may lose strength prior to tissue healing. Braided sutures are strong, hold well, and are easy to tie. However, they are more prone to infection than monofilament. Braided sutures may also cause tissue tearing as in the case of venous repairs. Monofilament sutures are smooth and resist infection but are less forgiving and require more knots to resist slippage.

Placement of sutures can also contribute to wound compromise. Simple interrupted sutures and vertical mattress sutures produce less wound edge ischemia than running and horizontal mattress sutures when tissue viability is in question. Horizontal mattress sutures placed under excessive tension can further impede blood supply to wound edges resulting in infection, necrosis, or dehiscence. Care must be taken not to incorporate or impinge vasculature pedicles when placing sutures.

NEW TECHNOLOGY TO IMPROVE WOUND HEALING

Hyperbaric Oxygen Therapy

Inherent to healing any surgical wound is the requirement for adequate perfusion and oxygenation of the tissues. Various technologies have been developed to increase the oxygenation of compromised wounds. In recent years, hyperbaric oxygen therapy has become a recognized modality to manage struggling wounds or wounds with compromised healing capacity. Hyperbaric oxygen therapy involves breathing 100% oxygen at pressures greater than atmospheric pressure, thereby delivering an increased partial pressure of oxygen to the tissues. This, in turn, stimulates the production of reactive oxygen species and reactive nitrogen species. At the cellular level, these reactive gas species serve as signaling molecules in transduction cascades for a variety of growth factors, cytokines, and hormones. Resultantly, wounds experience an increase in collagen synthesis, growth factor production, angiogenesis, fibroblast activation, improved cell migration, and stimulation of stem/progenitor cells. An evidence-based review of hyperbaric oxygen therapy on flaps and grafts in animal models identified a substantial amount of data supporting the application of hyperbaric oxygen. Unfortunately, to date, there are few well-designed clinical studies to provide guidelines for its clinical use. One recent review of eight trials looking at the use of hyperbaric oxygen for acute wounds found that seven of the eight trials supported the use of hyperbaric oxygen therapy in compromised acute wounds. Most wounds, regardless of cause, treated with hyperbaric oxygen therapy receive some degree of clinical benefit.

Laser-Assisted Indocyanine Green Fluorescent Angiography

Adequate perfusion of the wound is crucial for wound healing. Intraoperatively, clinical assessment of wound perfusion relies on subjective parameters including color, capillary refill, and dermal edge bleeding. These findings are difficult to quantitate and often rely on surgeon experience; however, recent advances in laser angiography can now allow for observation of real-time skin perfusion. Assessment of skin flap perfusion with intraoperative laser-assisted indocyanine green fluorescent angiography (LA-ICGA) allows for real-time visualization of skin perfusion providing the surgeon with an objective marker to facilitate surgical decision making. For example, if LA-ICGA shows minimal or no perfusion to the skin edges, the surgeon can either resect the underperfused skin or release and/or modify the closure to improve perfusion. This technology is based on the intravenous administration of indocyanine green dye, which absorbs light in the near-infrared spectrum. Various intraoperative imaging systems have been developed all of which contain an 806-nm diode laser to provide near-infrared illumination. The SPY System (LifeCell, New Jersey) is one such intraoperative imaging system commonly used in plastic and reconstructive surgery. A recent randomized controlled trial utilized the SPY System to evaluate the effect wound closure technique (running subcuticular, vertical mattress, or skin staples) had on perfusion of the wound edges following total knee arthroplasty. This study was able to show that running subcuticular suture technique had the least detrimental effect to wound edge blood flow and in concept could lead to fewer woundless problems following total knee arthroplasty. This information enables the surgeon to be proactive in preventing wound healing complications directly related to perfusion.

CONCLUSION

Prevention of wound complications starts with the preoperative evaluation, during which risk factors for wound healing are identified and modified prior to elective procedures. In the traumatic setting and in the established soft tissue deficit, patient factors such as glucose control and nutritional status can be optimized to maximize the patient's healing potential. With this chapter as an introduction, the following chapters will address evaluation of traumatic wounds followed by techniques for recruiting or mobilizing surrounding tissue to close large wounds and soft tissue deficits.

PEARLS AND PITFALLS

- Tight control of glucose in the perioperative period mitigates the postoperative complications seen in the diabetic patient. Preoperative hemoglobin A1C of less than 7% drastically decreases postoperative infections.
- Vitamin A has been shown to counteract the effects of steroids on wound healing in all areas except wound contraction and infection.
- Healing seems to proceed normally in patients who receive their chemotherapy 3 to 4 weeks after surgery, as the wound has been allowed to proceed through the first stages of healing.

- Following massive weight loss, patients can be at risk of wound complications due to malabsorption. Those at risk for wound complications include those with moderate weight loss, severe weight loss, and serum albumin of 3.2 to 2.5 g/dL.
- TcPO$_2$ levels greater than 30 mm Hg correlate with a high likelihood of healing, whereas levels less than 15 mm Hg rarely heal. CT angiograms can be used to evaluate the status of blood vessels within the zone of injury for evidence of occlusive disease.

RECOMMENDED READING

Anstead GM. Steroids, retinoids, and wound healing. *Adv Wound Care.* 1998;11(6):277–285.

Bratzler DW. The Surgical Infection Prevention and Surgical Care Improvement Projects: promises and pitfalls. *Am Surg.* 2006;72(11):1010–1016.

Bratzler DW, Houck PM, Richards C, et al. Use of antimicrobial prophylaxis for major surgery: baseline results from the National Surgical Infection Prevention Project. *Arch Surg.* 2005;140(2):174–182.

Christensen K, Klarke M. Transcutaneous oxygen measurement in peripheral occlusive disease. An indicator of wound healing in leg amputation. *J Bone Joint Surg Br.* 1986;68(3):423–426.

Cruse PJ, Foord R. The epidemiology of wound infection: a 10-year prospective study of 62,939 wounds. *Surg Clin North Am.* 1980;60(1):27–40.

Culver DH, Horan TC, Gaynes RP, et al. Surgical wound infection rates by wound class, operative procedure, and patient risk index. National Nosocomial Infections Surveillance System. *Am J Med.* 1991;91(3B):152S–157S.

Dauwe PB, Pulikkottil BJ, Lavery L, et al. Does hyperbaric oxygen therapy work in facilitating acute wound healing: a systematic review. *Plast Reconstr Surg.* 2014;33(2):208e–215e.

Dellinger EP, Hausmann SM, Bratzler DW, et al. Hospitals collaborate to decrease surgical site infections. *Am J Surg.* 2005;190(1):9–15.

Drake DB, Oishi SN. Wound healing considerations in chemotherapy and radiation therapy. *Clin Plast Surg.* 1995;22(1):31–37.

Dronge AS, Perkal MF, Kancir S, et al. Long-term glycemic control and postoperative infectious complications. *Arch Surg.* 2006;141(4):375–380.

Edwards PS, Lipp A, Holmes A. Preoperative skin antiseptics for preventing surgical wound infections after clean surgery. *Cochrane Database Syst Rev.* 2004;3:CD003949.

Eskes A, Ubbink DT, Lubbers M, et al. Hyperbaric oxygen therapy for treating acute surgical and traumatic wounds. *Cochrane Database Syst Rev.* 2013;12:CD008059.

Etter JF, Burri M, Stapleton J. The impact of pharmaceutical company funding on results of randomized trials of nicotine replacement therapy for smoking cessation: a meta-analysis. *Addiction.* 2007;102(5):815–822.

Falanga V. Wound healing and its impairment in the diabetic foot. *Lancet.* 2005;66(9498):1736–1743.

Friedman HI, Fitzmaurice M, Lefaivre JF, et al. An evidence-based appraisal of the use of hyperbaric oxygen on flaps and grafts. *Plast Reconstr Surg.* 2006;117(7 suppl):175S–190S.

Gislason H, Søreide O, Viste A. Wound complications after major gastrointestinal operations: the surgeon as a risk factor. *Dig Surg.* 1999;16:512–514.

Goonetilleke KS, Siriwardena AK. Systematic review of peri-operative nutritional supplementation in patients undergoing pancreaticoduodenectomy. *J Pancreas.* 2006;7(1):5–13.

Haley RW, Culver DH, White JW, et al. The efficacy of infection surveillance and control programs in preventing nosocomial infections in US hospitals. *Am J Epidemiol.* 1985;121(2):182–205.

Krueger JK, Rohrich RJ. Clearing the smoke: the scientific rationale for tobacco abstention with plastic surgery. *Plast Reconstr Surg.* 2001;108(4):1063–1073.

Kuri M, Nakagawa M, Tanaka H, et al. Determination of the duration of preoperative smoking cessation to improve wound healing after head and neck surgery. *Anesthesiology.* 2005;102(5):892–896.

Kurz A, Sessler DI, Lenhardt R. Perioperative normothermia to reduce the incidence of surgical-wound infection and shorten hospitalization. Study of Wound Infection and Temperature Group. *N Engl J Med.* 1996;334(19):1209–1215.

Mainous MR, Deitch ED. Nutrition and infection. *Surg Clin North Am.* 1994;74(3):659–676.

Manassa EH, Hertl CH, Olbrisch RR. Wound healing problems in smokers and nonsmokers after 132 abdominoplasties. *Plast Reconstr Surg.* 2003;111(6):2082–2087.

Mangram AJ, Horan TC, Pearson ML, et al.; Centers for Disease Control and Prevention (CDC) Hospital Infection Control Practices Advisory Committee. Guideline for prevention of surgical site infection, 1999. *Am J Infect Control.* 1999;27(2):97–132.

Marti A, Marcos A, Martinez JA. Obesity and immune function relationships. *Obes Rev.* 2001;2(2):131–140.

Mehrabi A, Fonouni H, Wente M, et al. Wound complications following kidney and liver transplantation. *Clin Transpl.* 2006;20(s17):97–110.

Mishriki SF, Law DJ, Jeffery PJ. Factors affecting the incidence of postoperative wound infection. *J Hosp Infect.* 1990;16(3):223–230.

Norgren L, Hiatt WR, Dormandy JA, et al. Inter-society consensus for the management of peripheral arterial disease (TASC II). *Int Angiol.* 2007;26(2):81–157.

Parvizi J, Trousdale RT, Sarr MG. Total joint arthroplasty in patients surgically treated for morbid obesity. *J Arthroplasty.* 2000;15(8):1003–1008.

Poulsen KB, Bremmelgaard A, Sørensen AI, et al. Estimated costs of postoperative wound infections: a case-control study of marginal hospital and social security costs. *Epidemiol Infect.* 1994;113(2):283–295.

Roeckl-Wiedmann I, Bennett M, Kranke P. Systematic review of hyperbaric oxygen in the management of chronic wounds. *Br J Surg.* 2005;92(1):24–32.

Schaffer M, Bongartz M, Hoffman W, et al. MHC-class-II-deficiency impairs wound healing. *J Surg Res.* 2007;138(1):100–105.

Shapiro M, Munoz A, Tager IB, et al. Risk factors for infection at the operative site after abdominal or vaginal hysterectomy. *N Engl J Med.* 1982;307(27):1661–1666.

Smiley DD, Umpierrez GE. Perioperative glucose control in the diabetic or nondiabetic patient. *South Med J.* 2006;99(6):580–589.

Springfield DS. Surgical wound healing. *Cancer Treat Res.* 1993;67:81–98.

Stadelmann WK, Digenis AG, Tobin GR. Physiology and healing dynamics of chronic cutaneous wounds. *Am J Surg.* 1998;176:26S–38S.

Thom SR. Hyperbaric oxygen: its mechanisms and efficacy. *Plast Reconstr Surg.* 2011;127(suppl 1):131S–141S.

Thornton AD, Winslet M, Chester K. Angiogenesis inhibition with bevacizumab and the surgical management of colorectal cancer. *Br J Surg.* 2006;93(12):1456–1463.

Tran NV, Evans GR, Kroll SS, et al. Postoperative adjuvant irradiation: effects on transverse rectus abdominis muscle flap breast reconstruction. *Plast Reconstr Surg.* 2000;106(2):313–317.

Van den Berghe G, Wouters P, Weekers F, et al. Intensive insulin therapy in critically ill patients. *N Engl J Med.* 2001;345(19):1359–1367.

Wicke C, Halliday B, Allen D, et al. Effects of steroids and retinoids on wound healing. *Arch Surg.* 2000;135(11):1265–1270.

Wilson JA, Clark JJ. Obesity: impediment to wound healing. *Crit Care Nurs Q.* 2003;26(2):119–132.

Windsor A, Braga M, Martindale R, et al. Fit for surgery: an expert panel review on optimising patients prior to surgery, with a particular focus on nutrition. *Surgeon.* 2004;2(6):315–319.

Wyles CC, Jacobson SR, Houdek MT, et al. The Chitranjan Ranawat Award: running subcuticular closure enables the most robust perfusion after TKA: a randomized clinical trial. *Clin Orthop Relat Res.* 2016;474(1):47–56.

Yablon SA, Novick ES, Jain SS, et al. Postoperative transcutaneous oxygen measurement in the prediction of delayed wound healing and prosthetic fitting among amputees during rehabilitation: a pilot study. *Am J Phys Med Rehabil.* 1995;74(3):193–198.

Zenn MR. Fluorescent angiography. *Clin Plast Surg.* 2011;38(2):293–300.

2 Initial Evaluation and Management of Complex Traumatic Wounds

Emily N. Morgan and George Nanos III

The principles in this chapter are forged from our experience with the treatment of high-energy contaminated wounds resulting from recent overseas military conflicts. The soft tissue injuries discussed within this chapter encompass a broad spectrum of clinical presentations, both acute and chronic. These treatment protocols reflect the ever-growing body of scientific knowledge and technological advances contributing to the successful treatment of our patients. In the following illustrations, we hope to point out the common mistakes and potential pitfalls of operative and perioperative wound management and provide surgeons with a framework for successful treatment of all types of wounds.

INITIAL EVALUATION

A thorough patient evaluation gives the surgeon the information by which to formulate a treatment plan with the best chance for success. A complete and accurate history must include the circumstances leading to the current wound presentation, the mechanism of injury if associated with trauma, underlying medical conditions, current occupational and socioeconomic status, and patient social habits that may have detrimental effects on reconstructive efforts, such as smoking.

In cases of trauma, the energy level, mechanism, location, and time course from injury to presentation are invaluable in predicting prognosis and planning treatment. Medical comorbidities such as underlying cardiopulmonary or peripheral vascular disease, endocrinopathy, neuropathic disease, immunocompromising conditions, psychiatric illness, nutritional deficits, and allergies can negatively impact the success of treatment if not identified and optimized. Medical consultation and comanagement are recommended in these cases. Tetanus status must be addressed in accordance with Centers for Disease Control and Prevention guidelines. Early antibiotics for open fractures are crucial for preventing infection.

Failure to fully recognize the scope of the wound and/or injury can have dire consequences on outcome. A detailed physical examination with critical assessment of vital signs, secondary survey, and multisystem examination is required in all cases to evaluate the wound and exclude other medical conditions or associated injury that may take greater priority in treatment.

In multisystem trauma, the Advanced Trauma Life Support (ATLS) approach, beginning with airway, breathing, and circulation (ABCs), is recommended. Traumatologists or critical care specialists should be the principal coordinators of all initial medical care to ensure appropriate global management of the patient.

Critical attention should be directed to vascular status. If capillary refill and/or pulses are abnormal or absent, or if the mechanism introduces suspicion for vascular injury, Doppler testing and/or perfusion studies must be obtained. Revascularization or repair of vessels should be completed prior to, or concurrent with, surgical wound treatment. A neurological examination should be performed and all deficits clearly documented. In cases of extremity trauma, the surgeon should have a high index of suspicion for compartment syndrome. Compartment pressure monitoring should be performed at regular intervals if the diagnosis is suspected. Emergent compartment release should be performed if indicated. Prophylactic release should be considered in trauma cases with revascularization procedures or in situations requiring transfer to a higher echelon for care during which compartments cannot be monitored or released in an expeditious manner.

Ancillary studies aid in full comprehension of the clinical situation. Plain radiographs should be routinely obtained to evaluate for associated fracture, foreign body, exostosis, osteomyelitis, soft tissue emphysema, vascular calcifications such as those associated with diabetes mellitus, or other factors contributing to or resulting from the overlying wound. CT scans and MRI may provide additional valuable information. Markers of hematologic and immune status, clotting factors, electrolyte and renal function, and adequacy of resuscitation must all be accounted for based on the clinical situation.

Careful documentation of every aspect of the evaluation and treatment must be made, and generous use of medical photography is helpful not only for documentation but also for preoperative planning purposes.

PREOPERATIVE PLANNING

Once the evaluation is complete, the surgeon can formulate a treatment plan and determine if surgical intervention is required. The most important question to consider is whether the surgeon and the facility possess the requisite experience, capability, equipment, and consultative and ancillary services to render optimal treatment (Figs. 2-1 and 2-2). The surgeon must have the technical ability and anatomic knowledge for the given location of the injury. The treating hospital and operating room must also be able to furnish the necessary instruments, implants, and wound treatment dressings. When confronted with cases of multisystem trauma, a multidisciplinary team involving traumatologists, intensivists, medical consultants, infectious disease specialists, and wound care support personnel is generally considered to be mandatory. If unable to meet these basic requirements, the clinical situation should be carefully reviewed and the strongest consideration should be given for referral to a higher level of care.

SURGERY

Patient positioning varies depending on the site of the wound in question. General or regional anesthesia may be employed, and consideration for peripheral nerve blocks should be considered for perioperative pain control. A sterile or nonsterile tourniquet is indispensable to ensure optimal visualization for meticulous, thorough debridement and protection of vital structures. Appropriate broad-spectrum antibiotics should be given as scheduled throughout the surgical procedure.

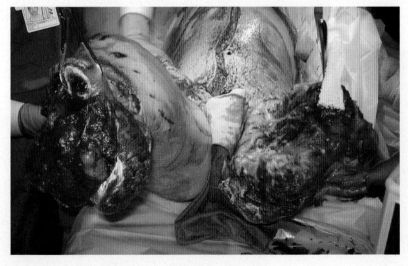

FIGURE 2-1

Injury to multiple extremities and organ systems changes surgical options, increases the risk for systemic problems, and has greater psychological impact. Options for flaps or skin grafts are far more limited. Proper room setup and a hospital team that is prepared to manage comorbidities will facilitate delivery of appropriate care and provide the greatest likelihood of success.

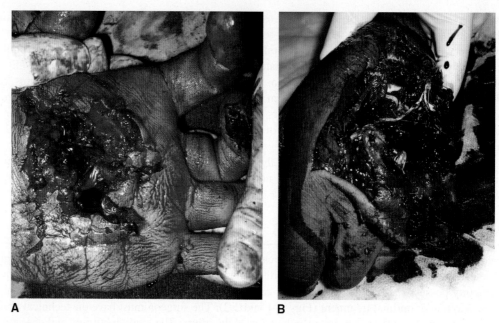

FIGURE 2-2

Palmar **(A)** and dorsal **(B)** views of an acute hand injury produced by an improvised explosive device. Jagged skin margins, necrotic tissue, foreign material, and hematoma are visible. (Courtesy of Dr. Dana Covey, CAPT, MC, USN.)

Debridement

Successful surgical treatment of wounds begins with the meticulous and complete removal of foreign material, infection, and devitalized tissue to create a healthy wound bed (Figs. 2-3 and 2-4). In chronic wounds, we attempt to create an acute wound to promote healing by removing fibrinous and necrotic tissue down to a healthy bleeding bed. In acute injury, wounds must be extended past the zone of injury to ensure complete treatment, and failure to do so significantly limits the effectiveness of debridement. Judicious use of lavage may help remove foreign matter, but care must be taken not to extend the zone of contamination by forcing debris into the surrounding tissue. Use of a tourniquet early in the case is important to best visualize all contaminants and devitalized tissue and avoid injury to vital structures such as nerves and blood vessels. The tourniquet should be released prior to closure or dressing application to confirm removal of all devascularized tissue and excellent hemostasis.

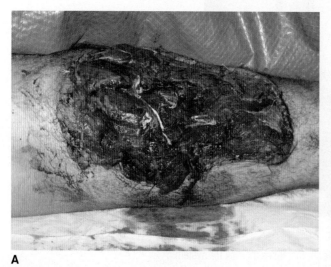

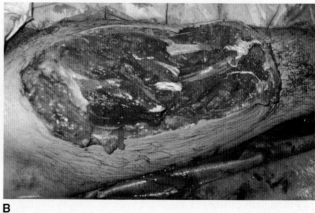

FIGURE 2-3

A: Contaminated lower extremity blast wound with gross contamination. **B:** The same wound after meticulous debridement and irrigation.

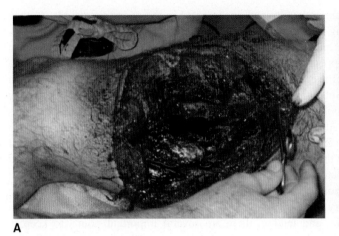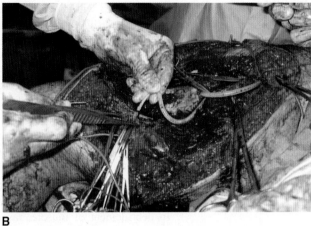

A   B

FIGURE 2-4

A: Lower extremity blast injury wound with gross contamination and associated femoral shaft fracture and segmental femoral artery laceration seen at a forward surgical hospital in a combat setting. **B:** Meticulous debridement of the wound with placement of a vascular shunt.

A systematic approach to wound debridement is required and sharp debridement is the cornerstone of this surgical technique. We prefer the centripetal approach working from superficial tissues to deep, from the margins to the center of the wound; starting at the skin edges, we meticulously work toward the deeper structures within the wound (Fig. 2-5). In general, we prefer excision of all devitalized tissue to a healthy tissue margin instead of a "wait and see" approach to suspect tissue as we feel this limits persistent contamination and infection. All nonviable or suspect tissue is sharply debrided from the wound until a healthy margin of viable tissue is achieved. Every effort to preserve nerves and blood vessels crossing the zone of injury is made, and if they are transected, these structures are

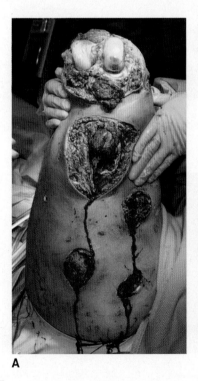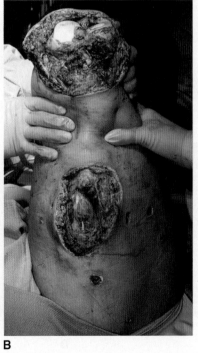

A   B

FIGURE 2-5

Injured by an improvised explosive device, this patient sustained bilateral lower extremity injuries **(A, B)**. Excellent serial wound debridement results in smooth margins, healthy skin and muscle ready for skeletal stabilization, and delayed primary wound closure for the lower extremities.

carefully tagged with dyed monofilament suture and documented in the operative records, so they may be more easily visualized during later wound debridements or reconstructive efforts.

Identification of nonviable tissue remains a challenge, and there is no substitute for experience. In general, nonbleeding skin that appears dusky or does not blanch should be excised, creating a smooth wound margin and avoiding the creation of a ragged skin edge that is difficult for subsequent skin grafting or closure (Fig. 2-6). Subcutaneous fat should be soft and yellow; hard, dusky, or gray fat should be excised. It is also important to keep this tissue moist during deeper debridement, as it will easily desiccate. Injured blood vessels or nerves must be carefully assessed for primary or delayed repair or grafting. Smaller sensory nerve branches may not be amenable to salvage, and if so, we like to pull gentle traction on the proximal end, cut sharply, and allow retraction into the soft tissues. If the stump cannot be retracted, we make every effort to bury it in muscle. To the greatest extent possible, local soft tissues should be used to cover exposed tendons, nerves, and vessels to prevent desiccation and further injury.

In debridement of muscle, fascia, and tendon, there are several important points to keep in mind. Muscle fascia should be stout, white, and shiny, while nonviable fascia will often appear gray or black, fragile, and stringy. When excising fascia, however, great care should be taken as

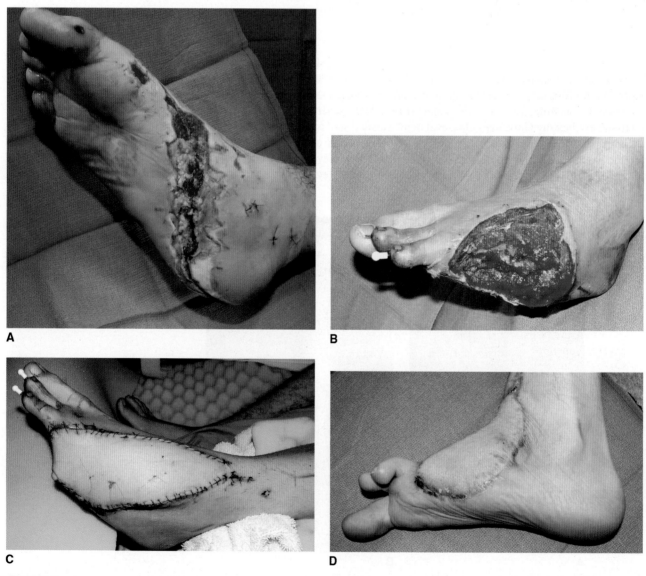

FIGURE 2-6

A: Plantar wound is not ready for closure or coverage; jagged skin and eschar at the wound edge need to be sharply debrided. Serial debridements allow the zone of injury to fully declare itself. **B–D:** In contrast to **(A)**, this foot wound was ready for a lateral thigh free flap as evidenced by the healthy wound bed and margins, minimal residual limb edema, and excellent flap healing.

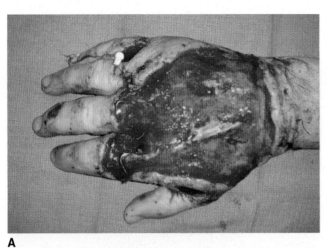
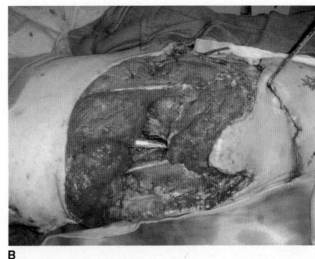

A   **B**

FIGURE 2-7

Right hand **(A)** and left hip **(B)** open wounds ready for further coverage. Note the healthy, smooth skin margins, clean granulating tissue bed, minimal edema, and skeletal stabilization.

neurovascular bundles may be in close proximity. Muscle should be red, shiny, of good consistency, contractile, and bleeding (Fig. 2-7). Squeezing muscle to assess for contractility provides a better assessment of viability than electrical stimulation. Anything to the contrary should be considered for debridement. Knowledge of anatomy and local blood supply is paramount in this endeavor as overly aggressive debridement within muscle compartments may devascularize previously viable tissue. Tendon debridement must be carefully considered due to potential loss of function. Tendons are also easily desiccated, especially if overlying paratenon or sheath is missing.

Devascularized bone fragments must be removed from the wound bed, with the exception of substantial articular fragments, which should be retained in an attempt to preserve the articular surface (Fig. 2-8). Curettes, rongeurs, and burs are useful to check for punctated bleeding indicative of healthy bone that should be preserved. Wound cultures in cases of frank infection can help guide antibiotic selection. In the past, wound cultures taken during serial debridements have been used to guide timing of wound closure; however, this practice has been disproven and is unnecessary in routine debridements.

Several tools have been developed for debridement of chronic wounds and burns that also show promise for acute wounds. One tool we find useful for very large wounds is the VersaJet99 Hydrosurgery System (Smith and Nephew). This device uses negative pressure from a high-speed stream of water across a small aperture at the tip to remove softer tissue and surface debris by suction. Additional lavage is not required when using this device. However, great care must be used around neurovascular structures to avoid injury. This device also can aerosolize bacteria and debris, and therefore, protective measures are required. Coblation devices such as the WoundWand (ArthroCare Corporation) utilize radiofrequency energy to excite electrolytes in saline, allowing the saline to then remove necrotic debris from wounds without causing thermal damage. Both devices have shown promise in reducing bacterial load in wound models, although their clinical efficacy remains unproven.

Strict hemostasis is critical to prevent hematoma and limit further infection and morbidity due to blood loss. Suture ligatures and surgical clips should be used for larger vessels and Bovie or bipolar cautery for smaller vessels. We avoid use of braided suture when possible to avoid harboring bacteria. Judicious use of a tourniquet is helpful to identify and control large bleeding vessels and includes release to assess hemostasis prior to closure, grafting, or dressing application. Adjunctive topical hemostatic agents are available and have been used successfully in some of our most severely war injured patients. Lavage is important for removal of foreign debris and lowering bacterial counts. Reflecting prior published research, we use plain saline for lavage without antibiotics. Based on our experience and the literature, we limit use of pulsatile lavage in the forearm and lower leg and almost never use it in the hand or foot. Pulsatile lavage can further damage delicate tissues, exacerbating the potential for adhesions and functional loss. Usually, bulb irrigation is sufficient when combined with careful debridement.

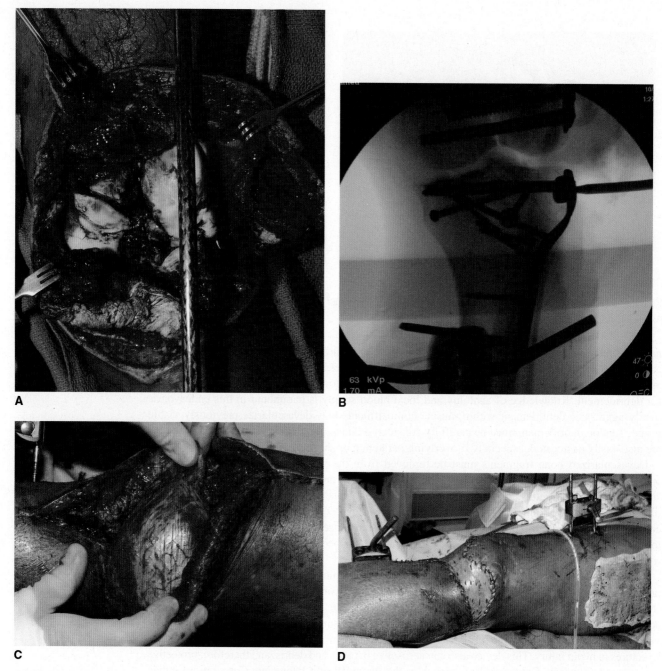

FIGURE 2-8

During serial debridements, every effort is made to preserve substantial articular cartilage fragments. This case also illustrates the value of a team approach, and after extensive surgical time to obtain the best possible open reduction internal fixation (ORIF) of this comminuted intra-articular knee injury **(A, B)**, the plastic surgery service performed a medial gastrocnemius pedicled rotation flap and split-thickness skin grafting **(C, D)**.

Temporary Coverage and Void Fillers

Negative pressure dressings are a great advance in the treatment of wounds not amenable to primary closure (Fig. 2-9). The wound VAC (vacuum-assisted closure) dressing is commonly employed at our institution. It reduces edema and promotes growth of healthy granulation tissue. It also eliminates the need for multiple daily dressing changes, thereby reducing the patient's discomfort and nursing staff workload. Studies regarding the wound VAC's ability to reduce bacterial counts within the wound have had mixed results. Wound VACs have demonstrated improvement in infection following treatment of open fractures in comparison to traditional wet-to-dry dressings. While a useful adjuvant to wound care, the wound VAC cannot substitute for appropriate and comprehensive surgical debridement.

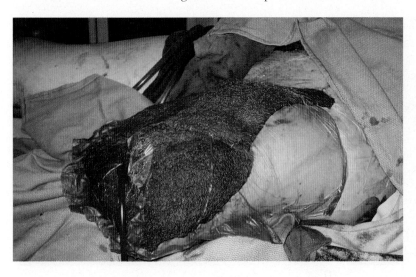

FIGURE 2-9

Use of serial debridements and negative pressure dressings prepare the wound for subsequent flap coverage.

We use portable suction devices supplied by the manufacturer set at the recommended 125 mm Hg intermittent suction. Wall suction can be used if a portable unit is not available, but care must be made to ensure the unit is calibrated to provide a true measurement of suction. We prefer to use less suction in the upper extremity due to the more delicate nature of the soft tissues and have found this to be effective. In the hand, use of the wound VAC is limited to avoid desiccation and injury to vital nerves, blood vessels, and tendons. It can be of benefit when the underlying tissue is robust such as the thenar or hypothenar eminence or when the more delicate tissues are absent due to the injury and debridements (Fig. 2-10). When neurovascular structures are exposed, we employ standard wet-to-dry dressings. In general, we try to limit exposure of blood vessels, nerves, or tendons to the wound VAC and try to rotate available local tissue to provide coverage prior to placement of the wound VAC. Multiple wounds can be treated with the same suction tube using a foam bridging technique. However, care must be taken to cover the skin with the supplied biofilm or Ioban to prevent local skin breakdown.

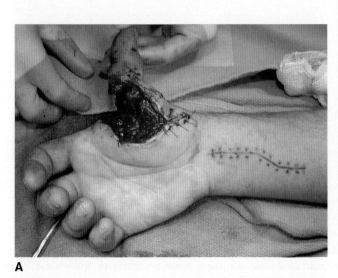

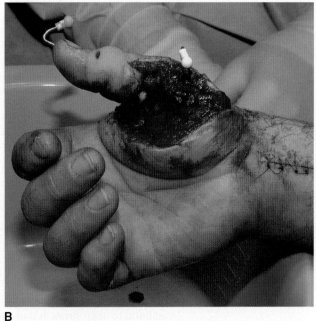

A   **B**

FIGURE 2-10

This case, of a patient who sustained an isolated injury to the thumb from an AK-47 rifle round, illustrates several principles of wound management: thorough debridement preserving vital structures **(A)** and provisional skeletal fixation with K-wires **(B),** the use of negative pressure dressings to prepare the wound for coverage **(C),** and attainment of a closed healthy soft tissue envelope prior to reconstruction **(D–H);** in this case, a local rotation flap and full-thickness skin graft were selected.

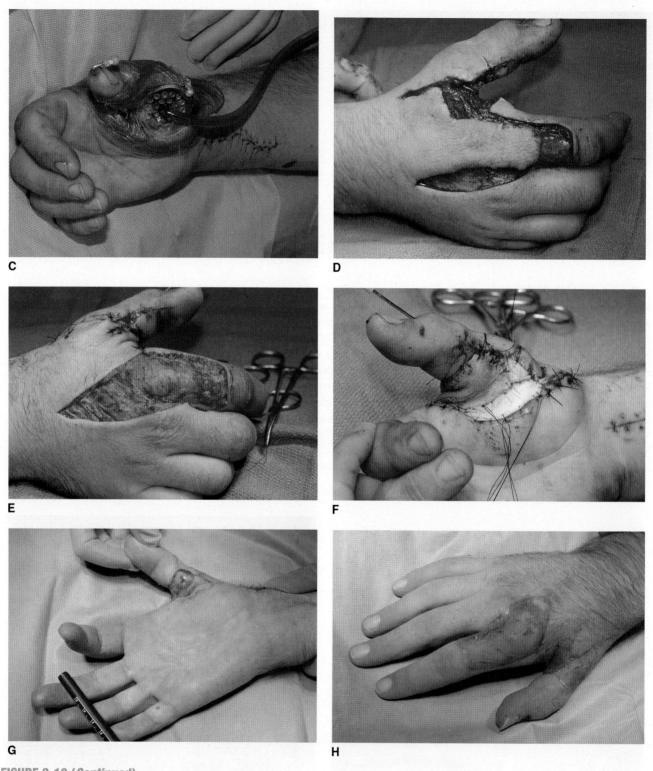

FIGURE 2-10 (*Continued*)

Adequately eliminating contamination and infection is essential to successful wound treatment. In addition to appropriate broad-spectrum antibiotic use, there are many different options available to provide local infection control that can be tailored to the clinical or surgical situation. Antibiotic bead pouches or fracture spacers have been used effectively to provide local infection control in cases of wounds with associated high-energy fracture patterns. The Masquelet technique provides stability and maintains soft tissue space in situations with traumatic bone loss while allowing the formation of a biomembrane, which provides growth factors to allow osseous integration of bone graft during a second-stage procedure, optimally performed at approximately 6 weeks (Fig. 2-11).

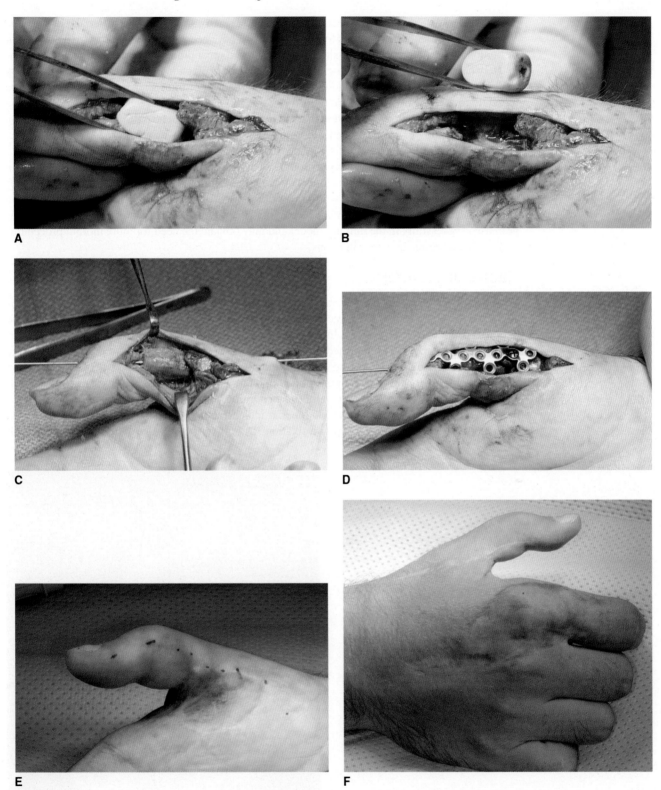

FIGURE 2-11

In cases of contaminated segmental bone loss (same patient as in Fig. 2-8), an antibiotic-impregnated cement spacer can be used to decrease infection risk and maintain space and alignment **(A, B)** until the wound is clean enough for soft tissue reconstruction with bone grafting **(C, D)**. **E, F:** A well-healed soft tissue envelope is necessary prior to performing nerve and tendon grafting.

In highly resistant bacterial infection, silver-impregnated films, colloidal materials, and wound VAC sponges are additional options for the surgeon and have been utilized with great frequency at our institution. Silver-impregnated dressings initially showed great promise in clinical models but unfortunately have not shown any decrease in subsequent wound infection in a recent prospective military trial. Given the increased cost of these dressings and the lack of trials showing clear superiority, we presently reserve the use of silver for refractory cases. For extremely large wounds with highly resistant bacterial colonization or infection that are not amenable to wound VAC treatment, Sulfamylon (mafenide acetate) or Dakin's soaked wet-to-dry dressings have proven effective and resulted in successful wound closure. Infectious disease specialty assistance is recommended in such cases.

Integra (Integra LifeSciences Corporation) has become a useful bridge to closure of wounds with exposed tendon, bone, or other structures that would not normally allow skin graft application following debridement. It provides a scaffold for fibroblasts to create a neodermis upon which a skin graft can successfully be applied. While its cost may be prohibitive to use in some institutions, it has been used successfully in the military model and may obviate the need for more morbid procedures such as flap coverage in many situations.

Choice of Fixation

When wounds are associated with fractures in the acute setting, provisional stabilization should be attempted to maintain soft tissue space, prevent mechanical agitation of the surrounding tissues, and optimize pain control (Fig. 2-12). In general, external fixators are preferred acutely with conversion to definitive fixation as indicated by the injury (Fig. 2-13). In the setting of blast injuries, large amounts of debris are forced into the wounds with tremendous energy and the level of contamination is typically higher than that seen in most blunt open trauma. Our experience has shown the significant potential for widespread osteomyelitis when intramedullary fixation is selected for blast-injured patients. For the distal extremity, as well as periarticular fractures, Kirschner wires are indispensable for temporary and sometimes definitive fixation. Definitive fixation that requires significant soft

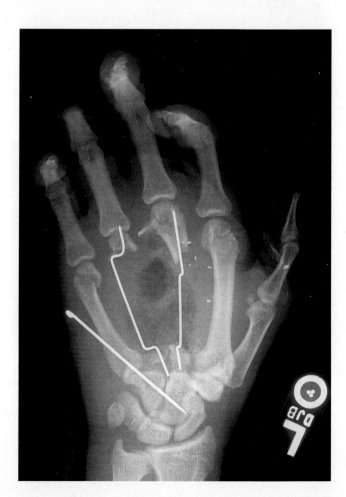

FIGURE 2-12

Fracture stabilization is required to assist in soft tissue management and to maintain structural relationships for subsequent reconstruction. K-wires are especially useful in traumatic, highly contaminated wounds.

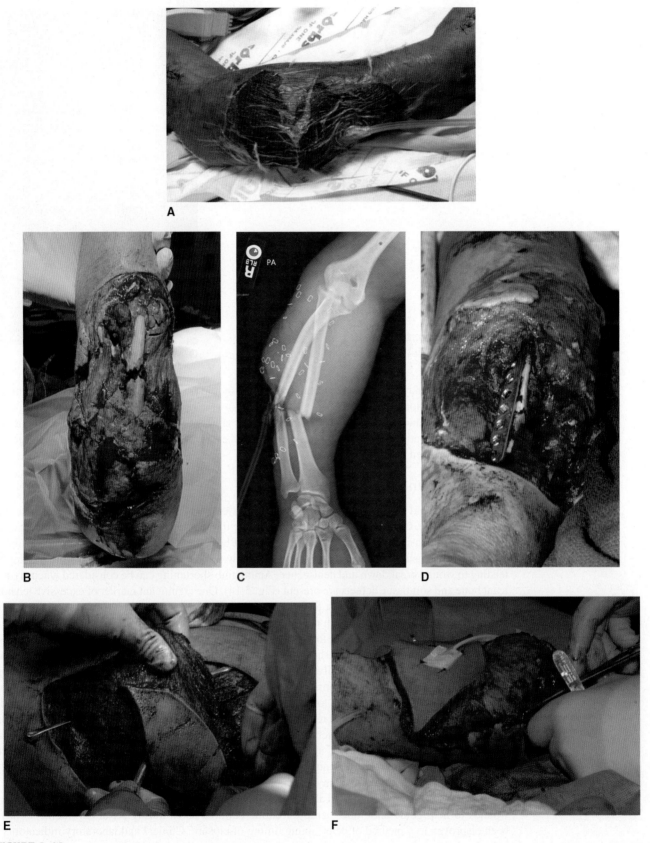

FIGURE 2-13

A–C: Young man with large forearm wound and radius and ulna fractures transferred to a large tertiary care hospital for definitive treatment. He had been treated with serial wound debridements, use of vacuum-assisted closure, and provisional external fixation. **D–F:** He underwent definite fracture fixation concurrent to free tissue transfer utilizing a latissimus dorsi muscle flap.

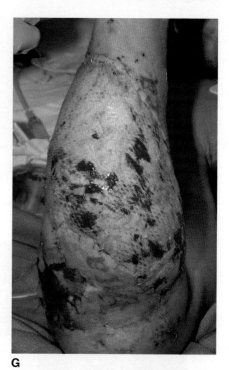

FIGURE 2-13 (*Continued*)
G: Wound after split-thickness skin grafting.   **G**

tissue stripping may only compound the injury and should be entertained with extreme caution as the clinical situation dictates.

For highly contaminated wounds, or when there is concern for viability in critical areas or structures, repeat operative debridement should be planned every 24 to 36 hours until a healthy, vascularized soft tissue bed is achieved.

Timing of Final Closure

When is the wound ready to close? There are several elements that must be present to ensure success of wound closure. Certainly, all nonviable or necrotic tissue must be absent from the wound. It cannot be overemphasized that good vascular flow must be present for healing of tissues. In addition, a tension-free closure must be achieved or blood flow will be compromised at the wound margins leading to wound breakdown and dehiscence. Acute limb shortening can be considered when significant bone and soft tissue defects are present (Fig. 2-14). One significant marker of excessive tension is blanching at the wound margins. Suture type, configuration, and binding tightness of the suture must all be considered. Mattress sutures can be tension relieving and provide nice eversion of wound edges, but one must also recognize that inappropriate orientation or overtightening of these sutures, especially in horizontal mattress fashion, can create ischemia at the wound edges. In wounds prone to tension in the closure, we typically choose nylon suture sized appropriately to the wound in vertical mattress fashion to distribute tension evenly. At times, we will also use "trauma retention"–type sutures using heavier gauge nylon to improve local tension. When excessive tension remains, it is better to leave the wound open and return to the operating room later when tension-free closure can be obtained. In these cases, we prefer a "Jacob's ladder"–type closure with staples and vessel loops, usually over or under a wound VAC sponge or gauze dressings to create gentle traction at the wound edges and promote future closure attempts. While commercial skin traction devices are available (Fig. 2-15), we have not found them to be more effective, and they are certainly more costly.

Absence of infection is also critical to wound closure. We routinely culture infected or suspicious wounds to help guide antibiotic therapy. Routine cultures taken during serial debridements have been disproven as a method of determining timing of closure. Clinical and laboratory indicators of infection such as fever, elevated white blood cell count, and elevated inflammatory markers such as C-reactive protein and erythrocyte sedimentation rate can help guide decision making. Examination of the wound may provide obvious clues like purulent material, unhealthy appearing sheen to the tissues, and foul smell. However, even in the most experienced hands, this determination can be exceedingly difficult; surgeons must rely on the clinical appearance and laboratory markers.

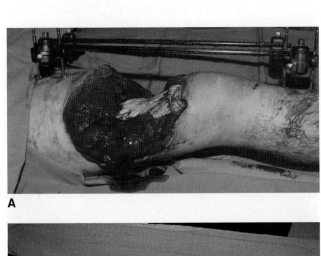

A

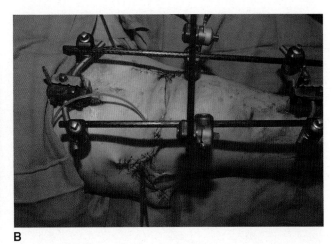

B

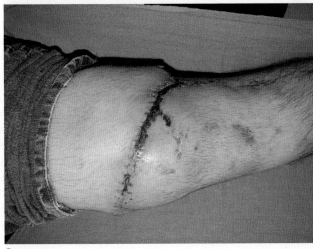

C

FIGURE 2-14

Large wound with a segmental femoral defect **(A)** and associated loss of the anterior thigh soft tissue was managed with acute femoral shortening **(B, C)**. Following soft tissue stabilization, the femur was subsequently lengthened.

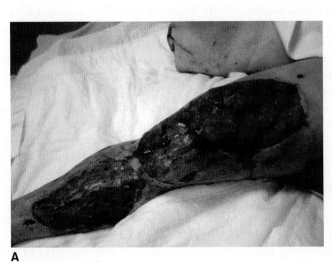

A

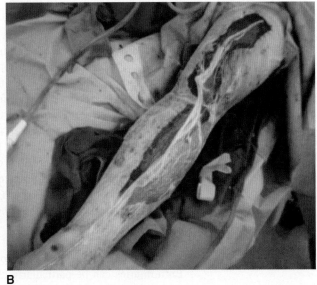

B

FIGURE 2-15

A: In some cases, tension-relieving devices can be used alone or in conjunction with negative pressure dressings to facilitate closure, as in this patient with a large wound involving the anterior aspect of the lower extremity. **B, C:** Serial debridements and use of a Jacob's ladder with a negative pressure dressing allowed eventual primary wound closure. **D:** Tension-relieving slits in the skin of the lower leg were also used in this case.

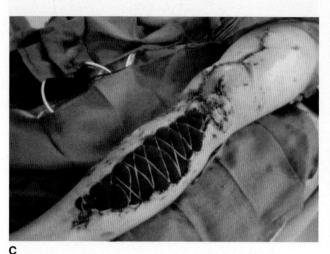

C

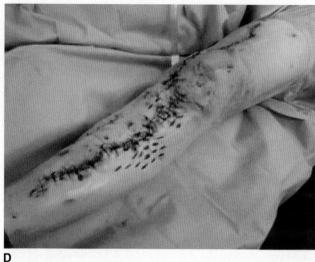

D

FIGURE 2-15 *(Continued)*

Unfortunately, even experienced trauma surgeons can be fooled by the appearance of a wound. During the recent conflict, we have found that severely injured soldiers exhibit systemic inflammatory dysregulation and relative immunosuppression. We believe this accounts for the increased rate of complications that we have seen during the treatment of our wounded warriors. In order to combat this, Forsberg et al. performed a study where serum, wound exudates, tissue samples, and clinical information were collated and analyzed looking at patients whose wounds were successfully versus unsuccessfully closed in order to create a treatment algorithm to help direct the timing of wound closure. This model was then found to be a successful predictive model for patients with similarly severe injuries who were treated at a civilian trauma institution. This algorithm and other research efforts may help provide assistance to surgeons' clinical judgment for determining the correct timing of wound closure in the future.

POSTOPERATIVE MANAGEMENT

Postoperative wound care focuses on protecting the healing wound and optimizing medical care to ensure success. Initially, after wound closure or flap coverage, complete soft tissue rest of the involved extremity by splinting or external fixation should be considered (Figs. 2-16 and 2-17). Care should be taken when splinting to ensure functional positions are maintained; the intrinsic plus position for the hand, full extension at the knee, and a plantigrade position for the ankle can facilitate return to function and reduce the need for secondary procedures. Provisional fracture fixation constructs must be checked to ensure integrity of the construct with modifications made as needed to control motion at the fracture site and ongoing tissue injury.

Elevation of the extremity is critical to reduce local swelling and edema formation. When an external fixation device is present, it can be tied to balanced suspension supported by an overhead trapeze. We avoid the use of slings on the lower extremity due to the potential for pressure necrosis. If an external fixator is not present and a sling is used under the calf, it should always be tied to balanced suspension, not the overhead frame, in this manner. As the patient moves, the pressure on the calf remains constant due to the hanging weights. The skin must be assessed periodically throughout each day (Fig. 2-18).

Mobilization and edema control of the digits should begin as early as possible. Once or twice daily motion begun within 7 days of injury can significantly reduce edema and long-term stiffness. Burn injuries can be particularly challenging due to pain, contracture, and poor durability of the grafted skin (Fig. 2-19). While consultation with physical and occupational therapists aids in maximizing return of function, a balance between early motion and soft tissue rest must be achieved to ensure proper wound healing. Effective communication with these vital specialists will ultimately benefit both the surgeon and patient.

Patient physiologic factors and comorbidities must continually be re-evaluated and optimized in the postoperative period (Figs. 2-20 and 2-21). Markers for infection, hemodynamic status, systemic

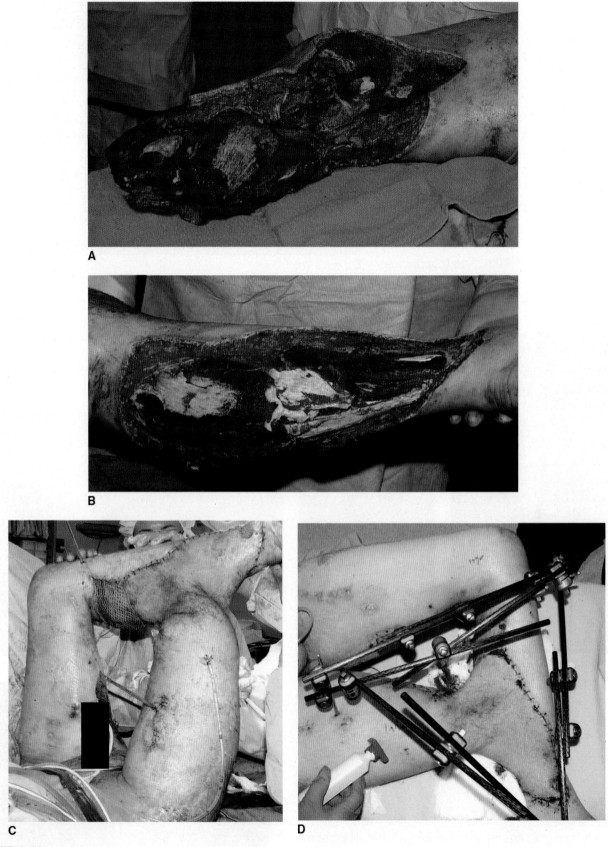

FIGURE 2-16

This patient presented with bilateral lower extremity wounds. His right below-knee amputation lacked adequate soft tissue for closure and prosthetic wear **(A)**; his left lower extremity had a large soft tissue wound **(B)**. The tissue that would have been discarded in a revision amputation to an above-knee level was used in a "cross-leg" flap **(C, D)** with an excellent clinical result **(E)**. Note the external fixator used to protect the flap after inset **(D)**.

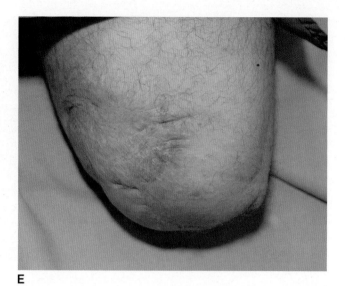

FIGURE 2-16 (*Continued*)   E

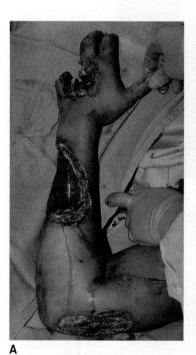

A

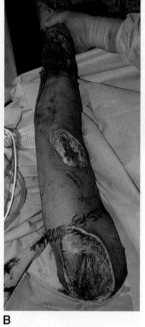

B

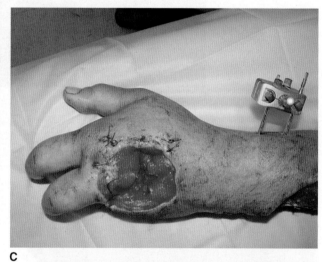

C

FIGURE 2-17

A, B: The same patient as in Figure 2-5 also experienced left upper extremity injuries. **C:** After continued treatment with VAC dressings and ORIF, the left upper extremity wounds are ready for definitive coverage. In this case, flap selection is limited by the injuries. **D:** Bilateral groin flaps were used to obtain coverage of both the hand and forearm wounds. To minimize tension on the pedicles, external fixators were used to stabilize the forearm to the pelvis.

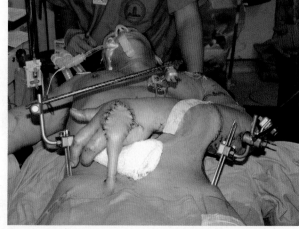

D

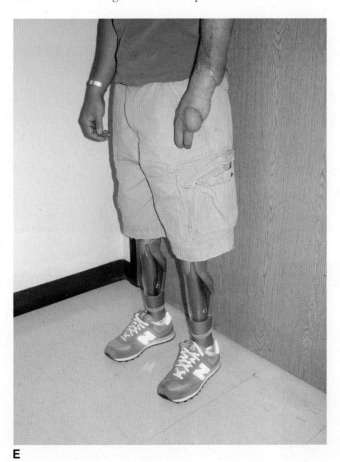

E

FIGURE 2-17 (*Continued*)
E: Healed wounds with durable, healthy coverage.

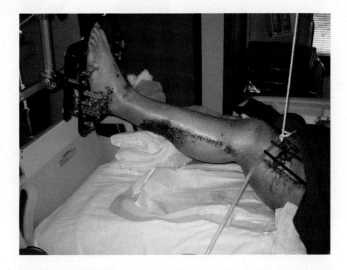

FIGURE 2-18

Elevation is a valuable tool for managing edema. Care must be taken when applying elevation, particularly in the ICU and polytrauma setting, where patients are often sedated and less mobile. This patient, with multiple bilateral lower extremity fractures eventually received a below-knee amputation after development of a full-thickness posterior pressure ulcer. The leg was initially elevated by a sheepskin sling tied directly to the overhead bed frame resulting in significant pressure over the posterior calf. Use of a balanced suspension device secured to an external ankle fixator, as demonstrated in the photo, may have prevented this complication.

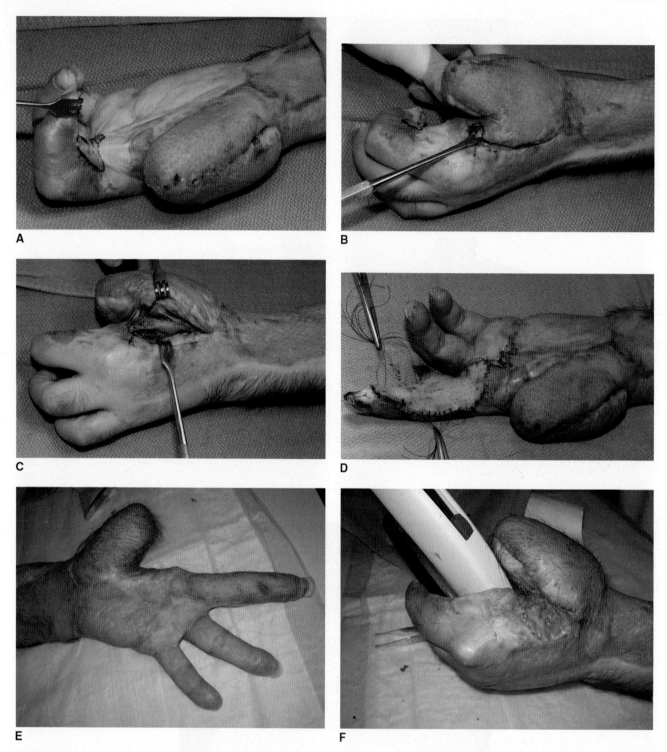

FIGURE 2-19

This patient received severe burns to the upper extremity and chest requiring groin flap to the thumb and multiple skin grafting procedures complicated by recurrent infections with methicillin resistant staphylococcus aureus. Upon presentation to us, he had severe contracture of the long finger **(A)**, erosion of the skin over the residual index metacarpal **(B)**, and essentially no use of the thumb or long finger. Staged reconstruction included thumb metacarpal lengthening, completion of the index ray amputation **(C)**, full-thickness skin grafting to the long finger **(D)**, first web space deepening, thumb carpometacarpal joint arthroplasty, and tendon transfer to the thumb metacarpal for abduction and opposition. **E, F:** The result: a supple, durable soft tissue envelope and functional hand. Attention to detail through all phases of care can reduce the need for additional procedures.

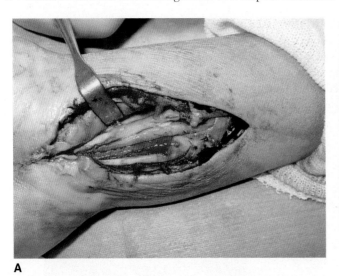
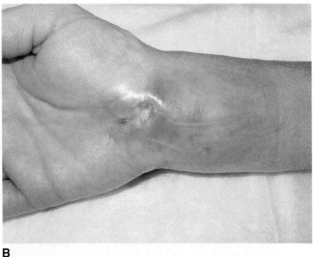

A   **B**

FIGURE 2-20

Underlying medical conditions where immunosuppression is present can lead to wound healing problems even after elective surgery. This rheumatoid arthritis patient underwent routine open carpal tunnel release with subsequent persistent wound drainage. Ultimately, she was diagnosed with Mycobacterium avium. The initial debridement and culture **(A)** failed to heal fully **(B)**. The gelatinous-appearing tenosynovium and indolent course are typical of mycobacterial infections. Successful wound healing followed appropriate antibiotic therapy and delayed primary closure.

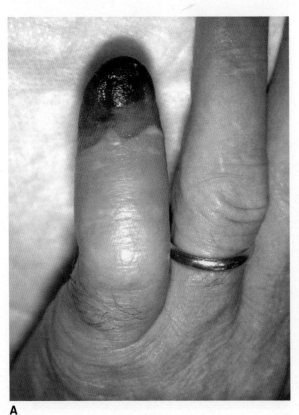
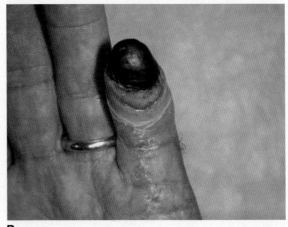

A   **B**

FIGURE 2-21

This patient had compromised sensation and vascularity following multiple surgeries to the small finger for Dupuytren's disease **(A)**. A burn to the distal phalanx occurred as a result of the moist heat pads used before therapy. The initial blister and mild erythema were followed by progressive distal tip necrosis **(B)**. Ultimately, the patient requested an amputation of the digit.

function, and nutritional status should be reassessed in accordance with the clinical picture. Wound cultures are checked, and antibiotic choices are re-evaluated in consultation with infectious disease specialists. When using the wound VAC system, special attention must be made to the pressure settings and quality of suction. Nursing and ancillary staff education is invaluable. Prominent bone or hardware, especially when combined with inadequate or marginal soft tissue coverage, can lead to wound breakdown and the need for additional surgery (Fig. 2-22).

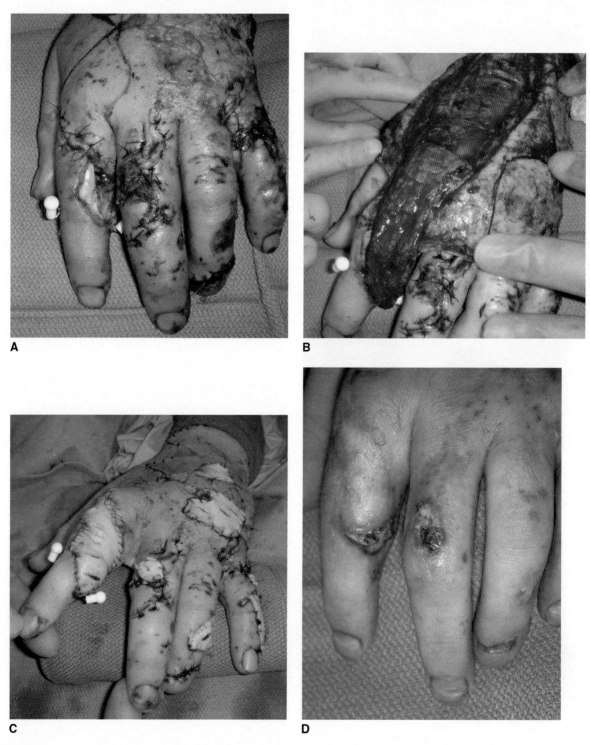

A

B

C

D

FIGURE 2-22

This patient's initial wounds were closed primarily, but there was inadequate coverage of the proximal interphalangeal joints dorsally **(A)**. A delayed adipofascial flap **(B)** and overlying full-thickness skin grafts taken from his amputated lower extremity **(C)** were not robust enough to cover over the dorsally applied plates **(D)**. Removal of the dorsal plates and primary closure lead to successful wound healing **(E)**.

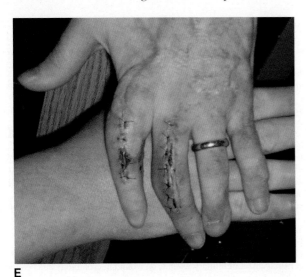

E   **FIGURE 2-22 (*Continued*)**

Pain management is not only humane, but we believe greatly it contributes to the success of treatment, especially in cases requiring frequent bedside dressing changes. Reuben et al. have shown a reduced incidence of complex regional pain syndrome with aggressive pain management. In many cases, especially trauma, our anesthesia colleagues on the pain service oversee medical management of pain and provide regional nerve blocks when appropriate. Anesthesiologists have been pushing the frontiers of regional anesthesia as close as possible to the initial encounter with the patient, with subsequent improvement in pain control and diminished opioid requirements. The mental health of the patient must also never be forgotten, especially in cases of traumatic injury, and appropriate consultation with psychiatric specialists and/or a chaplain should be considered to assist in the patient's overall well-being and ability to participate fully in their own recovery and rehabilitation.

PEARLS AND PITFALLS

- The most important question to consider is whether the surgeon and the facility possess the requisite experience, capability, equipment, and consultative and ancillary services to render optimal treatment.
- Failure to fully recognize patient medical conditions and the scope of the wound and/or injury can have dreadful consequences to the outcome.
- The surgeon must develop a stepwise system of debridement that ensures complete treatment of the wound.
- Successful surgical treatment of wounds begins with the meticulous and complete removal of foreign material, infection, and devitalized tissue to create a healthy wound bed.
- A sterile or nonsterile tourniquet is indispensable to ensure optimal visualization for meticulous, thorough debridement and protection of vital structures.
- When wounds are associated with fractures in the acute setting, provisional stabilization should be attempted to maintain soft tissue space, prevent mechanical agitation of the surrounding tissues, and optimize pain control.
- Tag important neurovascular structures for later repair or reconstruction.
- Use of VAC devices and dermal substitutes may simplify wound closure or coverage.
- Vascular compromise must be immediately recognized and promptly treated.
- In cases of extremity trauma, a high index of suspicion for compartment syndrome is essential.
- Negative wound dressings are not a substitute for formal debridement.
- Prominent bone or hardware can result in wound dehiscence.
- A tension-free closure must be achieved or blood flow will be compromised at the wound margins leading to wound breakdown and dehiscence.

Disclaimer. The views expressed in this chapter are those of the authors and do not necessarily reflect the official policy or position of the Department of the Army, the Department of the Navy, Department of Defense, or the U.S. Government.

RECOMMENDED READING

Aho OA, Lehenkari P, Ristiniemi J, et al. The mechanism of action of induced membranes in bone repair. *J Bone Joint Surg Am.* 2013;95(7):597–604.

Anglen JO. Wound irrigation in musculoskeletal injury. *J Am Acad Orthop Surg.* 2001;9(4):219–226.

Argenta LC, Morykwas MJ. Vacuum-assisted closure: a new method for wound control treatment: clinical experience. *Ann Plast Surg.* 1997;38(6):563–576.

Attinger CE, Janis JE, Steinberg J, et al. Clinical approach to wounds: debridement and wound bed preparation including the use of dressings and wound-healing adjuvants. *Plast Reconstr Surg.* 2006;117(suppl):72S–109S.

Buckenmaier C III, Mahoney PF, Anton T, et al. Impact of an acute pain service on pain outcomes with combat-injured soldiers at Camp Bastion, Afghanistan. *Pain Med.* 2012;13(7):919–926.

CDC. Preventing tetanus, diphtheria, and pertussis among adults: use of tetanus toxoid, reduced diphtheria toxoid and acellular pertussis vaccines. Recommendations of the Advisory Committee on Immunization Practices (ACIP) and Recommendation of ACIP, supported by the Healthcare Infection Control Practices Advisory Committee (HICPAC), for Use of Tdap Among Health-Care Personnel. *MMWR Morb Mortal Wkly Rep.* 2006;55(RR-17):1–37.

Couch KS, Stojadinovic A. Negative-pressure wound therapy in the military: lessons learned. *Plast Reconstr Surg.* 2011;127:117S.

Forsberg JA, Potter BK, Wagner MB, et al. Lessons of war: turning data into decisions. *EBioMedicine.* 2015;2(9):1235–1242.

Fries CA, Ayalew Y, Penn-Barwell JG, et al. Prospective randomized controlled trial of nanocrystalline silver dressing versus plain gauze as the initial post-debridement management of military wounds on wound microbiology and healing. *Injury.* 2014;45:1111–1116.

Gage MJ, Yoon RS, Egol KA, et al. Uses of negative pressure wound therapy in orthopedic trauma. *Orthop Clin North Am.* 2015;46(2):227–234.

Helgeson MD, Potter BK, Evans KN, et al. Bioartificial dermal substitute: a preliminary report on its use for the management of complex combat-related soft tissue wounds. *J Orthop Trauma.* 2007;21(6):394–399.

Henry SL, Ostermann PA, Seligson D. The antibiotic bead pouch technique: the management of severe compound fractures. *Clin Orthop Relat Res.* 1993;295:54–62.

Klein MB, Hunter S, Heimbach DM. et al. The Versajet water dissector: a new tool for tangential excision. *J Burn Care Rehab.* 2005;26(6):483–487.

Lenarz CJ, Watson JT, Moed BR, et al. Timing of wound closure in open fractures based on cultures obtained after debridement. *J Bone Joint Surg Am.* 2010;92(10):1921–1926.

Madhok BM, Vowden K, Vowden P. New techniques for wound debridement. *Int Wound J.* 2013;10(3):247–251.

Masquelet AC, Begue T. The concept of induced membrane for reconstruction of long bone defects. *Orthop Clin North Am.* 2010;41(1):27–37.

Micev AJ, Kalainov DM, Soneru AP. Masquelet technique for treatment of segmental bone loss in the upper extremity. *J Hand Surg Am.* 2015;40(3):593–598.

Morykwas MJ, Argenta LC, Shelton-Brown EI, et al. Vacuum-assisted closure: a new method for wound control and treatment: animal studies and basic foundation. *Ann Plast Surg.* 1997;38(6):553–562.

Mouës CM, Vos MC, Van Den Bemd GC, et al. Bacterial load in relation to vacuum-assisted closure wound therapy: a prospective randomized trial. *Wound Repair Regen.* 2004;12(1):11–17.

Nusbaum AG, Gil J, Rippy MK, et al. Effective method to remove wound bacteria: comparison of various debridement modalities in an in vivo porcine model. *J Surg Res.* 2012;176(2):701–707.

Plunkett A, Turabi A, Wilkinson I. Battlefield analgesia: a brief review of current trends and concepts in the treatment of pain in US military casualties from the conflicts in Iraq and Afghanistan. *Pain Manag.* 2012;2(3):231–238.

Reuben SS. Preventing the development of complex regional pain syndrome after surgery. *Anesthesiology.* 2004;101(5):1215–1224.

Reuben SS, Buvanendran A. Preventing the development of chronic pain after orthopaedic surgery with preventive multimodal analgesic techniques. *J Bone Joint Surg Am.* 2007;89(6):1343–1358.

Robson MC, Stenberg BD, Heggers JP. Wound healing alterations caused by infection. *Clin Plast Surg.* 1990;17(3):485–492.

Schlatterer D, Hirshorn K. Negative pressure wound therapy with reticulated open cell foam—adjunctive treatment in the management of traumatic wounds of the leg: a review of the literature. *J Orthop Trauma.* 2008;22(10):S152–S160.

Stannard JP, Volgas DA, Stewart R, et al. Negative pressure wound therapy after severe open fractures: a prospective randomized study. *J Orthop Trauma.* 2009;23(8):552–557.

Storm-Versloot MN, Vos CG, Ubbink DT, et al. Topical silver for preventing wound infection. *Cochrane Database Syst Rev.* 2010;17(3):CD006478. doi: 10.1002/14651858.CD006478.pub2.

Weed T, Ratliff C, Drake DB. Quantifying bacterial bioburden during negative pressure wound therapy: does the wound VAC enhance bacterial clearance? *Ann Plast Surg.* 2004;52(3):276–279.

3 Management of Simple Wounds: Local Flaps, Z-Plasty, and Skin Grafts

John B. Hijjawi and Steven L. Moran

S kin grafting and local flap coverage have remained a common means of covering traumatic wounds. Skin grafts, local flaps, and random flaps are not as simple as direct wound closure, nor are they are as "elegant" as procedures that are found higher on the reconstructive ladder such as pedicled flaps or free tissue transfer (Fig. 3-1). However, the procedures described in this chapter remain straightforward, reliable, and time-tested and should be an essential component of any surgeon's reconstructive armamentarium.

SKIN GRAFTS

Skin grafts are classified by source and thickness. By far the most common, durable, and successful skin grafts are autografts harvested from the patient's own skin. There are no immunologic issues, since the tissue comes from the patient's own body. Concerns over disease transmission are eliminated, and expense is minimal. The only disadvantage is the creation and care of a donor site.

Skin grafts are also available as cadaveric allografts, xenografts (typically porcine skin), and, most recently, cultured epithelial grafts. These materials are lifesaving sources of temporary wound coverage in the context of massive burns. Allografts and xenografts do have the disadvantage of immunogenicity and thus impermanence since they are bound to be rejected. However, if the quality of a wound bed is questionable, preserved porcine xenografts may be an excellent option for temporary wound coverage.

Currently available cultured epithelial grafts are expensive, require time to culture, and are not as durable as autografts. Additionally, studies have shown that they are significantly more susceptible to infection than standard autografts. Newer products have also been developed to create a neodermis upon which a skin graft may be placed. These new biologic dressings and dermal scaffolds are discussed further in Chapter 4.

Skin grafts are also classified based on thickness. The skin is composed of an outer epidermis and a deeper dermis, which is further subdivided into the reticular and papillary dermis (Fig. 3-2). All skin grafts consist of the entire epidermis and a variable amount of dermis. Split-thickness skin grafts contain only a portion of the dermis, whereas full-thickness skin grafts contain the entire dermis and dermal appendages. As a result, full-thickness skin grafts continue to support hair growth following transfer. This needs to be carefully considered when selecting donor sites in situations when a full-thickness skin graft is to be transferred to a conspicuous, previously hairless area.

Since full-thickness skin grafts include all dermal appendages, skin at the donor site will not spontaneously regenerate following harvest; therefore, these donor sites need to be closed primarily or with a split-thickness skin graft. Split-thickness donor sites retain the ability to generate epithelium and will be largely healed within several weeks if cared for properly.

Split-thickness and full-thickness skin grafts have quite different contractile characteristics on harvesting (primary contraction) and after they heal (secondary contraction). Primary contraction is the initial contraction of a graft when it is harvested. Due to the greater proportion of elastic fibers in a full-thickness skin graft (the dermis is the location of all elastic fibers in the skin), it will undergo more primary contraction than will a split-thickness skin graft when harvested. Similarly, a thicker

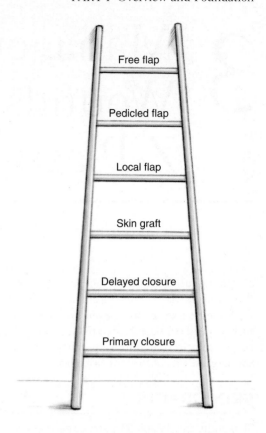

FIGURE 3-1

Reconstructive ladder. Historically, surgeons have closed wounds with the simple procedure first, moving up the rungs of the reconstructive ladder as wounds become larger and more complex.

split-thickness skin graft (e.g., 0.018 inch) will undergo more primary contraction than will a thin split-thickness skin graft. Most skin grafts can be stretched under minimal tension at inset to overcome this contraction, restoring their original size.

Conversely, split-thickness skin grafts undergo more secondary contraction than do full-thickness grafts. This can be exploited to provide gradual contraction of a wound over the course of several months. An example is a fasciotomy wound that is under too much tension to close primarily within the days following compartment release. A very thin split-thickness skin graft applied to the wound will undergo significantly more secondary contraction than would a full-thickness skin graft, resulting in contraction of the wound itself. After several months, this may result in a wound that is small enough to allow serial excision of the skin graft and primary closure under minimal tension.

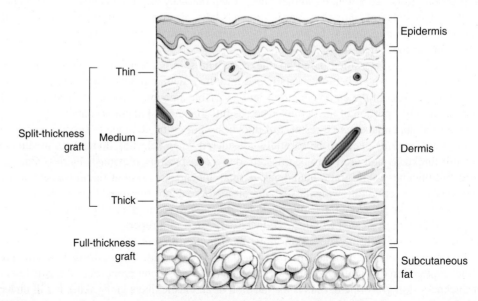

FIGURE 3-2

Skin anatomy.

In comparison, full-thickness skin grafts can be relied on to undergo virtually no secondary contraction in situations where this is not desirable, such as across a joint surface or in a web space.

Initial adhesion of a skin graft is the result of fibrin present between the graft and the recipient bed. Initial survival of a skin graft relies on plasmatic imbibition, which is the process of nutrient diffusion from the recipient site into the skin graft. Later, vascular channels within the graft line up with vascular channels in the recipient bed through the process of inosculation. Finally, long-term graft survival relies on neovascularization, or the process of new blood vessel growth into the skin graft from the recipient bed. Because skin grafts, both split thickness and full thickness, are completely reliant on the recipient bed for survival, the wound bed must be well vascularized and free of infection to support skin graft take. Split-thickness skin grafts have lower metabolic demands than do full-thickness grafts, and so they don't require recipient beds with as rich a blood supply. Along the same lines, full-thickness grafts take longer, from 7 to 10 days, to heal. Split-thickness grafts are generally considered healed by 5 days and should be left immobilized and dressed at least that long postoperatively. The time of healing in specific situations depends most on the quality of the recipient wound's blood supply.

Indications/Contraindications

Indications

Skin grafting may be indicated for any defect that cannot be closed primarily and that has a wound bed that can support skin graft take (Table 3-1). Skin grafts survive for the first several days through a process called imbibition. During this stage of skin graft healing, the graft obtains nutrients from the underlying wound bed through a process of diffusion. Wound beds devoid of blood flow, or with little vascularized tissue, will make for poor recipient sites. Exposed structures that will accept a graft include subcutaneous tissue, paratenon, and muscle. Other tissues, such as exposed bone, joint, tendon, and nerve, may be covered temporarily by graft used as a biologic dressing but will not support a graft for permanent coverage. Beds containing tissues of questionable viability, chronic granulation tissue, or frank infection can accept a skin graft but require thorough debridement prior to graft placement. Wounds that contain fewer than 10^5 bacteria per gram of tissue or that allow xenograft adherence within 24 hours allow successful skin grafting.

Contraindications

Skin grafts are contraindicated in areas that are exposed to repetitive trauma or that lie over osseous prominences. Bone, cartilage, and tendons denuded of periosteum, perichondrium, or paratenon cannot be covered with skin grafts as there is inadequate vascular supply to support healing of the skin graft. Controversy exists over whether skin grafts should be placed over bone, cartilage, or tendons with healthy periosteum, perichondrium, or paratenon. It is certainly possible to get skin-graft healing over such structures. However, skin grafts in these situations are rarely optimal for long-term durable coverage. In addition, skin grafting should be avoided in areas that may require secondary surgery for bone or nerve grafting, as adherence to underlying muscle, nerve, and tendon may complicate secondary surgery. All split-thickness grafts will undergo some component of contracture over time; thus, if these grafts are placed over large areas of the antecubital fossa, popliteal fossa, or olecranon, there is a risk of limitation in joint motion.

Preoperative Planning

The wound must be debrided and clean prior to attempts at skin grafting. Infection is one of the leading causes of skin graft failure. Since skin grafts are completely dependent on the wound bed they are transplanted to for nutrition, they possess no intrinsic ability to resolve infection. Quantitative wound cultures have been used for many years in some centers to determine the adequacy of a

TABLE 3-1   Wound Analysis
Is there too much tension across the wound for primary closure?
Is there adequate perfusion of the wound bed?
Are vital structures exposed at the base of the wound?
Is the wound infected or contaminated?
Is the wound geometry favorable for closure?

wound's microenvironment for closure. A quantitative culture revealing less than 10^5 bacteria per gram of tissue has been traditionally regarded as an acceptable level of colonization below which a wound can be closed by skin graft or local flap. However, such cultures are highly dependent on the experience of the technician performing them. A careful clinical evaluation and serial sharp debridement of clinically infected or contaminated wounds are advised.

Donor site selection must also be decided before surgery. Considerations when choosing a donor site for split-thickness skin grafts include cosmesis, the thickness of skin in the donor site region, and ease of care of the donor site after graft harvest. The most common split-thickness skin donor sites include the buttocks, lateral and anterior thighs, and lower abdomen. These sites are relatively easy to conceal, have thick skin resulting in less pigmentation once healed, and are readily accessible in even a bed-bound patient, easing postoperative care.

Full-thickness skin grafts are most commonly harvested from the groin, antecubital fossa, volar wrist crease, medial arm, postauricular sulcus, or lower abdomen. These donor sites all exist in areas where closure can be performed within preexisting skin creases, thus resulting in relatively inconspicuous donor sites. The hypothenar skin or plantar instep offers the unique quality of glabrous skin if needed for graft material. Always keep in mind that any amputated "spare parts" can provide a good source of viable skin graft with no added morbidity to the patient.

Surgery

Patient Positioning

The patient's position will depend on the location of the graft to be harvested. Most frequently, we harvest split-thickness grafts from the upper thigh area, where they may easily be concealed under clothing. A supine position with a roll underneath one hip is ideal. The majority of full-thickness grafts are harvested from the hairless skin of the groin crease, though the inner upper arm may be used as well. The patient is positioned supine for such harvests. For glabrous skin grafts, the instep of the foot may be positioned so as to allow ease of harvest. For wounds on the posterior aspect of the lower extremity or trunk, a lateral decubitus position readily exposes both the wound and a lateral thigh donor site. With careful planning, it is almost never necessary to reposition a patient after harvesting the skin graft.

Split-Thickness Grafts

Power dermatomes are the most common method of harvesting split-thickness skin grafts, although for very small split-thickness grafts, hand-driven Weck blades may be more convenient.

Measure the recipient wound and choose a dermatome guard based on that measurement (Fig. 3-3A). Set and check the dermatome thickness (usually 0.010 to 0.015 inch) with a no. 15 scalpel blade. The thin, beveled edge of the knife is about 0.010 inch, whereas the thickest portion of the blade is 0.015 inch thick (Fig. 3-3B).

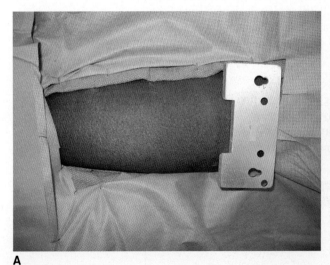
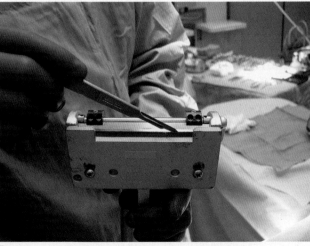

A   B

FIGURE 3-3

A: A dermatome guard of appropriate width is chosen. **B:** The thickness setting is double checked.

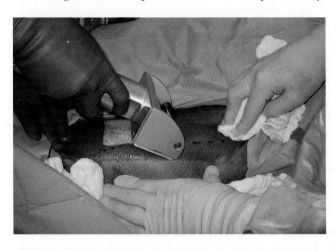

FIGURE 3-4

Countertraction is applied to avoid "skipping" along the skin.

Mark the donor site with a ruler so that you will know where the dermatome needs to "touch down" and "lift off." Relying on your memory or estimating how far you will have to drive the dermatome can lead to harvesting too little graft and having to reharvest, creating an unnecessary seam in the graft. In cases of overharvesting, the extra graft can be replaced onto the donor site, but this complicates the donor site dressing.

Clean the donor site to remove any sticky material that will cause the dermatome to stick, and apply copious amounts of mineral oil to the donor skin and the dermatome.

Apply countertraction to the skin in front of and behind the dermatome blade. Dermatomes, particularly when fitted with larger guards, function much more effectively on flat surfaces (Fig. 3-4).

Activate the dermatome before "touching down" on the skin and plan to keep it activated until after "lifting off" of the skin. Touch down at 45 degrees to the skin and then slightly flatten the angle between the dermatome and skin, maintaining constant firm pressure on the head of the dermatome.

Realize that if you need to reset a hand for countertraction, you can stop the blade without lifting off of the skin and reset countertraction. The harvest can then be continued without interrupting the continuous sheet of skin graft.

Transfer the harvested graft onto a dermal carrier with the dermis side up. This side is shinier and has less friction when rubbed than the epidermis side. If you become confused as to which side is the dermis side, realize that the skin graft edges will always roll toward the dermis side.

Either make several small slits in the skin graft with a scalpel ("pie crusting") to allow for drainage of accumulated fluid from the wound bed or run the graft and dermal carrier through a skin graft meshing device (Fig. 3-5). Most typically, grafts are meshed at a 1:1.5 ratio. This is done to allow drainage through the graft, to make grafts more conformable to the underlying wound bed, and to increase the area a graft can cover. It is not necessary, however, and many surgeons avoid it since the meshed appearance will be permanently obvious and will significantly compromise the final cosmesis.

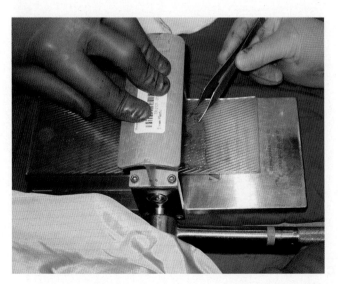

FIGURE 3-5

Meshing the skin graft dermis side up facilitates placement onto the wound.

Fix the graft dermis side down to the wound bed with either staples or absorbable sutures such as
5-0 chromic. Traditional bolster or "tie-over" dressings employ silk suture placed circumferentially
around the skin graft and left long. They are then tied over mineral oil–soaked cotton wrapped in
a nonadherent dressing and placed firmly onto the skin graft (Figs. 3-6). A very convenient bolster
dressing can be fashioned by placing a nonadherent Nterface dressing (Delasco, Council Bluffs,
IA) over the skin graft, followed by mineral oil–soaked cotton pushed firmly into the wound bed to
compress the skin graft. Finally, a Reston (3M, St. Paul, MN) sponge can be cut to conform to the
wound, placed adhesive side up, and stapled to the skin surrounding the wound. This is a very stable
bolster construct that resists shearing forces and provides firm compression. For skin grafts placed
on an extremity, an Ace wrap can be used to protect this entire dressing. Appropriate splints should
be applied to immobilize the recipient site until the skin graft is totally healed.

Full-Thickness Grafts

Full-thickness grafts are harvested after drawing an ellipse, which includes the necessary amount of
skin based on the wound measurements. Closure without dog-ears is best achieved when the length
of the ellipse is about four times the width of the ellipse. A scalpel is used to incise the skin just
through the dermis. One end of the ellipse is then lifted firmly with a single skin hook or toothed
forceps, and a fresh scalpel is used to elevate the skin graft just deep to the dermis, taking as little fat
as possible with the skin graft. Once harvested, the full-thickness graft can be rolled over a finger or
shot glass with the dermis side up, and a curved iris scissors is used to remove every bit of residual
fat from the dermis.

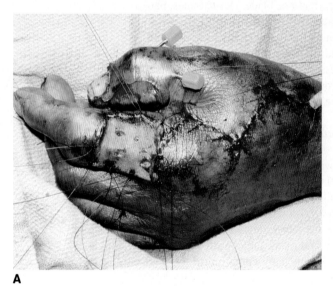
A

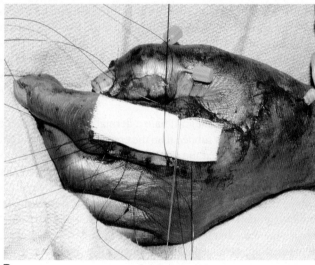
B

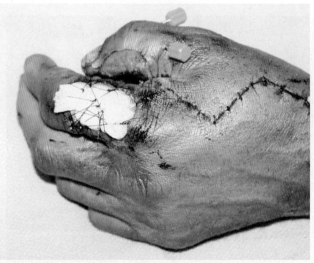
C

FIGURE 3-6

A: The bolster or "tie-over" dressing begins with placement of
long sutures along the edge of the skin graft. **B:** Cotton balls are
wrapped in a nonadherent dressing and compressed onto the skin
graft. **C:** The completed tie-over.

Full-thickness grafts are not typically meshed. Otherwise, they are fixed into position as described for split-thickness grafts. They should be left undisturbed for 7 to 10 days. Donor sites are best treated with primary closure after moderate undermining of the wound edge.

Postoperative Management

Split-thickness skin grafts should not be disturbed for a minimum of 5 days. The dressing can then be carefully removed to not disturb the healing skin graft, and once daily dressings are begun with an antibacterial ointment and a nonadherent dressing such as Adaptic (Johnson and Johnson, New Brunswick, NJ). Full-thickness grafts should remain covered for 7 to 10 days before removing the split or bolster.

Donor sites up to 100 cm² can be covered with Tegaderm (3M, St. Paul, MN) as long as care is taken to carefully dry the skin surrounding the donor site before applying the dressing. Serum will collect under the Tegaderm after several days and can be left alone. If the Tegaderm leaks, a patch can be placed over the hole. The benefit of Tegaderm is a completely isolated, moist environment that is virtually painless for the patient (Fig. 3-7). The donor site is typically re-epithelialized by 2 weeks at which point the Tegaderm can be removed and replaced with once daily application of a moisturizing cream and nonadherent dressing. Alternatively, the donor site can be covered with a Xeroform (Sherwood Medical Industries Ltd., Markham, Ontario, Canada), which will dry into an eschar when exposed to air. Once dry this will be painless but is extremely sensitive until the eschar develops.

Rehabilitation

Rehabilitation of the affected extremity can begin once the surgeon is assured of stable graft take. Grafts placed over joints may benefit from 7 to 10 days of immobilization before initiating motion across the joint. For grafts placed away from a joint, normal motion can begin almost immediately if the graft has been securely bolstered to its wound bed.

Complications

Skin graft necrosis or failure is the most common complication following split-thickness skin grafting. The formation of fluid under a skin graft, whether hematoma or seroma, is the most common cause of skin graft loss. As noted, the graft is completely reliant on the recipient bed for nutrition and so needs to be in complete contact with the recipient bed to survive. Therefore, precise hemostasis of the wound bed is critical before skin graft application as is firm compression of the graft onto the recipient bed through the use of bolster dressings.

Infection is the next most common cause of skin graft loss. This is best avoided by careful debridement before placement of the graft. Shearing forces can interrupt the formation of vascular connections between the graft and the recipient bed. This will ultimately lead to loss of a graft since healing relies on the formation of genuine vascular connections and is not possible through plasmatic imbibition alone. Therefore, firm immobilization of all skin grafts is critical to their healing.

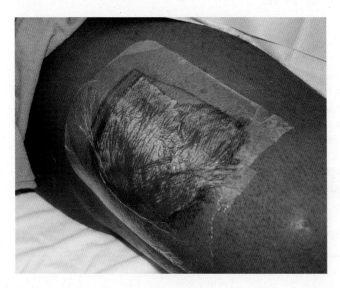

FIGURE 3-7

Donor site dressing.

Finally, an inadequately perfused recipient bed will certainly lead to skin graft loss. Common situations include patients with peripheral vascular disease, previously radiated tissues, and tendon or bone denuded of paratenon or periosteum.

RANDOM FLAPS

Random flaps, by definition, have no named or defined blood supply. They are raised in a subdermal plane and so rely on the subdermal vascular plexus of skin for circulation. To ensure adequate circulation, random flaps should be limited to a length no greater than 2.5 times the width of their base, which is the uncut border of the flap. This ratio may be even more limited in poorly perfused extremities.

Indications/Contraindications

Indications

The elasticity and slight redundancy of local tissue are critical to the success of most random flaps. They are based on local tissue so are typically contraindicated for wounds with significant surrounding soft tissue damage such as radiation wounds. The advantage of random flaps in comparison to skin grafts is that they can provide well-vascularized, full-thickness tissue for wound coverage. Far more durable to friction and repeated stress than skin grafts, local flaps are preferred for closure over vital structures such as tendons, nerves, and blood vessels. An added benefit is that they can be used to close wounds over vital structures denuded of paratenon, periosteum, or perineurium, since a well-vascularized wound bed is not required as it is for skin graft survival. Finally, despite the new scars made to raise random flaps, they are ideal in terms of color match, since they come from local skin.

Contraindications

Gross contamination or frank infection is an absolute contraindication to wound closure with local flaps. In fact, while free flaps and pedicled flaps have been shown to introduce enough independent new blood supply to overcome infectious processes like osteomyelitis, local flaps need to be placed over a clean, uncontaminated wound bed. Finally, local flaps are limited to small wounds usually less than 15 to 20 cm^2; wounds exceeding these dimensions should be covered with another method of soft tissue coverage.

Preoperative Planning

As mentioned previously, adequate surgical debridement is a must before any attempt at closure. Tissue culture is a useful adjunct, particularly in cases of significant blunt trauma with devitalized tissue or cases of gross contamination. Often, serial wound debridement every other day for several days is necessary to obtain negative cultures.

It may not be possible to completely resolve a patient's systemic medical issues, but they should be as optimized as much as possible. Tight control of blood glucose levels in patients with diabetes, management of extremity edema, and nutritional status can all be significantly improved in many patients with several days of focused inpatient care.

Surgery

Z-Plasty

Probably, the most familiar random flap to any surgeon, the Z-plasty is not actually indicated for the treatment of open wounds. Rather, the main indications for a Z-plasty include lengthening scars, interrupting linear scars with the transposition of unscarred tissue, and disrupting circumferential or constricting scars (Table 3-2). A common indication in hand surgery is to employ a Z-plasty in contracted web spaces in an effort to introduce healthy adjacent tissue relieving web contractures.

TABLE 3-2 Z-Plasty Indications

Lengthening scars
Interrupting linear scars
Disrupting circumferential or constricting scars

Z-plasties rely on limbs of equal length to facilitate closure. The most common Z-plasty design employs 60-degree angles, which theoretically results in a 75% increase in the length of the central limb of the Z-plasty (Fig. 3-8). Although clinically not feasible, a Z-plasty with angles of 90 degrees would result in the greatest theoretical gain of central limb length, approximately 120%.

Executing an effective Z-plasty is not simply a matter of elevating the triangular flaps and transposing them. Mobility and a tension-free closure are greatly facilitated when the tissue at the bases of the triangular flaps is also elevated.

Four Flap Z-Plasty

Most commonly used for first web space contractures, the four flap Z-plasty results in a 150% gain in length of the original central limb, or scar contracture. Essentially, a 120-degree standard Z-plasty is drawn. Each triangular flap is then bisected, resulting in four equivalent 60-degree triangles that are raised and interdigitated as shown (Fig. 3-9).

Rhomboid Flap

Executing a rhomboid flap begins with converting the defect (even if it is circular) into a rhomboid to better visualize the flap design. A line equivalent in length to the limbs of the rhomboid is then drawn perpendicular to the short axis of the rhomboid (Fig. 3-10). Next, a line (B–C) is drawn at 60 degrees to the A–B line. It will be parallel to one of the limbs of the original rhomboid.

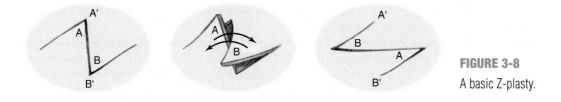

FIGURE 3-8

A basic Z-plasty.

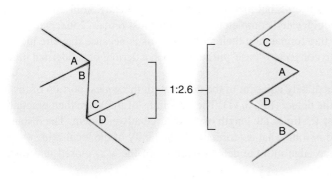

FIGURE 3-9

Four-flap Z-plasty.

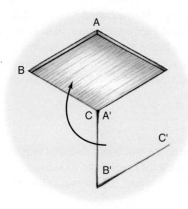
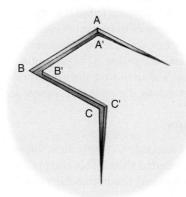

FIGURE 3-10

Rhomboid flap.

The flap is then elevated. It is also critical to elevate the skin around the base of the flap very liberally to facilitate transposition of the flap and closure of the wound. The flap should not be closed under tension; rather, further undermining of the base of the flap should be executed until the flap closes without tension.

Banner Flap

The banner flap is a type of transposition flap. A pendant or banner of skin is designed with one edge of the banner (near the base of the flap) running tangentially to the wound edge. The flap is elevated and transposed after which any redundant flap can be trimmed. It is important that the original design of the flap places the banner in an area of redundant skin. Since the banner can be designed along any border of the defect, it is helpful for eventual cosmesis if the original banner is designed within a relaxed skin tension line.

Rotational Flap

Rotational flaps are frequently employed on the dorsum of the hand, on the fingers, and in the scalp to close triangular defects. They are deceptively simple, and poor planning can lead to a large incision with an inadequate flap.

Unfortunately, relatively little advancement of the flap edge is possible without making a flap that is approximately four times greater in length than the defect length. Even with an adequately designed flap, tension can develop at a point opposite the pivot point in the base of the flap. This can be overcome by back-cutting the base of the flap or excising a Burow's triangle. The pitfall here is the risk of cutting into the base of the flap, which can reduce the circulation of the flap. This added tension in the flap can lead to tip necrosis.

One simple solution for a rotation flap that seems to be under excessive tension is to simply advance the leading edge of the flap into the defect, which results in a new defect at the opposite end of the flap. Since this donor defect should be well vascularized (the flap should be taken from an area of healthy tissue), the donor site can be skin-grafted rather than closed primarily. This strategy, while not elegant, is much less likely to result in excessive tension on the closure.

V-Y Advancement Flap

V-Y advancement flaps are extremely useful, but their execution differs greatly from transposition flaps. V-Y advancement flaps are not elevated completely but rather must remain connected to the subcutaneous tissue underlying the flap to maintain their viability. This is because they are incised along all skin borders and so have no connected "base" through which a dermal or subdermal blood supply can provide circulation.

A V-shaped flap is designed immediately adjacent to the defect with the widest portion of the V equivalent in width to the width of the defect (Fig. 3-11). The two limbs of the V are then gradually tapered so that their length is at least 1.5 times the length of the desired advancement. The distance the edge of the flap can be advanced is somewhat determined by the laxity of the local skin.

Following advancement of the flap edge into the defect, the base of the V is closed in a linear fashion, resulting in a Y.

Postoperative Management

On completion of the operation, a bulky, noncompressive dressing is applied to the wound, which may be supported with a plaster splint if immobilization is required. A small window can be left to monitor the flap for signs of ischemia or congestion. Sutures remain for an average of 10 to 14 days, depending on the status and tension of the surrounding tissue. Ideally, flaps are inset under minimal tension, allowing the patient to begin gentle range of motion exercises immediately following surgery. Once sutures are removed, the wounds may be kept moist with a petroleum-based product, which will prevent itching during the early postoperative period.

Complications

The most feared postoperative complication following local flap reconstruction is necrosis or partial necrosis of the transferred tissue. This complication occurs because of inadequate blood supply to the flap. Flap ischemia may result from flap closure under excessive tension, hematoma, or infection.

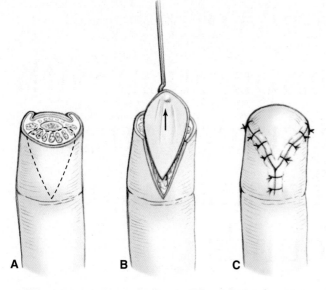

FIGURE 3-11

A–C: The Atasoy-Kleinert V-Y advancement flap. Note that the subcutaneous tissue has remained undisturbed to maintain blood supply. (Redrawn after Louis DS, Jebson PLJ, Graham TJ. Amputations. In: Green DP, Hotchkiss RN, Pederson WC, eds. *Operative Hand Surgery.* New York: Churchill Livingstone; 1999:48–94.)

If total flap loss develops, the wound will require closure by another means, either pedicled flap or skin graft. If partial necrosis has occurred, one can debride the necrotic portion of the flap and begin dressing changes to the underlying wound bed. Once the underlying tissues are clean of any infection and necrotic debris, the surgeon can consider allowing the wound to heal through secondary intention or attempt wound closure with an alternative reconstructive method.

PEARLS AND PITFALLS

- Use a VAC or Reston bolster to immobilize and compress skin grafts quickly.
- Exploit secondary contraction of thin split-thickness grafts (0.010 to 0.012 inch) to induce contraction of fasciotomy wounds.
- Employ Tegaderm for small donor sites (100 cm^2) to decrease pain and provide a moist wound-healing environment. Larger absorbent Tegaderm is available for larger donor sites.
- Splint extremities to help immobilize skin grafts.
- Salvage improperly planned local flaps by skin grafting the local flap donor site.
- Inadequate hemostasis and hematoma formation will result in skin graft failure.
- Seroma formation below a skin graft will result in skin graft failure. Seroma formation can be avoided with the use of a bolster or VAC dressing following skin graft placement.
- Inadequate immobilization of grafts or flaps while healing can lead to flap and graft failure.
- Meshing grafts on the hand produce a poor aesthetic outcome.
- Inadequate initial wound debridement will lead to skin graft failure.

RECOMMENDED READING

Ablove RH, Howell RM. The physiology and technique of skin grafting. *Hand Clin.* 1997;13:163–173.

Chao JD, Huang JM, Weidrich TA. Local hand flaps. *J Am Soc Surg Hand.* 2001;1:25–44.

Lin SJ, Hijjawi JB. Skin grafting. In: Lin SJ, Hijjawi JB, eds. *Plastic and Reconstructive Surgery Pearls of Wisdom.* New York: McGraw Hill; 2006:435–436.

Louis DS, Jebson PLJ, Graham TJ. Amputations. In: Green DP, Hotchkiss RN, Pederson WC, eds. *Operative Hand Surgery.* New York: Churchill Livingstone; 1999:48–94.

Tschoi M, Hoy EA, Granick MS. Skin flaps. *Clin Plast Surg.* 2005;32:261–273.

4 Integra Bilayer Wound Matrix in Combination with Negative Pressure Wound Therapy for Treatment of Extremity Wounds

Kanu Goyal and Ian L. Valerio

The management of large skin and soft tissue extremity defects after trauma, burns, or tumor resection can present difficult challenges in the restoration of extremity form and function. The traditional reconstructive ladder outlines progressively complex options for extremity soft tissue coverage, advancing from the "lower rungs" of primary closure, secondary intention, and skin grafts to "higher rungs" consisting of local flaps, distant flaps, tissue expansion, and free flaps. However, a number of adjunctive and useful tools, techniques, and regenerative medicine products have become incorporated into the traditional reconstructive ladder to provide additional solutions for today's extremity salvage and coverage problems. In this chapter, we focus on the application of a skin substitute/dermal regenerate, specifically the Integra Bilayer Wound Matrix (BWM) (Integra LifeSciences Corporation, Plainsboro, NJ), in combination with negative pressure wound therapy (NPWT) to achieve soft tissue restoration in challenging extremity injuries.

INDICATIONS/CONTRAINDICATIONS

Since its introduction to mainstream clinical practice, NPWT has become an extremely useful tool in managing extremity injuries. NPWT has been previously shown to decrease bacteria counts, improve the local blood flow and perfusion of the wound bed and tissue, as well increase the rate, quality, and quantity of granulation tissue formation within a wound bed. Given its versatility and ease in use, NPWT and its indications span from active management in acute wounds to certain subacute injuries as well as treatment of chronic wounds. The various indications for NPWT are extensive and include many of the following useful applications:

- Initial short-term treatment of traumatic wounds associated with soft tissue loss or having certain exposed vital structures (e.g., exposed adipose, fascia, muscle, tendon, ligament, or bone)
- Short-term treatment of wounds having exposed hardware until definitive coverage measures can be performed
- Assistance in wound healing, granulation formation, and contraction
- Edema and exudative control associated with certain wounds
- Potential reduction in odor, better tolerance, and decreased pain issues as compared to other topical wound care dressings such as wet-to-dry dressings, bandages, and dry techniques
- Temporizing wounds after appropriate debridement to aid in transport to definitive care facilities/ medical centers (especially pertinent to military trauma)
- Treatment of chronic nonhealing wounds and certain soft tissue ulcers or pressure sores
- Provides a bolster dressing, protective barrier, as well as minimizing of sheer forces to wound beds and soft tissue treatment strategies

- Allows for concurrent resumption of rehabilitation therapies in many cases
- Placement within postextirpative wound defects until pathological clearance prior to second stage or definitive reconstruction
- Aids in facilitating the incorporation of skin grafts or dermal substitutes/regenerates to their wound beds
- Reduction in wound care treatment costs for appropriately selected wound treatment regimen
- Appropriate for inpatient and outpatient wound treatment

Although the indications for NPWT are well recognized and outlined above, familiarity with various skin substitutes and dermal regenerates for extremity reconstruction is less so, although interest and use in extremity reconstruction for burn and traumatic injuries are growing. The indications for the application of Integra Bilayer Wound Matrix include partial- and full-thickness wounds, pressure, diabetic, and/or venous ulcers, surgically created wounds (e.g., fasciotomies, postoncologic extirpation defects, dehiscence), traumatic wounds, burn wounds, and certain exudative or transudative wounds. It comes in both a meshed and unmeshed type with a variety of sizes ranging from 5×5 cm (25 cm^2) to upward of 20×25 cm (500 cm^2) and can be fashioned to the size of the wound defect being treated.

While NPWT has numerous benefits and applications to a great variety of extremity wound types, there are cases in which its use is absolutely or relatively contraindicated. Current contraindications include avoidance in the following circumstances:

- Active infections, both soft tissue and osteomyelitis of bone
- Wounds associated with active or nonaddressed malignancies as it may stimulate cancer proliferation and/or expansion
- Nonexplored or nonenteric fistulae
- Direct application of sponge dressing over specific exposed vital structures such as arteries, veins, nerves, internal organs, brain, dura, as well as anastomotic sites
- Wounds having heavy contamination, necrotic tissue, fibrinous exudate, eschar, sloughing, or inadequately debrided foreign material

Additional care and precaution should also be taken in the following cases:

- Patients with wounds having active bleeding, having certain bleeding disorders, or on certain anticoagulation therapy regimens, which may predispose such patients to ongoing or uncontrolled potential hemorrhage
- Wounds with exposed blood vessels, vascular grafts, or vascular anastomoses, which may predispose the patient to vascular injury
- Wounds with exposed nerves, fascia, or bone in which the perivascular structures are not adequately protected and may be further stripped or injured by direct sponge contact
- Wounds or enteric fistulae having communication, contamination, or direct exposure to bowel contents or anastomoses
- Patients who may require various advanced studies or treatments such as MRIs, hyperbaric chamber/dives, or defibrillation
- Circumferential dressings of the extremities

The contraindications for application of skin substitutes and dermal regenerates such as Integra include those as listed above for NPWT use. Patients having known sensitivities to bovine collagen and/or chondroitin should not have their extremity wounds treated with this particular dermal substitute either. Additionally, those patients having untreated malnutrition or immunocompromised states may have issues with substitute incorporation secondary to impaired wound healing potential.

PREOPERATIVE PLANNING

The main concepts for preoperative planning for use of Integra dermal regeneration template (DRT) in combination with NPWT mainly stem from availability of the required materials (product, device, and sponge). Additional considerations should be taken in those patients with aversion to bovine or xenografts; patients with poor reliability or transportation access issues, which may affect compliance; patients unwilling or uninterested in undergoing multiple staged procedures; and patients having health care access issues, which may impact their ability to complete the serial procedures and NPWT changes necessary prior to undergoing definitive skin grafting procedure.

SURGERY

Anatomy

As one may recall, the primary functions of skin consist of protecting our body from the external environment, innate immunity measures, thermoregulation, and preventing our underlying tissues from fluid loss. It consists of the epidermis, dermis (composed of dense connective tissue, hair follicles, and sweat glands), and the hypodermis or subcutaneous tissue (composed of loose connective tissue and fat). In skin avulsion injuries without exposure of critical underlying structures such as tendon, fascia, nerve, or bone, skin grafting can be utilized to provide definitive coverage. Most skin substitutes and DRTs have been used to cover open wounds and function similar to dermis by creating a layer of tissue upon which the epidermis can adequately adhere and proliferate as well as can provide a viable, neovascularized construct over exposed critical structures. Integra BWM is an acellular membrane that consists of cross-linked bovine tendon collagen and chondroitin-6-sulfate. This bioartificial template has been shown to provide an extracellular matrix that facilitates the migration of host fibroblasts, macrophages, lymphocytes, as well as capillary ingrowth, thereby helping regenerate dermal tissue. Histologically after incorporation, the generated neodermis is composed of collagen, elastin, and host cellular elements, which aid in skin mobility and pliability. The silicone layer it possesses serves as a temporary synthetic "epidermis substitute" that helps protect the underlying dermal template from temperature variability, insensible fluid, and protein losses from the wound bed and protects the extracellular matrix against potential contamination especially when used in combination with NPWT.

Patient Positioning

As the described technique can be applied to nearly any location of the extremity, from proximal to distal, to both upper and lower extremity, or even multiple limb injuries, positioning of the patient should maximize the necessary exposure for the wound of interest to permit access for debridement, graft placement, and ease in NPWT dressing application. Patients may be placed within any acceptable position from supine to prone to lateral depending on the site of the extremity defect.

Technique

After it has been determined that a patient and his/her soft tissue extremity wound would benefit from Integra BWM, a stepwise approach should be performed before the graft is applied. First, sharp debridement to a healthy wound bed that is free of contamination and/or infection is performed typically within the operative setting (Fig. 4-1). Hemostasis is then obtained with an electrocautery

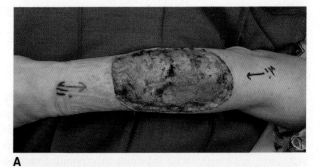

A

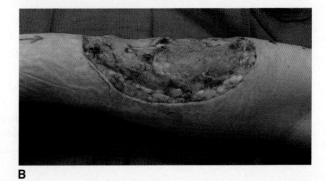

B

FIGURE 4-1

Case 1. A 41-year-old woman with a history of common variable immunodeficiency (CVID) and multiple prior cutaneous bacterial infections suffered a necrotizing soft tissue infection of her left dorsal forearm. She underwent operative debridement of the soft tissue infection down to the underlying fascia, which was viable. Wet-to-dry Dakins was performed for a few days prior to undergoing a wound debridement in preparation of graft placement.

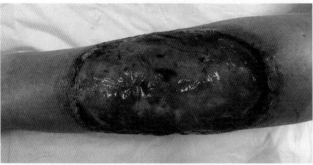

A

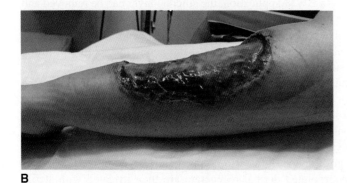

B

FIGURE 4-2

Case 1. After debridement, a 4 × 5-in. bilaminar unmeshed Integra DRT was applied to the prepared wound bed and sutured in place.

device to minimize potential for postoperative hematoma or seroma. Once the wound bed is surgically prepared, the appropriate size of Integra BWM is chosen and fashioned to completely cover the underlying wound bed (Fig. 4-2). Care is taken to ensure that the graft conforms to irregular wound surfaces as best as possible and is in optimal contact to the bed with the silicone layer (designated with a black line) facing away from the wound bed. After the Integra BWM is applied to the bed, it is secured with either skin staples or sutures (2-0 or 3-0 nylon typically) to the wound edges. Additional interrupted tacking sutures may be placed within the graft to better adhere the device to its underlying wound bed in an effort to avoid excessive elevation and potential shear forces. This step is important to improve incorporation and take especially if one desires to have the patient begin rehabilitation measures after surgery.

After securing the graft to its wound bed, the authors often place an antimicrobial silver dressing, such as Restore silver, Acticoat, etc., over the graft or skin substitute followed by a black GranuFoam sponge (Fig. 4-3). If the patient has a sensitivity to silver, then no additional antimicrobial dressing is used, and the black GranuFoam sponge is placed over an Adaptic nonadhering dressing or simply directly onto the silicone layer. Use of skin staples may be used to secure the sponge in place if one desires, and the NPWT occlusive dressings are secured to the extremity surrounding

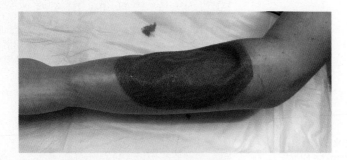

FIGURE 4-3

Case 1. A silver porous dressing (Restore silver) was placed onto the Integra DRT and NPWT initiated with a black GranuFoam sponge set at 125 mm Hg continuous pressure applied. The NPWT was changed at 1 and 2 weeks after placement, with the silicone layer removed once the DRT was incorporated to the wound. NPWT was reapplied directly to the neodermis for an additional week to aid in filling in the wound defect.

the wound. A negative continuous pressure of 75 to 100 mm Hg is typically applied, although pressures ranging from as low intensity as 50 mm Hg to upward of 125 mm Hg have been used with this technique without adverse outcomes. In our experience and the experience of others, application of NPWT over a bilaminar Integra BWM helps to not only improve take but also aid in reducing infection rates while also permitting the patient to begin certain rehabilitation measures. We then apply Kerlix, Ace wraps, and/or upper extremity splint or lower extremity splint/walking boot depending on the site of the wound being treated. After completion of the above first-stage surgery, the patient is usually discharged home with a home NPWT device and dressings with the first change scheduled in the office at 5 to 7 days postsurgery. We typically change the negative pressure wound dressing at 1-week intervals following the initial dressing change with home care assistance only if there is trouble with the device.

At approximately 2 weeks after Integra BWM application, the silicone layer can be removed and NPWT is then applied directly onto the incorporated neodermis of the substitute (see Case 1 videos). Our group has found that direct negative pressure therapy on the incorporated neodermis 2 weeks after initial Integra BWM application encourages hypertrophy of the neodermis, aiding in filling deeper defects and improving soft tissue contour (see Case 1 and 2 videos).

One week after the silicone layer has been removed and NPWT at 75 mm Hg reapplied over the dermal substitute, split-thickness skin grafting (STSG) can be performed for definitive soft tissue coverage and skin restoration (Fig. 4-4A). Since the underlying neodermis minimizes the number of migrating myofibroblasts, scar contracture is minimized. The patient is taken to the operating room, the NPWT is removed, and the incorporated dermal regenerate is prepped with Betadine or chlorhexidine solution, and the skin graft donor site is also prepped and draped in usual standard sterile technique. The wound and incorporated dermal regenerate are then irrigated with sterile saline, and a split-thickness skin graft at 12/1,000ths of an inch as a sheet or meshed graft can be

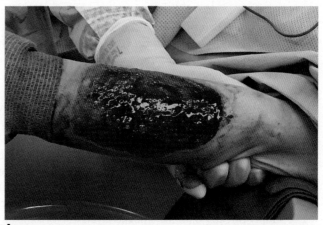

A

FIGURE 4-4

Case 1. At the 3-week post-DRT placement mark, when the NPWT dressing was removed, the neodermis exhibited near-normal contour and defect coverage. A pie-crusted STSG was then applied to the DRT and NPWT again applied for an additional week.

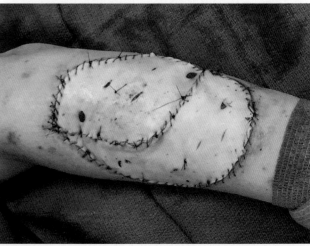

B

placed (Fig. 4-4B). The skin graft is secured into the wound bed with 3-0 or 4-0 chromic sutures. As described during the first-stage procedure, after securing the graft to its wound bed, the authors often place an antimicrobial silver dressing, such as Restore silver, Acticoat, etc., over the skin graft followed by a black GranuFoam sponge. If the patient has a sensitivity to silver, then no additional antimicrobial dressing is used and the black GranuFoam sponge is placed over an Adaptic nonadhering dressing. Use of skin staples is usually avoided when possible to allow ease in change of NPWT within the clinic setting. The NPWT occlusive one to two dressings are secured to the extremity surrounding the wound and a negative continuous pressure of 75 to 100 mm Hg is applied. At 5 to 7 days after skin graft placement, NPWT is discontinued and routine skin graft care with bacitracin and Adaptic daily along with Ace wrap, Kerlix, and splint or walking boot is performed for 2 additional weeks until the skin graft completely heals.

Figures 4-5 and 4-6 depict two additional cases, and the accompanying videos for all three cases show the stepwise approach.

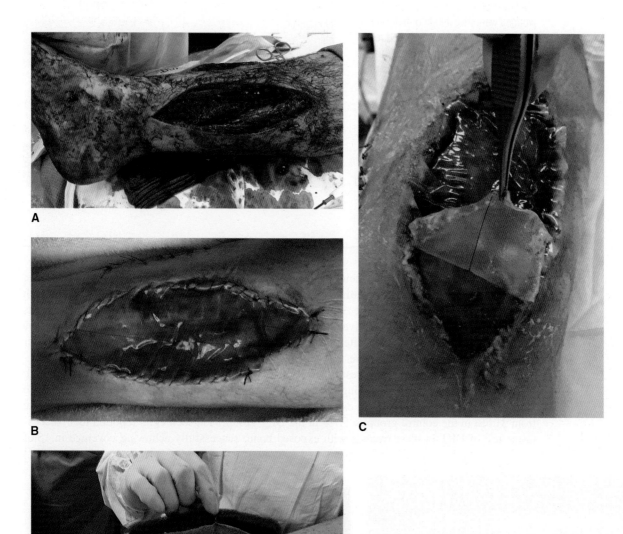

FIGURE 4-5

Case 2. A 40-year-old man who sustained an open distal tibial shaft fracture with an open medial leg wound that necessitated soft tissue coverage. **A:** The wound was debrided to healthy margins. Bilaminar Integra BWM was applied with accompanying NPWT. **B:** One week after bilaminar Integra BWM was applied. **C:** Two weeks after Integra BWM application, silicone layer was removed and NPWT was applied directly over the neodermis for one additional week prior to skin grafting. **D:** Meshed split-thickness skin graft applied with Restore silver nonadherent gauze and NPWT application for 1 week.

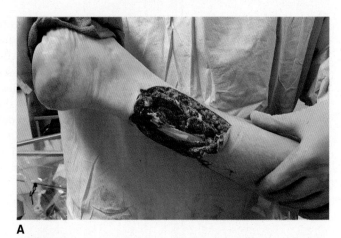

FIGURE 4-6

Case 3. A 33-year-old man sustained multiple gunshot wounds to his right posterior calf, left residual limb/below-knee amputation stump, and bilateral upper extremities. All of his gunshot wounds were irrigated and debrided, with local wound care performed to his upper limb wounds and left residual limb wound. The right lower extremity injury exhibited an exposed Achilles tendon, and after debridement, an Integra DRT was placed in conjunction with NPWT. Two weeks after the Integra DRT was placed, the patient returned to the OR to have the same procedures performed as outlined and as described for Case 1.

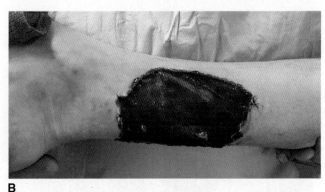

RESULTS

Figures 4-7 to 4-9 shows the results several months postoperatively for Case 1 to 3, respectively.

Valerio et al. recently reported their results with the use of Integra DRT in the setting of traumatic wounds sustained in the combat setting. Two hundred and fifty-one traumatic combat wounds with extensive contamination and a large zone of injury were treated with a median of three debridements before DRT placement, and definitive closure with skin graft was performed at a median of 15 days after DRT placement and 35 days after the initial injury. The authors report an 86% healing rate after the first attempt of definitive closure.

Others have shown promising results using dermal regeneration templates as well. Jeng et al. reported their 7-year experience using Integra DRT in various complex soft tissue wounds and were able to salvage several threatened extremities from amputation, decreasing their amputation rate from 31.5% in the control group to 5.7% in the DRT group. Helgeson et al. reported their success in the use of DRT in blast wounds with exposed bone, successfully achieving coverage in 15 of

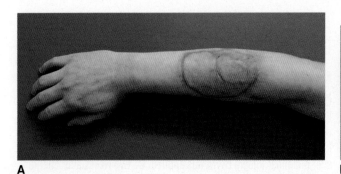

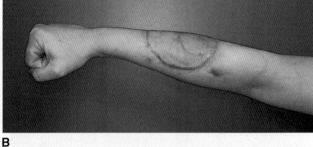

FIGURE 4-7

Case 1. At 6 months after completion of the reconstructive procedures, the patient's forearm exhibits near-normal contour with good skin pliability and tendon/muscle excursion.

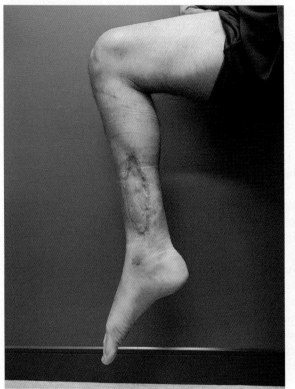 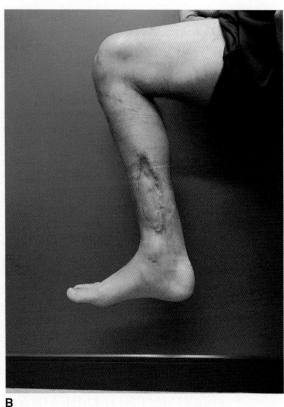

A   **B**

FIGURE 4-8

Case 2. A few months after reconstruction of a medial leg wound, the patient exhibits good ankle dorsiflexion and plantarflexion.

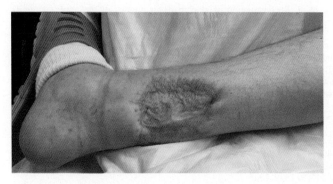

FIGURE 4-9

Case 3. Stable reconstruction 6 months after skin grafting procedure on the lower leg. The patient was able to successfully wear normal footwear on his right lower extremity and resume full ambulatory status including normal use of his left below knee amputation prosthetic.

16 patients. Muangman et al. showed that DRT can be helpful in the setting of severe burns. In 29 patients with mean total burn surface area of 43%, successful take of DRT occurred in 83% and delayed skin grafting in 92% despite having 90% of their wounds contaminated with bacteria on culture.

COMPLICATIONS

Complications with use have been reported but are relatively of low morbidity and include rash, skin tears, bleeding/hematoma, seroma, and infection. Loss of suction, inadequate vacuum pressures, and clogging of suction tubes can increase rates of DRT or graft shearing and nonadherence especially if early mobilization and rehabilitation measures are performed. These same issues also can increase infection rates and thus potential loss of DRT and increase the time to definitive coverage or prolonged delay in wound healing. In rare cases, NPWT has contributed to death, usually associated with hemorrhage and bleeding especially when used in wounds having major vessel injury, having vascular grafts, or on anticoagulation therapies. Wounds complicated by bacterial infections such as *Staphylococcus aureus* or *Pseudomonas aeruginosa* are the most common source of infection and partial/full loss of dermal substitutes and regenerates, followed by shearing of graft from its wound bed preventing incorporation.

PEARLS AND PITFALLS

- NPWT is a useful method to improve skin substitute, dermal regenerate template, and skin graft incorporation and take
- Care must be taken to ensure complete DRT/skin substitute and graft contact with the wound bed to maximize adherence. Tacking sutures and NPWT can aid in obtaining graft incorporation especially in irregular or nonconforming wound beds.
- NPWT in conjunction with DRTs and skin substitutes can reduce graft loss rates, aid in pain reduction, reduce infection rates, and, for extremity wounds, permit limited rehabilitation and controlled physical and occupational therapy measures by protecting and splinting the grafts.
- NPWT used for extremity wounds is often changed at 2- to 3-day intervals for active wound management whereas when used with a DRT or skin substitute may be left in place for 5 to 7 days after grafting and changed weekly without adverse outcomes in appropriately selected cases.
- DRTs and skin substitutes can be used in two-stage or single-stage soft tissue reconstructions to improve outcomes and wound treatment in extremity injuries.
- There are a variety of skin substitutes and DRTs that have an evolving role within the treatment of burn and traumatic and oncologic extremity defects and wounds and should be incorporated within algorithms for extremity reconstructive strategies.

RECOMMENDED READING

Apelqvist J, Armstrong DG, Lavery LA, et al. Resource utilization and economic costs of care based on a randomized trial of vacuum-assisted closure therapy in the treatment of diabetic foot wounds. *Am J Surg.* 2008;195(6):782–788.

Argenta LC, Morykwas MJ. Vacuum-assisted closure: a new method for wound control and treatment: clinical experience. *Ann Plast Surg.* 1997;38(6):563–576.

Chalmers RL, Smock E, Geh JL. Experience of Integra® in cancer reconstructive surgery. *J Plast Reconstr Aesthet Surg.* 2010;63(12):2081–2090.

Demiri E, Papaconstantinou A, Dionyssiou D, et al. Reconstruction of skin avulsion injuries of the upper extremity with Integra® dermal regeneration template and skin grafts in a single-stage procedure. *Arch Orthop Trauma Surg.* 2013;133:1521–1526.

Helgeson MD, Potter BK, Evans KN, et al. Bioartificial dermal substitute: a preliminary report on its use for the management of complex combat-related soft tissue wounds. *J Orthop Trauma.* 2007;21(6):394–399.

Henderson V, Timmons J, Hurd T, et al. NPWT in everyday practice made easy. *Wounds Int.* 2010;5(1). Available at http://www.woundsinternational.com/media/issues/375/files/content_9720.pdf. Accessed January 2016.

Janis JE, Kwon RK, Attinger CE. The new reconstructive ladder: modifications to the traditional model. *Plast Reconstr Surg.* 2011;127(suppl):205S–212S.

Jeng JC, Fidler PE, Sokolich JC, et al. Seven years' experience with Integra® as a reconstructive tool. *J Burn Care Res.* 2007;28(1):120–126.

Moiemen N, Yarrow J, Hodgson E, et al. Long-term clinical and histological analysis of Integra dermal regeneration template. *Plast Reconstr Surg.* 2011;127(3):1149–1154.

Molnar JA, DeFranzo AJ, Hadaegh A, et al. Acceleration of Integra incorporation in complex tissue defects with subatmospheric pressure. *Plast Reconstr Surg.* 2004;113(5):1339–1346.

Morykwas MJ, Argenta LC, Shelton-Brown EI, et al. Vacuum-assisted closure: a new method for wound control and treatment: animal studies and basic foundation. *Ann Plast Surg.* 1997;38(6):553–562.

Morykwas MJ, Simpson J, Punger K, et al. Vacuum-assisted closure: state of basic research and physiologic foundation. *Plast Reconstr Surg.* 2006;117(7S):121S–126S.

Muangman P, Deubner H, Honari S, et al. Correlation of clinical outcome of Integra application with microbiologic and pathological biopsies. *J Trauma.* 2006;61(5):1212–1217.

Nyame TT, Chiang HA, Leavitt T, et al. Tissue-engineered skin substitutes. *Plast Reconstr Surg.* 2015;136:1379.

Park CA, Defranzo AJ, Marks MW, et al. Outpatient reconstruction using Integra and subatmospheric pressure. *Ann Plast Surg.* 2009;62(2):164–169.

Rehim SA, Singhal M, Chung KC. Dermal skin substitutes for upper limb reconstruction: current status, indications and contraindications. *Hand Clin.* 2014;30(2):239.

Seavey JG, Masters ZA, Balazs GC, et al. Use of a bioartificial dermal regeneration template for skin restoration in combat casualty injuries. *Regen Med.* 2016;11(1):81–90.

Streubel PN, Stinner DJ, Obremskey WT. Use of negative-pressure wound therapy in orthopaedic trauma. *J Am Acad Orthop Surg.* 2012;20(9):564–574.

Valerio IL, Sabino JM, Dearth CL. Plastic surgery challenges in war wounded II: regenerative medicine. *Adv Wound Care.* 2016;5(9):412–419.

Wallis L. FDA warning about negative pressure wound therapy. *Am J Nurs.* 2010;110(3):16.

5 Management of Nerve Injuries Following Soft Tissue and Bony Trauma

Ida K. Fox and Amy M. Moore

Nerve injuries are common in the setting of upper extremity soft tissue and bony trauma. Timely recognition and repair of nerve injuries is essential for successful outcomes. A missed nerve injury or delay in treatment can result in the development of chronic pain and disability. Isolated nerve injuries can be challenging to diagnose and treat; devastating multisystem trauma adds further complexity. In this chapter, we provide an overview of the diagnosis and management of these complicated cases.

INDICATIONS

When to Operate?

Nerve injury may be seen with concomitant soft tissue and bony injury. It is critical to identify the mechanism and time course of the nerve injury. For open nerve transection injuries, immediate loss of function is seen and intervention is warranted. In blunt, closed nerve injuries, documentation of the timing and degree of dysfunction are critical to determine when and what to do surgically. The history and physical exam are critical when considering nerve injuries in the setting of soft tissue and bony trauma as it can give you clues to bigger issues. For example, the presence of retained near-normal nerve function after the initial injury, followed by progressive loss of function points to the development of compartment syndrome or acute nerve compression (acute decompression is critical to avoiding pain and potential limb loss and maximizing restoration of function; Fig. 5-1).

Loss of function after fracture manipulation and splinting or fracture fixation surgery should be recognized and treated. Often, the nerve injury is sustained at the time of injury. Although reduction can improve function, the more concerning scenario is loss of nerve function after manipulation or surgical intervention. Partial (and complete) nerve injury is a known risk with fracture reduction, pinning, placement of external fixators, and plating. Thus, it is important to document function both before and after intervention. If the nerve function is intact preoperatively and loss of function occurs postoperatively, one should remain concerned for possible sharp transection injury and follow patients closely and, depending on fracture type and associated symptoms, consider preemptively treating as such with exploration.

55

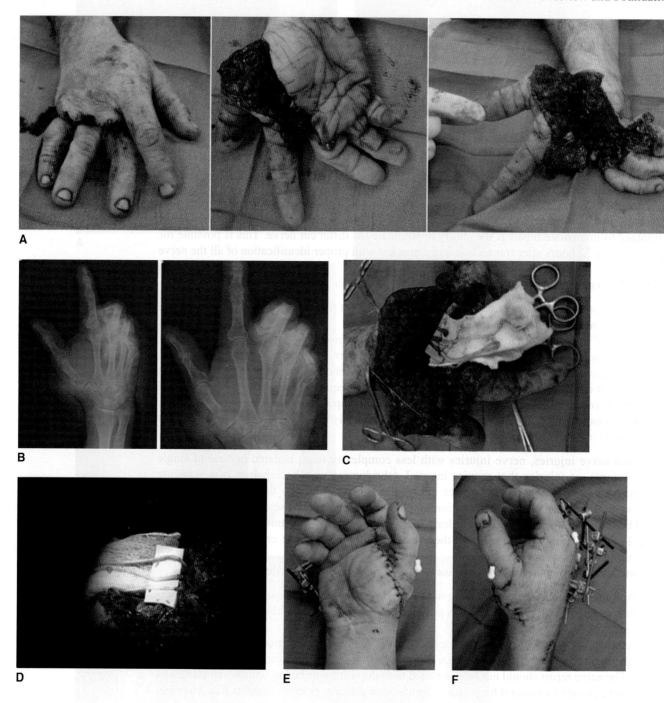

FIGURE 5-2

A, B: A 47-year-old man presented after table saw injury with digital nerve, tendon, and bony injuries. Although all of the digits were perfused, the patient was taken for urgent fracture washout and stabilization. **C, D:** Because of the unusual pattern of injury, acute repair of the thumb ulnar and radial and index radial digital nerve with interposition sural grafts were completed. The extensor tendons to the thumb, index, long, ring, and small fingers were repaired as were the flexor tendons to the thumb and index fingers. **E–G:** An external fixator was used to stabilize the intra-articular long, ring, and small finger fractures. **H:** At 2 years postinjury, he had recovered protective sensation and had returned to work doing highway maintenance. (Printed with permission ©2000 nervesurgery.wustl.edu.)

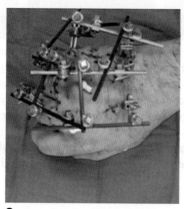

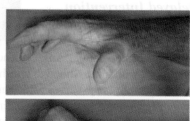

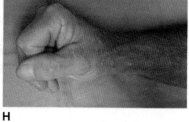

nerve transfer to restore function; early intervention may be warranted to begin nerve regeneration and maximize function. Further, in the setting of a large vessel repair, delayed intervention and re-exploration could risk injury to the recent vascular repair and lead to potential ischemic limb loss. In this case, proactive and aggressive debridement and grafting at the time of arterial repair is indicated.

CONTRAINDICATIONS

There are few contraindications to nerve repairs with trauma. Timing is the key determinant. For example, nerve repairs in the setting of closed or gunshot wound injuries should not be completed unless a lack of spontaneous recovery is noted. Also, nerve repairs and grafting should not be performed in a contaminated or devitalized field to avoid graft loss. Thorough debridement and definitive coverage should be completed prior to or at the time of nerve grafting (see Fig. 5-3).

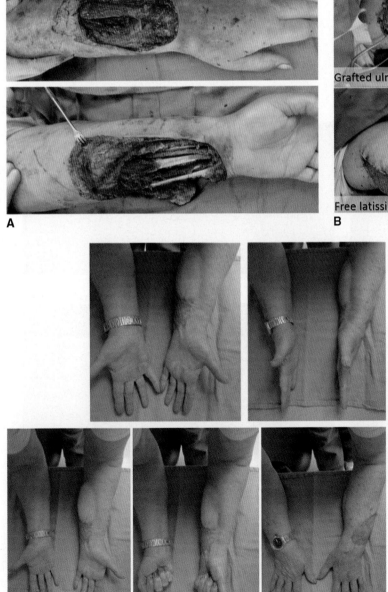

FIGURE 5-3

A 63-year-old woman presented after rollover motor vehicle accident with a left open ulnar fracture, disruption of the ulnar neurovascular bundle, and significant soft tissue trauma. **A:** After serial debridement and appropriate culture-specific antibiotic coverage with the assistance of the infectious diseases service. **B:** At 1 week postinjury, bony fixation, nerve grafting, and free flap (latissimus muscle) coverage were performed. The ulnar nerve was repaired using three cables of sural nerve graft material (length of 12 cm); distal decompression was also completed. **C:** At approximately 1 year, left-sided pinch and grip were 6 and 30 (right was 16 and 65). She had early ulnar intrinsic function with some adduction and abduction of the fingers but still had mild clawing and a positive Froment sign. She had return of sensation at the palm level but not yet at the fingertips. (Printed with permission ©2014 nervesurgery.wustl.edu.)

PREOPERATIVE PLANNING

A thorough preoperative exam that documents existing motor and sensory function is required. For open wounds with obvious transection of the nerve, history and physical exam provide the information necessary to create a preoperative plan. Further testing, beyond the standard imaging required for bony stabilization, is unnecessary. If immediate repair is not performed and/or multiple debridements are required for the concomitant trauma, it is helpful to tag the transected nerve ends with 4-0 Prolene suture or otherwise mark the nerve ends to allow for easier identification at the time of definitive repair (see Fig. 5-4).

In the case of closed blunt force trauma (with or without fractures) and gunshot wounds, multiple serial exams are required to assess nerve function over time. Electrodiagnostic testing can be helpful for managing these types of patients. We recommend this testing at 10 weeks from injury in order to determine severity of injury and to detect subclinical recovery. At 10 weeks postinjury, denervation and early muscle reinnervation can be identified.

If delayed intervention is warranted, imaging, to determine the extent of bony injury and fixation, confirm the patency of the vasculature (angiogram) or position of repaired vessels (ultrasound) is often useful to further developing the operative plan.

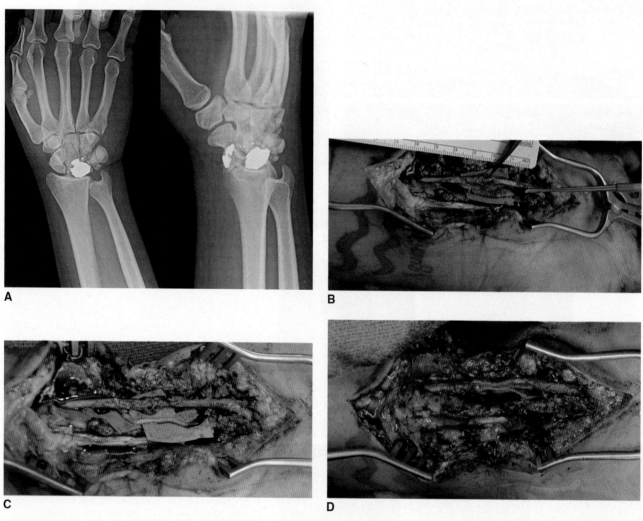

FIGURE 5-4

Gunshot wound to the right wrist. **A:** PA and lateral radiographs demonstrate lunate replaced with bullet remnant. Entrance site of bullet was ulnar just proximal to wrist crease. **B:** The patient was originally taken to the OR for carpal tunnel release and Guyon canal release at day of injury. Ulnar nerve ends were tagged, and a decellularized nerve allograft (Avance Nerve Graft, Axogen Inc.) was used to hold motor component at length. Three weeks later, definitive nerve reconstruction was performed. This image demonstrates the large zone of injury marked with blue lines. **C:** The motor component of the ulnar nerve was reconstructed with a 4-cm reversed sural nerve graft. The purple coloring on the nerve graft denotes the proximal aspect of the nerve ("purple marks proximal"). **D:** The sensory component was reconstructed with 3.5-cm reversed sural nerve cable grafts. (Printed with permission ©2015 nervesurgery.wustl.edu.)

Most importantly, complex extremity trauma with nerve injuries requires extensive preoperative discussions with the patients. Depending on the severity of the injury, it is often unknown what damage will be found intraoperatively. It is important to discuss broadly your goals for reconstruction (to restore function) and obtain a consent that allows for more fluid intraoperative decision making. For example, a consent could read "exploration of wound, possible direct nerve repair, possible nerve graft, possible decellularized allograft, possible nerve transfer, and possible soft tissue coverage of the grafted nerve with local or regional flap".

SURGERY

Careful preoperative planning for peripheral nerve surgery procedures prevents complications and frustration and improves the intraoperative decision making required of these complicated cases. Reports of the preoperative function and electrodiagnostic test results should be immediately available. Because stimulation of nerve donor and recipient pairs and partially intact or distal nerve ends is helpful, the anesthesiology team must avoid using long-acting paralytics. Extended use of a tourniquet (greater than 30 to 60 minutes) may also affect intraoperative stimulation and should be avoided. Finally, major nerve injury exploration and repair almost always takes an entire OR day. Particularly if multiple patient positioning changes are required, staging procedures (such as shoulder, posterior arm, and, separately, anterior arm nerve transfers) may be prudent.

Anatomy

Understanding the anatomy and course of the peripheral nerves is imperative for the nerve surgeon. We recommend identifying a good anatomic atlas and bringing it with you to the operating room when performing complex cases. A few pearls unique to the subject matter at hand will be briefly discussed.

Of primary concern is the proximity of nerves to other critical structures such as blood vessels. Delayed repair of nerve injury, such as a laceration of the median nerve, is potentially fraught with complication if a previous arterial repair should be disrupted. Furthermore, use of a tourniquet is also contraindicated after recent vascular repair making reoperation in a scarred bed even more challenging. For that reason, attention to the nerve injury at the time of arterial repair is helpful. For injuries that may require a delayed approach (to allow the zone of injury to become better defined), consideration of distal transfers and avoiding reoperation at the site of original trauma is helpful. Otherwise, tagging of the nerve ends to adjacent musculature away from the arterial repair may be helpful in the acute phase if the hand surgeon (ideally) is involved. In cases where there are multiple nerve injuries, an arterial repair, and poor soft tissue coverage (such as a skin graft); extra-anatomic grafting may be a useful strategy (Fig. 5-5). In this case, a clear working knowledge of the proximal and distal anatomy will allow proper identification of the appropriate nerve ends to coapt via interposition graft.

An understanding of the internal topography of the major peripheral nerves allows for more precise coaptation and matching of motor-to-motor and sensory-to-sensory fibers within the grouped epineural repair. For example, the median nerve at the antecubital fossa has a defined branch to the pronator teres that lies superficial on the nerve. This branch can be dissected free

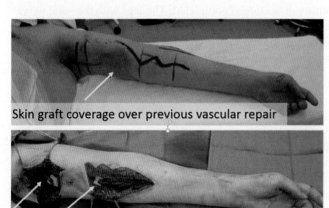

Skin graft coverage over previous vascular repair

Median nerve ends prepared for extranatomic grafting

FIGURE 5-5

A 33-year-old man presented 5 months after gunshot wound injuries to the left upper extremity. He had previously undergone exploration, repair of the brachial artery with interposition vein grafting, humeral fixation, and skin graft coverage of the medial arm. He had intractable pain, loss of median nerve function, and evidence of recovering ulnar and radial nerve function. Extra-anatomic grafting of the median nerve was completed to avoid reoperation in the area of previous skin graft and vascular repair. Staged decompression of the ulnar nerve at the elbow and the median and ulnar nerves at the wrist was completed. (Printed with permission ©2010 nervesurgery.wustl.edu.)

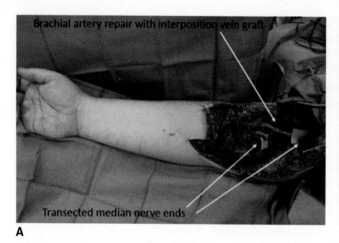
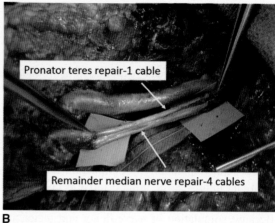

FIGURE 5-6

A 63-year-old man presented as a level 1 trauma patient with a right brachial artery injury and hemodynamic instability. After interposition vein graft repair of the arterial injury and resuscitation **(A)**, a grouped fascicular repair of the intimately associated median nerve injury was completed **(B)**. One sural cable graft was used to repair the pronator teres branch, and four additional cables were used to repair the remainder of the median nerve. At 2 years postinjury, he had recovered extrinsic median nerve function and had right- and left-sided pinch of 14 and 22 and grip of 50 and 87, respectively. He had a stationary Tinel sign at the carpal tunnel and absent intrinsic function but declined additional intervention due to comorbidities and the limited impact of these issues on the quality of his life (he had minimal pain and the ability to do all activities of daily living). (Printed with permission ©2012 nervesurgery.wustl.edu.)

and separately grafted with a single-cable graft if interposition graft is needed. The remaining median nerve can be separately repaired using three or four cables for a grouped fascicular or epineural repair (Fig. 5-6).

It is also important to recognize that with significant soft tissue trauma, the nerves may be "turned," rotated, or otherwise in an unusual position and harder to find or line up topographically. In these cases, a grouped fascicular repair should be performed.

Patient Positioning

For most of these surgeries, the patient is positioned in the supine position with the arm abducted at the shoulder and resting on a hand table. If nerve graft material (small or moderate amount) may be required, surgical prep to the axilla and use of a sterile tourniquet will permit use of both the medial and/or lateral antebrachial cutaneous nerves.

For more extensive nerve injuries where sural nerve graft harvests are required, prone positioning makes the sural nerve dissection and closure much easier (particularly in a more obese patient population or in cases where dissection proximal to the popliteal fossa is required to obtain additional graft length). For these more extensive cases, if it is unclear whether or not the entire nerve graft (or any) is needed, the nerve can be dissected out, vessel loops are placed to mark the proximal and distal ends, hemostasis and closure are obtained (except immediately at that vessel looped site), and the nerve is left in situ while the patient is in prone position. The patient is then repositioned into the supine position, and the upper extremity dissection is completed. The legs with the sural nerves "predissected" out are prepped into the field. Once it confirmed that nerve grafting is necessary and it is clear how much nerve material is required, the sural nerve harvest is completed—often a single stitch is required to close the remaining small incision, and the leg can be temporarily held up for this step to be completed.

Technique

Dissection of the nerves, identification of the proximal and distal ends, and nerve graft harvesting can all be completed using loupe magnification. The coaptation and final trimming of the nerve ends will benefit from the superior magnification of the operating room microscope. Toothed Adson forceps and tenotomy scissors are used for initial dissection. Microsurgical forceps should be used for directly grasping the nerve tissue (holding the epineurium or surrounding fat decreases the trauma to the fascicles themselves). Heparinized saline solution (100 units/mL in adults or 50 units/mL in children) can be used to irrigate as it prevents the suture and graft and adjoining tissue from sticking together.

For all nerve injuries, the nerve ends should be trimmed back to uninjured nerve tissue. Trimming may be done with good quality tenotomy or microscissors, but with larger caliber nerves, they create too much of a crushing injury. The peripheral nerve cutting device (manufactured by ASSI, Westbury, NY) or a fresh 11 blade used with a tongue depressor as a cutting board should be used for transecting larger nerves.

Determining the extent of nerve injury acutely can be challenging, and a number of factors may aid in this process, such as the mechanism of the injury (glass or other sharp mechanisms often require less nerve trimming then a blast or avulsion injury). Sequentially slicing the nerve back until the surgeon can see normal appearing bulging uninjured fascicles is the traditional approach. Nerve ends that are relatively firm and fibrotic feeling to palpation should be trimmed. Another adjunct technique it to lighten the anesthetic and serially trim back the proximal nerve until the heart rate or blood pressure increases—a matching length can also be trimmed from the distal insensate end. This requires close communication with the anesthesiology team, and several minutes should pass between each serial nerve slice to allow time for the blood pressure cuff to cycle. Of note, for young and large patients, this can be a somewhat dangerous technique as previously well-anesthetized patient may become quite combative with this noxious stimulus.

The nerve repair may be completed on top of a blue background, and the coaptations should be performed with 9-0 nylon microsuture. Use of neurosurgical patties (Cottonoid) or Weck-Cel sponges can help wick away blood to improve visualization. Irrigation using a small syringe can also be useful to see the anatomy particularly if there is bleeding of the vasa nervorum. We often seal the coaptations with fibrin glue once the coaptations have been performed under the microscope.

Decompression

Patients with significant edema associated with crush or significant bony trauma closed injury patterns may develop acute nerve compression and urgent decompression may be indicated (see Fig. 5-1). Also, in patients with vascular injury, subsequent reperfusion, and associated compartment syndrome, nerve decompression with specific release of the carpal tunnel and Guyon canal is often indicated with the fasciotomy procedure.

In addition, for cases of major peripheral nerve repair, the authors recommend distal decompression when proximal nerves are repaired. Also, in cases of closed nerve injury or gunshot wound injury, distal decompression alone can often be helpful to nerve recovery and/or pain management. With nerve regeneration, secondary compression can occur at known compression sites (such as carpal tunnel, Guyon canal), and decompression cannot only relieve pain but may, in fact, foster subsequent recovery. We think of this as opening the door to recovery.

Direct Repair

Direct repair means end-to-end approximation of the distal and proximal nerve stumps. A tension-free repair is critical to success as nerves repaired under tension have a higher rate of fibrosis and failure. A rule of thumb is that if the two nerve ends can be held together with two 8-0 nylon epineural sutures placed 180 degrees apart with full range of joint motion, no graft is required. Thus, the wrist is placed in slight extension when repairing the median or ulnar nerve and the finger is placed into extension when repairing a digital nerve. Repairing nerves with the joints at maximal stretch allows the patient to begin early upper extremity motion following surgery with little risk of nerve rupture or fibrosis.

Direct nerve repairs are indicated for nerve injuries that are performed in the acute setting and where minimal associated trauma has been sustained. Patients that are younger tend to have more elasticity to their tissue, and this may also allow direct coaptation. They can rarely be performed in the delayed fashion as the nerve ends retract and become stiff and edematous within 1 week. Direct repair can be advantageous because it minimizes the risk of neuroma, eliminates any nerve graft donor site morbidity, and minimizes the need for sensory or motor reeducation. However, with soft tissue trauma and bony injuries, the zone of injury affecting nerves can make a direct repair difficult.

For direct repair, it is often easiest to place two 180-degree sutures leaving one suture tail on each about 1 cm long to permit later manipulation and positioning. The anterior wall sutures are placed in the epineurium. At this point, it is easier to turn the nerve over and, using the suture tails to hold the nerve, perform the back wall repair.

TABLE 5-1	Strategies to Bridge or Bypass the Gap		
Graft Material or Operative Technique	Advantages	Disadvantages	Common Indication
All autografts	Best results	Donor site deficits	For any nerve gap requiring interposition grafting; best choice (some would say only acceptable choice) for motor or mixed nerve gap repair
Allograft nerve	Unlimited graft material	Requires immunosuppression	Described but rarely used
Decellularized allograft material	Unlimited graft material; does not require immunosuppression; superior to conduits or vein graft as nerve interposition material	Costly, not always available; effectiveness debated	For repair of nonessential sensory nerve territories, to prevent pain (e.g., repair of radial sensory nerve injury)
Conduits	Unlimited material	Moderately costly, effectiveness limited	For repair of nonessential sensory nerve gaps (such as digital nerve at a noncontact surface)
Vein grafts	Unlimited material	May require additional incision/dissection, effectiveness limited	Described but less commonly used
Nerve transfers	Gets out of zone of injury and closer to target, often can avoid interposition graft	Not an option if multiple nerves are involved—due to lack of donors; not an option if muscle is terminally denervated (typically this happens within about 1 y of injury)	To restore function when there is no proximal nerve end available—brachial plexus avulsion and/or in a timely fashion—proximal ulnar nerve injury (for intrinsic function), etc.
Tendon transfers	Can be done years after injury	Requires adequate donor and recipient tendons and reasonable soft tissue envelope	To restore function >1 y after nerve injury as motor reinnervation is no longer an option
Free muscle transfer	Can be done years after injury; can be used to "replace" muscle that is terminally denervated or absent from trauma	Technically challenging, limited amount of function can be restored with each free muscle transfer completed (e.g., composite finger flexion)	To restore function when muscle tissue is absent or donor muscles for tendon transfers are lacking

Printed with permission ©2015 nervesurgery.wustl.edu.

Repair with Interposition

When an end-to-end repair cannot be completed without tension, interposition of some conduit is required to bridge the gap. What this something should be is debatable and will be discussed further below. The most commonly described options include use of sensory (or, less commonly, motor) autograft (expendable nerve from the same patient), allograft nerve material (nerve obtained from a cadaver), synthetic conduits, and autologous vein graft material.

The gold standard continues to be autologous expendable, cabled nerve graft material for critical repairs—motor nerve repairs, mixed nerve repairs, and pure sensory nerves that provide critical sensation (such as the contact surfaces of the first webspace and ulnar border of the small finger).

While cadaveric processed or decellularized human nerve allograft is an attractive option due to the lack of additional surgery required and lack of a donor site morbidity, the effectiveness of this material is under debate. For critical motor, mixed, and sensory nerve gaps, until further definitive data are available, the authors recommend that autograft should be used.

See Table 5-1 for the advantages, disadvantages, and common indications for use of a variety of interposition materials to bridge a nerve gap. See Table 5-2 for the advantages, disadvantages, and common indications for use of the variety of autologous nerves available for use as cable graft material.

INTERPOSITION SINGLE-CABLE GRAFT. When a cable graft is used, the technique for the direct repair can be modified. It is often best to perform the more technically challenging repair first (such as at the distal coaptation site for a digital nerve repair). The anterior wall sutures are placed and then the graft can be flipped or turned back on itself as if turning the page of a book to expose the "back wall." Once the posterior repair is completed, the graft is brought back into position ("flipped back") to permit repair of the proximal coaptation site.

Use of slightly redundant single-cable grafts, particularly for digital nerve repairs in replantation and revascularization, is useful. The redundant graft can be tucked under the dorsal skin and protected so it is out of the way of the subsequent tendon repair and other procedures.

Decellularized allograft can be used in a similar fashion as indicated. This material can be more challenging to handle as the epineural layer is sometimes softer or less defined. If the size match is inappropriate, an internal neurolysis and trimming of any fascicle that is producing the size mismatch may be completed in a longitudinal fashion along the length of the graft material (Fig. 5-7).

TABLE 5-2   Autograft Options

Graft Material[a]	Advantages	Disadvantages	Common Indication
Sural nerve	Large amount available; long graft	Awkward to harvest (prone position preferred for bilateral and/or above knee harvest; obese patients)[a]	Large nerve gaps, multiple nerve gaps
MABC	Moderate amount available; more hidden scar	Can't keep tourniquet on when harvesting; be careful it is the correct nerve (not median) that you are harvesting; try and harvest anterior fascicle only to maintain sensation to posterior elbow contact surface	For short and moderate gaps, such as digital nerve injury(ies), short length of single major peripheral nerve injury
LABC	Moderate amount available; can keep TQ on	More noticeable scar and shorter length then MABC; also adjoining veins make dissection tedious	For shorter gaps; such as digital nerve injury

OTHER POSSIBLE GRAFTS

PIN	The terminal end of the nerve can be used, but it is relatively small in caliber (even for digital nerve repairs) and should only be considered if there is another reason dissection within the fourth extensor compartment is needed; it has essentially no donor site deficit however and transection may help decrease chronic wrist pain.		
Saphenous nerve	In cases in which the saphenous vein is being harvested for concomitant procedures, this nerve may be exposed and can be useful but is small and branches quite a bit.		
Other	Motor nerve (e.g., gracilis branch of obturator nerve, which might be indicated for specific high impact motor nerve repairs—deep motor branch of ulnar nerve or spinal accessory nerve repair) or (relatively speaking) spare parts nerves (e.g., use of the sensory component of the sciatic nerve to repair a more critical motor component of the nerve in the case where there is a paucity of available nerve graft materials)		

[a]Autologous nerve graft materials are listed in order of preference.
LABC, lateral antebrachial cutaneous nerve; MABC, medial antebrachial cutaneous nerve; PIN, posterior interosseous nerve.
Printed with permission ©2015 nervesurgery.wustl.edu.

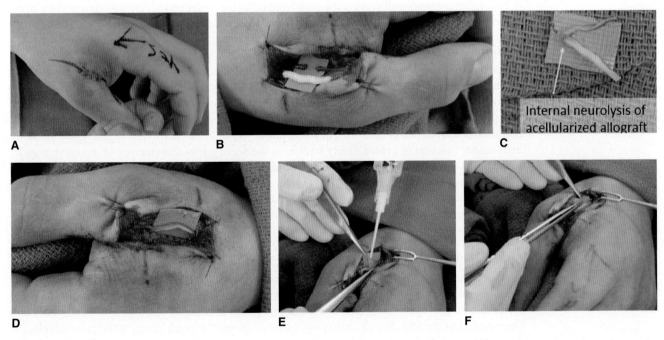

FIGURE 5-7

A: A 13-year-old presented with an accidental stab injury to the left hand; sutures were placed in the ER. Inconsistent distal sensation and a high index of suspicion prompted exploration. At 5 days postinjury, repair of a lacerated branch of the radial sensory nerve with decellularized nerve allograft (Avance Nerve Graft, Axogen Inc.) and repair of the adductor at its tendinous insertion were completed. Because of a size mismatch **(B)**, the nerve allograft material was divided longitudinally (neurolysed) to allow for a technically easier repair **(C)**. The neurolysed allograft was sewn into place **(D)**, fibrin glue was used to reinforce the sutures **(E)**, and the *blue* background was held around the nerve graft repair sites during the setting up of the fibrin glue to keep it from adhering to the underlying soft tissue **(F)**. The thumb interphalangeal joint was left free after surgery and formal therapy was begun at 1 week to avoid painful nerve tethering but protect the tendon repair. (Printed with permission ©2015 nervesurgery.wustl.edu.)

INTERPOSITION MULTIPLE-CABLE GRAFT. Using multiple cables of nerve graft material is often needed to repair the major peripheral nerves of the extremity. In the following section, detailed practical pearls for preparing the cable grafts will be outlined (Fig. 5-8).

- To save time, the graft material can be prepared on the back table while another team turns and positions the patient (if sural grafts were harvested in the prone patient position) or when the second team is dissecting and preparing the proximal and distal transected nerve ends.
- Use of a piece of the Esmarch as a platform is helpful, and the grafts should be occasionally irrigated to prevent desiccation.
- Snake the long cable on itself in a zigzag-type pattern over the nerve gap length (adding a centimeter of extra length is a good idea to build in extra redundancy), then cut the turns to create the multiple cables (reverse the graft segments if there are branches—in most cases, this is unnecessary).
- Sew the cables to each other in a side-to-side fashion using 9-0 nylon epineural stitches to create a "log raft."
- Roll up the log raft to make into a tubular construct but try and preserve the linear organization of the cables and do not allow the cables to crisscross or twist around each other.
- Drip a small amount of fibrin glue onto the construct and quickly fold up and pinch the Esmarch around the nerve graft construct to maintain the tubular shape.
- Allow the fibrin to set, then unroll the Esmarch, trim the nerves ends and excess fibrin glue, then take the construct and insert it into the defect.
- Avoid twisting the construct of cable grafts; lay it into place and coapt it in a position that attempts to line up the proximal and distal internal topography of the native injured nerve ends (this can be identified by examining and matching the proximal and distal fascicular anatomy of the nerve end viewed en face).
- Epineural sutures between the transected nerve ends and the cable graft construct can be reinforced by the use of additional fibrin glue.
- Keeping an Esmarch or blue background under the nerve graft coaptation sites until the added fibrin glue congeals will prevent the graft from adhering to the underlying and surrounding structures and will promote nerve gliding and, hopefully, reduce pain.

Repair with Distal Nerve Transfers

Nerve transfers can be useful in the treatment of complex nerve injuries with associated soft tissue and bony injuries. Nerve transfers have a number of advantages that may make them an attractive reconstructive choice. They can be used to "get out of the zone of injury" as in the case of a significant proximal soft tissue, bony, and/or vascular injury. Nerve transfers allow you to avoid operating in a hostile scarred bed (Fig. 5-9). They also allow you to get closer to the target, restoring motor and sensory function in a more timely fashion as the nerve grows from the site of the nerve transfer to the target end organ. Additionally, nerve transfers often obviate the need for use of interposition grafts and can be done specifically from motor-to-motor nerve or from sensory-to-sensory nerve, avoiding fascicle mismatch. If multiple nerves are injured, then distal nerve transfer may not be a viable option due to the lack of expendable donor nerves. In these cases, direct repair and/or interposition nerve grafting is needed.

Other Techniques

Tendon transfers and free functioning muscle transfers can also be considered in cases of chronic nerve injuries or when there has been direct injury to the motor end plates or muscle itself. If a nerve repair fails to get regenerating fibers to motor end plates in a timely fashion, motor end plates will deteriorate and the muscle will undergo permanent fibrosis. In such cases, subsequent attempts at reinnervation of the muscle will fail, and other methods of improving joint motion must be considered. When contemplating whether nerve repair will be successful in restoring motor function, one should remember that reinnervation must occur within 12 to 24 months of injury to be successful. One must also remember that nerve regeneration occurs at an inch a month, thus late presentation of proximal nerve injuries producing distal motor weakness may be not be amenable to primary repair due to the time required for the regenerating nerve to reach the motor end plates prior to muscle fibrosis.

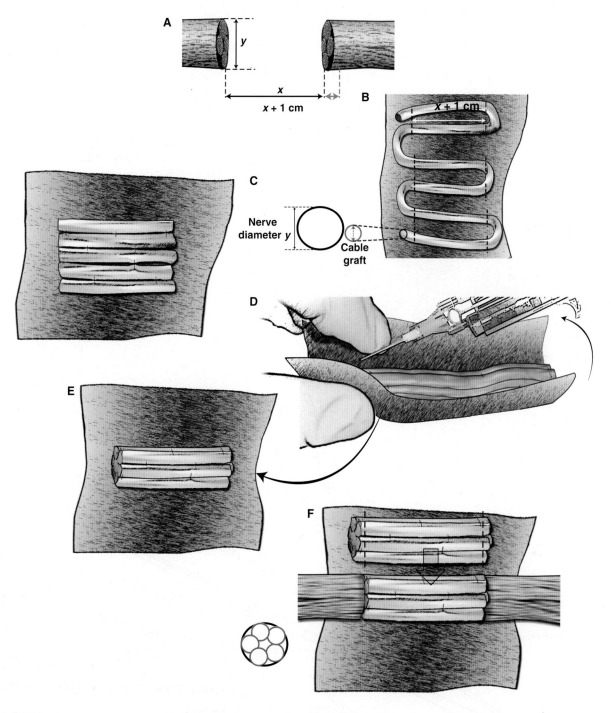

FIGURE 5-8

Schematic depicting preparation of multiple cable grafts. To save time, the graft material can be prepared on the back table while another team turns and positions the patient (if sural grafts were harvested in the prone patient position) or when the second team is dissecting and preparing the proximal and distal transected nerve ends. Use of a piece of the Esmarch as a platform is helpful, and the grafts should be occasionally irrigated to prevent desiccation. **A:** Measure length of gap (*x*) and add about 1 cm. **B:** Coil graft to get, for example, five equal lengths of *x* + 1 cm, then cut and lay out like a log raft (reverse the graft segments if there are branches; in most cases, this is unnecessary). The number of cable grafts required to match the native nerve diameter (*y*) can be more difficult to estimate and may be better judged by eye balling the cross-sectional area of both the native nerve and cables simply by temporarily placing the cable folded up on itself next to the native nerve to see if it "measures up" in terms of the width. **C:** Place a few scattered side-to-side 9-0 nylon epineural sutures to hold together raft. **D:** Roll raft up in Esmarch and add fibrin glue to make a more tubular construct. Preserve the linear organization of the cables and do not allow the cables to crisscross or twist around each other. **E:** Unroll and trim ends and excess glue. **F:** Insert into nerve gap, avoid twisting the construct of cable grafts, lay it into place, and coapt it in a position that attempts to line up the proximal and distal internal topography of the native injured nerve ends (this can be identified by examining and matching the proximal and distal fascicular anatomy of the nerve end viewed en face) and perform coaptation. Add additional fibrin glue to reinforce coaptation site. Keeping an Esmarch or blue background under the nerve graft coaptation sites until the added fibrin glue congeals will prevent the graft from adhering to the underlying and surrounding structures and will promote nerve gliding and, hopefully, reduce pain.

POSTOPERATIVE MANAGEMENT

Management of pain after nerve repair is critical. Most adults benefit from starting gabapentin in addition to narcotics. Other approaches for pain control include the use of long-acting local anesthetics or placement of indwelling supraclavicular anesthetic catheters. Pain management specialists can also be recruited early to assist with long-term pain control. Indwelling supraclavicular catheters can be used to manage pain in the perioperative period.

Early motion to promote nerve gliding and reduce pain from tethering of the repaired nerves is recommended. Even if concomitant bony or tendon repairs preclude movement in all areas, motion

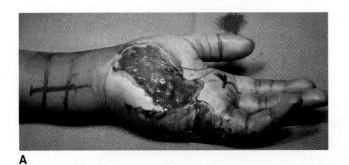

A

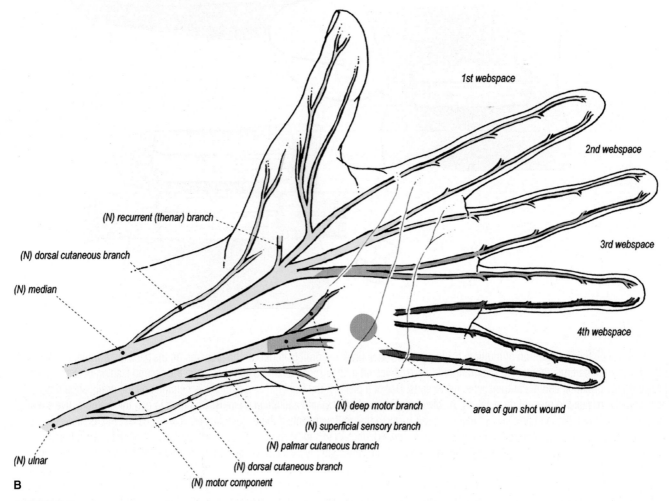

B

FIGURE 5-9

A 5-year-old girl presented with gunshot wound injuries to the ulnar hand. **A:** A washout and amputation of the devascularized small finger was completed. **B:** The following was noted: intact ulnar motor function, segmental loss of the sensory ulnar nerve, and need for soft tissue coverage.

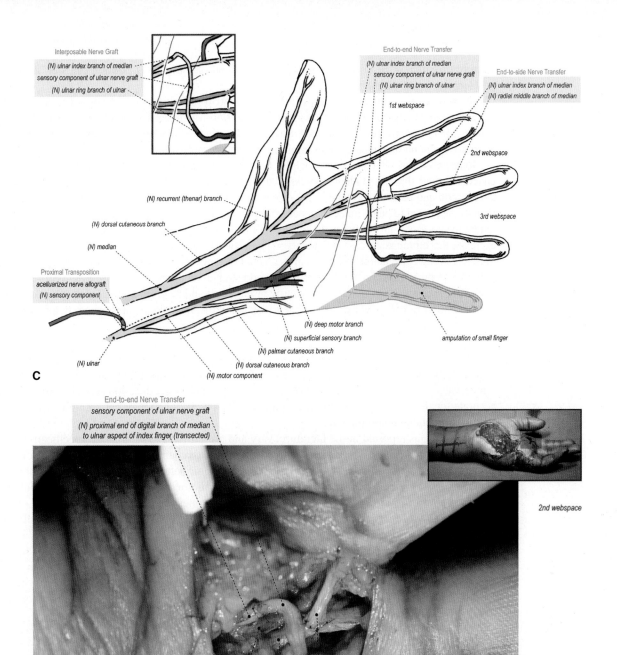

Interposable Nerve Graft
(N) ulnar index branch of median
sensory component of ulnar nerve graft
(N) ulnar ring branch of ulnar

End-to-end Nerve Transfer
(N) ulnar index branch of median
sensory component of ulnar nerve graft
(N) ulnar ring branch of ulnar

1st webspace

End-to-side Nerve Transfer
(N) ulnar index branch of median
(N) radial middle branch of median

2nd webspace

3rd webspace

(N) recurrent (thenar) branch

(N) dorsal cutaneous branch

(N) median

Proximal Transposition
acelluarized nerve allograft
(N) sensory component

amputation of small finger

(N) deep motor branch

(N) superficial sensory branch

(N) palmar cutaneous branch

(N) ulnar

(N) dorsal cutaneous branch

(N) motor component

C

End-to-end Nerve Transfer
sensory component of ulnar nerve graft
(N) proximal end of digital branch of median to ulnar aspect of index finger (transected)

2nd webspace

3rd webspace

(A) common digital

End-to-side Nerve Transfer
(N) distal end digital branch of median to ulnar aspect of index finger (transected)
(N) digital branch of median to radial aspect of long finger

D

FIGURE 5-9 (*Continued*)

C: To avoid the use of long nerve grafts and a complex coverage procedure, a combination of nerve transfers, spare parts surgery, and skin grafting was used for reconstruction. **D:** Specifically, the ulnar digital nerve to the index finger was transferred to the new ulnar border of the hand (ring finger) and then to restore rudimentary sensation back to the donor nerve sensory territory, an end-to-side nerve transfer to the median sensory branch to the radial aspect of the long finger was also performed. The ulnar nerve sensory component in the forearm was harvested as a "spare part" to bridge the gap. A decellularized nerve allograft (Avance Nerve Graft, Axogen Inc.) was used as an extender to allow proximal transposition of the ulnar nerve sensory component intramuscularly at the forearm to prevent painful neuroma formation. At 7 months, sensation was intact at the ring and index fingers to 2.83 Semmes-Weinstein filament, which is indicative of normal light touch. Locognosia was intact in the index and ring fingers to moving and static touch. Further details could not be elicited due to the young age of the patient. (Printed with permission ©2014 nervesurgery.wustl.edu.)

at more proximal or distal joints can still be beneficial (see Fig. 5-7). Motion can start 2 to 3 days postsurgery, when edema is decreasing.

For most nerve graft harvest sites, a limited airstrip dressing is removed and normal showering can begin 2 days postsurgery. For the lower extremity, depending on the presence of vascular, venous, or lymphatic disease, support hose, nondissolvable stitches, less-restrictive footwear, and aggressive edema management can minimize wound complications.

Motor and sensory reeducation is helpful both for nerve transfer and nerve repair patients. Guiding patients through the very gradual progression that occurs after reinnervation is extremely helpful for both the surgeon and patient who tend to get discouraged by the slow time course of recovery. Patients are initially instructed to begin bilateral upper extremity exercises to promote co-contracture of the muscles within the zone of injury. After a "twitch" of motion is appreciated, therapy can be advanced to include exercises that eliminate friction and gravity so that patients may more easily move the joint with the weak muscle. Setting expectations is important as gradual resumption of antigravity motion and strengthening will take months. Coordination, incorporation, and strength continue to improve even years after nerve transfer or repair. Patients that are temporarily insensate should be given tips and tricks on managing the injured extremity and should also start desensitization of the nerve donor site territory if applicable.

RESULTS

Patients who have undergone nerve repair and grafting can achieve individual control over these reinnervated muscle groups given proper retraining. Sensory reeducation can also produce quite accurate localization of sensation. More importantly, a well-done repair can minimize scarring and prevent intractable neuroma pain.

The results, as reported in the literature, vary and are difficult to summarize specifically because the mechanism of injury, type of nerve injured, age, time to repair, and many other factors affect outcomes. Overall, nerve injuries due to simple lacerations fair better than missile/blast and more blunt mechanisms of injury. Younger patients have improved motor and sensory recovery. Proximal injuries have inferior return of both motor and sensory outcomes than distal injuries. Results of injury treated by direct repair compared to interposition grafting are not necessarily dramatically better until the gap exceeds approximately 5 cm. Overall, results with respect to motor function are good for median and radial nerve return of function and ulnar nerve extrinsic muscle return of function. Proximal ulnar nerve injuries are perceived as being the most devastating in terms of return of function and other patient-perceived factors. This may be ameliorated by the use of distal nerve transfers in proximal nerve injury patterns such as the distal anterior interosseous nerve to deep motor branch of ulnar nerve transfer for ulnar nerve injuries proximal to the elbow.

COMPLICATIONS

Nerve pain is a potential complication following any nerve repair. Pain can develop because a nerve injury has been missed or inadequately treated resulting in neuroma formation. It is common to have pain and discomfort in the setting of any major nerve injury; however, this pain will subside as the nerve regenerates. During the regenerative process, nerve pain may flare again as the nerve endings get close to the motor end plates, producing a sensation of "soreness" at the muscle belly. It is important to recognize symptoms of "normal" recovering nerve pain from those of *complex regional pain syndrome*. Complex regional pain syndrome may be associated with abnormal skin color changes, abnormal sweating, pain extending outside the dermatome zone of nerve injury, swelling, and joint stiffness. Management of complex regional pain syndrome is beyond the scope of this chapter, but is best managed using a multidisciplinary approach, including pain specialists, the surgeon, and physical and occupational therapists.

Infection can lead to nerve graft loss (or even limb loss). Aggressive treatment of infection with debridement, antibiotics, and local wound care is the mainstay of treatment. Aggressive initial debridement prior to nerve repair is always the best means of preventing postoperative infections (Fig. 5-10). When nerve repairs lie in an area of compromised or devitalized skin, one may need to consider immediate flap coverage.

Finally, nerve repairs may not function. This could be due to repair rupture if inadequate postoperative immobilization is not utilized or neuroma formation at the repair site. Prior to assuming that this is the most likely possibility, however, it is important to make sure that enough time has passed and that adequate therapy and motor reeducation have been completed. Imaging modalities such as

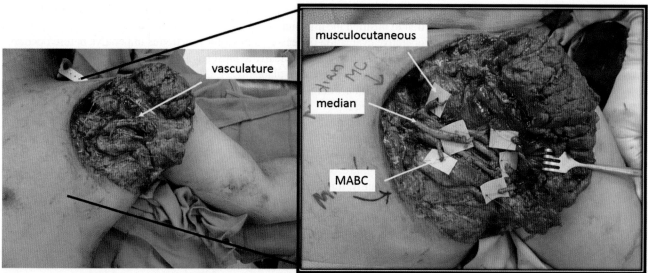

A

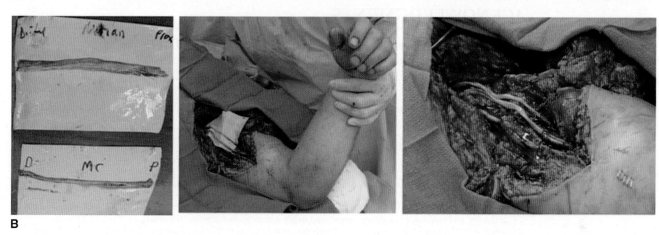

B

FIGURE 5-10

A: A 30-year-old presented after motor vehicle crash with an open brachial plexus injury, clavicular fracture, and shoulder injury. **B:** He underwent staged washouts and tagging of the identified nerve ends with 4-0 Prolene sutures, bony fixation, and rotator cuff repair, and then, nerve transfer (thoracodorsal to suprascapular nerve transfer) and grafting (of the median and musculocutaneous nerves) were performed. Five months postinjury, he presented with infection with *Mycobacterium* requiring hardware removal and wide debridement. Painful shoulder instability remained a significant issue. (Printed with permission ©2009 nervesurgery.wustl.edu.)

MRI and ultrasound can make the definitive diagnosis in these cases. Consideration of rerepair may need to be considered if rupture has occurred.

PEARLS AND PITFALLS

- Identify mechanism of nerve injury, that is, crush, sharp laceration, or gunshot wound.
- Pain trumps all—if you don't manage the pain of nerve injury, it doesn't matter what else you do. A repair or surgery may help the pain, but you need to keep this up front and center when treating these patients. Simply acknowledging nerve pain goes a long way toward building a patient-physician relationship.
- Record time course of functional loss and recovery, that is, motor function was intact until fracture was reduced.
- Don't let the sensory exam confuse you. Patients with multisystem and multistructure trauma can be challenging to examine. Patients want to feel their hands. In the setting of trauma, they will often inaccurately report that sensation is normal. The physical exam is critical.
- Don't let gravity confuse you. Patients with nerve injury often figure out how to position their arms and hands to produce useful movement by substituting one motion for another. For example,

it may seem that triceps function is intact when in fact it is not, and the patient is simply using shoulder abduction to position the arm and gravity to extend the elbow.

- A thorough preoperative evaluation of sensory and motor function is imperative before operative intervention. This should be documented clearly at presentation. You have to know what is in and what is out. This determines the operative plan.
- In cases of penetrating trauma where there is high index of suspicion for nerve injury, err on the side of early exploration and repair.
- Perform nerve repairs in a healthy tissue bed and with stable soft tissue coverage.
- Get out of the zone of nerve injury. The surrounding soft tissue zone of injury will help determine the amount of nerve trimming required. Wide debridement and interposition grafting are often required.
- Don't cut a nerve that might recover; manage most closed injuries (and gunshot wounds without clear transection) expectantly. It is never appropriate to jump in and do distal nerve transfers until lack of recovery is confirmed with serial exams and electrodiagnostic testing.
- Be patient. Nerve recovery is unlike a vascular repair (where flow and reperfusion of the tissue occur almost instantaneously) and even unlike bony healing (where callus formation, diminished pain, and subsequent definitive radiologic healing can take place in just a few months). Nerves take time on the order of months to years to see maximal recovery.

ACKNOWLEDGMENTS

Ida K. Fox, MD, has current funding from the Craig H. Neilsen Foundation for her book, *Nerve Transfers to Restore Hand Function in Cervical Spinal Cord Injury*. Craig H. Neilsen Foundation Spinal Cord Injury Research on the Translational Spectrum (SCIRTS) grant.

Amy M. Moore, MD, has current funding from the Department of Defense for her *Macroscopic Management of Neuromas in Residual Limbs* Peer Reviewed Orthopaedic Research Program (PRORP) Translational Science Award.

RECOMMENDED READING

Boyd KU, Nimigan AS, Mackinnon SE. Nerve reconstruction in the hand and upper extremity. *Clin Plast Surg.* 2011;38(4):643–660.

Brooks DN, Weber RV, Chao JD, et al. Processed nerve allografts for peripheral nerve reconstruction: a multicenter study of utilization and outcomes in sensory, mixed, and motor nerve reconstructions. *Microsurgery.* 2012;32(1):1–14.

Campbell WW. Evaluation and management of peripheral nerve injury. *Clin Neurophysiol.* 2008;119(9):1951–1865.

Clark WL, Trumble TE, Swiontkowski MF, et al. Nerve tension and blood flow in a rat model of immediate and delayed repairs. *J Hand Surg Am.* 1992;17(4):677–687.

Fox IK, Mackinnon SE. Adult peripheral nerve disorders: nerve entrapment, repair, transfer, and brachial plexus disorders. *Plast Reconstr Surg.* 2011;127(5):105e–118e.

Kahn KC, Moore AM. Donor activation focused rehabilitation approach (DAFRA): maximizing outcomes after nerve transfers. *Hand Clin.* 2016;32(2):263–277.

Ljungquist KL, Martineau P, Allan C. Radial nerve injuries. *J Hand Surg Am.* 2015;40(1):166–172.

Moore AM, Novak CB. Advances in nerve transfer surgery. *J Hand Ther.* 2014;27(2):96–104.

Moore AM, Wagner AJ, Fox IK. Principles of nerve repair in complex wounds of the upper extremity. *Semin Plast Surg.* 2015;29(1):40–47.

Pederson WC. Median nerve injury and repair. *J Hand Surg Am.* 2014;39(6):1216–1222.

Poppler LH, Davidge K, Lu JC, et al. Alternatives to sural nerve grafts in the upper extremity. *Hand (NY).* 2015;10(1):68–75.

Post R, de Boer KS, Malessy MJ. Outcome following nerve repair of high isolated clean sharp injuries of the ulnar nerve. *PLoS One.* 2012;7(10):e47928.

Rochkind S, Strauss I, Shlitner Z, et al. Clinical aspects of ballistic peripheral nerve injury: shrapnel versus gunshot. *Acta Neurochir (Wien).* 2014;156(8):1567–1575.

Safa B, Buncke GM. Autograft substitutes: conduits and processed nerve allografts. *Hand Clin.* 2016;32(2):127–140.

Sameem M, Wood TJ, Bain JR. A systematic review on the use of fibrin glue for peripheral nerve repair. *Plast Reconstr Surg* 2011;127:2381–2390.

Schreiber JJ, Strauss I, Shlitner Z, et al. Preoperative donor nerve electromyography as a predictor of nerve transfer outcomes. *J Hand Surg Am.* 2014;39(1):42–49.

Schwartzman RJ, Maleki J. Postinjury neuropathic pain syndromes. *Med Clin North Am.* 1999;83(3):597–626.

Stewart JD. Peripheral nerve fascicles: anatomy and clinical relevance. *Muscle Nerve.* 2003;28(5):525–541.

Toby EB, Meyer BM, Schwappach J, et al. Changes in the structural properties of peripheral nerves after transection. *J Hand Surg Am.* 1996;21(6):1086–1090.

Tse R, Ko JH. Nerve glue for upper extremity reconstruction. *Hand Clin.* 2012;28(4):529–540.

Upton AR, McComas AJ. The double crush in nerve entrapment syndromes. *Lancet.* 1973;2(7825):359–362.

Wang JP, Rancy SK, Lee SK, et al. Shoulder and elbow recovery at 2 and 11 years following brachial plexus reconstruction. *J Hand Surg Am.* 2016;41(2):173–179.

Woo A, Bakri K, Moran SL. Management of ulnar nerve injuries. *J Hand Surg Am.* 2015;40(1):173–181.

6 Management of Vascular Injuries Following Soft Tissue and Bony Trauma

Randall R. DeMartino and Gustavo S. Oderich

Accidental injuries affect 2.6 million people in the United States each year. Mechanisms of injury include penetrating, blunt, and iatrogenic trauma. It is estimated that vascular trauma affects 0.2% to 4% of all injured patients. Over 80% of these vascular injuries will be located in extremities. Ninety percent of all vascular injuries are associated with penetrating trauma, of which 70% are due to gunshot injuries, 20% are due to stab wounds, and 10% are due to blunt trauma. Combined vascular and orthopedic trauma is relatively uncommon, accounting for less than 1% of all cases of traumatic injuries. Vascular injuries can occur because of the superficial location of vessels, their proximity to bones, and their relatively fixed position across joints. Patients sustaining combined injuries are exposed to substantially increased risk of amputation and limb dysfunction. This chapter focuses on the indications, contraindications, preoperative planning, operative approach, and results of repair of the most common combined vascular and orthopedic injuries.

INDICATIONS/CONTRAINDICATIONS

Primary repair of arterial and venous injuries is indicated to control bleeding and/or to relieve limb or organ ischemia. Life-threatening injuries should be recognized early during the resuscitation phase and prioritized before proceeding with vascular and orthopedic repair. Arterial injuries affecting only one of the tibioperoneal or forearm arteries may be treated conservatively provided that there is no evidence of distal ischemia. Nonocclusive arterial injuries (e.g., small intimal flaps or dissections) incidentally found on imaging studies can be safely observed. The benign natural history of these injuries is well documented in several large series; operative repair is required in less than 1% of patients.

Extremity trauma with complex soft tissue, vascular, and skeletal injuries poses one of the most difficult management problems. These patients should be evaluated by a multidisciplinary team. Coordinated interaction of various specialists including a vascular, orthopedic, and plastic surgeon is of paramount importance to optimize outcome. Injuries of the head, chest, and abdomen may require additional neurosurgical and general trauma consultation. Every effort is made to balance the potential success of an arterial reconstruction and correction of the orthopedic injury with the overall clinical status of the patient and the potential for complete functional recovery. In general, once life-threatening injuries are stabilized, treatment priorities are control of bleeding and restoration of arterial inflow, fracture reduction and stabilization, and soft tissue coverage.

Vascular repair should be prioritized over definitive orthopedic repair. Any delay in vascular reconstruction is a gamble and may risk the only opportunity for limb salvage. Patients with stable fractures or dislocations in which minimal manipulation and length discrepancy are anticipated should be treated with immediate definitive arterial revascularization. However, patients with severely comminuted fractures and dislocations, segmental bone loss causing limb discrepancy, or severe soft tissue disruption and contamination should be treated initially with temporary intra-arterial shunts. In these cases, it is wise to delay the definitive vascular reconstruction until wide debridement and initial skeletal repair are accomplished.

TABLE 6-1	Factors Associated with Poor Functional Recovery or Need for Primary Amputation after Combined Vascular and Orthopedic Extremity Trauma

Transected sciatic or tibial nerve
Transection of two of the three upper extremity nerves
Gustilo III-C orthopedic injury
Below-knee arterial injury with two of the three arteries injured
Prolonged limb ischemia >12 h
Cadaveric limb
Multiple comminuted fractures
Extensive soft tissue loss
Crush injury
Severe contamination
Elderly patients or multiple medical comorbidities
Shock or other life-threatening injuries

Contraindications for vascular repair include presence of other life-threatening injuries requiring immediate attention or causing hemodynamic instability. Several predictive factors should be taken into consideration when deciding to perform revascularization versus primary amputation (Table 6-1). Overall, approximately 10% to 20% of patients with complex extremity injuries have nonsalvageable limbs and require primary amputation. Assessment of these patients should be individualized. Several factors should be taken into consideration, including the overall clinical status; severity of the arterial, neurologic, and orthopedic trauma; and expected functional recovery. A primary amputation is considered in cases of dysvascular extremity with complex fractures and extensive soft tissue and nerve damage. Patients with major nerve transections (e.g., tibial nerve transection) and open comminuted tibiofibular fractures with arterial injuries (Gustilo III-C) have very poor functional outcome and high amputation rates; these patients are generally treated with primary amputation. Major nerve transections should be confirmed by direct visualization. Other indication for amputation is prolonged ischemia time (greater than 12 hours) with evidence of a cadaveric extremity (e.g., mottled with absence of motor function, arterial, or venous Doppler signals).

PREOPERATIVE PLANNING

Prolonged ischemia time is the most important factor associated with limb dysfunction or amputation. A high index of suspicion coupled with accurate neurovascular examination is necessary for prompt diagnosis of a vascular injury. Accurate diagnosis of vascular injuries is an essential aspect in the preoperative evaluation of patients with complex extremity trauma. Prompt restoration of arterial blood flow within 6 hours from the time of initial extremity injury is the most critical factor that determines limb salvage and function.

Complete history including the mechanism of trauma, associated injuries, medical history, medications, and allergies should be recorded. In older patients, history should include any previous claudication symptoms or known peripheral vascular disease. Extremity vascular trauma is immediately apparent because of external bleeding, hematoma, or obvious limb ischemia. Physical examination includes inspection of the injured limb for open wounds, obvious deformities, and signs of ischemia. Distal ischemia is manifested by the five Ps: pallor, paresthesia, paralysis, pain, pulselessness, and poikilothermia. A thorough sensory and motor examination and pulse examination should be noted. The presence of hematoma, pulsatile or not, bruit, and thrill must be documented. If distal pulses are diminished or absent, the ankle-brachial index (ABI) should be determined using a handheld Doppler device. An ABI of less than 0.9 is considered abnormal and requires further testing. Patients with known vascular disease may also be evaluated with an ankle-ankle index, where less than 0.9 is abnormal.

Signs of arterial injury have been traditionally classified into "hard" and "soft" signs (Table 6-2). These correlate with the presence of a hemodynamically significant arterial lesion. "Hard" signs include absence of distal pulses, pulsatile bleeding, expanding hematoma, palpable thrill, and audible bruit. "Soft" signs include proximity to the vessel, peripheral nerve deficit, history of moderate hemorrhage, and *diminished* distal pulses.

TABLE 6-2 Clinical Signs of Vascular Injury	
Hard Signs	**Soft Signs**
Absent distal pulses	Diminished distal pulses or ABI < 0.90
Active pulsatile bleeding	Unexplained hypotension or large blood loss at the scene
Expanding hematoma	Small or moderate nonexpanding hematoma
Bruit	Injury in proximity to a major vessel
Thrill	Neurologic injury in proximity to vessel

The general recommendation is that patients with hard signs associated with uncomplicated penetrating trauma should undergo immediate operative exploration, without need for arteriography or duplex ultrasound. The indications for arteriography are summarized in Table 6-3. Patients with multiple penetrating injuries should be evaluated with arteriography to determine the exact location and extent of arterial lesions. Arteriography is also advised in patients with combined arterial and orthopedic trauma, even in the absence of hard signs. While the presence of hard signs predicts major vascular injury in nearly 100% of patients with uncomplicated penetrating trauma, less than 15% of patients with complex blunt injuries will require vascular repair. The inaccuracy of hard signs in this subgroup is explained by a combination of multiple other factors that ultimately lead to diminished pulses, including fractures, soft tissue disruption, compartment syndrome, and extrinsic arterial compression. Therefore, we generally recommend arteriography in all patients with complex skeletal trauma and hard signs of vascular injury.

We generally prefer a one-shot intraoperative arteriography technique. This avoids the 1- to 3-hour time delay required to obtain a formal arteriography in the angiography suite. An antegrade or retrograde approach in the affected limb is used for most cases. The availability of a portable C-arm and fluoroscopy permits localization of bony landmarks, selective catheterization of arterial branches, and endovascular treatment of arterial lesions. However, because fluoroscopy is usually not readily available in the emergency setting, we usually use ultrasound guidance and a micropuncture set for arterial access. The target artery (e.g., common femoral artery or brachial artery) is accessed with a micropuncture needle (18 gauge) in an antegrade or retrograde fashion. A 0.018-in. guidewire is advanced to allow placement of a sheath. The sheath can be used for contrast injection. Alternatively, the 0.018-in. wire is exchanged into a 0.035-in. wire and a 4-French sheath is advanced. The arterial inflow proximal to the access site should be manually compressed during contrast injection using digital pressure or a tourniquet. A single-hand injection of 30 mL of diluted (50:50) iso-osmolar contrast allows adequate visualization of the area of concern and distal runoff vessels.

Other noninvasive imaging modalities are duplex ultrasound, computed tomography angiography (CTA), and magnetic resonance angiography. CTA is now available in most centers, is quite expeditious, and permits excellent image of the arterial circulation, soft tissue, and bone. This is particularly useful for planning operative approach in patients with centrally located lesions (e.g., aorta, subclavian, or iliac arteries). However, limitations are the relatively large contrast load (150 mL) in a patient who may potentially require additional angiography.

We recommend duplex arterial ultrasound in patients with "soft" signs of vascular injury, including those with an ABI of less than 0.90. Arterial imaging is not required in patients with normal pulses and no other sign of arterial injury. Physical examination excludes significant arterial injuries as reliably as arteriography or surgical exploration. This is also true for patients with

TABLE 6-3   Indications for Preoperative or Intraoperative Diagnostic Arteriography in Patients with Combined Extremity Trauma
Multiple penetrating injuries
Unclear location or extent of arterial injuries
Extensive soft tissue injury
Fracture or dislocations with hard signs of vascular injury
Trajectory parallel to artery
Underlying peripheral arterial disease

posterior knee dislocations, in whom arteriography used to be obtained routinely in the 1980s. Results of a recent series show that in the absence of hard signs, less than 5% of patients had abnormalities on the arteriography and none required operative treatment or had amputation. On the other hand, the incidence of significant vascular injuries is 70% in the presence of hard signs. In patients with normal pulse examination, nonocclusive lesions include small intimal flaps, dissections, contusions, or small pseudoaneurysms; these lesions should be treated with antiplatelet therapy only.

SURGERY

Patient Positioning and General Approach

All vascular injuries can be accessed using the supine anatomic position (Fig. 6-1). Although prone position and a posterior approach may be used for isolated popliteal artery injuries, which do not extend into the superficial femoral or tibioperoneal arteries, this approach limits access to the great saphenous vein if harvesting is necessary and may require excessive manipulation of the fractured limb. A generous sterile field should be prepared and draped to allow adequate exposure, proximal and distal control, and options of extra-anatomic reconstruction if indicated. The wise surgeon should always consider the "worst case scenario" (e.g., axillofemoral graft). A noninjured lower extremity should be prepped circumferentially for possible vein harvesting. The ideal conduit is an autologous great or small saphenous vein. Preoperative intravenous antibiotics (e.g., a first-generation cephalosporin) should be administered. Based on the planned approach, prior imaging, and the acuity of the injury, intraoperative angiography should be strongly considered and made available. In many centers, this can be performed in a hybrid operating room with fixed imaging equipment or a room large enough for mobile fluoroscopy units. In some situations, an endovascular approach may be feasible and/or preferable for treatment or proximal vascular control.

Open Surgical Technique

Repair of vascular injuries can be one of the most challenging aspects of trauma management. Some basic principles of vascular repair are applicable to all vascular injuries (Table 6-4).

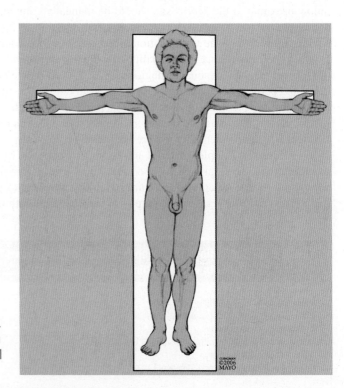

FIGURE 6-1

Patients should be positioned supine with one or both upper extremities abducted. At least one unaffected lower extremity should be circumferentially prepped for vein harvesting if indicated. (By permission of the Mayo Foundation for Medical Education and Research. All rights reserved.)

TABLE 6-4   Basic Principles of Repair of Vascular Injuries
Manual pressure for vascular control
Access using standard vascular exposure
Ensure proximal and distal control prior to entering a hematoma
Carefully enter the hematoma, avoiding injury to adjacent structures
Assess the extent of injury and presence of concomitant venous injury
Use systemic heparinization whenever possible
Determine type of vascular repair
Debridement of vessel edges
Proximal and distal Fogarty catheter thromboembolectomy
Instill regional heparin after two "clean" passes
Perform vascular anastomosis in a tensionless fashion
Allow prograde and retrograde bleeding prior to completing the anastomosis
Complete suture line, remove distal and proximal clamp sequentially
Assess distal circulation with pulse examination and handheld Doppler
Obtain completion arteriography
Consider need for fasciotomy
Ensure adequate soft tissue coverage of vascular reconstruction

The operative sequence consists of access, exposure, control, and repair. Initial control of external hemorrhage is usually obtained with simple digital or manual pressure. Use of surgical instruments such as hemostats not only is ineffective but also risks iatrogenic injury of adjacent nerves or veins. Manual compression is maintained by a member of the surgical team until definitive proximal and distal control of the injured vessel is obtained.

The hematoma should not be entered without first obtaining proximal and distal control away from the site of injury. Access is gained using the standard exposure techniques described in the following discussion. Vascular clamps should not be applied forcefully and blindly; instead, the artery should be completely dissected, looped with a silastic vessel loop, and clamped under direct vision. One important adjunct is the use of balloon occlusion catheters. This facilitates control in areas of difficult access and avoids excessive dissection. In addition, pressure cuff tourniquets may be used in the extremities to achieve prompt vascular control.

Once control is gained, the hematoma is explored with careful attention to avoid injury to adjacent structures. The extent of vascular injury is assessed and clamps are moved closer to the vascular wound.

The injured vessel should be debrided and cleaned using tenotomy scissors. The extent of debridement should take into consideration the mechanism of injury, with more extensive debridements for high-velocity gunshot wounds and blast or crush injuries. One should avoid excising the adventitia of the vessel while dissecting or debriding the artery.

Distal and proximal thrombectomy using a Fogarty balloon thromboembolectomy catheter should be performed even in the presence of relatively good prograde or retrograde bleeding. The size of the catheter is generally a 4 or 5 for the iliacs, 4 for the superficial femoral, 3 or 4 for the deep femoral, 2 or 3 for the tibials, and 2 for the pedal and smaller arteries of the forearm. Passage of thromboembolectomy catheters into the deep femoral, tibials, and smaller arteries should be done gently because of risk of arterial rupture, dissection, or intimal injury due to excessive balloon inflation. At least two "clean" passes should be made with brisk prograde and retrograde bleeding before considering the artery free of thrombus.

Preoperative and intraoperative systemic heparinization (80 mg/kg bolus) should be used unless there is a contraindication (e.g., head injury). An activated clotting time above 250 seconds is considered optimal. Liberal regional heparinization should be used with flushes of heparinized saline proximally and distally to prevent propagation of any thrombus.

Restoration of extremity perfusion does not always require definitive arterial reconstruction. Another important adjunct is a temporary arterial shunt placed in the proximal and distal arterial ends. This promptly controls hemorrhage and re-establishes inflow. Our preference is to use either a short or long Sundt intraluminal arterial shunt (Fig. 6-2). The shunt is secured to the artery using silk suture or a Rummel tourniquet. Although systemic heparinization is preferred, this is not an absolute requirement for shunt placement. The main advantage of temporary shunts is the avoid-

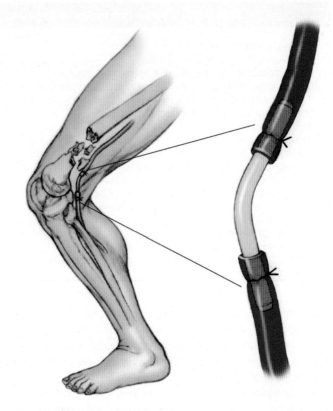

FIGURE 6-2

Intra-arterial Sundt shunt for temporary
control and restoration of blood flow.
(By permission of the Mayo Foundation
for Medical Education and Research.
All rights reserved.)

ance of damage to a fresh arterial repair during subsequent orthopedic manipulations in cases of comminuted, unstable skeletal injuries.

The injured vessels are set up for the reconstruction using stay sutures and clean white towels. The anastomosis should be performed without any tension using optic magnification and small monofilament suture (e.g., Prolene). In general, a 4-0 or 5-0 monofilament suture is used for the femoral arteries, and 6-0 or 7-0 for the popliteal, tibials, and smaller arteries. The type of reconstruction varies and should be tailored to both the patient condition and extent of injury (Fig. 6-3). Simple repair entails a lateral arteriorrhaphy or venorrhaphy. One should avoid excessive narrowing of the lumen and use patch angioplasty if there is any question. A segment of saphenous vein or bovine pericardium can be used for vascular patches. Vessels with injuries involving less than 1.5 cm in length can usually be reapproximated using end-to-end anastomosis. Mobilization of the artery or vein may require ligation of multiple side branches to gain enough length to allow a tensionless anastomosis. The vessel ends should be spatulated to prevent anastomotic narrowing. A running anastomosis is used in most cases, but interrupted sutures may be required in smaller vessels or pediatric cases. Before completion of the anastomosis, the proximal and distal clamps are temporarily removed to ensure adequate prograde and retrograde bleeding. Absence of back bleeding indicates thrombus formation or a technical defect and warrants further catheter embolectomy or revision. Approximately 80% of all vascular extremity injuries that occur in association with orthopedic trauma can be repaired using one of these three techniques: simple closure, end-to-end anastomosis, or patch angioplasty.

Insertion of an interposition or bypass graft is required in approximately 20% of cases. Vessels with more extensive injuries of greater than 1.5 cm in length cannot be reapproximated without tension. The preferred conduit in these cases is the great saphenous vein harvested from the contralateral noninjured extremity. The ipsilateral saphenous vein should be avoided due to a high incidence of concomitant deep venous injuries (50%) and postoperative deep venous thrombosis. The great saphenous vein is ideal for vessels 6 mm or smaller. Some size mismatch is acceptable. However, for injuries of larger vessels, a larger conduit should be selected. Spiral or panel vein grafts, or femoral vein grafts, are acceptable options. For arterial injuries of the aorta and major branches, polytetrafluoroethylene (PTFE) or Dacron grafts have been used extensively with excellent results. Obviously, contamination of the surgical field represents a limiting factor in these cases. Every attempt should

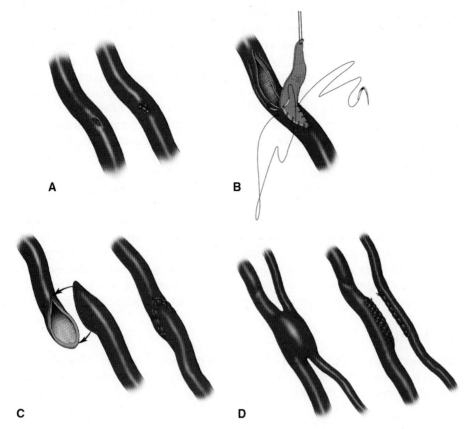

FIGURE 6-3

Types of vascular injuries and repair: simple laceration treated with arteriorrhaphy **(A)**, use of patch angioplasty for longer lesions **(B)**, end-to-end anastomosis **(C)**, and lateral arteriorrhaphy **(D)**.

be made to repair both the arterial and venous injury. Although venous repair has limited patency, improved outflow decreases edema and may affect patency of the arterial repair. The traditional recommendation is that all venous injuries involving the popliteal, common femoral, axillary, and portal veins should be repaired because of poor collateral flow. This recommendation has now been extended to all major named veins.

After the vascular reconstruction is complete, the surgeon should assess the adequacy of the repair for any residual stenosis or kinks. The limb should be examined and distal perfusion documented with pulse and handheld Doppler examination. The goal in a patient without preexisting vascular disease is to obtain normal distal pulses at the end of the operation. Completion arteriography is important to detect any technical abnormalities that may cause early thrombosis of the repair, as well as to assess the patency of the distal runoff vessels. Finally, the vascular reconstruction should be covered with viable soft tissue. Occasionally, flaps are required to bring vascularized tissue over the reconstruction.

Endovascular Technique

Endovascular approaches have become more common for treatment of arterial trauma, particularly in blunt injuries. The appeal of an endovascular approach is that it can reduce the morbidity of the operation and treat the injury in a rapid and expedient fashion. Additionally, since many patients may need diagnostic arteriography, much of the arterial access is already established for intervention. Endovascular treatment refers to several therapeutic options such as stent graft treatment of arterial occlusions or embolization of bleeding vessels. It may also serve as proximal control for vessels with difficult exposure, such as the proximal subclavian artery.

Basic vascular access technique includes the use of ultrasound imaging of the access vessel (i.e., femoral) for cannulation with a micropuncture needle (18 gauge) in an antegrade or retrograde fashion. A 0.018-in. guidewire is advanced, and using a Seldinger technique, this is exchanged for a larger 0.035-in. wire and 5-French sheath to allow for stable access. The use of shaped catheters and guidewires permits selective catheterization of the target artery. If possible, heparin should be given. However, lower doses may be used (i.e., 5,000 units intravenous) compared to open reconstructions that typically require higher anticoagulation parameters. In the setting of blunt injury with vessel occlusion, the occlusion may be crossed with a hydrophilic wire. If the vessel is not in continuity, this may not be possible and open repair is needed. Successful crossing of an occlusion with confirmatory arteriogram is mandatory to ensure true lumen re-entry has occurred and no dissection has been created before proceeding to treatment. In a penetrating trauma setting, once the vessel injury is delineated and the injury traversed, stent graft placement may then proceed. Placement of an appropriately sized (roughly 10% oversized) stent graft is then placed across the injury and deployed with attempts to preserve any patent collaterals. Post–stent grafting angioplasty should be performed to ensure seal and deployment to stent graft profile. Completion arteriography is performed to ensure no residual dissections or arterial defects persist and no embolization has occurred. Treatment with aspirin and clopidogrel, if not contraindicated, is usually necessary after stent graft placement. As with open reconstructions, attention to development of compartment syndrome is important. In some setting, such as deep femoral artery branch bleeding, embolization with coil or glue may be used for treatment with little long-term sequelae. If proximal control is anticipated to be difficult, an appropriately sized balloon may be used for inflow control to permit open surgical repair.

Specific Injuries

Penetrating injuries can affect any arterial segment. Specific patterns of blunt orthopedic and arterial trauma are well recognized (Table 6-5). The surgical anatomy and exposure of the most common arterial injuries are outlined in the following paragraphs.

Upper Extremity Injuries

SUBCLAVIAN ARTERY. The right subclavian artery originates from the innominate artery, and the left subclavian from the aorta (Fig. 6-4). The subclavian artery is divided into three parts in relation to the anterior scalene muscle: proximal, middle, and distal. The proximal subclavian artery gives off the vertebral, internal thoracic, and thyrocervical trunk. The middle subclavian artery contains the costocervical trunk and the dorsal scapular artery. The distal subclavian artery has no branches. A supraclavicular incision one fingerbreadth above the clavicle allows excellent exposure of the middle and distal subclavian artery (Fig. 6-5). For exposure of the proximal subclavian artery, median sternotomy is required for right-sided injuries and left anterolateral thoracotomy for left-sided injuries.

Subclavian artery injuries are uncommon and represent less than 5% of all vascular injuries. Blunt injuries may occur in association with clavicular or first rib fracture. Over 50% of patients present with massive bleeding. Subclavian artery occlusion is well tolerated in 85% of patients because of a rich collateral system. Amputation is rarely required. Arterial repair usually requires end-to-end anastomosis or a small interposition graft using autologous vein. Overall, the mortality rate for subclavian artery injuries is 16%.

AXILLARY ARTERY. The axillary artery extends from the lateral border of the first rib to the lateral border of the teres major muscle (see Fig. 6-4). The artery is divided into three parts in relation to the

TABLE 6-5   Patterns of Combined Orthopedic and Vascular Trauma

Orthopedic Injury	Arterial Injury Location
Supracondylar humeral fracture	Brachial artery
Clavicular fracture	Subclavian and axillary artery
Shoulder dislocation	Axillary artery
First rib fracture	Subclavian artery and aorta
Femoral shaft fracture	Superficial femoral artery and above-knee popliteal artery
Posterior knee dislocation	Popliteal artery
Proximal tibiofibular fracture	Popliteal and tibioperoneal arteries

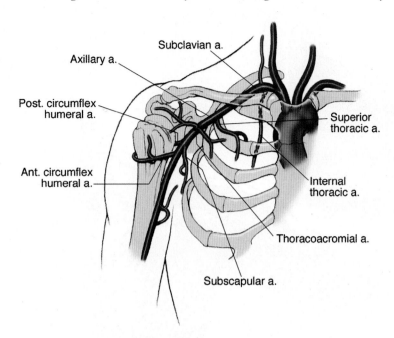

FIGURE 6-4

Surgical anatomy of the subclavian and axillary arteries. (By permission of the Mayo Foundation for Medical Education and Research. All rights reserved.)

pectoralis minor muscle: proximal, middle (beneath), and distal. The first part of the axillary artery gives off one branch (supreme thoracic), the second part gives off two branches (thoracoacromial and lateral thoracic), and the third part gives off three branches (subscapular, anterior, and posterior humeral circumflex). The artery lies in close proximity to the axillary vein and to the brachial plexus.

Axillary artery injuries represent 5% to 10% of all arterial injuries. The vast majority (95%) are due to penetrating trauma. Although blunt injuries are rare, these occur in 1% of the patients presenting with either a fracture of the proximal humerus or anterior dislocation of the shoulder. In addition, patients who chronically use crutches may develop stenosis or occlusion from repetitive trauma. Patients with axillary artery injuries often sustain associated nerve trauma.

Exposure of the axillary artery is best achieved using an infraclavicular incision one fingerbreadth below the clavicle (see Fig. 6-5). Most injuries can be repaired with end-to-end anastomosis or a small interposition graft. The mortality and amputation rates are exceedingly low for axillary injuries. However, two-thirds of the patients have significant neurologic dysfunction or persistent neuralgia from associated trauma to the brachial plexus.

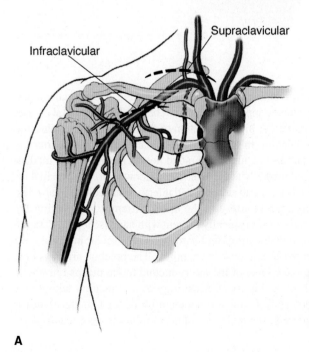

FIGURE 6-5

Preferred surgical approaches for exposure of the subclavian (supraclavicular, **A**) and axillary (infraclavicular, **B**) arteries. (By permission of the Mayo Foundation for Medical Education and Research. All rights reserved.)

A

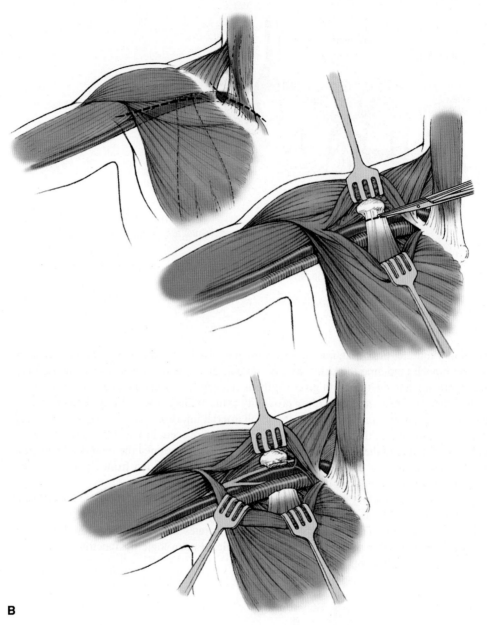

B

FIGURE 6-5 *(Continued)*

BRACHIAL ARTERY. The brachial artery is a continuation of the axillary artery (Fig. 6-6). It starts at the lower edge of the teres major muscle and terminates approximately 2 cm below the antecubital crease, where it bifurcates into the radial and ulnar arteries. A high bifurcation of the brachial artery above the antecubital crease is found in 20% of the population. In the upper and midarm, the brachial artery is accompanied by the median nerve laterally and by the ulnar and radial nerves medially. The median nerve crosses anterior to the artery and is located medially at the level of the elbow joint. The brachial artery has three important branches: deep brachial artery and superior and inferior ulnar collateral arteries.

The brachial artery is the most commonly injured artery of the upper extremity, accounting for 15% to 30% of all peripheral vascular injuries. Patients typically present with hand ischemia. Patients with supracondylar humeral fractures or elbow dislocations and hard signs of vascular injury should be further evaluated with arteriography to rule out brachial artery injury. The brachial artery is best exposed using a longitudinal incision along the course of the artery medial to the biceps muscle or an S-shaped incision across the antecubital fossa (Fig. 6-7). Most injuries are repaired with either end-to-end anastomosis or interposition vein graft. Clinical outcome after repair is better than for injuries of the axillary or subclavian artery because the incidence of nerve injury is significantly less. Amputation or death is rare.

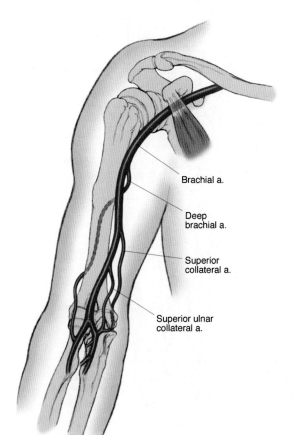

Brachial a.

Deep
brachial a.

Superior
collateral a.

Superior ulnar
collateral a.

FIGURE 6-6

Surgical anatomy of the brachial artery. (By
permission of the Mayo Foundation for Medical
Education and Research. All rights reserved.)

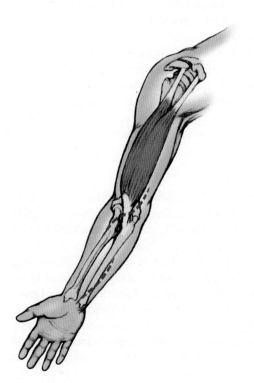

FIGURE 6-7

Preferred surgical approaches for exposure of the distal
brachial artery and forearm vessels. (By permission
of the Mayo Foundation for Medical Education and
Research. All rights reserved.)

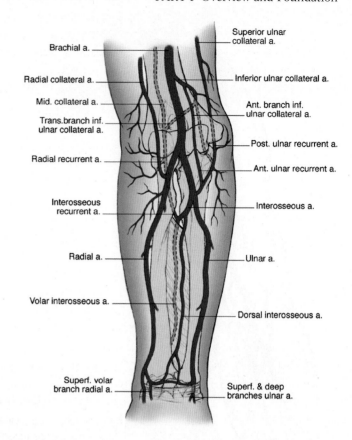

FIGURE 6-8

Surgical anatomy of the forearm arteries. (By permission of the Mayo Foundation for Medical Education and Research. All rights reserved.)

RADIAL AND ULNAR ARTERIES. The ulnar artery is the larger branch of the brachial artery and gives off the ulnar recurrent arteries and the common interosseus artery (Fig. 6-8). The ulnar artery terminates in the superficial palmar arch. The radial artery gives off the radial recurrent artery, which anastomoses to the deep brachial artery. Distally, the brachial artery gives off a small branch to the superficial palmar arch and terminates in the deep palmar arch.

Injuries to the radial and ulnar artery are also common but most often result from penetrating trauma. Complete occlusion or transection of either the radial or ulnar artery will often have no adverse effect on the circulation of the hand because of rich collateral circulation. However, patients with marked hematoma in the forearm may develop compartment syndrome requiring fasciotomy. Distal thrombectomy catheters should be handled gently because these arteries are prone to rupture or intimal injury. Repair often requires simple closure, end-to-end anastomosis, or small interposition grafts. Amputation is rare.

Lower Extremity Injuries

COMMON, PROFUNDA, AND SUPERFICIAL FEMORAL ARTERIES. The common femoral artery originates at the level of the inguinal ligament as a continuation of the external iliac artery (Fig. 6-9). The common femoral artery is located adjacent to the femoral nerve (laterally) and common femoral vein (medially). The first branch of the common femoral artery is the superficial circumflex iliac artery, which marks the transition from external iliac to common femoral artery just below the inguinal ligament. The second branch is the superficial epigastric artery. Approximately 5 cm distal to the inguinal ligament, the common femoral artery bifurcates into the superficial and deep femoral arteries. The deep (profunda) femoral artery is located in a posterolateral position. This artery gives off the medial and lateral femoral circumflex arteries and four to five perforator branches in the thigh. The superficial femoral artery follows its course underneath the sartorius muscle (Hunter canal) and terminates in the popliteal artery at the level of the adductor hiatus. The artery is adjacent to the saphenous nerve and femoral vein.

Injury to the femoral vessels accounts for one-third of all peripheral vascular injuries in civilian and military series. The most common mechanism of injury is penetrating trauma. Anterior dislocation of the femoral head is a rare cause of blunt injury. The superficial femoral artery is

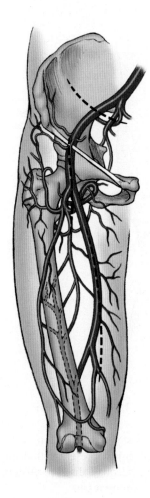

FIGURE 6-9

Surgical anatomy and preferred surgical approaches for exposure of the common, superficial, and deep femoral arteries. (By permission of the Mayo Foundation for Medical Education and Research. All rights reserved.)

injured in 5% of the patients presenting with femoral shaft fracture. Bleeding is the most common presentation in cases of penetrating trauma, whereas distal limb ischemia predominates in patients with blunt injury.

Exposure of the common femoral artery and femoral bifurcation is best obtained using a longitudinal incision two fingerbreadths lateral to the pubic tubercle (see Fig. 6-9). The incision extends from the level of the inguinal as far distally as necessary, depending on how extensive the injury is to the proximal deep and superficial femoral arteries. Rarely, a suprainguinal curvilinear incision is required for retroperitoneal exposure of the external iliac artery to achieve proximal control. Exposure of the superficial femoral artery can be achieved through a longitudinal incision along the course of the sartorius muscle. Patients with small, clean injuries of the femoral arteries may be treated with primary closure, end-to-end anastomosis, or patch angioplasty. Longer lesions require an interposition graft using autologous saphenous vein from the contralateral thigh. Long-term patency rates approach 100% for interposition grafts. Lower extremity function is predominantly determined by the extent of skeletal and neurologic injury.

POPLITEAL AND TIBIOPERONEAL ARTERIES. The popliteal artery is the continuation of the superficial femoral artery and originates at the adductor magnus hiatus (Fig. 6-10). The popliteal artery gives off multiple genicular collateral branches at the above- and below-knee level. The artery bifurcates in 90% of individuals and gives off the anterior tibial artery and the tibioperoneal trunk. The tibioperoneal trunk gives off the posterior tibial artery and the peroneal artery. The anterior tibial artery follows an anterior and lateral course, perforates the interosseous membrane, and is located in the anterior compartment of the leg along with the deep peroneal nerve. The peroneal artery is the middle branch of the three, follows its course in the deep posterior compartment, and bifurcates into the perforating branch to the anterior artery and communicating artery to the posterior tibial

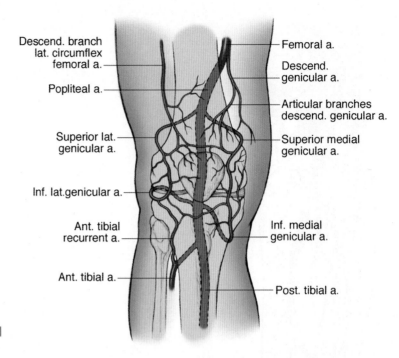

FIGURE 6-10

Surgical anatomy of
the popliteal artery. (By
permission of the Mayo
Foundation for Medical
Education and Research. All
rights reserved.)

Labels in figure:
Descend. branch lat. circumflex femoral a.
Popliteal a.
Superior lat. genicular a.
Inf. lat.genicular a.
Ant. tibial recurrent a.
Ant. tibial a.
Femoral a.
Descend. genicular a.
Articular branches descend. genicular a.
Superior medial genicular a.
Inf. medial genicular a.
Post. tibial a.

artery. The posterior tibial artery is the most medial branch of the three tibioperoneal arteries and terminates as the common plantar artery below the ankle joint.

Popliteal artery injuries often result from blunt trauma. Fracture or posterior dislocation of the knee is a known mechanism of injury. Most patients with popliteal artery injury present with distal ischemia because the genicular collaterals are not effective in maintaining adequate distal perfusion. Occlusion of a single tibioperoneal artery is well tolerated and does not require repair.

Most popliteal and tibioperoneal artery injuries can be exposed using a generous medial approach above and/or below the knee level depending on the extent of injury (Fig. 6-11). The great saphenous vein should be identified and protected. Division of the semimembranous and semitendinous

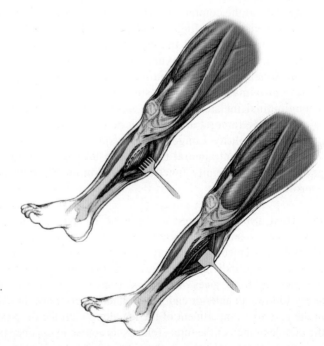

FIGURE 6-11

Preferred medial knee approach for
exposure of the below-knee popliteal
artery and proximal tibioperoneal vessels.
(By permission of the Mayo Foundation
for Medical Education and Research. All
rights reserved.)

muscles is often required for adequate exposure. The posterior tibial and peroneal arteries are also exposed using a medial incision along the posterior margin of the tibia. The soleus muscle is incised longitudinally allowing exposure of the mid- and distal portions of the posterior tibial and peroneal arteries. Although the origin of the anterior tibial artery can be exposed through a medial incision, an incision in the anterior compartment two fingerbreadths lateral to the tibia is required for exposure of the anterior tibial artery.

Injury to the popliteal and tibioperoneal arteries is associated with significant morbidity. Clinical outcome is affected by the extent of skeletal and neurologic trauma, time of ischemia, and adequacy of runoff through the tibial and peroneal arteries.

VENOUS INJURIES   The management of venous injuries is essentially identical to that for any arterial injury. Although venous repair does not yield the same satisfactory results of arterial repair and there is a higher incidence of early thrombosis, current recommendations are to attempt venous repair of any named major vein whenever possible. Large veins such as the inferior vena cava and iliac veins pose a problem in terms of conduit size mismatch. Options in these cases are use of spiral or paneled vein grafts or externally supported PTFE grafts. Injuries affecting minor veins or patients with other life-threatening injuries should be managed with primary ligation. Major veins can be exposed using the same incisions as for their arterial counterpart. Direct pressure using sponge sticks or pressure cuff tourniquets are excellent means of obtaining control in cases of bleeding. Techniques for repair should be the same as for arterial injuries with the caveat that catheter embolectomy often cannot be used because of competent valves.

MANGLED EXTREMITY   One should use clinical judgment in cases of severe trauma with complex soft tissue, skeletal, and vascular injuries. Although there are scoring systems to quantify the degree of injury, cases should be individualized. The Mangled Extremity Severity Score grades skeletal/soft tissue damage, limb ischemia, shock, and age. However, this scoring system is inaccurate in identifying the irretrievable limb requiring primary amputation. Factors associated with need for amputation after below-knee fractures are injury of more than three muscle compartments, occlusion of more than two tibial arteries, and presence of cadaveric changes at initial presentation. When more than two of these predictive factors are present, none of the extremities were salvageable. Primary amputation should be considered early in patients with a dysvascular extremity and extensive soft tissue loss, as the chance of functional recovery is minimal.

POSTOPERATIVE MANAGEMENT

Patients should be continuously evaluated for bleeding, distal limb perfusion, and development of compartment syndrome. Following massive bleeding and coagulopathy, one should aggressively resuscitate the patient and monitor laboratory results every 4 hours (complete blood count, platelets, prothrombin and partial thromboplastin times, and fibrinogen levels). We recommend that laboratory levels are kept within normal limits during the first 48 hours. Parameters include hemoglobin above 10 g/dL, platelet count above 100,000, international normalized ratio of less than 1.2, and partial thromboplastin time of less than 40 seconds. Mild abnormalities contribute to postoperative "oozing," large hematoma, and initiate a cascade of coagulopathy that ultimately may lead to bleeding requiring re-exploration. Assessment of vascular pulses should be done routinely with serial examination and handheld Doppler interrogation. This is repeated every 2 hours for the first 24 hours and every 4 hours thereafter.

The injured extremity should be checked for any signs of infection. Early wound infection, particularly if associated with soft tissue necrosis, is one of the most important determinants of delayed amputation. Aggressive perioperative antibiotic therapy is recommended.

Compartment syndrome is a common occurrence in patients with combined vascular and orthopedic trauma. Patients with ischemic limbs for more than 4 hours can be expected to have some degree of compartment syndrome. Presentation can be delayed up to 12 to 24 hours after reperfusion of the ischemic limb. Early or prophylactic fasciotomy in this setting may be associated with improved outcome. If fasciotomy is deferred at the time of arterial reconstruction, physical examination and compartment pressure measurements should be repeated frequently. Compartment pressures of higher than 30 cm H_2O strongly indicate fasciotomy.

COMPLICATIONS

The most common complications after vascular reconstructions are bleeding, infection, early thrombosis, and compartment syndrome. Medical complications involving cardiac, pulmonary, renal, and neurologic systems are also common. Amputation can result because of early technical failure, venous outflow problems, infection, and fracture instability. Deep venous thrombosis is a common occurrence after combined vascular and orthopedic trauma. Aggressive prophylaxis should be instituted in the early postoperative period. Postoperative duplex ultrasound is indicated for any sign of worsening limb edema or pain. Patients need to be followed regularly because of the potential for late complications. Arterial stenosis or thrombosis, aneurysmal degeneration of vein grafts, and chronic venous insufficiency after primary venous ligation or thrombosis of venous repair can be identified using duplex ultrasound surveillance. We generally re-evaluate patients with combined injuries 6 months after dismissal or earlier if the patient develops symptoms of chronic limb ischemia (e.g., claudication).

RESULTS

The three most important factors affecting clinical outcome in patients with combined vascular and orthopedic trauma are the mechanism of injury, the time interval from injury to restoration of arterial inflow, and the extent of damage to soft tissue, bone, and nerves. Whereas military trauma is almost universally associated with high-velocity penetrating injuries, the majority of civilian injuries are due to blunt mechanisms. In general, penetrating injuries are associated with better outcome. Blunt injuries with complex fractures, dislocations, and extensive soft tissue damage are associated with much worse results. The results of contemporary clinical series of combined vascular and orthopedic extremity trauma are summarized in Table 6-6. Overall, the amputation rate in combined series

TABLE 6-6	**Results of Contemporary Series of Combined Orthopedic and Vascular Trauma**		
Author	**Year**	**n**	**n (%) Amputation**
Penetrating Trauma			
Bishara et al.	1986	29	0
Swetnam et al.	1986	24	8 (33)
Bongard et al.	1989	11	2 (18)
Russell et al.	1991	35	1 (2.8)
Norman et al.	1995	30	0
Attebery et al.	1996	29	0
Granchi et al.	2000	13	1 (10)
McHenry et al.	2002	27	0
Total		198	12 (6)
Blunt Trauma			
Lange et al.	1985	20	12 (60)
Swetnam et al.	1986	10	8 (80)
Bishara et al.	1986	22	1 (4.5)
Howe et al	1987	16	6 (37.5)
McNutt et al.[a]	1989	17	6 (35)
Drost et al.	1989	14	4 (28.5)
Bongard et al.	1989	26	3 (11.5)
Johansen et al.	1990	26	12 (46)
Odland et al.	1990	28	11 (39)
Russell et al.	1991	35	18 (51)
Alexander et al.	1991	29	9 (31)
Schlickewei et al.	1992	113	50 (45)
Attebery et al.	1996	12	3 (25)
Rozycki et al.	2002	59	11 (18.5)
Hossny[b]	2004	17	4 (23.5)
Menakuru et al.	2005	90	7 (12.8)
Total		534	165 (31)

[a]All patients had tibial fractures.
[b]All patients had knee dislocation with associated popliteal artery injury.

was 6% for penetrating injuries and 31% for blunt trauma. Although there are few series reporting long-term outcomes, use of endovascular approaches appears to be associated with shorter hospital stay and complications. Patency rates appear reasonable, but stent graft occlusions or stenosis occurs that require mandatory follow-up.

PEARLS AND PITFALLS

- All hard signs of vascular trauma mandate emergent intervention.
- Soft signs of vascular trauma mandate further evaluation.
- In some situations, angiography may be diagnostic and therapeutic and the information obtained from angiography ensures that equipment and expertise are available when proceeding to the operating room for intervention.
- Proximal and distal control is paramount for repair of vascular injuries.
- Autogenous material is preferred for vascular repair if possible.
- Use of an intra-arterial shunt can be beneficial to reperfuse the extremity while awaiting definitive arterial repair.
- All patients with arterial trauma must be followed closely with neurovascular exams.
- Delay in recognition or treatment for arterial trauma carries increased risk of amputation.
- If fasciotomies are not performed, close observation is needed to monitor for compartment syndrome. It is a clinical diagnosis with no single test or sign to determine it. Loss of a pulse is a late finding associated with muscle necrosis and nerve ischemia. Increased pain and fullness should mandate consideration for fasciotomy regardless of ischemia time.
- Reconstruction of a mangled extremity with little chance of functionality may offer little benefit and consideration of primary amputation should be considered preferably through a multidisciplinary team.

RECOMMENDED READING

Alexander JJ, Piotrowski JJ, Graham D, et al. Outcome of complex orthopedic and vascular injuries of the lower extremity. *Am J Surg.* 1991;162:111.

Attebery LR, Dennis JW, Russo-Alesi F, et al. Changing patterns of arterial injuries associated with fractures and dislocations. *J Am Coll Surg.* 1996;183:377.

Bandyk DF. Vascular injury associated with extremity trauma. *Clin Orthop Relat Res.* 1995;(318):117–124.

Bishara FS, Pasch AR, Lim LT, et al. Improved results in the treatment of civilian vascular injuries associated with fractures and dislocations. *J Vasc Surg.* 1986;3:707.

Bongard FS, White GH, Klein SR. Management strategy of complex extremity injuries. *Am J Surg.* 1989;158:151.

Drost TF, Rosemurgy AS, Proctor D, et al. Outcome of treatment of combined orthopedic and arterial trauma to the lower extremity. *J Trauma.* 1989;29:1331.

Howe HR, Poole GV, Hansen KJ, et al. Salvage of lower extremities following combined orthopedic and vascular trauma: a predictive salvage index. *Am Surg.* 1987;53:205.

Johansen K, Daines M, Howey T, et al. Objective criteria accurately predict amputation following lower extremity trauma. *J Trauma.* 1990;30:568.

Lange RH, Bach AW, Hansen ST, et al. Open tibial fractures with associated vascular injuries: prognosis for limb salvage. *J Trauma.* 1985;25:203.

Lin C-H, Weif C, Levin LS, et al. The functional outcome of lower extremity fractures with vascular injury. *J Trauma.* 1997;43:480.

McCready RA, Logan NM, Dangherty ME, et al. Long-term results with autogenous tissue repair of traumatic extremity vascular injuries. *Ann Surg.* 1997;206:804.

McNutt R, Seabrook GR, Schmitt DD, et al. Blunt tibial artery trauma: predicting the irretrievable extremity. *J Trauma.* 1989;12:1624–1627.

Miranda FE, Dennis JW, Veldenz HC, et al. Confirmation of the safety and accuracy of physical examination in the evaluation of knee dislocation for injury of the popliteal artery: a prospective study. *J Trauma.* 2002;52:247–251.

Norman J, Gahtan V, Franz M, et al. Occult vascular injuries following gunshot wounds resulting in long bone fractures of the extremities. *Am Surg.* 1995;61:146.

Odland MD, Gisbert VL, Gustilo RB, et al. Combined orthopedic and vascular injury in the lower extremities: indications for amputation. *Surgery.* 1990;108:660.

Palazzo JC, Ristow AB, Cury JM, et al. Traumatic vascular lesions associated with fractures and dislocations. *J Cardiovasc Surg.* 1986;121:607.

Schlickewei W, Kuner EH, Mullaji AB, et al. Upper and lower limb fractures with concomitant arterial injury. *J Bone Joint Surg.* 1992;74:181.

Swetnam JA, Hardin WD, Kerstein MD, et al. Successful management of trifurcation injuries. *Am Surg.* 1986;52:585.

Treiman GS, Yellin AE, Weaver FA, et al. Examination of the patient with a knee dislocation: the case for selective angiography. *Arch Surg.* 1992;127:1056.

Van Wijngaarden M, Omert L, Rodriguez A, et al. Management of blunt vascular trauma to the extremities. *Surg Gynecol Obstet.* 1993;177:41.

SURGERY

Patient Positioning

The patient is positioned in the lateral decubitus position on a standard operating room table, with the hand and forearm placed in a dynamic arm holder.

Technique

A vertical incision is made starting 2 cm medial to the medial aspect of the scapular spine extending 5 to 7 cm inferiorly. The lower trapezius is exposed with sharp skin and subcutaneous dissection (Fig. 7-3). The lower trapezius is exposed laterally by following the fibers medial to the scapular border to its insertion on the medial 2 to 3 cm of the spine of the scapula. The lower trapezius tendon is triangular in shape at this level. The superior border of the lower trapezius can be identified by following the horizontal fibers of the upper portion of the tendon medially. The interval between the lower and middle trapezius is developed using blunt and sharp dissection between muscle fibers without penetrating the deep fascia. This will protect the neurovascular bundle, which is located deep to the deep fascia of the trapezius muscle. The spinal accessory nerve can be located two fingerbreadths medial to the medial spine of the scapula (Fig. 7-4). If needed, a nerve stimulator may

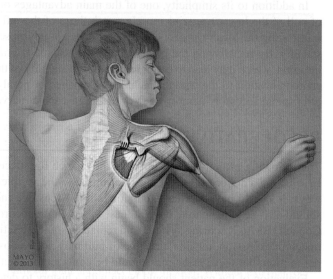

FIGURE 7-3

Medial incision is performed to expose the lower trapezius tendinous insertion. (From Elhassan B. Lower trapezius transfer for shoulder external rotation in patients with paralytic shoulder. *J Hand Surg Am.* 2014;39(3):556–562. Used with permission of Mayo Foundation for Medical Education and Research, all rights reserved.)

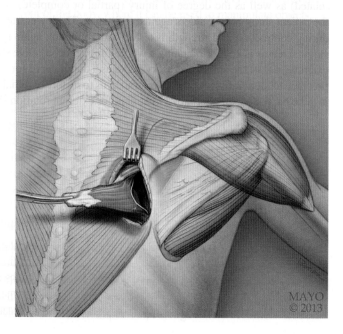

FIGURE 7-4

Lower trapezius detached and separated from middle trapezius. The spinal accessory nerve is shown, which is usually located around 2 cm medial to the medial border of the scapula. (From Elhassan B. Lower trapezius transfer for shoulder external rotation in patients with paralytic shoulder. *J Hand Surg Am.* 2014;39(3):556–562. Used with permission of Mayo Foundation for Medical Education and Research, all rights reserved.)

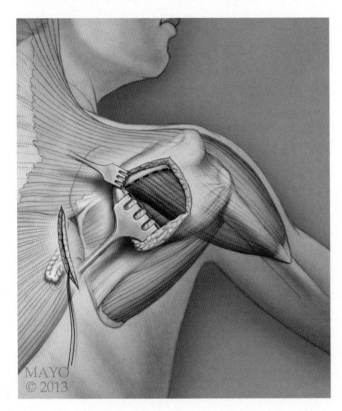

FIGURE 7-5

Exposure of the infraspinatus. A subdeltoid exposure may be used; however, we prefer to detach the posterior deltoid to have better exposure of the infraspinatus tendon. (From Elhassan B. Lower trapezius transfer for shoulder external rotation in patients with paralytic shoulder. *J Hand Surg Am.* 2014;39(3):556–562. Used with permission of Mayo Foundation for Medical Education and Research, all rights reserved.)

aid in identifying its location. Next, a Krakow stitch with no. 2 nonabsorbable suture is placed along the tendon and musculotendinous portion of the lower trapezius.

Next, the posterior insertion of the rotator cuff is exposed through a subdeltoid approach (Fig. 7-5). The infraspinatus tendon is inspected to ensure it is still well attached to the greater tuberosity. If the tendon is insufficient, augmentation with tendon allograft may be needed. (This technique is described in Chapter 8.) A subcutaneous tunnel is created using blunt dissection between the medial and lateral wounds (Fig. 7-6). The muscle is wrapped in TenoGlide (Integra LifeSciences, Plainsboro,

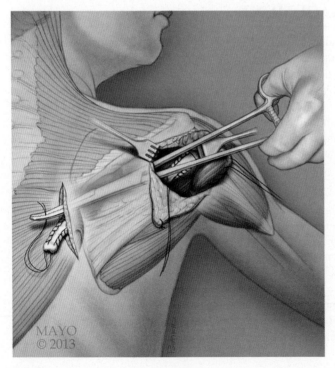

FIGURE 7-6

A deep tunnel is created between the lateral and medial wound through which a grasping clamp is passed to allow retrieval of the lower trapezius to the lateral wound to prepare it for transfer to the infraspinatus. (From Elhassan B. Lower trapezius transfer for shoulder external rotation in patients with paralytic shoulder. *J Hand Surg Am.* 2014;39(3):556–562. Used with permission of Mayo Foundation for Medical Education and Research, all rights reserved.)

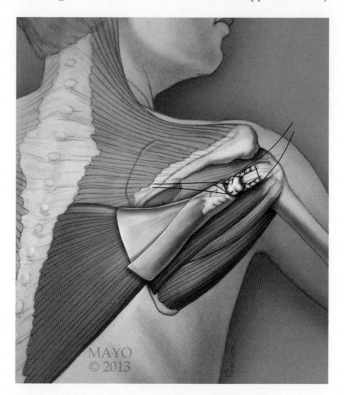

FIGURE 7-7

The lower trapezius tendon is repaired to the infraspinatus tendon. TenoGlide is used to wrap the tendon transfer site to decrease the risk of adhesion and scarring. (From Elhassan B. Lower trapezius transfer for shoulder external rotation in patients with paralytic shoulder. *J Hand Surg Am.* 2014;39(3):556–562. Used with permission of Mayo Foundation for Medical Education and Research, all rights reserved.)

NJ) and the tendon is passed through the tunnel using a blunt clamp. We believe TenoGlide reduces the risk for adhesion formation around the transfer. The tendon is repaired directly to the infraspinatus tendon using no. 2 nonabsorbable sutures while the shoulder is placed in maximal external rotation (Fig. 7-7). After the tendon is secured, the spinal accessory nerve is inspected for impingement on the medial spine of the scapula. If impingement is noted, 1 to 2 cm of medial spine is shaved and TenoGlide is interposed to eliminate any risk of impingement of the spinal accessory nerve. While the shoulder in maintained in external rotation, the wound is irrigated and a deep drain is placed in the posterior wound. Both wounds are closed in a layered fashion.

POSTOPERATIVE MANAGEMENT

The patient is placed in a custom-made shoulder spica brace that is adjusted to match the position used while performing the tendon transfer (45 degrees of abduction and 50 degrees of external rotation). The drain is removed when output is less than 30 mL in 24 hours. Patients remain in their brace for 6 weeks postoperatively. Passive forward flexion and external rotation are allowed with therapist assistance while patients are in the brace between weeks 6 and 8. Active assisted range of motion is started after the immobilization is discontinued and continued for 6 weeks. We recommend additional aquatherapy and no passive stretching during this period. The patient is then started on gentle strengthening and swimming exercises. Unrestricted activity is allowed 6 months postoperatively.

COMPLICATIONS

This transfer has a low complication rate. Hematoma may occur if the drain is removed prematurely. It is managed with observation with no expected sequelae. Infection is rare; we have had two wound infections out of 200 cases. In both cases, the patients were obese and had undergone multiple tendon transfers. The salvage of infection after appropriate medical and surgical treatment is almost always shoulder fusion. Tendon rupture could happen mostly after aggressive therapy or trauma during the early recovery period. If the muscle is still salvageable, revision transfer may be performed with tendon allograft augmentation. Other options include contralateral lower trapezius origin transfer or fusion.

PEARLS AND PITFALLS

- When defining the interval between the middle and lower trapezius, avoid penetrating the deep fascia, which protects the neurovascular bundle from damage.
- Inspect the spinal accessory nerve for impingement on the medial spine of the scapula prior to closure, and if necessary, use a burr to shave down the bone to prevent impingement.
- Be sure to have an Achilles allograft available in case the infraspinatus tendon is found to be insufficient.
- Patient understanding of and compliance with the postoperative bracing and rehabilitation protocol are essential to success.

RECOMMENDED READING

Elhassan B. Lower trapezius transfer for shoulder external rotation in patients with paralytic shoulder. *J Hand Surg Am.* 2014;39(3):556–562.

Elhassan B, Bishop A, Shin A, et al. Shoulder tendon transfer options for adult patients with brachial plexus injury. *J Hand Surg Am.* 2010;35(7):1211–1219.

Spinner RJ, Shin AY, Hébert-Blouin MN, et al. Traumatic brachial plexus injury. In: Wolfe SW, Hotchkiss RN, Pederson MH, et al., eds. *Green's Operative Hand Surgery.* 6th ed. St. Louis, MO: Elsevier Churchill Livingstone; 2011:1235–1292.

8 Rotational Flaps for Rotator Cuff Repair

Kathleen M. Kollitz and Bassem T. Elhassan

Massive, irreparable rotator cuff tears can lead to pain and loss of function. Loss of the rotator cuff leads to eccentrically applied loads during glenohumeral motion, which lead to eventual arthritis. In low-demand patients and the elderly, massive rotator cuff tears can be managed with reverse total shoulder arthroplasty; however, this is not an appropriate option for younger, high-demand patients. For younger patients, arthroscopic debridement and repair with the use of allograft to augment retracted tendons may offer some benefit for both pain relief and improvement of motion. Tendon transfer for reconstruction of an irreparable rotator cuff tear has been reported to lead to good outcomes.

Traditionally, transfer of the latissimus dorsi has been described for posterior-superior irreparable cuff tears, while transfer of the pectoralis major has been described for anterior-superior irreparable cuff tears. Additional transfer options include transfer of the pectoralis minor, teres major, and lower trapezius. The purpose of this chapter is to review basic shoulder anatomy and biomechanics in order to understand the rationale behind different types of reconstructive procedures. Then, we will report on the different types of tendon transfers performed for posterior-superior and anterior-superior irreparable rotator cuff tears. In addition, our preferred tendon transfer options are described, and the techniques are detailed.

ANATOMY AND BIOMECHANICS

Shoulder motion is a combination of motion at the scapulothoracic articulation and the glenohumeral joint with contributions from the acromioclavicular joint, sternoclavicular joint, and subacromial articulation. There are 14 muscles that act as dynamic stabilizers and contribute to motion in 3 planes. According to Goldner, the muscles around the shoulder can be thought of in four functional categories: prime movers, stabilizers, depressors, and accessory stabilizers. The prime mover group includes the clavicular head of the pectoralis major and deltoid. The stabilizer group includes the subscapularis, supraspinatus, and infraspinatus. The depressors include the teres major, biceps, latissimus dorsi, pectoralis major, and triceps. Finally, the accessory stabilizers include the trapezius, serratus anterior, pectoralis minor, levator scapula, and rhomboids. The scapula serves as a mobile base for the glenoid and must be stable enough to allow for force transmission through the arm.

The glenohumeral joint is the most mobile joint in the body, with six degrees of freedom for translation and rotational motion. Stability is generated primarily by the rotator cuff, which pulls the humeral head into the glenoid during motion. The rotator cuff consists of four muscles that originate about the scapula and insert on the humerus in one large, blended tendon. The supraspinatus originates from the scapula in the supraspinatus fossa and passes below the acromion and on to the superior greater tuberosity. The infraspinatus and teres minor contribute to external rotation, and both insert on the posterior aspect of the greater tuberosity. The infraspinatus originates from the infraspinatus fossa and is innervated by the suprascapular nerve, while the teres minor originates from the posteroinferior aspect of the scapula and is innervated by the axillary nerve.

The subscapularis is the primary internal rotator of the humerus. It originates on the ventral surface of the scapula and inserts on the lesser tuberosity, passing under the coracoid process. It is innervated by the upper and lower subscapular nerves. It acts as a dynamic stabilizer from 0 to 45 degrees of abduction.

In patients with massive rotator cuff tears, whether anterior-superior or posterior-superior, the stabilizing effect of the rotator cuff will be jeopardized, which in turn leads to proximal migration of the humeral head. These changes significantly alter the biomechanics of the shoulder and lead to severely reduced shoulder motion that may manifest as pseudoparalysis.

INDICATIONS/CONTRAINDICATIONS

Our preferred tendon transfer for posterosuperior rotator cuff tear is the lower trapezius transfer. The primary indication for this procedure is the loss of active external rotation due to an irreparable tear or a failed primary repair of the posterosuperior rotator cuff in a patient who is dissatisfied with the level of pain or disability resulting from conservative management. Loss of passive external rotation and forward elevation are contraindications for this tendon transfer, as is loss of function of the lower trapezius.

For anterosuperior rotator cuff tears, our preferred transfer is the latissimus dorsi to subscapularis with or without teres major transfer. The primary indication for this transfer includes an irreparable subscapularis tear with retraction and fatty atrophy of the muscle belly. Anterosuperior escape of the humeral head is also an indication for latissimus transfer to the supraspinatus footprint. Contraindications to this transfer include a paralytic latissimus dorsi and loss of passive range of motion at the shoulder.

PREOPERATIVE PLANNING

The history and physical exam are essential in diagnosis and assessment of the nature of the rotator cuff tear. Often, the patient complains of pain or dysfunction with an insidious onset. Other times, the patient complains of fatigue during forward elevation or external rotation of the shoulder. The physical examination of the shoulder begins by inspection of both shoulders. Deformity associated with anterior-superior escape of the humeral head indicates anterosuperior rotator cuff tear. Spinati muscle atrophy is noted and often indicates that an irreparable rotator cuff tear is present. A defect of the deltoid is a relative contraindication for tendon transfer. Manual motor testing of shoulder forward elevation, abduction, external rotation, and internal rotation is recorded.

The *hornblower's sign*, or external rotation lag sign (discrepancy between active and passive external rotation of greater than 30 degrees), is important to recognize. A positive sign is highly suggestive of massive rotator cuff tear, amenable to lower trapezius tendon transfer or latissimus dorsi to infraspinatus footprint transfer.

Another physical examination finding that is important to recognize is the *lift-off test* (the inability to actively lift the dorsum of the hand off from a resting position on the lower back) or the *belly press test* (the inability to actively maintain the elbow anterior to the midline of the trunk as viewed from the side). An inability to perform these maneuvers is highly suggestive of involvement of the subscapularis in the rotator cuff tear. When present and irreparable, the latissimus dorsi or pectoralis major transfer to the subscapularis footprint is indicated.

MRI is the imaging modality of choice for the diagnosis of rotator cuff tears. Rotator cuff tears are quite common; 34% of asymptomatic individuals will have some degree of rotator cuff tearing. The incidence increases with age, with 50% of patients over age 50 and up to 80% of patients over age 80 having rotator cuff lesions detectable by ultrasound. Of these, up to 40% are "massive," meaning two or more tendons are involved with up to 5 cm of the muscle insertion footprint. Up to 30% of all rotator cuff tears are not primarily reparable.

There are no strict criteria for diagnosis of irreparable rotator cuff tears. Proximal migration of the humeral head, advanced fatty atrophy of the involved rotator cuff muscles, and loss of most of the tendon of the involved muscle are considered poor prognostic indicators for repair. In symptomatic patients with massive rotator cuff tears that are determined to be irreparable, selection of the donor muscle to transfer should follow the principles of tendon transfer outlined in Chapter 7.

POSTEROSUPERIOR ROTATOR CUFF TEARS

Tendon transfer options to reconstruct posterosuperior rotator cuff tear include latissimus dorsi (Fig. 8-1), teres major, and lower trapezius. Outcomes for the latissimus dorsi tendon transfer have been reported as 74% to 86% of patients being satisfied with the outcome at 9 to 10 years of follow-up. The failure rate was 10% at an average of 9 years of follow-up, and 4% of patients went on to shoulder arthroplasty. Poor function was correlated with a loss of function of the subscapularis.

Though latissimus transfer is the most commonly reported transfer, Hartzler et al. showed in a biomechanical study a significantly higher moment arm in external rotation using the lower

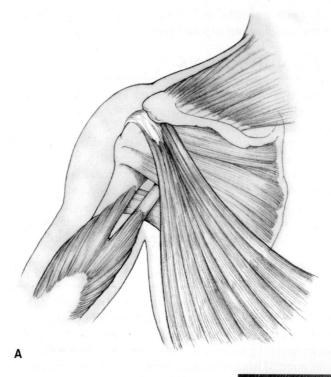

A

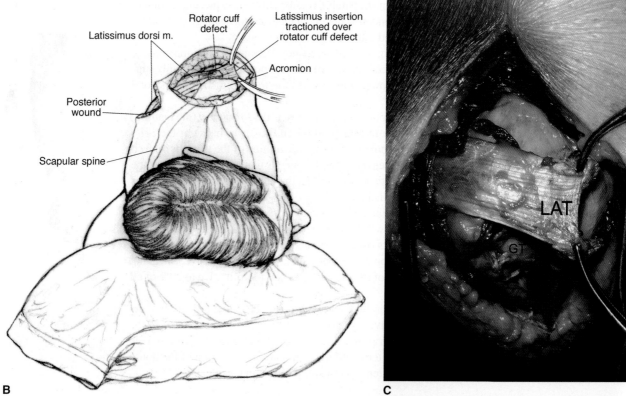

Rotator cuff defect

Latissimus insertion tractioned over rotator cuff defect

Latissimus dorsi m.

Acromion

Posterior wound

Scapular spine

B

C

LAT

GT

FIGURE 8-1

A–C: The latissimus tendon (LAT) has been passed under the posterior deltoid, up into the superior wound, and over the posterior aspect of the humeral head. The teres major can be passed similarly. Note that the deltoid muscle has been removed for illustrative purposes. (Used with permission of Mayo Foundation for Medical Education and Research, all rights reserved.)

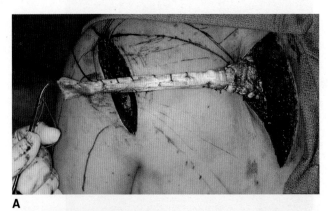

A

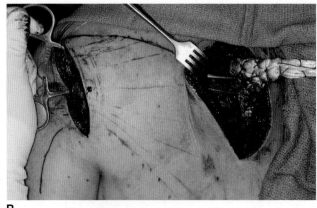

B

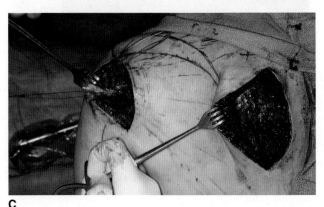

C

FIGURE 8-2

A: An Achilles tendon allograft is wrapped and sutured to the tendinous and musculotendinous portions of the lower trapezius using multiple no. 2 Orthocord. Notice that the suture that was placed originally in the muscle was further threaded through the tendon allograft to reinforce and strengthen the repair of the Achilles tendon on the lower trapezius. **B:** A soft tissue tunnel is created deep to the deltoid using a Carmalt, which is passed from the lateral to the medial wound to retrieve the tendon allograft. **C:** The Achilles tendon is passed through the tunnel from medial to lateral.

trapezius transfer as compared to the latissimus or teres major. In another biomechanical study, Omid et al. showed that the lower trapezius transfer to reconstruct posterior-superior rotator cuff tear led to better restoration of shoulder joint kinematics when compared to latissimus transfer. For these reasons, our tendon transfer of choice to reconstruct posterosuperior rotator cuff tear is lower trapezius prolonged with Achilles tendon graft.

The surgical technique of the lower trapezius to the rotator cuff is similar to the one described in Chapter 7 for brachial plexus injury but with a few modifications. In this technique, tendon allograft is needed to prolong the lower trapezius tendon because the posterior-superior rotator cuff tendons are deficient and require reconstruction. The steps to harvest the lower trapezius are similar to those described in Chapter 7, but exposure of the posterior-superior rotator cuff is modified. The lateral 5 mm of the acromion is osteotomized, and the middle deltoid is mobilized and reflected to allow for inspection of the posterior-superior rotator cuff footprint. A partial repair is performed if possible. The footprint of the supraspinatus and infraspinatus is debrided to bleeding bone. At this time, the lower trapezius tendon is augmented with an Achilles tendon allograft (Fig. 8-2A). The wide, thin portion of the allograft is sutured securely to the lower trapezius tendon, and then the tendon is passed from the medial wound to the lateral wound, deep to the posterior deltoid (Fig. 8-2B, C). The tendon allograft is repaired with transosseous sutures to the prepared footprint while the shoulder is in maximum external rotation. The transferred tendon is wrapped with TenoGlide. The acromial osteotomy is then repaired anatomically with multiple no. 2 nonabsorbable, transosseous sutures.

ANTEROSUPERIOR ROTATOR CUFF TEARS

The pectoralis major transfer is the most commonly performed transfer for anterosuperior rotator cuff deficiency (Fig. 8-3). It is indicated in cases of subscapularis tears, which are associated with anterosuperior escape of the humeral head. Results of pectoralis major tendon transfer have been inconsistent. This may in part be accounted for by the dissimilar line of pull between the pectoralis major and the subscapularis. While both muscles exert a medializing force on the

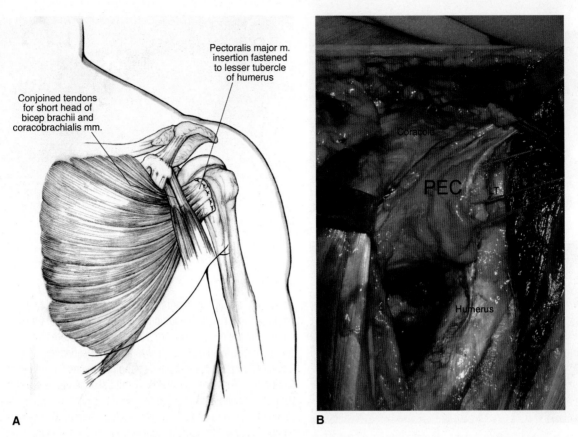

Conjoined tendons for short head of bicep brachii and coracobrachialis mm.

Pectoralis major m. insertion fastened to lesser tubercle of humerus

A

B

FIGURE 8-3

A: The pectoralis major muscle is advanced behind the conjoined tendon in front of the musculocutaneous nerve. For illustrative purposes, the inferior half of the pectoralis tendon is not shown. **B:** The tendon is attached to the lesser tuberosity using transosseous repair, with the arm in neutral rotation. For illustrative purposes, the inferior half of the pectoralis tendon is not shown. (Used with permission of Mayo Foundation for Medical Education and Research, all rights reserved.)

humerus, the pectoralis major is relatively anterior while the native subscapularis exerts a relatively posterior force on the humerus. The pectoralis major exerts a force roughly 90 degrees to that of the subscapularis, making it a suboptimal tendon transfer in our minds. Our preferred tendon transfer for anterosuperior rotator cuff dysfunction is the latissimus dorsi, with or without the teres major. The origin of the latissimus, posterior to the chest wall, more closely mimics that of the subscapularis.

LATISSIMUS DORSI TO SUBSCAPULARIS TRANSFER

Patient Positioning

The patient is positioned in a similar fashion to the pectoralis major transfer, upright in a beach chair position. A standard deltopectoral approach is used, with a skin incision of approximately 5 to 7 cm (Fig. 8-4A). The subscapularis tendons are exposed and evaluated for reparability (Fig. 8-4B, C).

Technique

Through the same exposure, the proximal third of the pectoralis tendon is incised with a small cuff of tendon left attached to the bone to facilitate repair during closure. The latissimus tendon lies immediately deep to the pectoralis major tendon. Dissection of the tendinous insertion of the latissimus is performed, and the tendon may be harvested with or without a segment of its boney insertion. A Krakow stitch is placed in the tendon using nonabsorbable suture and is used to help mobilize the muscle for transfer and tendon repair. The neurovascular bundle is identified and protected.

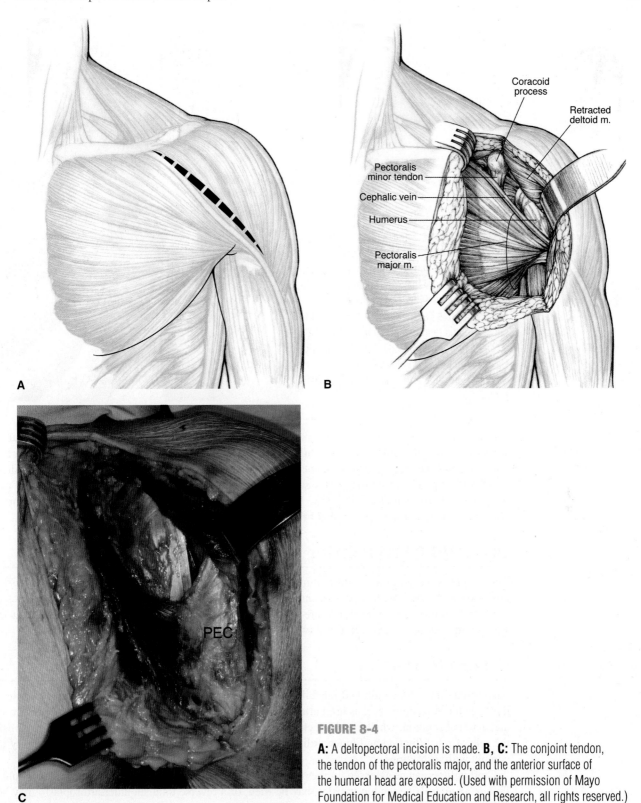

The tendon is then transferred to the lesser tuberosity using transosseous, no. 2 nonabsorbable suture (Fig. 8-5). In patients with proximal migration of the humeral head due to supraspinatus insufficiency, we aim to transfer the tendon to the anterior aspect of the greater tuberosity at the level of the footprint of the supraspinatus.

Alternatively, the teres major may be harvested and transferred along with the latissimus. If this double transfer is performed, we recommend transferring the latissimus proximally to the

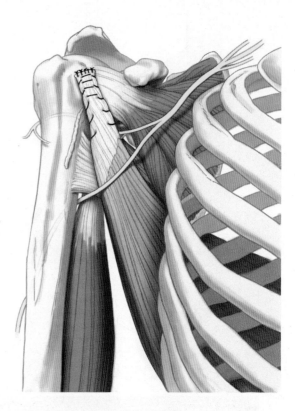

FIGURE 8-5

Relationship between the axillary nerve and radial nerve and final placement of the transferred latissimus dorsi to the lesser tuberosity. (From Elhassan B, Christensen TJ, Wagner ER. Feasibility of latissimus and teres major transfer to reconstruct irreparable subscapularis tendon tear: an anatomic study. *J Shoulder Elbow Surg.* 2014;23(4):492–499. Used with permission of Mayo Foundation for Medical Education and Research, all rights reserved.)

subscapularis insertion and the teres major distally. The reason of this transfer pattern is because we have shown in a prior anatomic study that transfer of the teres major more proximally on the humeral head may lead to impingement on the axillary nerve (Fig. 8-6). The indication of this dual transfer is for patients with irreparable subscapularis tear associated with anterior subluxation of the humeral head. In such cases, when the latissimus transfer alone is determined to be insufficient to reduce the joint, additional teres major transfer is recommended.

POSTOPERATIVE CARE

The patient is placed in a shoulder immobilizer with the shoulder in internal rotation for 6 weeks postoperatively. At 4 weeks, passive shoulder exercises are begun with external rotation restricted to neutral. Active-assisted exercises are begun at 8 weeks, with gentle strengthening starting at 16 weeks with a slow progression over 2 to 3 months to unrestricted activities after 6 months.

COMPLICATIONS

Appropriate immobilization and rehabilitation are keys to bone-tendon junction healing after tendon transfer. A custom brace is used after external rotation procedures to hold the arm in abduction and external rotation, which can be a challenge for patient compliance. It is important to establish the role of rehabilitation and brace utilization prior to surgery to assess for the patient's ability to comply with restrictions.

Graft failures can be assessed for the possibility of reoperation/rerepair. In the case of catastrophic failure, an alternative tendon transfer may be tried, or a reverse total shoulder arthroplasty may be indicated. Shoulder fusion is viewed as a last resort; however, patients often maintain acceptable range of motion via the scapulothoracic articulation.

Transfers for anterosuperior rotator cuff dysfunction involve dissection near the brachial plexus, which may place the musculocutaneous, axillary, radial, or long thoracic nerves at risk during surgery. The treating physician is urged to identify the musculocutaneous and axillary nerves pre-emptively in order to protect these structures. The same principles apply for transfers for posterosuperior cuff dysfunction, namely, identification of the axillary nerve in the quadrilateral space and careful attention to the radial nerve location. After all transfers are completed, at-risk structures should be

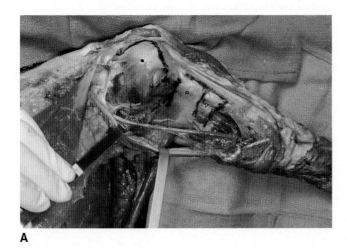
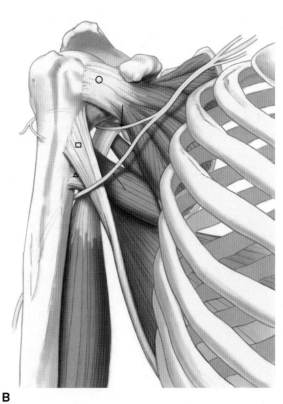

A   **B**

FIGURE 8-6

Photograph **(A)** and drawing **(B)** of the subscapularis insertion (*circle*), latissimus dorsi insertion (*square*), and teres major insertion (*triangle*). *Arrows* indicate the axillary nerve (*black arrow*) and radial nerve (*blue arrow*). (From Elhassan B, Christensen TJ, Wagner ER. Feasibility of latissimus and teres major transfer to reconstruct irreparable subscapularis tendon tear: an anatomic study. *J Shoulder Elbow Surg.* 2014;23(4):492–499. Used with permission of Mayo Foundation for Medical Education and Research, all rights reserved.)

evaluated for possible compression. Finally, the neurovascular supply to the donor muscles must be mobilized so that they are not under tension after transfer.

Rarely, frozen shoulder may develop after tendon transfer. We recommend conservative management with physical therapy.

PEARLS AND PITFALLS

- Tendon transfers that most closely replicate the original muscle line-of-pull are most successful in our experience.
- For exposure of the posterosuperior rotator cuff, an acromial osteotomy and reflection of the middle deltoid allow for a bone-to-bone repair during closure, which in our experience produces more reliable healing than attempts to reattach the muscle to its origin on the acromion directly.
- For anterosuperior rotator cuff tears with superior escape, the latissimus should be transferred to the anterior aspect of the greater tuberosity.
- If a double transfer of the teres major and latissimus dorsi is to be undertaken for anterosuperior cuff tears, the latissimus should be transferred to the lesser tuberosity at the subscapularis footprint, while the teres major should be transferred more distally in order to protect the axillary nerve from impingement.

RECOMMENDED READING

Bedi A. Massive tears of the rotator cuff. *J Bone Joint Surg.* 2010;92(9):1894.

El-Azab HM, Rott O, Irlenbusch U. Long-term follow-up after latissimus dorsi transfer for irreparable posterosuperior rotator cuff tears. *J Bone Joint Surg Am.* 2015;97(6):462–469.

Elhassan B, Christensen TJ, Wagner ER. Feasibility of latissimus and teres major transfer to reconstruct irreparable subscapularis tendon tear: an anatomic study. *J Shoulder Elbow Surg.* 2014;23(4):492–499.

Elhassan B, Ozbaydar M, Massimini D, et al. Transfer of pectoralis major for the treatment of irreparable tears of subscapularis: does it work? *J Bone Joint Surg Br.* 2008;90(8):1059–1065.

Gerber C, Rahm SA, Catanzaro S, et al. Latissimus dorsi tendon transfer for treatment of irreparable posterosuperior rotator cuff tears: long-term results at a minimum follow-up of ten years. *J Bone Joint Surg Am.* 2013;95(21):1920–1926.

Goldner JL. Strengthening of the partially paralyzed shoulder girdle by multiple muscle-tendon transfers. *Hand Clin.* 1988;4(2):323–336.

Hartzler RU, Barlow JD, An K-N, et al. Biomechanical effectiveness of different types of tendon transfers to the shoulder for external rotation. *J Shoulder Elbow Surg.* 2012;21(10):1370–1376.

Jost B, Puskas GJ, Lustenberger A, et al. Outcome of pectoralis major transfer for the treatment of irreparable subscapularis tears. *J Bone Joint Surg Am.* 2003;85-A(10):1944–1951.

Milgrom C, Schaffler M, Gilbert S, et al. Rotator-cuff changes in asymptomatic adults: the effect of age, hand dominance and gender. *J Bone Joint Surg Br.* 1995;77(2):296–298.

Omid R, Heckmann N, Wang L, et al. Biomechanical comparison between the trapezius transfer and latissimus transfer for irreparable posterosuperior rotator cuff tears. *J Shoulder Elbow Surg.* 2015;24(10):1635–1643.

Resch H, Povacz P, Ritter E, et al. Transfer of the pectoralis major muscle for the treatment of irreparable rupture of the subscapularis tendon. *J Bone Joint Surg Am.* 2000;82(3):372–382.

Sher JS, Uribe JW, Posada A, et al. Abnormal findings on magnetic resonance images of asymptomatic shoulders. *J Bone Joint Surg Am.* 1995;77(1):10–15.

Warner JJ. Management of massive irreparable rotator cuff tears: the role of tendon transfer. *Instr Course Lect.* 2001;50:63–71.

9 Surgical Exposure of the Elbow Following Bony and Soft Tissue Trauma

Julie E. Adams and Scott P. Steinmann

INDICATIONS/CONTRAINDICATIONS

The soft tissue surrounding the elbow is thin and pliable, allowing it to withstand the stretch produced by the elbow's large arc of motion. Following elbow trauma, this skin can be compromised by lacerations, abrasions, edema, and relative ischemia making it prone to breakdown. Optimal functional recovery in the setting of elbow trauma is best achieved with early motion protocols, which can further subject elbow incisions to tension and possible dehiscence; however, properly planned incisions can allow for excellent exposure of the elbow and minimize the risks of postoperative wound complications.

Historically, many surgeons have favored a "universal" posterior incision. A single posterior incision allows for access to both the medial and lateral sides of the elbow by elevation of a full-thickness skin flap on each side; however, the down sides include the necessity of a long incision, substantial soft tissue stripping, the possibility of seroma formation, and soft tissue complications from excessive skin traction. Currently, the authors favor making separate medial and lateral incisions. This technique allows for direct exposure of the injury and obviates the need for a large incision and large skin flaps. Prior surgical incisions should be carefully noted preoperatively. Previous incisions may need to be incorporated in order to avoid creating narrow skin bridges, which are susceptible to skin necrosis and potential wound complications.

SURGERY

Patient Positioning

Depending on the procedure and the presence of support staff for retraction, the patient may be positioned prone, supine, or in the lateral decubitus position. The prone position may be problematic for anesthesia staff and presents problems with patient positioning so we generally avoid this position. The lateral position is helpful in situations in which retraction help may be limited, but this approach is useful for distal humerus fractures and some humeral shaft fractures. The arm may be supported by a knee holder or other padded bolster placed under the proximal arm. It is best to confirm that adequate films can be obtained with the fluoroscopy unit before prepping and draping the patient. In our practice, the patient is frequently placed in the supine position with a small stack of towels placed underneath the ipsilateral scapula and the arm draped across the chest after sterile preparation. The operating table should be slightly tilted away from the surgeon to help with visualization and exposure. This positioning is good for fixation of distal humeral fractures, radial head fractures, and medial or lateral ligament reconstruction. For medial ligament or coronoid fracture fixation, the supine position is used, but a sterile and well-padded Mayo stand is utilized to position the arm for medial elbow exposure. Hip rests or a beanbag, along with safety straps or belts across the patient, may provide additional stability.

Intraoperative fluoroscopy, if indicated, is placed on the ipsilateral side, and the elbow may be brought out laterally from the chest for the fluoroscope intermittently during the procedure. A mini fluoroscopy unit provides excellent visualization, is mobile and readily manned by the surgeon and team, and minimizes radiation exposure. Typically, the arm is prepped and draped from the fingertips to the axilla, and a sterile tourniquet is used. This allows for removal if more proximal exposure of the humerus is needed.

Posterior Approaches

Indications

- Triceps repair
- Combined medial and lateral approach
- Distal humerus ORIF
- Total elbow arthroplasty

Contraindications

Prior medial or lateral incisions represent a relative contraindication.

INCISION. The bony landmarks, including the olecranon process and the subcutaneous border of the proximal ulna, are marked (Fig. 9-1). The incision starts about 5 cm proximal to the olecranon process centered on the triceps tendon and slightly medially. It is then taken distally to the medial side of the olecranon and ends distally following the subcutaneous border of the ulna. Full-thickness skin flaps are then developed with a deep plane being established above the triceps fascia and epitenon proximally and the forearm fascia and ulnar periosteum distally. Care is taken in the region of the cubital tunnel in order to avoid injuring the ulnar nerve and the medial antebrachial cutaneous nerve.

DEEP DISSECTION. The ulnar nerve is most easily found proximally between the medial intermuscular septum and the medial head of the triceps muscle. If the nerve is going to be transposed, it should be mobilized, typically working from proximal to distal to identify and preserve the motor branches (Fig. 9-2). Articular branches can be sacrificed. One centimeter of the distal medial intermuscular septum is removed to prevent impingement on the ulnar nerve if an anterior transposition is to be

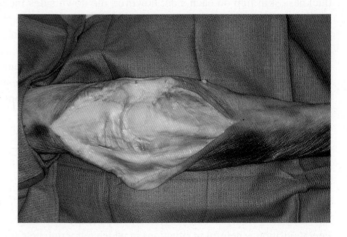

FIGURE 9-1

The skin is incised posteriorly with full-thickness flaps raised as needed.

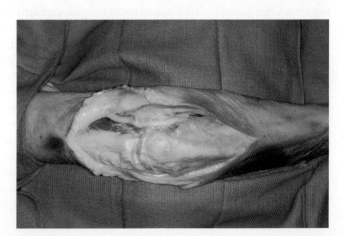

FIGURE 9-2

The ulnar nerve is carefully released from the cubital tunnel.

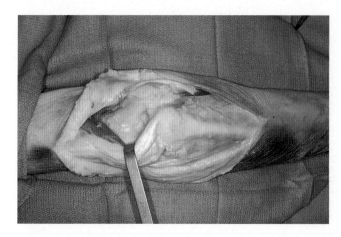

FIGURE 9-3

The medial and lateral sides of the triceps muscle are released in order to fully visualize the posterior fossa and the ulnohumeral articulation.

performed at the end of the case. If the nerve is transposed anteriorly, it is placed into a subcutaneous pocket anterior to the medial epicondyle. A suture is placed in the subcutaneous tissue and secured to the fascia to create a sling and prevent posterior subluxation of the nerve.

PARATRICIPITAL APPROACH. This approach is useful for exposure of distal humerus fractures when there is limited intra-articular involvement. The approach involves making a window for exposure on either side of the triceps, while keeping the triceps attached to the olecranon. On the medial side, the medial column of the humerus and the ulnar nerve are the landmarks. The ulnar nerve is identified and protected. Posteriorly, the triceps tendon is elevated from the humerus along the medial column. Working on the lateral side, the lateral column of the humerus is identified, and a cautery is used to divide the fascial attachments of the triceps off of the humerus. The triceps is then elevated from lateral to medial taking care to avoid injury to the ulnar nerve (Fig. 9-3). The exposure of the joint is limited, and occasionally, the approach may need to be extended with an olecranon osteotomy or other exposure.

OLECRANON OSTEOTOMY. An olecranon osteotomy may be performed to gain full visualization of the articular surface of the distal humerus. It is often helpful to provisionally place the hardware that will be used to fix the olecranon, prior to making the osteotomy. Options for fixation include intramedullary rods, tension band techniques using screw and washer, tension band fixation with K wires or plate fixation.

After identification and protection of the ulnar nerve, a capsulotomy is made at both the medial and lateral sides of the olecranon at the apex of the greater sigmoid notch to locate the olecranon "bare area." This is the area of the olecranon where the articular cartilage narrows and is the optimal location for the osteotomy. A sponge can be inserted into the joint under the olecranon in order to protect the distal humeral articular cartilage from inadvertent damage.

The osteotomy can be created in a chevron configuration, with the apex usually pointed distally (Fig. 9-4A), or more commonly a simple transverse osteotomy will suffice. The initial cuts are made using an oscillating saw, followed by an osteotome (Fig. 9-4B), and finally, the last third of the bone is cracked or fractured open with an osteotome to create the completed osteotomy (Fig. 9-4C).

One variation of a simple olecranon osteotomy is an anconeus flap transolecranon approach. In this approach, the anconeus is detached as a flap from distally to proximally, contiguous to the triceps, and the triceps, proximal olecranon osteotomy fragment, and the anconeus are retracted proximally as a group.

BRYAN-MORREY TRICEPS-REFLECTING APPROACH. After identification and protection of the ulnar nerve, a periosteal elevator is used to dissect the triceps muscle, including the medial and lateral margins of the triceps muscle, from the posterior humeral cortex. The triceps tendon is sharply dissected through Sharpey's fibers directly off of the olecranon starting medially and extending laterally. The fascia overlying Kocher's interval is identified and longitudinally split. The triceps tendon and anconeus should be reflected medially to laterally, ending at Kocher's interval. The triceps may be removed with a thin wafer of bone, which some surgeons believe may facilitate healing. At the

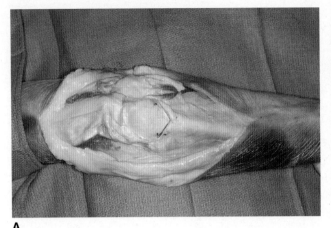

A

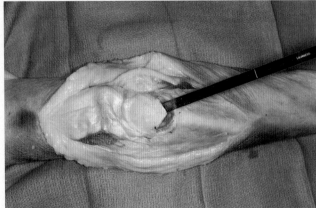

B

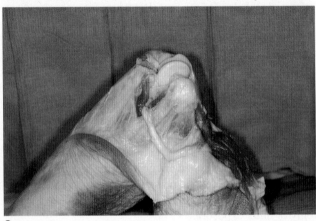

C

FIGURE 9-4

A: The olecranon osteotomy is best located at the small area of olecranon that is devoid of cartilage. A lap sponge may be threaded between the humerus and ulna to avoid inadvertent cartilage damage. **B:** The osteotomy is started with a reciprocating saw and then finished with an osteotome. Hardware may be predrilled to facilitate final osteotomy repair. **C:** After osteotomy, the olecranon is retracted with the triceps tendon, allowing near full visualization of the articular spool.

end of the procedure, the triceps tendon is repaired back to the olecranon using two transosseous drill holes placed in a cruciate configuration and one additional drill hole placed in a transverse orientation with nonabsorbable suture or alternatively suture anchors. The repair should be protected postoperatively by avoiding active elbow extension against resistance for a minimum of 6 weeks.

VAN GORDER APPROACH. After identification and protection of the ulnar nerve, the triceps tendon is identified several centimeters proximal to its insertion on the olecranon, and a chevron-shaped transection of the tendon is performed with the apex proximal. This is repaired at the end of the procedure with nonabsorbable suture. The repair should be protected postoperatively by avoiding active elbow extension against resistance and avoiding passive stretching in positions of terminal elbow flexion for a minimum of 6 weeks.

TRAP APPROACH. The TRansAnconeus Pedicle (TRAP) flap approach requires a longer skin incision distally along the subcutaneous border of the ulna. The anconeus muscle is identified along the lateral aspect of the subcutaneous border of the ulna and released by subperiosteal dissection from its insertion on the ulna. The muscle is released in its entirety distally to proximally. It is reflected proximally to afford visualization of the distal humerus.

Medial Approach

Indications

- Ulnar nerve pathology
- Capsular release for stiffness
- Need to preserve the lateral ulnohumeral ligamentous complex

Contraindications

- Need for access to radial head or lateral ligaments

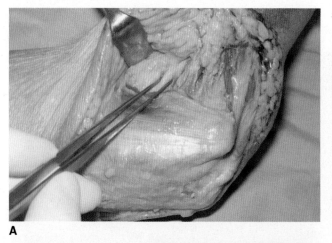

A

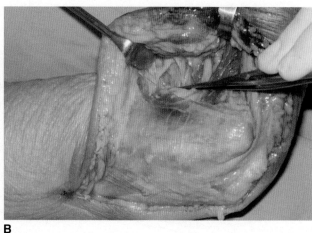

B

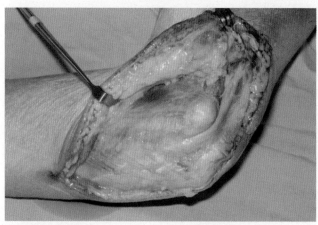

C

FIGURE 9-5

A: After the skin incision is made, the subcutaneous fat is elevated from the forearm fascia. Care is taken to protect the medial antebrachial cutaneous nerve that lies in the subcutaneous adipose tissue. **B, C:** The median nerve is found lateral and deep to the flexor pronator group, with the lateral antebrachial cutaneous nerve lying even more lateral.

INCISION. A medially or posteromedially based skin incision is made (Fig. 9-5A). Care is taken to identify and preserve the medial antebrachial cutaneous nerve (Fig. 9-5B, C). This nerve has a variable course and may cross the surgical field above or below the elbow and may have several branches.

The ulnar nerve is identified proximally and dissected distally. In revision surgery and cases with a prior transposition, it is especially helpful to identify the nerve in a normal area proximal to the scarred region.

If access is needed to the anterior portion of the joint, the medial supracondylar ridge and the intermuscular septum are identified. The ulnar nerve is mobilized and retracted, while a portion of the intermuscular septum is excised. A cautery is used to separate the brachial fascia and the superior portion of the flexor pronator group. An elevator is then used to elevate subperiosteally to expose the anterior joint. If additional distal exposure is needed, the flexor pronator group may be split leaving the inferior 1.5 cm or so of the flexor carpi ulnaris (FCU) attached to the epicondyle and elevating the superior portion to gain exposure to the joint.

The dissection is subperiosteal, deep to the brachialis so that the brachial artery and median nerve are protected.

Medial Coronoid Approach

Indications

● Fixation of coronoid fractures

INCISION. The medial coronoid can be easily exposed through the "floor" of the cubital tunnel. The ulnar nerve is identified and mobilized so it can be retracted safely (Fig. 9-6A, B). At the completion of the case, the nerve can be anteriorly transposed as previously described or the nerve may be left

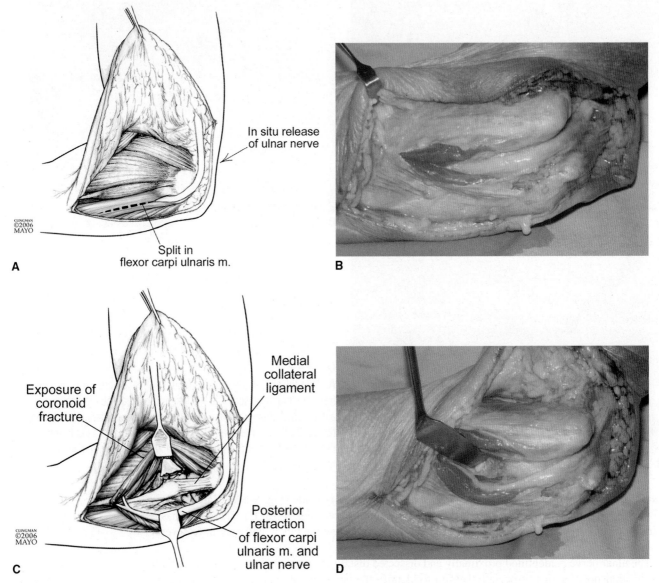

CLINGMAN
©2006
MAYO

In situ release
of ulnar nerve

Split in
flexor carpi ulnaris m.

A

B

Exposure of
coronoid
fracture

Medial
collateral
ligament

CLINGMAN
©2006
MAYO

Posterior
retraction
of flexor carpi
ulnaris m. and
ulnar nerve

C

D

FIGURE 9-6

A: The ulnar nerve is released from the cubital tunnel, and the FCU is split in line with its two heads. **B:** In this photograph, Osborne's ligament overlying the cubital tunnel has been released. **C, D:** The nerve is gently retracted posteriorly, and the ulnar head of the FCU is carefully dissected off of the MCL, exposing the coronoid.

in place if there are no concerns for irritation at the native site and as long as it is not destabilized. After the nerve is mobilized, the two heads of the FCU are split, and it is through this interval that one will expose the coronoid (Fig. 9-6C, D).

The dissection proceeds from distal to proximal. The surgeon will palpate for the sublime tubercle ridge on the medial side, being aware that this is the attachment site of the important anterior band of the medial collateral ligament (MCL) (Fig. 9-7A). By palpating and identifying the distal attachment of the ligament, one can then expose from distal to proximal without violating the ligament (Fig. 9-7B). As the surgeon works more proximally, he or she can thus be aware of the ligament's location and gradually expose the coronoid (Fig. 9-7C).

Lateral Approaches

Indications

- Radial head ORIF, resection, or replacement
- Lateral epicondylitis debridement

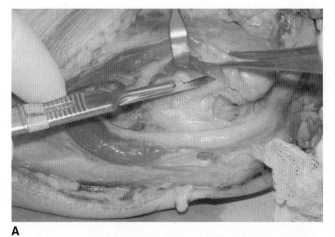

A

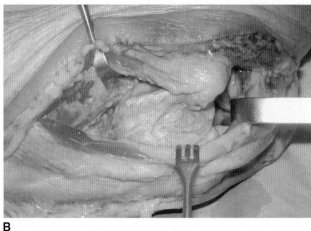

B

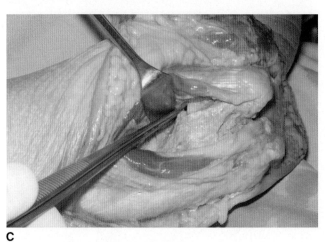

C

FIGURE 9-7

A: The MCL is better visualized by peeling the humeral head off the FCU laterally and superiorly. **B:** Using the full extent of this exposure affords access to the coronoid, the MCL, and portions of the posterior fossa. **C:** The entire coronoid can be seen. A full view of the MCL can be achieved including the medial epicondyle as well as the sublime tubercle.

- Repair of lateral ulnar collateral ligament
- Release of contractures

Contraindications

- The need to approach medial pathology
- Ulnar nerve involvement
- Medial humeral condyle fractures

INCISION. The lateral approach to the elbow is most useful to address radial head and capitellum fractures, lateral-sided instability, or lateral approaches to contracture release.

A laterally based, gently curved incision is made centered over the radial head and lateral epicondyle (Fig. 9-8). Alternatively, the posterior utilitarian approach may be used but requires a large incision and large skin flap. The deep dissection can proceed through Kocher's interval, or more commonly, via an extensor digitorum communis (EDC)-splitting approach.

EXTENSOR-SPLITTING APPROACH. This approach is favored in most cases when the lateral ulnar collateral ligament (LUCL) is intact. In addition, it is useful for exposures of the lateral joint for addressing lateral-sided pathology including capitellum fractures and radial head fractures and contracture release. The lateral epicondyle is identified and the lateral supracondylar ridge palpated. Distally, the radial head is palpated and the anterior and posterior extent noted. Identification of the midline of the radial head is the most important step of this exposure. The deep dissection proceeds by incising the lateral common extensor origin off of the supracondylar ridge and then proceeding through a split in the EDC tendon origin at the level of the midline (or equator) of the radial head (Fig. 9-9). Care is taken to avoid splitting or dissecting inferior to the midline of the radial head distally, to avoid iatrogenic injury to the LUCL. Pronation of the forearm will allow the posterior

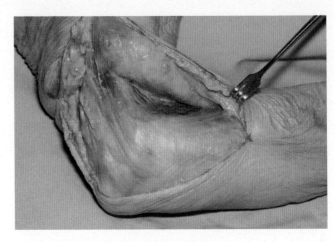

FIGURE 9-8

An example of a lateral or posterior skin incision. The skin and subcutaneous tissues are carefully removed from the investing fascia. Special attention should be taken to avoid damage to the lateral antebrachial cutaneous nerve, which will travel within the fat at the distal aspect of this incision.

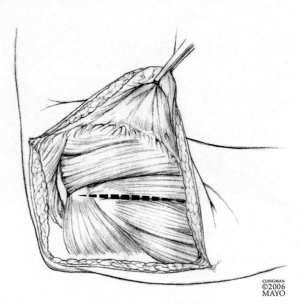

FIGURE 9-9

An alternative to the Kocher's approach is to split the common extensor group at the equator of the radiocapitellar joint. This decreases the likelihood of disrupting the lateral collateral complex.

Incision in common extensor tendon

CLINGMAN
©2006
MAYO

interosseous nerve (PIN) to move further away from the surgical field; however, the surgeon should be aware that the PIN is within 2 to 5 cm of the radiocarpal joint depending on the forearm size and relative position of the forearm with regard to pronosupination.

KOCHER'S INTERVAL. This approach is most useful for lateral-sided instability in the acute or chronic setting, as the interval takes the surgeon directly to the LUCL. In the setting of an acute radial head fracture, it is important to palpate for defects in the lateral extensor musculature, as occasionally the LUCL may be avulsed, providing a window for exposure that the surgeon should exploit. In the absence of elbow instability, the surgeon must exercise care to avoid iatrogenic injury to the LUCL.

For this approach, the interval between the extensor carpi ulnaris (ECU) and the anconeus is identified. The fascia is incised from the lateral epicondyle distally following the borders of the ECU and anconeus. Care is taken to elevate the ECU anteriorly and the anconeus posteriorly. The capsule is incised along the anterior border of the lateral ulnar collateral ligament, about 1 cm above the crista supinatoris (Fig. 9-10A), and the extensor origin is dissected from the lateral collateral ligament (LCL) complex (Fig. 9-10B). If the elbow is not already unstable, care is taken to preserve the LCL complex and avoid destabilizing the elbow (Fig. 9-11). This approach achieves excellent exposure of the radial head and neck (Fig. 9-12). When retracting the anterior structures, remember to pronate the forearm, which will reduce tension on the PIN.

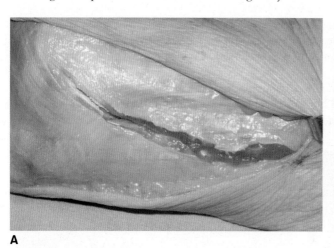
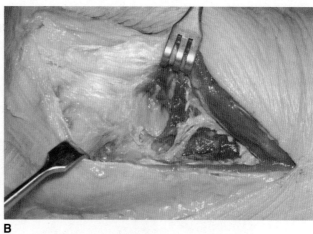

A   **B**

FIGURE 9-10

A: A traditional Kocher's incision is made between the anconeus and the ECU. Care is taken to develop this interval between the LCL and the ECU. **B:** The extensor origin is dissected from the LCL.

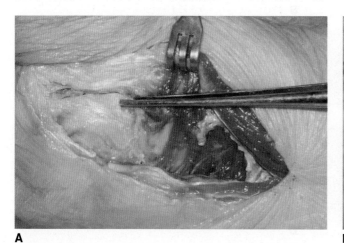
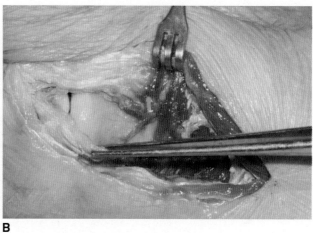

A   **B**

FIGURE 9-11

A, B: The capsule is incised anterior to the equator of the radial head in order to preserve the LCL complex.

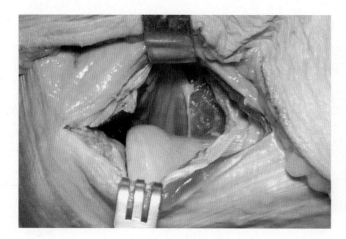

FIGURE 9-12

Excellent exposure of the radial head and neck is achieved with this approach.

DEEP DISSECTION. Proximally, the radial nerve is usually found as close as 8 cm (four finger-breadths) above the lateral epicondyle, or on average 10 cm from the articular surface (Fig. 9-13). Distally, the PIN will be found in the area of the radial neck about 4 cm (two fingerbreadths) distal to the radiocapitellar joint.

The lateral approach can be extended by continuing the dissection proximally in both the anterior and posterior sides of the lateral humerus, while always mindful of the LCL complex origin (Fig. 9-14). Elevation of the brachioradialis anteriorly allows for full visualization (Fig. 9-15).

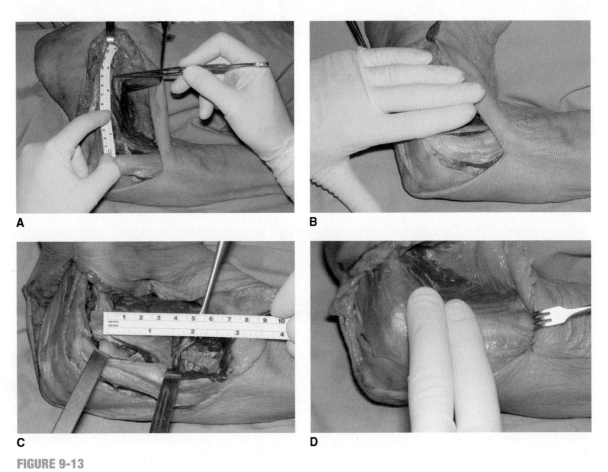

FIGURE 9-13

A, B: The radial nerve can be found at the level of the elbow 9 cm (four fingerbreadths) proximally from the lateral epicondyle. **C, D:** The safe zone for avoiding injury to the PIN is within 4 cm (two fingerbreadths) distal of the radial head.

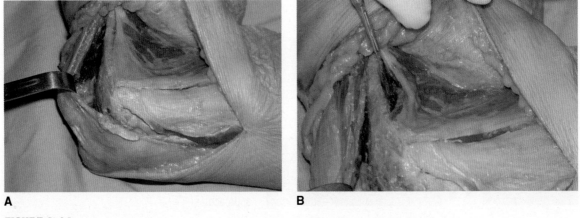

FIGURE 9-14

A, B: The lateral approach can be extended by continuing the dissection proximally on both the anterior and posterior side of the lateral humerus.

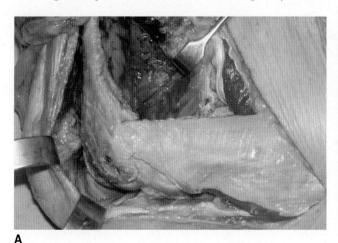
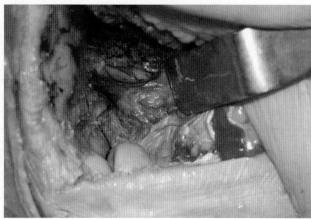

A   **B**

FIGURE 9-15

A, B: The brachioradialis is elevated anteriorly, allowing for improved visualization of the coronoid.

POSTOPERATIVE MANAGEMENT

Elbow rehabilitation is determined by fracture stability and concomitant ligamentous injury.

COMPLICATIONS

Flap necrosis, dehiscence, and wound infection are potential complications of surgical incisions about the elbow, particularly in the setting of trauma or in patients with wound healing comorbidities. Small areas of partial skin loss may be treated with local wound care, dressing changes, and immobilization to limit shear stresses. In cases where there is exposure of hardware, prosthesis, or nerve, we would recommend coverage with a local flap or a free flap for significant soft tissue loss.

PEARLS AND PITFALLS

- Properly planned incisions are critical to gaining adequate exposure and limiting complications.
- Full-thickness skin flaps are critical to limit tissue necrosis.
- Separate medial and lateral exposures to address pathology on either side of the elbow are often most helpful rather than a single large incision posteriorly.
- Preoperative planning and careful review of the patient's prior incisions, radiographic studies, and history are important to choose the most appropriate approach.

RECOMMENDED READING

Cheung EV, Steinmann SP. Surgical approaches to the elbow. *J Am Acad Orthop Surg.* 2009;17(5):325–333.

Cohen MS, Hastings H. Posttraumatic contracture of the elbow. Operative release using a lateral collateral ligament sparing approach. *J Bone Joint Surg Br.* 1998;80(5):805–812.

Hotchkiss RN. Elbow contracture. In: Green DP, Hotchkiss RN, Pederson WC, eds. *Green's Operative Hand Surgery.* Philadelphia, PA: Churchill-Livingstone; 1999:667–682.

O'Driscoll SW. The triceps-reflecting anconeus pedicle (TRAP) approach for distal humeral fractures and nonunions. *Orthop Clin North Am.* 2000;31(1):91–101.

Ring D, Gulotta L, Chin K, et al. Olecranon osteotomy for exposure of fractures and nonunions of the distal humerus. *J Orthop Trauma.* 2004;18(7):446–449.

Ring D. Fractures of the coronoid process of the ulna. *J Hand Surg Am.* 2006;31(10):1679–1689.

Taylor TKF, Scham SM. A posteromedial approach to the proximal end of the ulna for the internal fixation of olecranon fractures. *J Trauma.* 1969;9:594–602.

Tornetta P III, Hochwald N, Bono C, et al. Anatomy of the posterior interosseous nerve in relation to fixation of the radial head. *Clin Orthop Relat Res.* 1997;345:215–218.

Uhl RL, Larosa JM, Sibeni T, et al. Posterior approaches to the humerus: when should you worry about the radial nerve? *J Orthop Trauma.* 1996;10(5):338–340.

10 Radial Forearm Flap for Elbow Coverage

Sean R. Cantwell and Brian T. Carlsen

The elbow's extensive range of motion requires that its soft tissue envelope be pliable and durable. Soft tissue loss in and around the elbow is common and can occur for a variety of reasons including trauma, tumor, infection, olecranon bursitis, and pressure sores. Due to the superficial course of the neurovascular structures surrounding the elbow, soft tissue injury often results in exposure of critical structures. In these cases, primary closure and skin grafting may not be adequate for reliable soft tissue coverage. Various options exist for the treatment of elbow wounds, including local and free tissue transfer options; however, for many surgeons, the radial forearm flap has become the workhorse flap for elbow coverage.

The antegrade pedicled radial forearm flap is a fasciocutaneous flap based on perforators from the radial artery. The flap's popularity for elbow coverage stems from its reliable vascular pedicle, ease of dissection, and generous arc of rotation. It is one of the thinnest fasciocutaneous flaps, making it ideal for elbow coverage. Additionally, it can be harvested as a sensate flap when the medial or lateral antebrachial cutaneous nerves are preserved within the flap. For more complex cases, composite radial forearm flaps may be elevated to incorporate portions of the radius bone, palmaris longus tendon, flexor carpi radialis (FCR) tendon, and/or brachioradialis tendon or muscle. Finally, a great advantage of the flap is its ability to be re-elevated for secondary surgical procedures such as bone grafting, hardware removal, or nerve grafting.

INDICATIONS/CONTRAINDICATIONS

The flap is primarily indicated for soft tissue defects of the posterior elbow distal to the olecranon. Historically, more proximal wounds extending over the distal humerus can be covered with a pedicled latissimus flap. Exposed bone, nerve, tendon, and joint are all indications for radial forearm flap coverage. The size of the defect that can be covered by the flap is defined by the size of the patient's forearm. Flaps as large as 15 cm × 25 cm have been described; however, the larger the flap, the larger the resultant donor site and risk of donor site complications.

The flap can be used in a prophylactic manner for patients who have undergone multiple previous elbow procedures and have tenuous skin coverage prior to or at the time of a subsequent elbow operation. It may also be used prophylactically in patients with a high risk for wound complications, such as revision arthroplasty cases in patients with rheumatoid arthritis. Prophylactic flap coverage can also be considered in patients with underlying hardware if the overlying skin looks compromised, requires significant undermining to close, or is closed under significant tension. In these patients, even if primary closure of the wound may be possible under tension, flap coverage should be considered to avoid the catastrophic complication of an infected prosthesis resulting from wound dehiscence (Fig. 10-1).

The contraindications for flap use include the absence of or injury to the ulnar or radial artery. Use of the flap requires that there is satisfactory collateral flow through the ulnar artery into the palmar arches to maintain perfusion to the hand. A small percentage of patients are reliant upon the radial artery to perfuse a part or the entirety of the hand. In these patients, blood flow to the thumb is dependent upon the radial artery; therefore, radial forearm flaps cannot be performed without concurrent vein graft to reestablish the normal radial artery flow pattern. In such cases, an alternative flap is indicated. Additionally, if the patient has a history of radial artery harvest (for coronary bypass grafting), radial artery injury (from arterial line placement or catheterization using the radial artery), or trauma to the radial artery, an alternative means of elbow coverage should be chosen.

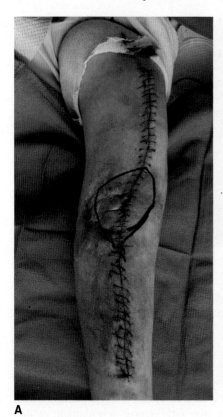
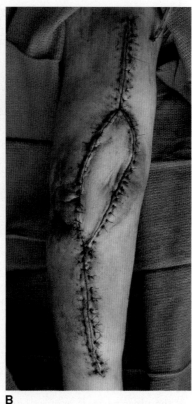

FIGURE 10-1

This tenuous closure of a posterior wound has excessive risk of wound breakdown **(A)**. Such cases may benefit from radial forearm flap coverage to minimize the risk of dehiscence and/or infection of underlying hardware **(B)**.

Though not technically a contraindication, postoperative donor site aesthetics can be a disadvantage and should be carefully considered. Surgeons are obliged to counsel patients regarding postoperative cosmesis so that they fully appreciate potential cosmetic outcomes. Split-thickness skin grafting is often used to cover the forearm donor site defect, but forearm contour and volume deformities may persist. There are ways to minimize evidence of the donor site defect, such as limiting the radial extent of the flap design so that it does not cross the radial border of the forearm. This modification has the added benefit of preventing exposure of the superficial branch of the radial nerve, maintaining coverage of this important structure with healthy, native skin. Fascia-sparing flap harvest can also improve the final appearance, as can initial coverage with bilaminar skin substitute and a negative pressure wound dressing for 3 to 4 weeks. For improvement in donor site aesthetics, we recommend covering the donor site with a non-meshed, split-thickness skin graft. Nevertheless, imperfect cosmetic results due to hyperpigmentation, hypertrophic scarring, and distorted forearm silhouette may still prove too bothersome for some patients. Patient factors that may contribute to poorer aesthetic outcomes include elevated body mass index and a hirsute volar forearm.

PREOPERATIVE PLANNING

Preoperatively, the patency of the radial artery, ulnar artery, and palmar arch is evaluated with the modified Allen test. While the radial artery is occluded, confirmation of perfusion via the ulnar artery may also be obtained using a Doppler ultrasound over the pulp of each digit. Particular consideration should be directed to obtaining a strong Doppler signal over the volar aspect of the first metacarpal, the location of the princeps pollicis artery. The princeps pollicis artery represents the most distal branch of the deep palmar arch relative to the ulnar artery and is the primary means of perfusion for the thumb. The Allen test remains a subjective assessment of hand and forearm perfusion. Equivocal test results should be critically interpreted and prompt more thorough investigation via angiography or formal noninvasive Doppler studies.

Preoperative evaluation should also include inspection of the elbow recipient site. Dirty wounds resulting from elbow trauma should be thoroughly debrided (Fig. 10-2). Fractures should be

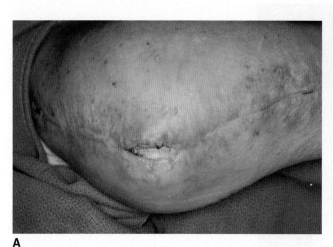

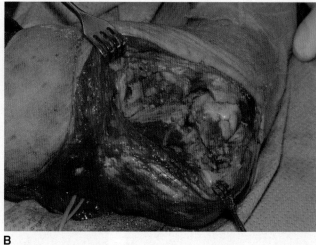

A   B

FIGURE 10-2

This 51-year-old woman had a history of elbow trauma requiring multiple operations complicated by infection. She ultimately underwent allograft-prosthesis composite reconstruction. **A:** Attempted primary closure of the wound lead to dehiscence with allograft bone exposure. **B:** After debridement of the wound.

stabilized prior to flap coverage, as fracture reduction following flap transfer may result in pedicle damage. Segmental bone loss should be addressed with an antibiotic spacer and spanning fixation prior to flap coverage. If the ulnar nerve is exposed, either by elbow wound debridement or flap elevation, we will transpose the nerve anteriorly. Protection of the nerve via transposition may prevent future discomfort and neural injury caused by fibrosis or compression. A careful review of the patient's previous operative notes is important. In many cases, the patient has already undergone transposition of the ulnar nerve. If the transposition was in the subcutaneous plane, it could be at risk if the flap is tunneled over the medial epicondyle to reach the defect. In such cases, the nerve is identified early in the course of the operation and marked with a vessel loop for easy identification during the operation.

SURGERY

Anatomy

The brachial artery bifurcates into the radial and ulnar arteries approximately 1 cm distal to the elbow. In up to 15% of patients, the radial artery can originate from the proximal part of the brachial artery near the axilla and run parallel to the brachial artery in the arm. In the forearm, the radial artery supplies the recurrent radial artery before it travels along the anterior aspect of the radius. The artery lies superficial to the pronator teres, flexor pollicis longus, and pronator quadratus. The brachioradialis overlies the artery on the proximal half of the forearm. Distally, the artery runs between the FCR and brachioradialis tendons. This consistent anatomy proves a reliable means to identify the location of the radial artery. The sensory branch of the radial nerve travels radial to the artery, deep to the brachioradialis until it courses dorsal to the brachioradialis approximately 8 cm proximal to the radial styloid.

Numerous branches of the radial and ulnar arteries form a delicate vascular plexus, which supplies the forearm muscles and skin. There are 9 to 17 septocutaneous branches that emerge from the radial artery as it travels down the forearm (Fig. 10-3). The branches are found within the intermuscular septum that separates the brachioradialis from the FCR, with a greater number of arterial branches originating from the distal part of the artery.

Upon reaching the wrist, the radial artery forms a palmar carpal branch and superficial palmar branch (Fig. 10-4). The artery then wraps around the carpal bones posteriorly, passing through the anatomic snuffbox where it gives off the dorsal carpal artery. It then pierces the two heads of the first dorsal interosseous muscle as it returns to the palmar surface of the hand. The artery finally divides into the deep palmar branch, princeps pollicis artery, and radial digital artery to the index finger.

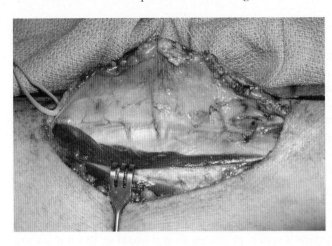

FIGURE 10-3

Perforators coursing from the artery to the overlying skin are found between the FCR and brachioradialis tendons distally.

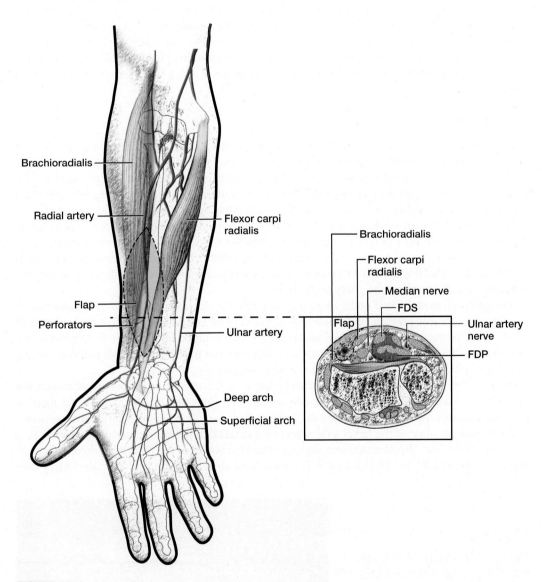

FIGURE 10-4

Radial artery anatomy demonstrating its relationship to the brachioradialis and FCR tendons at the wrist and its anatomic course.

The superficial and deep palmar branches anastomose with analogous branches of the ulnar artery to supply the common digital arteries.

There are two venous comitantes that run with the radial artery. These veins, one on each side of the radial artery, regularly communicate with one another and join the superficial forearm veins in draining the skin and fascia of the radial forearm flap. The cephalic vein also provides venous drainage to the territory supplied by the radial artery. This vein can be included within the flap to aid in venous drainage. As it courses proximally, it frequently runs with the lateral antebrachial cutaneous nerve. At the antecubital fossa, the cephalic vein often communicates with the basilic vein via the median cubital vein. In the arm, the cephalic vein runs anterolateral to the biceps brachii muscle before coursing through the deltopectoral groove.

Patient Positioning

To facilitate flap harvest, the patient is positioned supine on the operating table with the arm abducted and externally rotated. The patient's arm is placed on an arm board so that the anterior surface of the forearm is facing the ceiling. Both the upper extremity and the ipsilateral thigh (for skin graft harvest) are prepped and draped in a sterile manner. The surgeon often sits facing the volar aspect of the forearm. When it is time for flap inset, the patient's upper extremity may be internally rotated for better visualization of periolecranon defects. The surgeon may then choose to orient him or herself toward the posterior surface of the arm. Concomitant shoulder mobility issues are not uncommon due to rheumatoid arthritis or trauma, and occasionally, prone positioning is indicated to allow simultaneous access to the volar forearm and posterior elbow in patients who lack external rotation of the shoulder.

Technique

The course of the radial artery is identified using a handheld Doppler probe and traced from the antecubital fossa to a point at the wrist crease between the FCR and radial styloid. Flap design is not limited by the traditional width-to-length ratio; the flap may potentially include all skin from the entire volar forearm, and flaps as large as 15 cm × 25 cm have been reported. Surgeons often find it helpful to use a template of the elbow wound to accurately approximate the required flap dimensions and pedicle length. A skin island 10% to 15% larger than the measured defect is outlined on the forearm to allow for less tension during flap inset. Markings for the flap may be centered over the radial artery; however, as previously mentioned, the radial border of the forearm may be chosen to serve as the radial flap margin for cosmetic reasons. In this circumstance, the flap may be slightly eccentric over the course of the artery (Fig. 10-5).

The operation is performed under tourniquet control. The degree and method of exsanguination vary based on surgeon preference. Some surgeons prefer minimal exsanguination of the extremity to better visualize the septocutaneous perforators during the operation (see Fig. 10-3). Others (author included) prefer to use the Esmarch wrap to completely exsanguinate the limb prior to flap elevation. In cases of malignancy or infection, no wrap exsanguination is performed.

Once the recipient site has been appropriately prepared, flap dissection begins distally where the radial artery is superficial and anatomic landmarks are consistent and easy to localize. An incision is made along the distal-ulnar aspect of the forearm flap markings. Suprafascial dissection is carried out from the ulnar to the radial side. Great care is taken to protect the perforators to the skin island emerging from the intermuscular septum. When the border of the FCR is reached, dissection proceeds subfascially. The FCR tendon is retracted in an ulnar direction, and the radial artery with

FIGURE 10-5

Patient shown in Figure 10-2. A radial forearm flap is designed eccentrically over the radial artery (marked) with care to avoid crossing the radial border of the forearm.

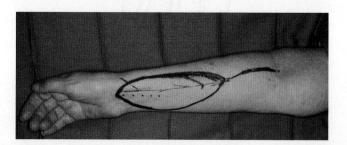

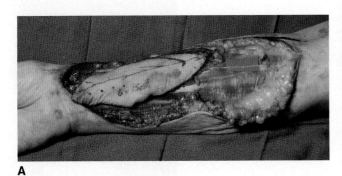
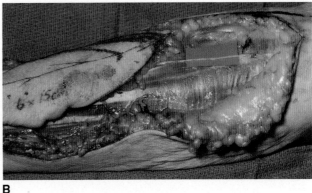

A   **B**

FIGURE 10-6

Patient shown in Figure 10-2 after complete flap mobilization. **A:** A branch of the lateral antebrachial cutaneous nerve is highlighted by the green background. This flap was innervated to provide protective posterior elbow sensation. **B:** Close-up image.

its venae comitantes is visualized. At this point, a final assessment of hand perfusion can be made. To do so, a vascular clamp is placed on the distal radial artery, the tourniquet is released, and a hand-held Doppler is used to evaluate the pulp of each digit for a Doppler signal. Alternatively, capillary refill of less than 2 seconds in each finger also can verify adequate circulation. If hand perfusion is normal, the artery is ligated and divided at this distal location. If perfusion is not normal, the surgeon must decide if he or she will proceed with flap elevation and subsequent reconstruction of the radial artery with a vein graft or move to another flap choice for elbow coverage.

If arterial flow in the ulnar artery is adequate for hand perfusion, dissection then proceeds along the flap's distal-radial border. Depending on flap design, identification and protection of the superficial branch of the radial nerve may be necessary. Suprafascial dissection is again performed until the ulnar border of the brachioradialis is visualized, at which point dissection proceeds subfascially. Subfascial dissection continues along the muscle's ulnar border and exposes deep muscular branches of the radial artery. These branches are ligated using vascular clips. These branches can tether the elevation of the radial artery during dissection. During this portion of the case, upward traction can be applied to the flap, but care must be taken not to avulse the artery from its fine perforators to the skin. The radial artery can be carefully sutured to the skin distally to prevent this.

Flap dissection proceeds from distal to proximal, alternating between the radial and ulnar sides to ensure the dissection includes the radial artery and venae comitantes with the flap. If a sensate flap is desired, the surgeon should take care to preserve the medial and/or lateral cutaneous nerves that supply the flap (Fig. 10-6). Paratenon overlying the FCR and brachioradialis is preserved to facilitate healing following skin grafting.

The proximal border of the flap incision is extended to allow for dissection of the radial artery to where it branches from the brachial artery. Diligence is required to avoid injuring the ulnar artery at its origin. The venae comitantes, medial and lateral antebrachial cutaneous nerves, and cephalic vein are also traced proximally. The flap is now completely mobilized, and caution is employed to avoid traction to the pedicle with any further manipulation of the extremity.

A generous subcutaneous tunnel is created between the proximal end of the donor site and the elbow recipient site (Fig. 10-7). The tunnel's preferred location is on the medial elbow because in this situation, the brachial artery is less of a tether to flap rotation and inset. Great care is taken when

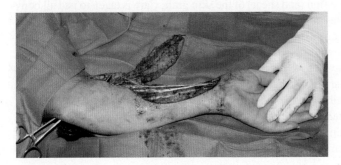

FIGURE 10-7

A tunnel is carefully created by working from both the donor site and the elbow wound to gently pass the flap medially with care to avoid injury to the ulnar nerve or medial antebrachial cutaneous nerves.

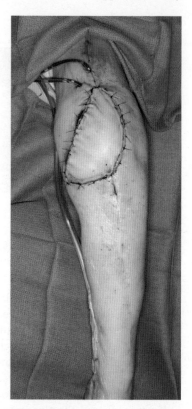

FIGURE 10-8

Patient shown in Figure 10-2. Posterior view of the elbow and forearm after flap rotation and inset. The flap nicely covers the soft tissue defect without tension.

making the tunnel to avoid injury to the medial antebrachial cutaneous nerve or ulnar nerve (in its native or transposed position). The flap is temporarily secured to the forearm and the tourniquet taken down. Flap and hand perfusion are confirmed before proceeding with passing the flap into the defect site. The flap is passed via the subcutaneous tunnel to the elbow wound (see Fig. 10-7). Extreme care is taken to ensure that the vascular pedicle remains tension free and does not kink as it is passed through the tunnel. The flap is then inset over a drain (Fig. 10-8).

Attention is now directed to the donor site. If the superficial radial nerve is exposed, it may benefit from coverage via imbrication of the skin or brachioradialis muscle with buried sutures. The forearm wound is closed as much as possible using nonabsorbable vertical mattress sutures at the wound's proximal and distal ends. An absorbable suture can then be used to purse-string the remaining defect. Radial and ulnar skin edges are marsupialized to the remaining antebrachial fascia. The remaining donor site wound is covered with a split-thickness skin graft or bilaminar skin substitute bilayer dressing (Fig. 10-9A). In our experience, bilaminar skin substitute can improve donor site morbidity by creation of a "neodermis" of granulation tissue (Fig. 10-9B). If bilaminar skin substitute is used, the patient will require a skin graft to the donor site in 2 to 3 weeks, after the bilaminar skin substitute is vascularized (Fig. 10-9C).

POSTOPERATIVE MANAGEMENT

A bulky dressing is applied with a window for flap observation. The elbow is immobilized in extension with a volar plaster slab, unless contraindicated based on orthopedic issues. The wrist is immobilized in neutral position to prevent motion (and shear) of the skin graft. Care is taken to pad all bony prominences and to ensure that the plaster does not compress any part of the flap or its pedicle. The extremity is elevated above the level of the heart to minimize edema. Typically, a negative pressure bolster is placed over the donor site, securing either the skin graft or bilaminar skin substitute. The bolster is maintained in place for 5 days, at which point the dressing and splint are first removed. At that time, a removable Orthoplast splint is fabricated, and the patient is allowed to initiate active range-of-motion exercises of the wrist and elbow at the reconstructive and orthopedic surgeon's discretion.

Anticoagulation is not routinely used as a part of postoperative pedicled flap management. Drains are typically removed once they drain less than 30 mL a day. Antibiotics are used to address any preexisting elbow infection; however, antibiotic prophylaxis is not routinely used in cases where there is no preexisting infection.

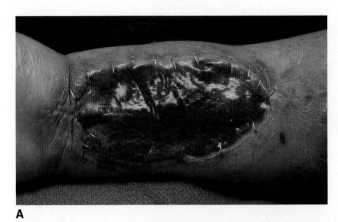
A

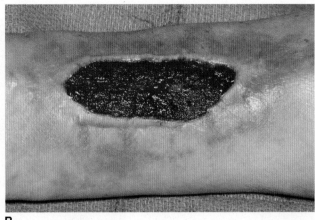
B

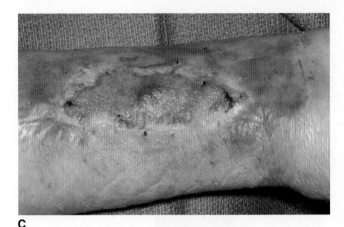
C

FIGURE 10-9

Patient shown in Figure 10-2. **A:** Bilaminar skin substitute is secured over the radial forearm donor site to minimize donor site morbidity as discussed in the text. **B:** Appearance of the flap donor site after 4 weeks of bilaminar skin substitute and negative pressure wound therapy. **C:** Two weeks after split-thickness skin graft coverage of the flap donor site.

RESULTS

The radial forearm flap was first described by Yang et al. in 1978 and popularized by Song et al. in 1982. Several subsequent case series serve to validate the efficacy and safety of the pedicle radial forearm flap for elbow coverage for a spectrum of indications, ranging from osteoradionecrosis to olecranon bursitis. Many authors conclude that for posterior elbow defects, the radial forearm flap represents the ideal flap for coverage (Fig. 10-10).

The flap, by definition, sacrifices radial artery perfusion of the hand. Contrary to previous reports, recent studies have demonstrated the radial artery to be the dominant arterial inflow to the hand. Despite this, several studies have demonstrated no detrimental change in hand perfusion following radial artery harvest. Still, one must consider the potential for vascular compromise to the hand after this procedure, including future cold intolerance. The unsightly donor site is the other considerable disadvantage of this flap. While techniques are employed to mitigate this morbidity, it remains a drawback of this reconstructive option.

Concerns regarding protection of the flap's vascular supply initially led surgeons to carry out a subfascial dissection during flap harvest. However, more recent evidence has demonstrated that a suprafascial vascular plexus located in the adipose tissue provides sufficient perfusion for skin flap survival. Maximizing the fascial integrity of the forearm is beneficial in terms of improved aesthetic outcomes, minimizing unnecessary flap bulk and decreasing donor site tendon adhesion to the overlying skin graft.

COMPLICATIONS

As with all other pedicled flaps, the radial forearm flap is at risk for seroma or hematoma formation, superficial skin necrosis, wound dehiscence, infection, scar contraction, and partial or total flap loss. Patients may also complain of decreases in hand sensation, wrist and hand strength, and wrist and finger range of motion. Superficial radial nerve injury during dissection has been reported and

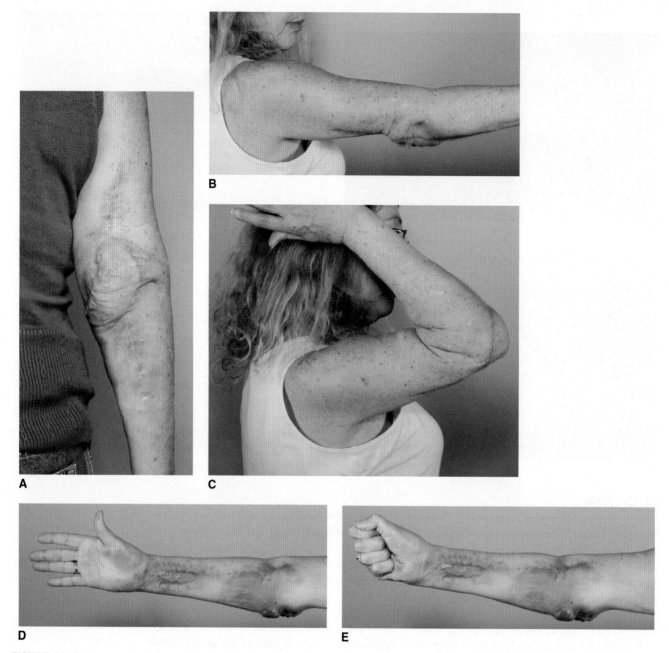

FIGURE 10-10

Patient shown in Figure 10-2. **A:** Several months after the flap procedure, the elbow wound is nicely healed and no evidence of active infection. **B:** In full elbow extension with minimal lag, demonstrating minimal loss of motion. **C:** In full elbow flexion without lag, demonstrating no loss of motion. **D:** With full hand opening, without loss of motion. **E:** With fully closed hand, without loss of motion.

results in loss of sensation over the dorsum of the hand. Finally, cold intolerance can also result following flap harvest.

Flap breakdown over the elbow can pose a difficult problem and often requires subsequent free flap coverage. In cases of recurrent elbow exposure in the setting of hardware or joint infection, flap failure is associated with significant morbidity and may lead to limb amputation.

Hand ischemia following radial artery ligation represents the most severe complication following elevation of the radial forearm flap. In cases where the flap has already been raised, saphenous vein grafting is required to reconstruct the radial artery and restore blood flow to the hand. Several case reports document instances where patients develop delayed hand ischemia despite normal preoperative Allen testing and Doppler ultrasound. Long-term vascular consequences of radial artery harvest remain unknown.

PEARLS AND PITFALLS

- A vascular exam, including an Allen test and Doppler ultrasound, should precede the decision to use the radial forearm flap.
- Before designing a radial forearm flap, the wound should be clean and completely debrided so that the proposed flap is of sufficient size to cover the entire wound.
- Inclusion of the medial or lateral antebrachial cutaneous nerves within the flap can provide protective sensation to the elbow.
- Limiting the radial extent of the flap to the radial border of the forearm can minimize the visibility of the donor site and decrease morbidity by leaving native skin overlying the superficial radial nerve.
- After transferring the flap, the surgeon should verify that there is no kinking, twisting, tension, or compression of the pedicle as any of these factors can cause partial or total flap loss.
- Creation of the subcutaneous tunnel for flap transfer should be performed carefully, while being mindful of the locations of cutaneous nerves and the (potentially transposed) ulnar nerve.

RECOMMENDED READING

Adkinson JM, Chung KC. Flap reconstruction of the elbow and forearm: a case-based approach. *Hand Clin.* 2014;30(2):153–163.

Bardsley AF, Soutar DS, Elliot D, et al. Reducing morbidity in the radial forearm flap donor site. *Plast Reconstr Surg.* 1990;86(2):287–292.

Chim H, Bakri K, Moran SL. Complications related to radial artery occlusion, radial artery harvest, and arterial lines. *Hand Clin.* 2015;31(1):93–100.

Choudry UH, Moran SL, Li S, et al. Soft-tissue coverage of the elbow: an outcome analysis and reconstructive algorithm. *Plast Reconstr Surg.* 2007;119(6):1852–1857.

Ciria-Llorens G, Gomez-Cia T, Talegon-Melendez A. Analysis of flow changes in forearm arteries after raising the radial forearm flap: a prospective study using colour duplex imaging. *Br J Plast Surg.* 1999;52:440–444.

Dumanian GA, Segalman K, Buehner JW, et al. Analysis of digital pulse-volume recordings with radial and ulnar artery compression. *Plast Reconstr Surg.* 1998;102(6):193–198.

Heller F, Wei W, Wei FC. Chronic arterial insufficiency of the hand with fingertip necrosis 1 year after harvesting a radial forearm free flap. *Plast Reconstr Surg.* 2004;114(3):728–731.

Higgins JP. A reassessment of the role of the radial forearm flap in upper extremity reconstruction. *J Hand Surg.* 2011;36A:1237–1240.

Ip TC, Jones NF. Treatment of chronic infected olecranon bursitis by radical excision and radial forearm flap coverage. *Tech Hand Up Extrem Surg.* 2001;5(2):112–116.

Jensen M, Moran SL. Soft tissue coverage of the elbow: a reconstructive algorithm. *Orthop Clin North Am.* 2008;39(2):251–264, vii.

Jones NF, Jarrahy R, Kaufman MR. Pedicled and free radial forearm flaps for reconstruction of the elbow, wrist, and hand. *Plast Reconstr Surg.* 2008;121(3):887–898.

Kasten SJ, Chung KC, Tong L. Simultaneous revascularization and soft tissue coverage in the traumatized upper extremity with a flow-through radial forearm free flap. *J Trauma.* 1999;47(2):416–419.

Kolker AR, Coombs CJ, Meara JG. A method for minimizing donor site complications of the radial forearm flap. *Ann Plast Surg.* 2000;45(3):329–331.

Lutz BS, Wei FC, Chang SC, et al. Donor site morbidity after suprafascial elevation of the radial forearm flap: a prospective study in 95 consecutive cases. *Plast Reconstr Surg.* 1999;103:132–137.

Meland NB, Clinkscales CM, Wood MB. Pedicled radial forearm flaps for recalcitrant defects about the elbow. *Microsurgery.* 1991;12(3):155–159.

Muhlbauer W, Herndl E, Stock W. The forearm flap. *Plast Reconstr Surg.* 1982;70:336–344.

Mullett H, Hausman M, Zaidemberg C. Recalcitrant distal humeral and proximal forearm nonunion: salvage using an extended pedicled radial forearm osseous flap. *J Trauma.* 2008;64(4):E60–E64.

Orgill DP, Pribaz JJ, Morris DJ. Local fasciocutaneous flaps for olecranon coverage. *Ann Plast Surg.* 1994;32(1):27–31.

Patel KM, Higgins JP. Posterior elbow wounds: soft tissue coverage options and techniques. *Orthop Clin North Am.* 2013;44(3):409–417.

Richardson D, Fisher SE, Vaughan ED, et al. Radial forearm flap donor-site complications and morbidity: a prospective study. *Plast Reconstr Surg.* 1997;99(1):109–115.

Schaverien M, Saint-Cyr M. Suprafascial compared with subfascial harvest of the radial forearm flap: an anatomic study. *J Hand Surg Am.* 2008;33(1):97–101.

Sherman R. Soft-tissue coverage for the elbow. *Hand Clin.* 1997;13(2):291–302.

Slade IJF, Gilbert RS, Mahoney JD. Soft tissue coverage of complex elbow wounds. *Tech Orthop.* 2000;15(2):79–92.

Stevanovic M, Sharpe F, Itamura JM. Treatment of soft tissue problems about the elbow. *Clin Orthop Relat Res.* 2000;370:127–137.

Yun TK, Yoon ES, Ahn DS, et al. Stabilizing morbidity and predicting the aesthetic results of radial forearm free flap donor sites. *Arch Plast Surg.* 2015;42(6):769–775.

11 Anconeus Muscle Flap and Flexor Carpi Ulnaris Muscle Flap for Soft Tissue Coverage of Elbow

Morad Askari, Bassem T. Elhassan, and Steven L. Moran

Soft tissue defects surrounding the elbow can result from multiple causes and can pose difficult reconstructive problems. Among the flaps used to cover the elbow, the anconeus muscle flap and flexor carpi ulnaris (FCU) muscle flap are two reliable local options that should be present in the armamentarium of any upper extremity surgeon. This chapter details the perioperative planning and surgical technique for these two flaps.

ANCONEUS MUSCLE FLAP

Indications/Contraindications

The anconeus flap is used as a muscle-only flap for coverage of small defects (6 to 7 cm^2) in close proximity to the muscle's origin or insertion. This flap can cover defects overlying the olecranon process as well as the lateral elbow. It is a useful flap in cases of chronic open olecranon bursitis and small defects following trauma or open reduction and internal fixation of the olecranon or distal humerus. In addition to wound coverage, the anconeus muscle flap can play a role in the treatment of refractory lateral epicondylitis as well as serving as an interposition flap in the prevention and management of proximal radioulnar synostosis.

Contraindications to use of anconeus muscle flap are injury to the muscle or disruption of its blood supply. In patients with a history of previous elbow surgery, proximal ulnar fractures, or prior anconeus elevation for exposure of the elbow, the surgeon may need to consider another option for wound coverage. Identification of muscle injury may not be apparent until the muscle is exposed intraoperatively; fortunately, it is easy to convert to the FCU flap should the anconeus appear inadequate for elbow coverage.

Anatomy

The anconeus muscle is a triangular fan-shaped muscle in the distal aspect of posterior elbow (Fig. 11-1). It originates from distal humerus posterior to the lateral epicondyle and inserts on the posterolateral surface of proximal ulna. It functions as an accessory muscle to the triceps while providing a small degree of stability to the elbow during forearm rotation; it can be sacrificed without resultant elbow instability or weakness.

The muscle is supplied by three pedicles: the recurrent posterior interosseous artery (RPIA), medial collateral artery (MCA), and posterior branch of radial collateral artery (PBRCA) (Fig. 11-2). Among these, MCA and RPIA are most consistent. To allow proper mobilization of the flap to cover areas over the radiocapitellar joint or olecranon, the muscle flap is based on MCA and the other pedicles are ligated. To allow coverage of more medial elbow defect, the proximal muscle may be mobilized using "anconeus slide" by splitting distal triceps fascia.

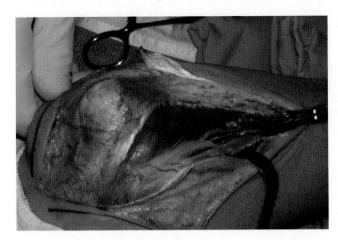

FIGURE 11-1

The anconeus muscle is a thin triangular muscle that extends from the proximal ulna to the radius in the posterior elbow.

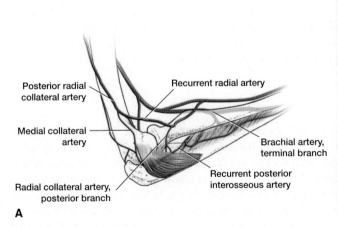

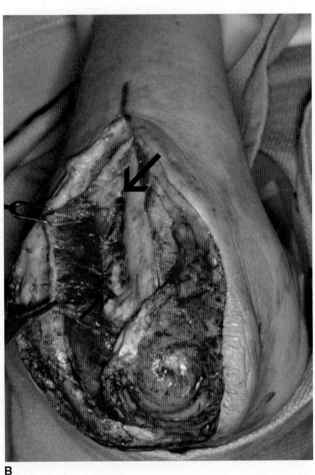

A   **B**

FIGURE 11-2

A: The blood supply to the muscle consists of posterior branch of radial collateral artery (a terminal branch of the profunda brachii), medial collateral artery, and recurrent posterior interosseous artery branch. **B:** Example of anconeus being elevated from the ulnar. On the deep surface of the muscle, the recurrent posterior interosseous artery (*large arrow*) can be seen connecting with the posterior branch of the radial collateral artery (*small arrow*). Both of these vessels will combine more proximally with the medial collateral artery. The flap is most commonly isolated on the medial collateral artery so it can reach the olecranon.

Surgery

Patient Positioning

The patient is positioned to allow wide access to the posterior elbow. Depending on the circumstance and preference, the patient may be placed in lateral decubitus position with ipsilateral shoulder elevated and the elbow flexed and supported anteriorly. A tourniquet may be used to allow for bloodless field. The lateral epicondyle is marked and a 6-cm line is drawn on the proximal posterolateral edge of the ulna to estimate the location of the insertion and origin of the muscle.

Technique

A longitudinal skin incision is made along the ulnar border of the ulna. If there is a previous posterior skin incision from previous surgery, this may be used for exposure of the muscle (Fig. 11-3A, B). The incision is connected to the defect in the elbow. Skin flaps are raised in the suprafascial plan medially and laterally to expose the ulnar shaft and extensor muscles. An incision is made on the ulnar aspect of the ulna, and the antebrachial fascia is incised to identify the broad attachment of anconeus muscle to posterior surface of ulna. The fascia may then be elevated as a flap to expose the muscle belly. The muscle is carefully elevated off the shaft of the ulna and the underlying fascia of the radiocapitellar joint capsule (Fig. 11-3C). Similarly, on the lateral side, the fascia is incised in the border of extensor carpi ulnaris (ECU). The muscle may now be divided distally leaving a small portion of the terminal tendon attached to the muscle to aid in insetting. The muscle is now elevated away from the ulna (Fig. 11-3D). The RPIA will be seen running on the floor of the fascia and radiocapitellar joint capsule (see Fig. 11-2B) and can be divided distally. As the muscle is elevated distal to proximal, the proximal segment of RPIA is preserved in the mobilized flap as this pedicle anastomoses with MCA in the anconeus muscle. The muscle is carefully raised completely based on MCA near the triceps as all other branches and perforators are ligated. To allow further mobilization of the muscle, it is necessary to detach it from lateral epicondyle. As this step is completed, PBRCA is ligated. Depending on the degree of mobility, the pedicle containing MCA can be further dissected and carefully skeletonized by allowing the flap to reach to the target area (Fig. 11-3E, F).

Following the inset of the flap, if feasible, the flap of antebrachial fascia is repaired over the donor bed and exposed ulnar shaft (Fig. 11-3G). The skin flaps are reapproximated and closed in layers. Drains may be used per discretion of the surgeon. Primary closure is often possible in nontrauma cases. In the setting of trauma, however, the muscle is skin grafted following insetting.

A soft compressive dressing is used over the donor site as well as the flap; alternatively, a negative pressure sponge may be applied to the skin graft. If a wound VAC is used, immediate motion may be initiated if fracture fixation allows for motion. Alternatively, the elbow may be splinted in whatever position is most appropriate for fracture healing. Any splint or cast should be carefully fitted to avoid putting pressure onto the muscle or vascular pedicle. If a skin graft is used, the wound is inspected at 5 days to ensure skin graft take. Sutures are removed at 2 weeks (Fig. 11-3H). Following this period, the patient is started on a therapy regimen to restore full range of motion of the elbow.

A second case is shown in Figure 11-4.

Results

In a cadaveric dissection of the anconeus flap, it was noted that when the muscle was elevated on the MCA, defects up to 7.3 cm^2 could be covered over the radiocapitellar joint, while defects up to 6.1 and 7.2 cm^2 could be covered over the distal triceps and olecranon, respectively. The same authors reported no compromise in elbow stability, range of motion, or elbow extension strength in a series of nine patients who had the anconeus flap used for elbow coverage. In a series of 20 patients with posterior elbow wounds covered with the pedicled anconeus muscle flap, wounds were healed on average 3 weeks after surgery with no cases of flap loss. At 17 months after surgery, there were significant improvements in Mayo Elbow Performance Scores (MEPS). All patients in this study regained full range of motion of the elbow and expressed satisfaction with the results. Fleager and Cheung used a modified sliding anconeus muscle technique for coverage of medial elbow defects in the context of primary or revision total elbow arthroplasty. In their series of 20 patients, which included four patients with wound complications following arthroplasty and one patient with open distal humerus, all wounds healed completely. Similar reports have shown reliability in use of the anconeus muscle for moderate soft tissue defects following total elbow arthroplasty.

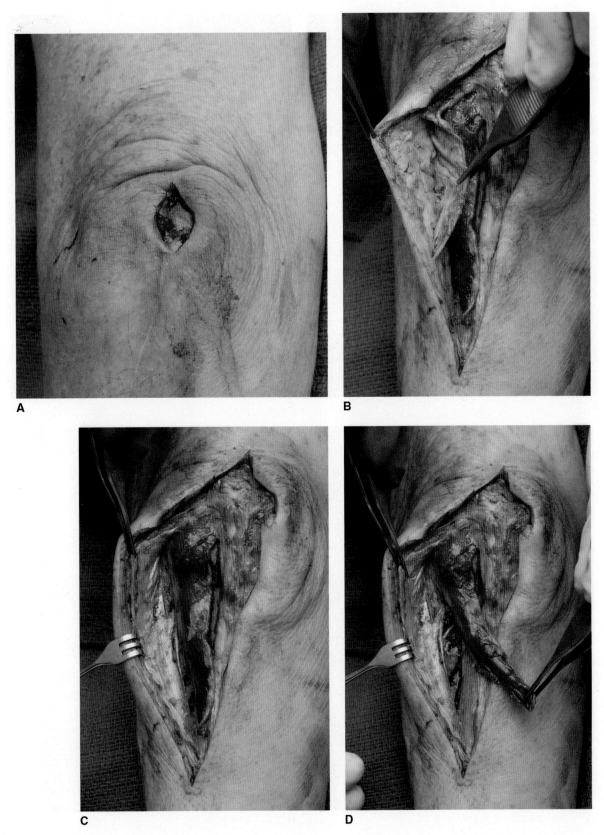

FIGURE 11-3

Technique for elevation of anconeus flap. **A:** A 68-year-old woman with a chronic draining elbow wound due to infected olecranon bursitis. **B:** The old posterior incision is used to expose the posterior fascia of the extensor compartment. **C:** The muscle can be visualized by elevating the fascia off the muscle lateral to the ulna. **D:** The flap is then mobilized off the ulna taking care to protect the underlying vessel.

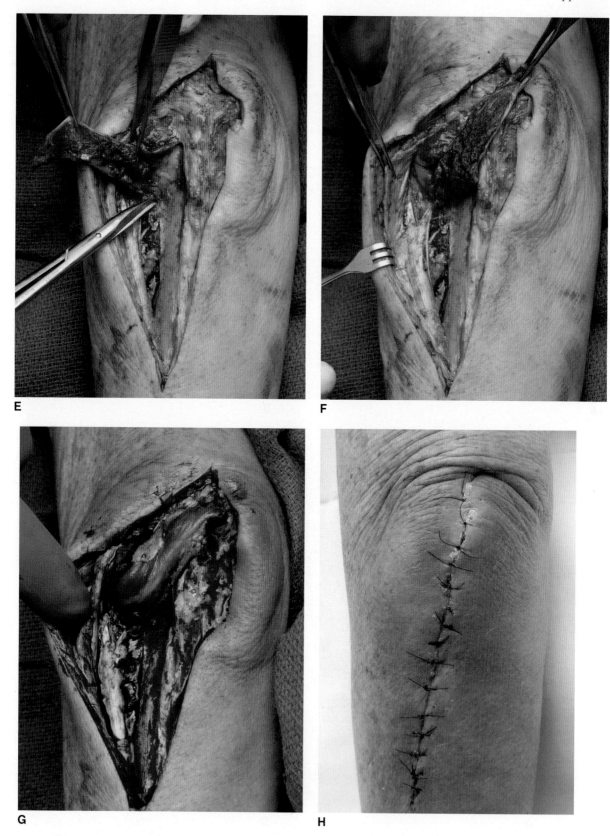

FIGURE 11-3 (Continued)

E: The medial collateral vessels can be dissected from the surrounding fascia to gain more pedicle length. **F:** When based on the medial collateral artery or posterior branch of the radial collateral artery, the anconeus muscle flap can be transposed to cover small posterior elbow wounds. **G:** The flap is well perfused with tourniquet released. **H:** Appearance of the elbow at 2 weeks.

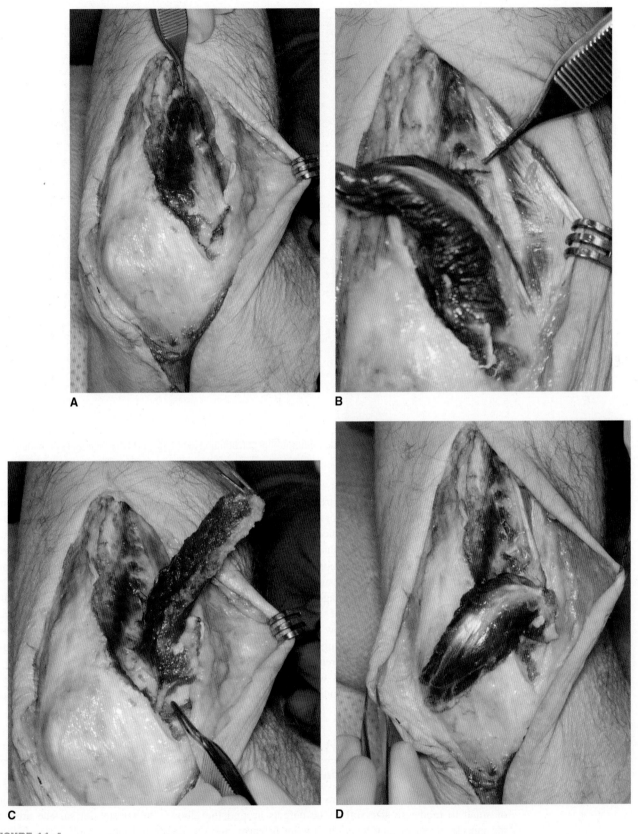

FIGURE 11-4

A: A case of a 54-year-old man with recurrent infected olecranon bursitis treated with an anconeus muscle flap. **B:** The distal branch of the recurrent posterior interosseous artery is divided, and the flap is isolated on the medial collateral artery. **C:** The medial collateral artery is seen at the tip of the forceps. **D:** The flap easily covers the olecranon.

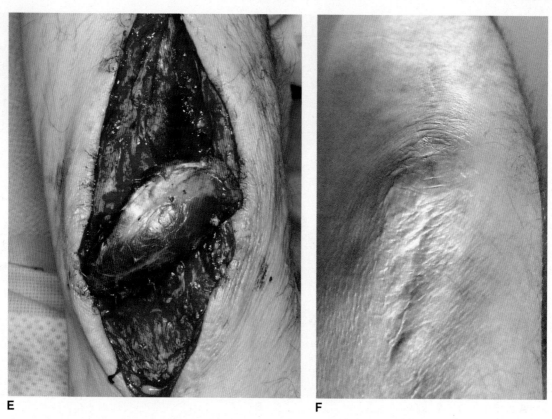

FIGURE 11-4 (Continued)

E: The flap is well perfused following release of tourniquet. With undermining of the surrounding skin flaps, primary closure is possible.
F: Final result at 1 year shows well-healed wound.

The flap has also been used for treatment of refractory lateral epicondylitis. In a study comparing patients undergoing debridement of the common extensor origin to those undergoing anconeus muscle flap coverage of the lateral epicondyle following debridement of the common extensor origin, those who underwent anconeus muscle flap coverage achieved better Disabilities of Arm, Shoulder, and Hand (DASH) scores than those with debridement alone. There was no difference in elbow stability, range of motion, or grip strength between the two groups.

In summary, the major advantage of the anconeus muscle flap is that it is a reliable flap with minimal morbidity for coverage of small areas in posterolateral and posteromedial elbow. The anconeus muscle functions as an elbow extensor that aids in the terminal 15 degrees of extension and forearm supination; thus, sacrificing the muscle for use as surgical flap does not produce noticeable decrease in range of motion or strength. The reported series of use of local anconeus muscle flaps for purposes of coverage of elbow wounds, treatment of lateral epicondylitis, or as an interposition flap in treatment of proximal radioulnar synostosis show improvement in outcomes with a high rate of flap success.

FLEXOR CARPI ULNARIS MUSCLE FLAP

Indications/Contraindications

The FCU muscle is a reliable flap that can be designed as a proximally based flap for coverage of small to moderate size soft tissue defects around the elbow. The substantial surface area of the muscle, its superficial location in volar forearm, and its consistent blood supply allow for the FCU muscle flap to be a practical option for coverage of elbow defects. This flap may be used as muscle-only flap or myocutaneous flap for coverage of soft tissue defects over all areas of elbow and proximal forearm. Defects as large as 8×16 cm^2 surrounding the elbow joint may be covered with FCU muscle flap.

Historically, concerns over potential forearm weakness from the detachment of the FCU from the pisiform (weakness of wrist flexion and stability) have made this flap a second-line option for elbow coverage. Use of this flap should be avoided in patients with absent or nonfunctioning flexor carpi radialis muscle (as in cases of high median nerve palsy) or weak wrist flexion due other etiologies. Its use should also be avoided in any patient who could potentially benefit from an FCU transfer for restoration of absent muscle function, as in the case of a radial palsy. This flap should be used with caution in the presence of ongoing infection or prior injury or damage to the ulnar artery.

Anatomy

The FCU is a bipennate muscle in superficial volar forearm. It is innervated by the ulnar nerve and perfused by branches from ulnar artery and branches of recurrent ulnar artery. The muscle has two heads, one attached to distal humerus and the other to proximal ulna. The muscle inserts into the pisiform bone, with some additional attachments that may continue onto the volar base of the fifth metacarpal and hook of the hamate. It functions primarily as a wrist flexor and is an important stabilizer of the wrist especially during dart-thrower–type movement.

The muscle is described as a Mathes type II muscle (one major pedicel and additional minor pedicles). The dominant perforator is a branch of the posterior ulnar recurrent artery entering the muscle approximately 6 cm from the medial epicondyle. The other minor pedicles (there can be from one to three minor pedicles) are described as arise from the ulnar artery; one of these usually occurs 2 to 3 cm distal to the most proximal pedicle, and another occurs at the midpoint of the muscle belly (Fig. 11-5).

Surgery

Patient Positioning

The patient is positioned supine with the entire arm prepped. If posterior elbow is to be accessed, the extremity is flexed at the elbow and internally rotated over the patient's chest and maintained in this position. Following debridement and irrigation, the elbow is extended and the forearm is supinated on the hand table to expose the volar aspect of the forearm. The tourniquet is used to improve visualization of the pedicle. Loupe magnification aids in pedicle dissection.

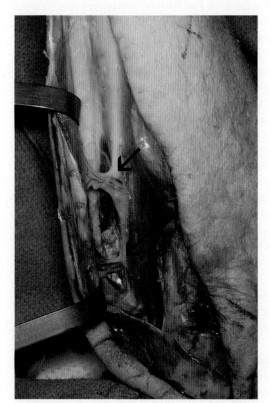

FIGURE 11-5

Intraoperative image of major proximal two pedicles going to FCU muscle (*arrows*). The most proximal pedicle is routinely identified 6 cm proximal to the medial epicondyle and originates from the recurrent ulnar artery. The more distal pedicle is a branch of the ulnar artery.

Technique

The incision is designed in a straight line over the ulnar border of the forearm and connected to the soft tissue defect in the elbow (Fig. 11-6A). The incision extends distally to the wrist crease. The muscle belly is initially identified in the middle third and traced distally. The proximal portion of the muscle is not dissected until the distal tendon is divided to protect the proximal vascular pedicles. The FCU tendon is identified and traced to its insertion on the pisiform (Fig. 11-6B). The ulnar neurovascular bundle is located deep and radial to the tendon. Just distal to the myotendinous junction of FCU, the tendon is transected while the neurovascular bundle is protected (Fig. 11-6C). The muscle is then elevated proximally. Small distal perforators are safely ligated (Fig. 11-6D). Within the proximal third of the forearm, more care is taken while dissecting deep to the muscle (Fig. 11-6E). The dominant arterial perforator from ulnar artery is frequently encountered at approximately 6 cm from the tip of the olecranon. Cadaveric dissections have shown this pedicle to be an average distance of 5.7 cm from the medial epicondyle (Fig. 11-6F). The dominant perforator marks the pivot point for the rotation of the muscle to its target site. If muscle rotation is possible without division of the most proximal minor pedicle, the minor pedicle should be left intact. The tourniquet is released prior to insetting of the muscle to verify that the full extent of the muscle is perfused. If the distal margin does not appear well vascularized, this portion should be excised until bleeding is seen coming from the muscle edges.

The distal aspect of the muscle is then inset in the defect while assuring that the pedicle is subject to minimal tension (Fig. 11-6G). The donor site in the forearm is closed primarily, while a split-thickness skin graft is used to cover FCU (Fig. 11-6H, I). Alternatively, a skin paddle could be designed over the muscular portion of FCU in the middle third of volar forearm; however, we have no experience with this technique. The width of the skin paddle should be as only as wide as the muscle, thus allowing incorporation of myocutaneous perforators as well as primary closure of the donor site. Postoperative management of FCU muscle flap is similar to that previously described for anconeus muscle flap.

Results

Despite the potential donor site morbidity from use of FCU muscle as surgical flap, there are several studies showing that sacrificing FCU does not adversely affect wrist function. In a series of 17 patients who underwent the use of FCU as a turnover flap for posterior elbow wound coverage, grip strength and wrist flexion peak torque strength were 97% and 89% of nonsurgical arm, respectively. The degree of wrist flexion fatigue was similar between the two sides as well. Similarly, Raskin and Wilgis, in long-term follow-up, have shown no difference in grip strength, peak torque flexion, and fatigue time following harvest of FCU in the treatment of radial nerve palsy.

Use of the FCU as a split muscle flap has been described and allows for preservation of the humeral origin of the muscle and thus maintenance of some muscle function. Recent evidence points toward a dual innervation of the humeral head as well as the ulnar head of FCU, thus allowing for use of ulnar portion while preserving the humeral origin and the function of FCU. At present, no comparative studies or large case series are available to verify this claim.

The distal extent of FCU allows for wider and larger defect coverage in the periphery of the elbow including the anterior elbow and defects as proximal as 9 cm above olecranon. The anconeus flap has a more limited reach due to the length of its pedicle but is an adequate choice for coverage of smaller posterior or lateral defects. Minimal morbidity has been associated with use of the anconeus muscle. Despite evidence pointing toward minimal morbidity from harvesting the FCU muscle, it is important to ensure this muscle will not be required for future tendon transfers or contribute to forearm weakness if there are concomitant injuries to other forearm flexor muscles.

PEARLS AND PITFALLS

- Closure of any elbow defect starts with a thorough debridement.
- The anconeus muscle flap is adequate for coverage of defect as large as 7 cm^2 over the olecranon region and lateral elbow.
- The MCA serves as a reliable pedicle for elevation of the anconeus muscle.
- The FCU muscle flap allows for coverage of moderate size defects in all aspect of the elbow including those proximal to the olecranon process.

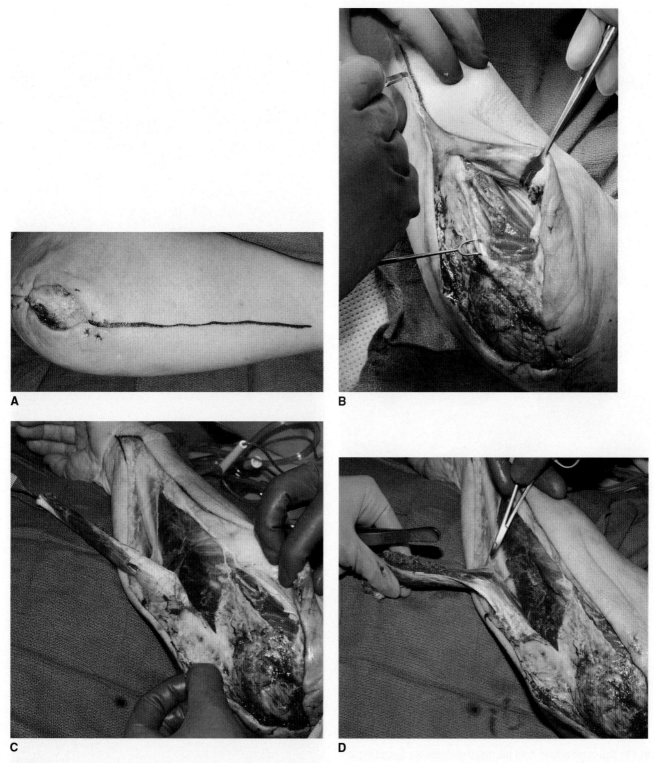

FIGURE 11-6

Technique for elevation of FCU flap. **A:** A case of a 62-year-old man with rheumatoid arthritis with a chronic infected elbow wound. **B:** The FCU flap is elevated through an incision over the radial border of the ulna, in line with the FCU muscle belly. **C:** The tendon is divided proximal to its insertion on the pisiform. The flap is then dissected proximally to its major pedicle. **D:** Smaller pedicles (tip of hemostat) in the distal and middle third of the forearm need to be divided to gain adequate length for elbow coverage.

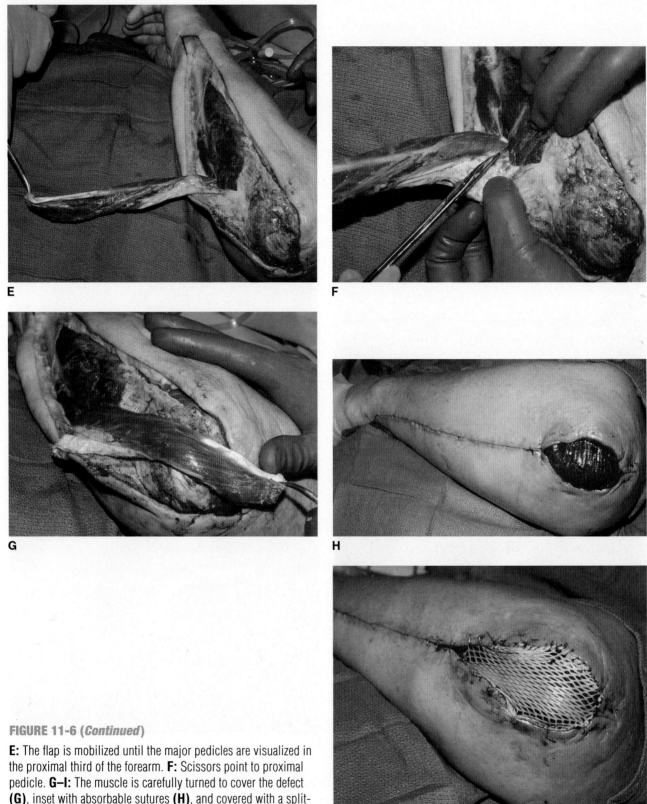

FIGURE 11-6 (Continued)

E: The flap is mobilized until the major pedicles are visualized in the proximal third of the forearm. **F:** Scissors point to proximal pedicle. **G–I:** The muscle is carefully turned to cover the defect **(G)**, inset with absorbable sutures **(H)**, and covered with a split-thickness skin graft **(I)**.

- The FCU muscle flap may be elevated based on the recurrent ulnar collateral artery located approximately 6 cm distal to medial condyle. The location of the perforator determines the extent of muscle elevation and pivot point for coverage.
- While reported experience points toward minimal functional loss following harvest of the FCU flap, one should approach this flap with caution if the patient has had any additional injury to the remaining muscles of the forearm, as the FCU could be used for future tendon transfer procedures.

RECOMMENDED READING

Bayne CO, Slikker W, Ma J, et al. Clinical outcomes of the flexor carpi ulnaris turnover flap for posterior elbow soft tissue defect. *J Hand Surg Am.* 2015;40:2358–2363.

Daluiski A, Schreiber JJ, Paul S, et al. Outcomes of anconeus interposition for proximal radioulnar synostosis. *J Shoulder Elbow Surg.* 2014;23:1882–1887.

Elhassan B, Karabekmez F, Hsu C, et al. Outcome of local anconeus flap transfer to cover soft tissue defects over the posterior aspect of the elbow. *J Shoulder Elbow Surg.* 2011;20:807–812.

Fleager KE, Cheung EV. The "anconeus slide": rotation flap for management of posterior wound complications about the elbow. *J Shoulder Elbow Surg.* 2011;20:1310–1316.

Gleason TF, Goldstein WM, Ray RD. The function of the anconeus muscle. *Clin Orthop Relat Res.* 1985;192:147–148.

Jensen M, Moran SL. Soft tissue coverage of the elbow: a reconstructive algorithm. *Orthop Clin North Am.* 2008;39:251–264.

Lingaraj K, Lim AY, Puhaindran ME, et al. Case report: the split flexor carpi ulnaris as a local muscle flap. *Clin Orthop Relat Res.* 2007;455:262–266.

Mathes S, Nahai F. *Clinical Applications for Muscle and Musculocutaneous Flaps.* St. Louis, MO: CV Mosby; 1982.

Nishida K, Iwasaki N, Minami A. Anconeus muscle flap for the treatment of soft tissue defects over the olecranon after total elbow arthroplasty. *J Hand Surg Eur.* 2009;34:538–539.

Payne DE, Kaufman AM, Wysocki RW, et al. Vascular perfusion of a flexor carpi ulnaris muscle turnover pedicle flap for posterior elbow soft tissue reconstruction: a cadaveric study. *J Hand Surg Am.* 2011;362:246–251.

Pereira BP. Revisiting the anatomy and biomechanics of the anconeus muscle and its role in elbow stability. *Ann Anat.* 2013;195:365–370.

Raskin KB, Wilgis EF. Flexor carpi ulnaris transfer for radial nerve palsy: functional testing of long-term results. *J Hand Surg Am.* 1995;20:737–742.

Ruch DS, Orr SB, Richard MJ, et al. A comparison of debridement with and without anconeus muscle flap for treatment of refractory lateral epicondylitis. *J Shoulder Elbow.* 2015;24:236–241.

Schmidt CS, Kohut GN, Greenberg JA, et al. The anconeus muscle flap: its anatomy and clinical application. *J Hand Surg.* 1999;24A:359–369.

Sharpe F, Barry P, Lin SD, et al. Anatomic study of flexor carpi ulnaris muscle and its application to soft tissue coverage of the elbow with clinical correlation. *J Shoulder Elbow Surg.* 2014;23:82–90.

Wysocki R, Gray R, Fernandez J, et al. Posterior elbow coverage using whole and split flexor carpi ulnaris flaps: a cadaveric study. *J Hand Surg Am.* 2008;33:1807–1812.

12 Bipolar Latissimus Dorsi Rotational Flap for Functional Reconstruction of Elbow Flexion

Frances Sharpe and Milan Stevanovic

Flexion of the elbow is critical for positioning the hand in space, as well as for reach and grasp. Loss of elbow flexion results in limitations in activities such as feeding, dressing, and personal hygiene. Loss of elbow flexion can occur for a variety of reasons following trauma including direct loss of bicep and brachialis muscle, direct injury to the musculocutaneous nerve, brachial plexus injury, and fractures of the humerus. Flexion may also be absent in cases of arthrogryposis and congenital absence of the biceps. For patients where elbow function is not recovered following repair of the initial trauma, muscle transfers (or flexorplasties) are an option to restore elbow flexor function. The goal of elbow flexorplasty is to achieve at least 90 degrees of elbow flexion against some resistance. One of the most common and reliable elbow flexorplasty reconstructions is the latissimus dorsi (LD) transfer, which can reliably produce approximately 0.5 to 4 kg of flexion force against gravity.

The LD is a versatile flap that can be harvested as a muscle or musculocutaneous flap. The length and proximal location of the neurovascular pedicle provides a wide arc of rotation for muscle transposition. The use of the LD as a functional muscle transfer for elbow flexion was first described by Schottstaedt et al. in 1955 and subsequently popularized by Zancolli and Mitre in 1973. They presented a series of eight patients with weakness or absence of elbow flexion treated with anterior transposition of the LD muscle. They described this as a "bipolar" muscle transfer, where both the origin and insertion of the muscle were relocated. Since that time, it has become one of the standard transfers for reconstruction of elbow flexion.

ANATOMY

The LD is a broad, thin, fan-shaped muscle originating from the thoracolumbar fascia and iliac crest (Fig. 12-1). It also has origins on the spinous processes of T7-L5, inferior three to four ribs, and variably on the inferior angle of the scapula. It inserts on the proximal medial humerus between the insertions of pectoralis major and teres major. (One can remember this important anatomical relationship by recalling the expression: "a miss between two majors.") It is a strong fan-shaped muscle with parallel muscle fibers. Its major blood supply comes from the thoracodorsal artery; however, there are several smaller segmental vascular pedicles near the muscle's origin entering the deep surface of the muscle just lateral to the paraspinal musculature, which also contribute to the medial perfusion of the muscle. The thoracodorsal pedicle has an average length of 12 cm from its origin at the subscapular artery. The arterial diameter is between 2 and 2.5 mm and the concomitant vein between 2.5 and 3 mm. It is supplied by a single motor nerve, the thoracodorsal nerve, which arises as a terminal branch from the posterior cord (C6, C7, and C8). It primarily functions as a shoulder adductor, extender, and internal rotator. It also helps to stabilize the scapula and contributes to pelvic and spinal stability.

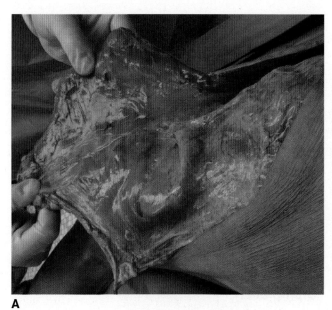
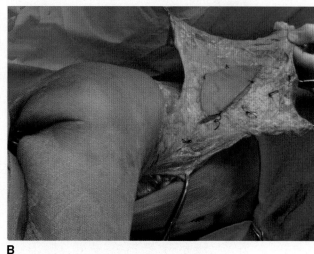

A   B

FIGURE 12-1

The latissimus dorsi is a thin, fan-shaped muscle, broad at its caudal origin and narrowing toward its insertion. **A:** Deep surface of the latissimus dorsi (LD). **B:** Thin fan-shaped muscle after release from the thoracodorsal fascia. (Copyright Frances Sharpe and Milan Stevanovic.)

INDICATIONS/CONTRAINDICATIONS

Indications

Several procedures have been described for reconstruction of elbow flexion. These include nerve transfers, Steindler flexorplasty, triceps tendon transfer, pectoralis major transfer, LD muscle transfer, and functional free muscle transfer (Table 12-1). The first pedicled LD transfer was described for patients with loss of elbow flexion due to the sequelae of poliomyelitis. Since that time, the LD has been used to reconstruct elbow flexion in the setting of brachial plexus injury; isolated neurologic injury; soft tissue loss due to trauma, tumor, severe electrical burn; and congenital absence of elbow flexion. It has the particular advantage of providing both soft tissue coverage and functional reconstruction (Fig. 12-2). Despite the versatility and availability of this muscle, it is an infrequent muscle transfer, with the literature consisting of case reports or small series of 10 or fewer patients.

TABLE 12-1	**Procedures for Reconstruction of Elbow Flexion**		
Procedure	**Indications**	**Disadvantages**	**Comments**
Nerve transfer to musculocutaneous nerve	Denervation of biceps from BPI or isolated nerve injury	Timing Unable to do in setting of muscle loss	Nerve donors: intercostal nerve, spinal accessory nerve, fascicles of ulnar nerve
Steindler flexorplasty	Intact and strong flexor-pronator and not candidate for other options	Weak transfer, flexion-pronation contracture	Limited mechanical advantage therefore weak elbow flexion
Pectoralis major transfer	Strong pectoralis major function and other options not available	Cosmetically disfiguring, especially in women Indirect line of transfer	
Triceps tendon transfer	Strong elbow extension and poor candidate for other procedures Requires limited dissection and local muscle source	Results in loss or weakness of elbow extension	Not a good choice for patients who need elbow extension for assistance in ambulation Indirect line of transfer
Latissimus dorsi muscle transfer (bipolar or unipolar)	Strong latissimus muscle Can be used to reconstruct soft tissue deficit in addition to restoring flexion	Can weaken shoulder girdle muscles	Distal attachment to biceps is thin muscle tissue rather than tendon
Functional muscle transfer	No local tissue available Also reconstructs soft tissue loss Ultimate reconstructive option	Requires available donor vessel and donor nerve. Sometimes not available in global BPP	Requires microsurgical skills and careful technique

BPI, brachial plexus injury; BPP, brachial plexus palsy.

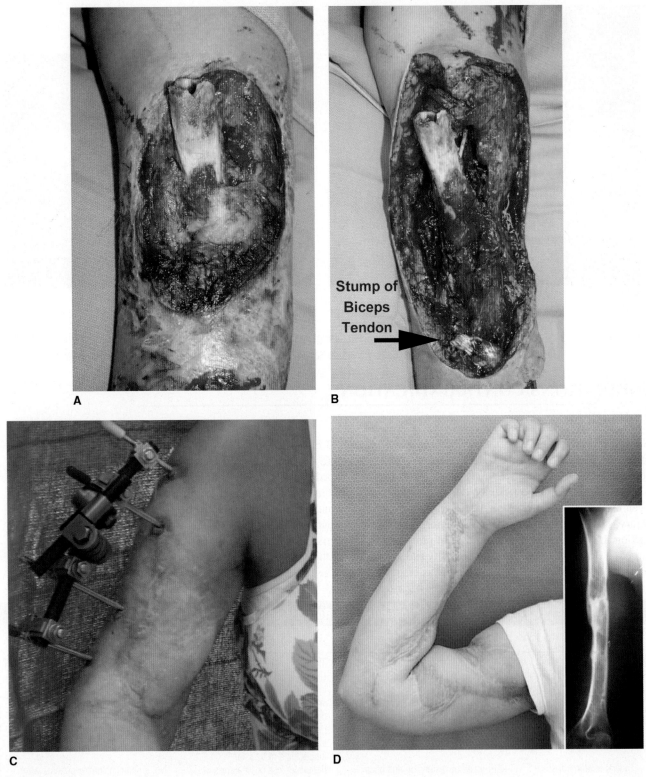

FIGURE 12-2

A 22-year-old presented with an isolated right upper extremity injury from a motor vehicle accident. She sustained a brachial plexus traction neuropraxia and an open humeral shaft fracture with a large soft tissue loss of her anterior arm compartment. She had a compartment syndrome of the forearm. Her initial treatment at an outside hospital included a fasciotomy of the forearm and splinting of the open humerus fracture. At the time of presentation 3 weeks after her injury, she had a necrotic-appearing anterior arm wound with exposed humerus fracture. **A:** Appearance of arm at presentation. Necrotic-appearing skin masks the underlying necrotic muscle. **B:** Appearance of the arm after debridement. **C:** Appearance of the arm after functional LD transfer, which provided both functional reconstruction and soft tissue coverage. The external fixator was used for fracture stabilization due to the chronicity of the open fracture. The fixator remained in place for 3 months. **D:** Elbow flexion at 6 months and healed humerus fracture. (Copyright Frances Sharpe and Milan Stevanovic.)

Contraindications

For most patients, the LD is an expendable muscle, as there are synergistic muscles for shoulder girdle function. However, it provides more critical shoulder girdle function for patients with severe lower extremity injuries or paraplegia. These patients need shoulder strength for bed-to-chair transfers, use of crutches or a walker, or use of a manual wheelchair. The role of the latissimus in stabilization of the spine and pelvis should be considered in patients with weakness of lower extremity function and patients at higher risk of developing scoliosis (younger patients and those patients with congenital anomalies of the spine). Ipsilateral shoulder girdle weakness, previous surgeries about the shoulder girdle, previous trauma affecting the subclavian or axillary artery, tumor resection, or lymph node dissection in the area of the thoracodorsal artery and nerve are further contraindications. Relative contraindications include patients with family history of breast cancer that might need future breast reconstruction using the latissimus muscle. A patient with a high body mass index (BMI) is a relative contraindication if the weight of the arm is too much for the transferred muscle to adequately move. Significant truncal obesity may prevent the use of a skin paddle but does not preclude the use of the latissimus if the arm size is appropriate.

Congenital deficiencies of the upper extremity can be associated with absence or weakness of the latissimus. The patients require a careful preoperative workup to determine if a functioning latissimus is present.

PREOPERATIVE PLANNING

Preoperative planning begins with a clinical history and examination. Patients should be asked about ipsilateral arm or chest injury, previous breast surgery, or radiation therapy, as these all could have potentially injured the thoracodorsal nerve. Clinical examination should evaluate any previous traumatic or surgical scars from breast reconstruction or thoracotomy scars. Patients with a history of brachial plexus injury should have a thorough motor examination. Assessment of preoperative shoulder range of motion and shoulder girdle strength helps identify shoulder pathology that may affect postoperative recovery. Preoperative elbow range of motion should be evaluated. Preexisting flexion or extension contractures of the elbow may need to be treated with therapy, stretching splints, or surgical contracture release prior to planned flexorplasty. Preoperative flexion less than 110 degrees compromises the final outcome of any flexorplasty.

Specific examination of the LD includes palpation of the size and bulk of the muscle as well as strength testing. It is helpful to compare this with the contralateral side (if normal). The LD can be palpated along the posterior axillary fold and along the chest wall (Fig. 12-3). This is best done with the patient sitting or lying on his contralateral side. Testing for latissimus contraction can be done in several ways. The examiner's hands are placed on bilateral LD muscles, and the patient is asked to cough. Contraction of the latissimus is frequently palpable with this maneuver.

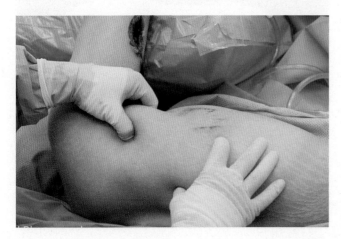

FIGURE 12-3

Palpation of the latissimus dorsi muscle. (Copyright Frances Sharpe and Milan Stevanovic.)

LD contraction and strength can be tested by having the patient in a sitting position with the elbow flexed at his side and having him press his elbow down (caudad) against the examiner's hand (shoulder depression). Another examination technique is to have the arm at the side with the arm in internal rotation and the shoulder and elbow in extension. The examiner then tests resisted shoulder adduction strength. One of the examiner's hands rests on the latissimus to palpate muscle contraction. Resistive strength of shoulder extension can also be used to assess the latissimus. Again, the elbow is held in extension to help isolate the latissimus from the contributions of the long head of the triceps.

Patients with congenital deficits of biceps function such as arthrogrypotics or patients with longitudinal deficiencies that include the upper arm may require additional investigation with a preoperative magnetic resonance imaging (MRI) of the chest and abdomen to evaluate the size and quality of the LD muscle. Comparison with the contralateral side (if normal) is useful to establish quantitative differences in muscle cross-sectional area (Fig. 12-4). These patients may also have a deficient biceps tendon. In this setting, the planned reconstruction of elbow flexion will have the distal insertion on the ulna (Fig. 12-5).

We do not routinely use electromyography (EMG) for preoperative assessment of latissimus function but rely on clinical examination; however, EMG can be obtained if there is any question about the status of the thoracodorsal nerve. Angiography that may be indicated in the setting of vascular trauma to the chest wall or axilla; other options for visualization of the thoracodorsal vessel include CT angiography or vascular ultrasound.

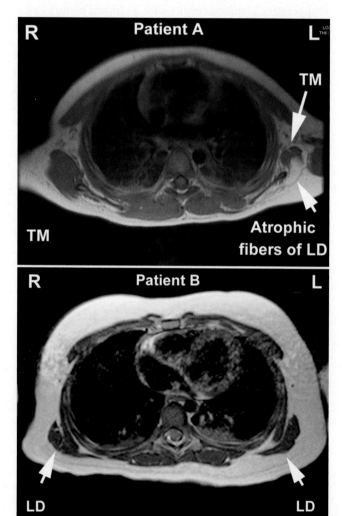

FIGURE 12-4

MRIs of the chest from two patients with arthrogryposis. *Patient A* had congenitally deficient latissimus dorsi bilaterally. A functional free muscle transfer was done for this patient to regain elbow flexion. *Patient B* has latissimus dorsi muscles on both sides, with the right slightly more robust than the left. (Copyright Frances Sharpe and Milan Stevanovic.)

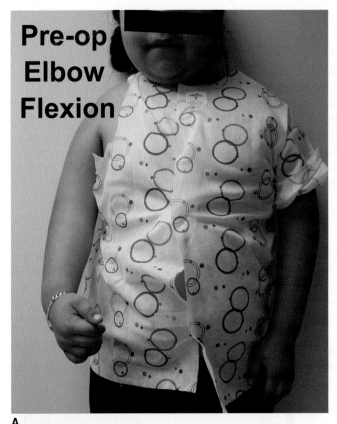

Pre-op Elbow Flexion

A

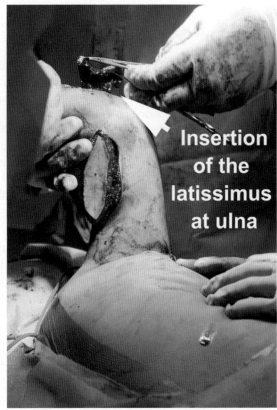

Insertion of the latissimus at ulna

B

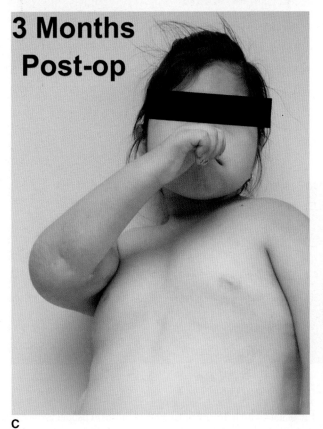

3 Months Post-op

C

FIGURE 12-5

This 10-year-old arthrogrypotic patient had no active elbow flexion, but good shoulder and hand function. She had good passive elbow flexion but no active flexion. She was reliant on others for feeding and hygiene. She underwent a bipolar latissimus rotational transfer. Since she did not have a biceps tendon, the latissimus was passed on the medial side of the elbow and anchored to the proximal ulna. At 3 months, she is able to bring her hand to her mouth. **A:** Preoperative attempt at elbow flexion. **B:** Intraoperative photo showing latissimus passed to medial proximal ulna. **C:** Three months after bipolar latissimus transfer. (Copyright Frances Sharpe and Milan Stevanovic.)

SURGERY

Positioning

The patient is positioned in the lateral decubitus position. The entire lateral side from the ilium to the shoulder girdle and affected arm are included in the surgical preparation site. Dorsally, this should include the spinous processes and, ventrally, the midumbilical line. The operative arm can be supported on a sterile Mayo stand. Prolonged abduction of the arm can cause a traction neuropraxia to the brachial plexus, and periodic repositioning of the arm should be performed. The donor site for harvesting split-thickness skin graft (if needed) should be considered in the surgical site preparation and is most conveniently harvested from the ipsilateral lateral thigh. The contralateral side should be well padded. An axillary roll should be placed to prevent compression of the brachial plexus and to prevent circulatory compromise to the contralateral limb.

Incision

The position of the latissimus is marked out on the chest wall, and a skin paddle that begins 6 to 8 cm caudad to the axillary fold is designed over the LD on the chest wall. The skin paddle should be elliptical in shape. The length of the skin paddle should approximate that of the biceps muscle belly approximately from the distal aspect of the deltopectoral groove to the area of the musculotendinous junction of the biceps above the antecubital fossa. The skin paddle should be 4 to 6 cm in width (Fig. 12-6).

The skin incision begins in the posterior axillary fold and follows the course of the latissimus along its midline axis. The incision extends from the axilla to approximately four fingerbreadths

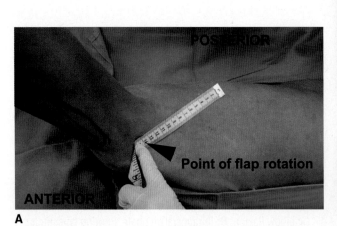
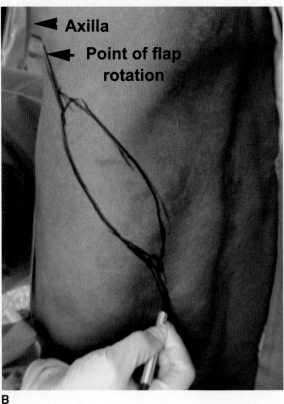

FIGURE 12-6

The desired position of the skin paddle is marked on the anterior arm. The distance from the proximal edge of this skin paddle is measured to the point of rotation (pedicle position) just posterior and proximal to the axilla. This distance is then measured from the point of rotation to the chest wall, and the skin paddle on the chest wall is then marked to match the desired size on the anterior arm. **A:** Length from the point of rotation to the position of the skin paddle on the chest wall. **B:** Skin paddle marked on the chest wall. (Copyright Frances Sharpe and Milan Stevanovic.)

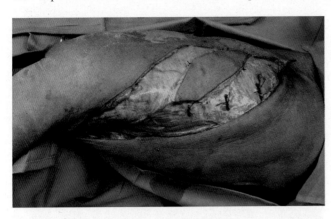

FIGURE 12-7

Appearance of the latissimus after dissection on the superficial surface before deep mobilization. (Copyright Frances Sharpe and Milan Stevanovic.)

cephalad to the posterior iliac crest (Fig. 12-7). The inclusion of a skin paddle for a functional muscle transfer is to reduce muscle adhesion and improve gliding of the transferred muscle. The skin paddle also increases the soft tissue envelope and decreases the risk of postoperative muscle compression, which can lead to compartment syndrome of the transferred muscle.

Dissection

During the dissection of the skin paddle, the incision is beveled away from the skin incision. The incision is carried down to the muscle fascia. The muscle fascia is left on the latissimus as skin flaps are elevated in the suprafascial plane first toward the anterior margin of the latissimus and then toward the posterior margin. The anterior margin of the latissimus is most easily identified and separated from adjacent muscles in the midpoint of the muscle. The anterior margin is mobilized and traced toward its caudal origin (Fig. 12-8).

After exposing the muscle in the suprafascial plane, and prior to release of the muscle origin and insertion, the muscle resting length is marked. The arm is positioned in maximum abduction and forward flexion, and the resting length is marked with sutures placed at 5-cm intervals from the musculotendinous junction toward the caudal origin (Fig. 12-9). If there is any question of latissimus function preoperatively (brachial plexus injury, associated trauma, or congenital hypoplasia of the muscle), the quality and bulk of the muscle is inspected and if thought to be inadequate for biceps reconstruction, the procedure is aborted. Additionally, the neurovascular pedicle can be exposed early with as little detachment of the proximal origin as possible to allow visualization of the pedicle. Direct stimulation of the thoracodorsal nerve can help in assessment of muscle function.

At the iliac crest, the fibrous origin of the latissimus must be carefully dissected from the fibers of the abdominal oblique muscles at the thoracodorsal fascia. The fibrous origin of the latissimus is released from the thoracodorsal fascia, and the muscle is elevated along its deep surface from caudad to cephalad. Deep perforating branches should be identified and cauterized or ligated. As the dissection continues cephalad, care should be taken to identify and protect the distal slips of the serratus anterior and the teres major muscle. The latissimus may be tightly adherent to the chest wall origin of the serratus anterior and to the scapular origin of the teres major, making it difficult to distinguish between the muscle planes. Electrical stimulation of the muscle fibers of the latissimus can help distinguish between the fibers of the latissimus and adjacent muscles.

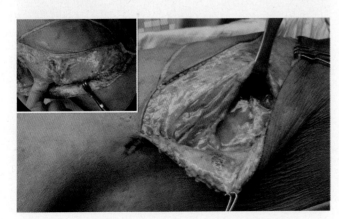

FIGURE 12-8

The latissimus is most easily separated from the deeper structures at its midpoint on the anterior border of the muscle. (Copyright Frances Sharpe and Milan Stevanovic.)

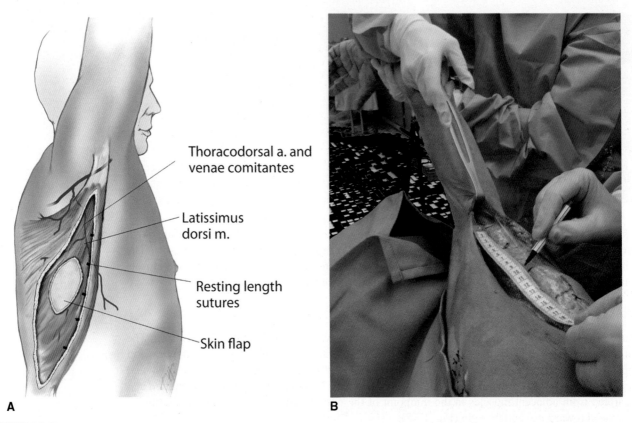

A   **B**

FIGURE 12-9

Marking of the latissimus resting length is done with the arm in full abduction. This must be done prior to dividing the muscle origin.
A: Schematic representation. **B:** Intraoperative appearance. (Copyright Frances Sharpe and Milan Stevanovic.)

During the dissection toward the axilla, the branch of the thoracodorsal artery that supplies the distal slips of the serratus anterior should be identified (Fig. 12-10). The branch origin is variable in location but is large and easy to identify. The serratus branch is ligated close to its takeoff from the thoracodorsal artery. During this portion of the dissection, the long thoracic nerve lies deep

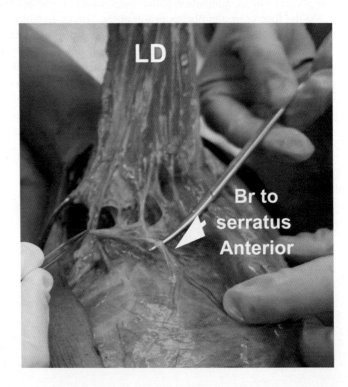

FIGURE 12-10

Dissection of the branch of the thoracodorsal artery to the serratus anterior muscle. LD, latissimus dorsi muscle; Br, arterial branch.

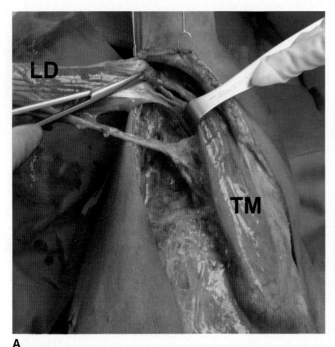

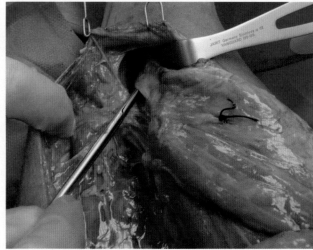

A

B

FIGURE 12-11

A: Separation of the tendinous portion of the latissimus dorsi (LD) from the muscle fibers of the teres major (TM) near the axilla.
B: Dissected latissimus dorsi tendon, ready for division. (Copyright Frances Sharpe and Milan Stevanovic.)

and medial to the thoracodorsal pedicle. It should be identified and protected. For ligation of the serratus branch, we recommend the use of a 2-0 suture ligature rather than hemoclips. Hemoclips may loosen or dislodge and lead to significant bleeding. As dissection continues toward the axillae, small perforating branches of the thoracodorsal artery to the scapula and teres muscles should also be ligated. Fascial bands around the thoracodorsal nerve should be released. The thoracodorsal pedicle must be protected from stretching or twisting during the remainder of the dissection. Complete mobilization of the pedicle reduces the chance of kinking the pedicle as it is transposed to the anterior surface of the arm.

Once the pedicle is completely mobilized, attention is directed cephalad to the insertion of the latissimus on the proximal humerus. The tendinous portion of the latissimus is identified and dissected along its anterior surface toward its insertion on the humerus. The tendinous insertion of the LD and teres major is in close proximity to each other; special attention is necessary to release only the insertion of the LD (Fig. 12-11). It is important to remember that the axillary nerve lies just superior and medial to the latissimus insertion. In addition, the radial nerve lies in the triangular space just inferior to the tendon of the latissimus. Careful dissection in this area is necessary to avoid injury to these nerves. Once the tendon is released, two parallel Krackow sutures are placed in the tendon using 2-0 braided nonabsorbable suture.

The muscle is now completely free and will be secured to the chest only by the neurovascular pedicle. The pedicle should not be twisted, and there should be no tension on the pedicle at the time of insetting.

Muscle Insetting

A 3- to 5-cm transverse or deltopectoral incision is made over the coracoid, and a separate longitudinal incision is placed over the biceps from the distal deltopectoral groove to the AC fossa to completely expose the biceps muscle and tendon. Four mattress sutures are placed in the biceps tendon—medial and lateral at the musculotendinous junction and medial and lateral more distally at the tendinous portion of the biceps—in preparation for securing the LD to distal biceps tendon.

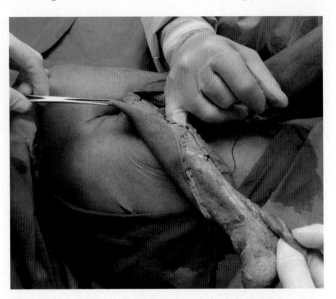

FIGURE 12-12

Tubularization of the latissimus dorsi. (Copyright Frances Sharpe and Milan Stevanovic.)

Skin flaps are elevated medially and laterally along the course of the biceps. The medial skin flap is developed, and a wide tunnel is created into the axilla to connect to the posterior incision. The tunnel is created in the plane superficial to the axillary fascia. The tunnel should be wide enough that four fingers can be easily passed through the tunnel. Any fascial band within this tunnel must be released. The muscle is then tubularized and secured with fascial sutures placed every 2 to 3 cm (Fig. 12-12).

Before passing the muscle through the tunnel, the LD insertion is transferred to the coracoid, which will now become the neobiceps origin. Blunt finger dissection below the tendon of pectoralis major is used to create a tunnel to the coracoid (Fig. 12-13). The tendon insertion of LD will be passed through this tunnel and secured to the coracoid (Fig. 12-14A). We try to maintain the width of the latissimus tendon by securing the tendon to the central, medial, and lateral sides of the coracoid. Periosteal sutures or sutures passed through bone tunnels in the coracoid are used to secure the LD tendon (Fig. 12-14B).

The LD muscle is then passed through the previously created subcutaneous tunnel to the anterior aspect of the arm (Fig. 12-15). The muscle is rotated on the pedicle with care to avoid twisting or kinking of the pedicle. Inspection of the pedicle and release of any additional perforators or fascia that can cause compression are important for the patency of the pedicle.

The muscle is stretched to restore the previously marked resting length; this is confirmed by noting a 5-cm interval between the previously placed marking sutures. The elbow should be fully

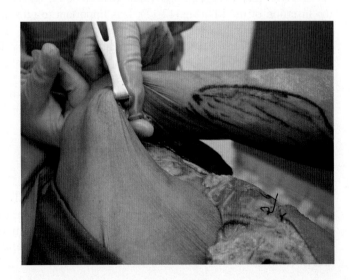

FIGURE 12-13

Creation of a tunnel connecting the incision over the coracoid to the axilla. The tunnel passes below the pectoralis major. (Copyright Frances Sharpe and Milan Stevanovic.)

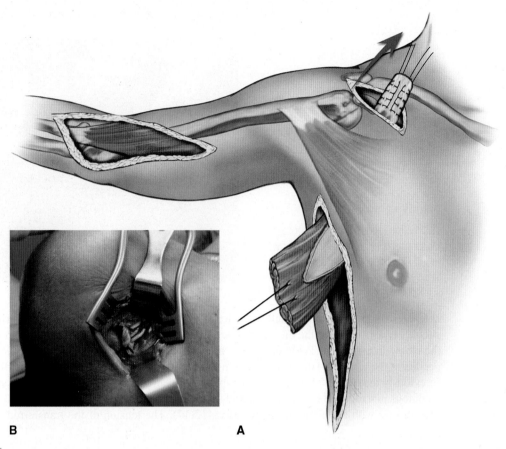

B   **A**

FIGURE 12-14

A: Diagrammatic representation of passing the tendon of the latissimus dorsi from the axilla to the coracoid below the pectoralis major, becoming the neobiceps origin. Placing the Krackow sutures in the tendon of the latissimus must be done prior to passing the tendon to the coracoid. **B:** Latissimus dorsi tendon is secured to the coracoid. (Copyright Frances Sharpe and Milan Stevanovic.)

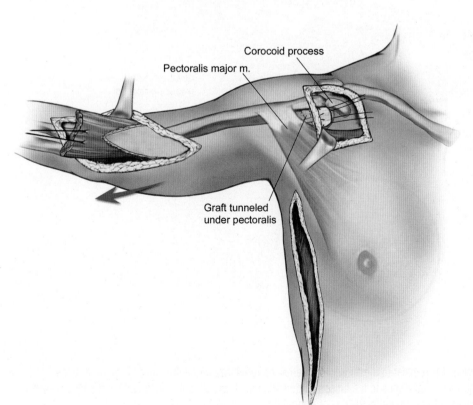

Corocoid process

Pectoralis major m.

Graft tunneled
under pectoralis

FIGURE 12-15

Diagrammatic representation of the latissimus dorsi transposed to the anterior arm. The tendon of latissimus has been secured to the coracoid. The distal portion of latissimus will be trimmed and wrapped circumferentially around the biceps tendon. (Copyright Frances Sharpe and Milan Stevanovic.)

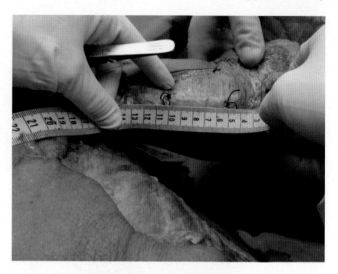

FIGURE 12-16

The resting length of the transposed latissimus is restored with the elbow in full extension. (Copyright Frances Sharpe and Milan Stevanovic.)

extended when the resting length is restored (Fig. 12-16). Proximally, the tubularized latissimus should lay superficial to the biceps muscle. The latissimus resting length is preliminarily reset with the elbow in extension. The muscle length of the transposed latissimus is usually longer than that needed at the recipient site. Excess length from the caudad origin is excised. The distal latissimus (previously the caudad origin) is then wrapped 360 degrees around the distal biceps at the musculo-tendinous junction and biceps tendon and secured to the LD with the previously placed nonabsorb-able sutures with the elbow in flexion (Fig. 12-17). The tension of the transferred muscle should

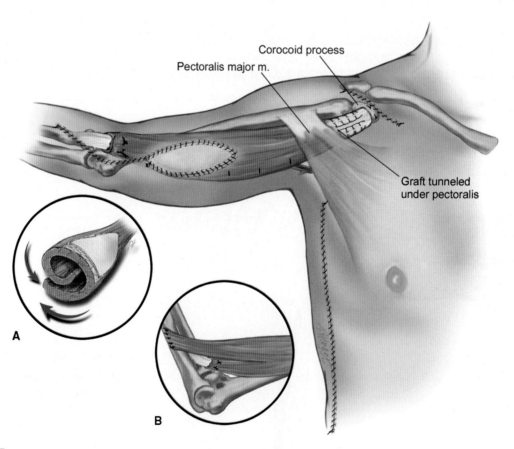

FIGURE 12-17

Diagrammatic representation of the latissimus after transfer to the anterior humerus. **A:** Tubularization of the muscular portion of the latissimus. **B:** Alternative attachment of one-half of latissimus to the biceps tendon and the other half to the distal ulna. If the biceps tendon is absent, the entire latissimus can be inserted onto the proximal ulna. (Copyright Frances Sharpe and Milan Stevanovic.)

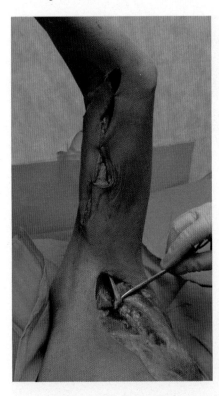

FIGURE 12-18

After the latissimus is inset, the pedicle is examined in the posterior axilla. There should be no tension on the pedicle as the arm is brought from adduction to full abduction. (Copyright Frances Sharpe and Milan Stevanovic.)

hold the elbow in at least 90 degrees of flexion. If the transfer is not maintaining at least 90 degrees of elbow flexion, the distal insertion of the LD should be advanced and retensioned. The attachment of the latissimus to the biceps tendon is through the thin muscular tissue of the latissimus, which does not hold suture well. Therefore, attempts at overtensioning the latissimus may result in suture pullout through the muscle.

An alternative insertion for the transposed latissimus is to secure the latissimus to the proximal ulna. This may be done in the setting of a congenitally absent biceps, where no biceps tendon is present for coaptation to the transferred latissimus. Even when the biceps tendon is present, the latissimus may be split distally, and half of the distal latissimus may be secured to the biceps tendon and the other half secured to the proximal ulna. By advancing the insertion of the latissimus more distally on the ulna, there is a theoretical mechanical advantage of the transferred latissimus that could potentially improve flexion strength. Surgically, a subcutaneous tunnel is created superficial to the flexor-pronator mass on the medial side of the elbow. A separate longitudinal incision is placed along the subcutaneous border of the ulna, and the latissimus or one-half of the latissimus is secured to the proximal third of the ulna using bone tunnels or bone anchors or to periosteum (see Figs. 12-5 and 12-17B).

Before skin closure, the pedicle should be checked both with the Doppler and by direct visualization. Any dark blood in the vein would indicate stretching or compression of the pedicle. If there is nothing compressing the pedicle, but the venous outflow appears dark, then the pedicle should be further mobilized in the axilla. There should be no tension on the pedicle as the arm is moved from adduction to abduction (Fig. 12-18).

One small silastic drain is placed below the transferred latissimus. Two large silastic drains are placed at the latissimus donor site. A quilting technique is used to secure the elevated skin flaps to the fascia of the underlying chest wall with 2-0 absorbable suture. This is done at 5-cm intervals. Fibrin glue may be used adjunctively below the skin flaps to further reduce the chance of seroma formation. Subsequent deep dermal and skin layer closure is performed at the donor site.

POSTOPERATIVE MANAGEMENT

The patient should be kept well hydrated and warm in a monitored setting during the first 48 hours. The skin paddle is monitored for color, temperature, turgor, and Doppler signal. Small petechial changes in the skin paddle can be a harbinger of compromised vascularity to the flap and requires emergent re-exploration in the operating room, even in the setting of good Doppler signal. Any

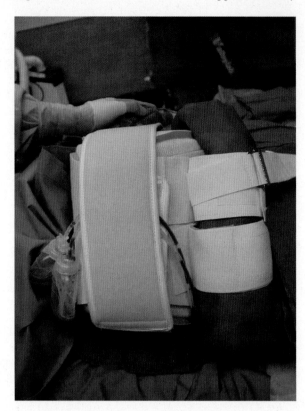

FIGURE 12-19

Postoperative immobilization for at least 8 weeks postoperatively in 90 degrees of elbow flexion. (Copyright Frances Sharpe and Milan Stevanovic.)

vascular compromise in the postoperative period may affect final functional recovery of the transferred muscle.

The drain below the transferred latissimus is removed at 24 to 48 hours postoperatively. The donor site drains are left in place until output is less than 25 mL in 24 hours. It is common to leave drains in place for up to 2 weeks.

The arm is kept immobilized in a sling with an abduction pillow for 8 to 9 weeks (Fig. 12-19). During this time, the patient is encouraged to maintain active and passive wrist and finger motion. At 4 weeks, the patient can start isometric contraction of the biceps while at 90 degrees of elbow flexion. After 9 weeks, the patient begins working on regaining extension at a rate of 10 to 20 degrees per week. A hinged elbow brace with adjustable flexion and extension stops is used to control the arm position. Elbow flexion and extension exercises are best done from a supine position with the posterior arm supported. Light and progressive strengthening may begin at 3 months, progressing to unrestricted activity by 6 months (Fig. 12-20).

COMPLICATIONS

Procedure-specific complications begin with intraoperative positioning. Placement in the lateral position requires careful padding of bony prominences. An axillary roll is used to reduce pressure on the contralateral brachial plexus and axillary artery. Patients with prolonged surgery and/or higher BMI may note postoperative contralateral thigh pain from sustained pressure on the muscle compartment. A theoretical risk of compartment syndrome exists. On the operative arm, prolonged hyperabduction of the arm can cause a traction neuropraxia of the ipsilateral brachial plexus. Episodic repositioning of the arm throughout the procedure can reduce this risk.

Complications can be divided into acute and long-term complications and also between donor and recipient sites.

Recipient Site

Acute complications at the recipient site include flap loss or partial flap loss (either skin paddle or partial muscle loss). Although it is less common with a rotational transfer, vascular compromise can occur through kinking of the vascular pedicle during rotation of the muscle. Postoperative swelling

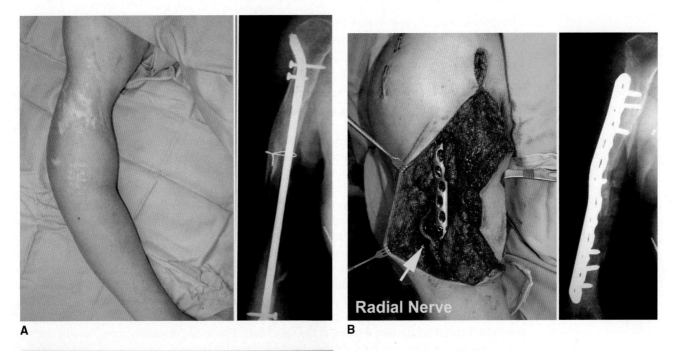

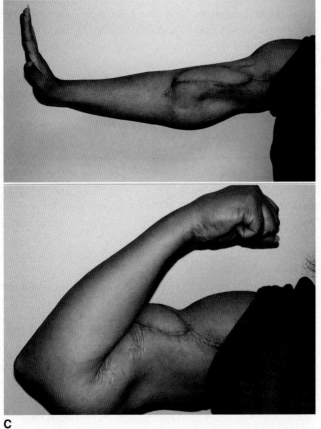

FIGURE 12-20

This 40-year-old woman sustained a crush injury to her right arm. She was treated with an intramedullary rod for a humerus fracture. She was referred 6 months after her injury for bone reconstruction. She was also noted to have absent elbow flexion, weak elbow extension, and absent radial nerve function. Reconstruction of the bone was performed by 3 cm shortening of the humerus, plating, and iliac crest bone grafting. Her radial nerve was explored and in continuity. A neurolysis was performed. A functional bipolar latissimus transfer was performed to reconstruct elbow flexion. Full radial nerve recovery was noted at 2 months and bone healing at 3 months, and the patient had full active flexion against gravity of her elbow at 3 months. **A:** Soft tissue and bone appearance at 3 months after injury and prior to reconstruction. **B:** Intraoperative neurolysis of the radial nerve and transposed latissimus. **C:** Elbow flexion and extension at 6 months postinjury, with full recovery of the radial nerve. (Copyright Frances Sharpe and Milan Stevanovic.)

may lead to compression of the pedicle in the subcutaneous tunnel. Postoperative hematoma or infection can occur. Any complication at the recipient site may cause changes in the muscle leading to decreased power of flexion.

Long-term complications at the recipient site include scaring and tendon adhesions that may require revision surgery. Attenuation at the tendon repair site shortens the muscle resting length and decreases power and excursion of the transferred latissimus. Pediatric patients may experience more rapid bone growth than growth of the transferred muscle. This can lead to joint contracture with growth. Rarely, patients may fracture at the neo-origin or recipient site related to the presence of stress risers from bone tunnels created for tendon attachment.

Donor Site

Early donor site complications include hematoma or seroma formation. These complications can be reduced with careful hemostasis to prevent hematoma formation. Quilting of the subcutaneous tissue layer to the chest wall fascia and the use of fibrin glue have been shown to decrease seroma formation. We also maintain one to two drains at the donor situ until the output has decreased to less than 25 mL in a 24-hour period. Correlations have been established between seroma formation and increased BMI, age, and smoking. Interestingly, a recent article identified decreased postoperative hemoglobin, decreased postoperative serum calcium, and the use of selective serotonin reuptake inhibitor antidepressant medications to be correlated with the incidence or volume of postoperative seroma formation. Seromas can usually be managed with serial aspirations. Surgical excision of the seroma capsule may be necessary for long-standing seromas. Hematomas require urgent surgical evacuation to reduce chances of wound dehiscence or skin necrosis.

Long-term complications at the donor site include tight, painful, or cosmetically displeasing scars. Loss of range of motion in shoulder forward flexion and abduction is common but improves with time and therapy. Functional loss of mobility is rare. Several studies have documented isolated loss of strength in the functions performed by the latissimus (extension, adduction, and internal rotation of the arm at the shoulder). The most frequently noted loss of strength is in extension of the arm through the shoulder. Despite isolated weakness in muscle testing, global shoulder function scores remain high due to compensation for LD function by synergistic muscle groups (predominantly teres major, pectoralis major, and subscapularis). Weakness was noted with specific activities such as ladder climbing, overhead painting, and pushing up from a chair.

Lumbar hernia, which may be misdiagnosed as a lumbar seroma, is an extremely rare complication. Careful preservation of the fascia underlying the latissimus at the aponeurotic origin is important in preventing this complication.

PEARLS AND PITFALLS

- Dissect in the suprafascial plane to maintain the integrity of the LD muscle and improve muscle gliding in its transposed position.
- Muscle resting length must be restored to maximize function of the transposed muscle.
  - Mark resting length prior to LD harvest with the arm in a position of maximum abduction and forward flexion.
  - Reset muscle resting length at the transposition site with the elbow in full extension. Once set, the elbow is then flexed to reduce tension at the repair site.
- Use muscle stimulation to separate fibers of the LD from the fibers of serratus anterior and teres major.
- Ligating the vascular branch to the serratus anterior and more proximal perforating branches will improve length and mobility of the vascular pedicle.
- The latissimus insertion is released as close as possible to its insertion.
- Inadequate preoperative assessment of muscle power leading to transfer of a weak muscle. Prevention: The LD can be difficult to assess preoperatively due to overlapping functions of other muscles. Careful clinical examination and preoperative MRI when indicated can help in identifying a compromised muscle.
- Failure to restore resting length can lead to compromised muscle function. Understretching can lead to decreased muscle power. Overtensioning can compromise muscle circulation and overstretch myosin-actin filaments that will also decrease muscle power.
- Pedicle compromise can occur as a result of overstretching or fascial compression and can lead to decreased arterial or venous compromise. Prevention: Make a wide soft tissue tunnel and release any fascial bands that can compress the pedicle. Release the arterial branch to serratus to improve pedicle length and decrease tension on the pedicle.
- Injury of the long thoracic nerve can occur during dissection of the cephalad portion of the LD muscle and can result in dysfunction of the serratus anterior and scapular winging.

RECOMMENDED READING

Bailey SH, Oni G, Guevara R, et al. Latissimus dorsi donor-site morbidity: the combination of quilting and fibrin sealant reduce length of drain placement and seroma rate. *Ann Plast Surg.* 2012;68:555–558.

Button J, Scott J, Taghizadeh R, et al. Shoulder function following autologous latissimus dorsi breast reconstruction: a prospective three year observational study comparing quilting and non-quilting donor site techniques. *J Plast Reconstr Aesthet Surg.* 2010;63:1505–1512.

Cambon-Binder A, Belkheyar Z, Durand S, et al. Elbow flexion restoration using pedicled latissimus dorsi transfer in seven cases. *Chir Main.* 2012;31:324–330.

Chuang D-C, Epstein M, Yey M-C, et al. Functional restoration of elbow flexion in brachial plexus injuries: results in 167 patients (excluding obstetric brachial plexus injury). *J Hand Surg Am.* 1993;18A:285–291.

Eggers IM, Mennen U, Matime AM. Elbow flexorplasty: a comparison between latissimus dorsi transfer and Steindler flexorplasty. *J Hand Surg Br.* 1992;17:522–525.

Gruber S, Whitworth AB, Kemmler G, et al. New risk factors for donor site seroma formation after latissimus dorsi flap breast reconstruction: 10-year period outcome analysis. *J Plast Reconstr Aesthet Surg.* 2011;64:69–74.

Kawamura K, Yajima H, Tomita Y, et al. Restoration of elbow function with pedicled latissimus dorsi myocutaneous flap transfer. *J Shoulder Elbow Surg.* 2007;16:84–90.

Lee KT, Mun GH. A systematic review of functional donor-site morbidity after latissimus dorsi muscle transfer. *Plast Reconstr Surg.* 2014;134:303–314.

Moneim MS, Omer GE. Latissimus dorsi muscle transfer for restoration of elbow flexion after brachial plexus disruption. *J Hand Surg Am.* 1986;11:135–139.

Pearle AD, Kelly BT, Voos JE, et al. Surgical technique and anatomic study of latissimus dorsi and teres major transfers. *J Bone Joint Surg Am.* 2006;88:1524–1531.

Rajoo R, Mennen U, Stevanovic M. Compartment syndrome in transferred muscle: an unusual complication. *J Hand Surg [Br].* 1991;16(1):75–77.

Russell RC, Pribaz J, Zook EG, et al. Functional evaluation of latissimus dorsi donor site. *Plast Reconstr Surg.* 1986;78:336–344.

Schoeller T, Wechselberger G, Hussl H, et al. Functional transposition of the latissimus dorsi muscle for biceps reconstruction after upper arm replantation. *J Plast Reconstr Aesthet Surg.* 2007;60:755–759.

Schottstaedt ER, Larsen LJ, Bost FC. Complete muscle transposition. *J Bone Joint Surg Am.* 1955;37-A(5):918–919.

Stern PJ, Caudle RJ. Tendon transfers for elbow flexion. *Hand Clin.* 1988;4:297–307.

Zancolli E, Mitre H. Latissimus dorsi transfer to restore elbow flexion: an appraisal of eight cases. *J Bone Joint Surg Am.* 1973;55:1265–1275.

13 Fasciotomies for Forearm and Hand Compartment Syndrome

Laura K. Tom and Jeffrey B. Friedrich

INDICATIONS/CONTRAINDICATIONS

Indications

Fasciotomies in the upper extremity are performed to treat compartment syndrome or prophylactically in cases where there is a high risk for the development of compartment syndrome. The diagnosis of upper extremity compartment syndrome is made with a combination of clinical presentation, examination, and objective diagnostic measurements.

The most common cause of compartment syndrome in adults is a fracture of the distal radius, whereas in children, the most common cause is a supracondylar fracture of the humerus. Other common causes of compartment syndrome include blast or crush injuries, two-bone forearm fractures, electrical injuries, and extended muscle ischemia. It should be emphasized that any situation where with a period of ischemia followed by reperfusion can lead to muscle necrosis and swelling, which can develop into compartment syndrome. Examples of reperfusion injury include prolonged use of a tourniquet prior to hospital arrival, a brachial arterial injury, upper arm replants, and patients found lying on their arms in the field. External pressure or rigid structures such as casts or splints can also lead to compartment syndrome and pressure necrosis of soft tissue.

The first step in diagnosing compartment syndrome is having a heightened suspicion for its presence. The very young, very old, and unresponsive patients are most vulnerable to its development. Before beginning the physical exam, always remove any casts, splints, dressings, or devices potentially causing external compression. On physical exam, the forearm and hand suffering from compartment syndrome will typically be very tense and swollen (Fig. 13-1). Skin changes such as blistering and a "shine" due to significant swelling are common findings (Fig. 13-2). Clinical findings for compartment syndrome traditionally are taught as the five Ps:

- Pain out of proportion of injury or increased pain with passive extensive extension of the fingers
- Paresthesia or decreased sensation
- Paralysis or decreased ability to move
- Pallor or pale appearance
- Pulselessness

The most reliable finding is decreased sensation, specifically a decrease in two-point discrimination or glove paresthesia. Contrary to previous teaching, pulselessness is a very late or potentially nonexistent finding in the patient who has a compartment syndrome. It should be emphasized that not all of the 5 Ps need to be present to diagnose compartment syndrome.

Objective data are obtained to help corroborate the clinical suspicion of compartment syndrome, usually in the form of intracompartmental pressure measurements. These can be taken by a variety of techniques including saline infusion pressure transducers, slit or wick catheters, or even arterial pressure monitors. There are newer diagnostic tools to diagnose compartment syndrome including near-infrared spectroscopy, electromyography, myotonometry, and laser Doppler; however, these modalities are experimental and can only be used as correlative measures at best. Objective data are

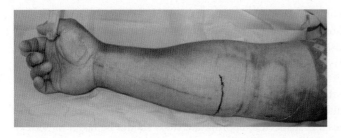

FIGURE 13-1
Patient with classic tense forearm edema and ecchymosis.

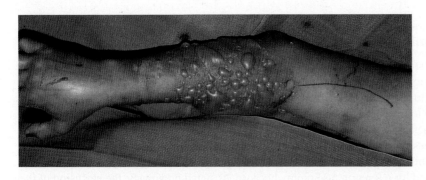

FIGURE 13-2
Patient with forearm compartment syndrome demonstrating typical cutaneous findings including tense edema and blistering.

not always necessary to make the diagnosis of compartment syndrome but can be useful for following an exam or making the diagnosis in the presence of a confusing or inconclusive physical exam.

If a patient is at risk for compartment syndrome, but does not have overt evidence of increased compartment pressures, compartment syndrome must be ruled out by close observation and serial physical exams. This is especially true for patients who cannot provide a reliable or responsive physical exam—examples include intubated patients, intoxicated patients, patients with polytrauma and distracting injuries, and children. If compartment syndrome is suspected but cannot be ruled out, it is essential that intervention be implemented quickly to lessen injury to the underlying muscles and nerves. Increased pressure on muscle can lead to irreversible ischemia and eventual necrosis. Late sequela of untreated compartment syndrome of the forearm produces contractures of the volar forearm muscles commonly known as Volkmann's ischemic contracture. In general, prompt intervention with surgical decompression of the hand and forearm compartments will adequately treat compartment syndrome and can leave a patient with minimal residual dysfunction.

Contraindications

While one can argue that hemodynamic instability is a relative contraindication to upper extremity fasciotomies, it is recommended that this not be viewed as an absolute contraindication. Once a patient is stabilized, the surgical team should proceed with forearm and/or hand fasciotomies as soon as the patient has stabilized. In the worst-case scenario, fasciotomies can be performed at the bedside in the intensive care unit if a patient cannot tolerate being transferred to the operating room. Upper extremity compartment syndrome is an emergency, and there should be no absolute contraindications to fasciotomies.

PREOPERATIVE PLANNING

When planning for surgical intervention for upper extremity compartment syndrome, the previously mentioned clinical and diagnostic findings should be used to document the diagnosis of compartment syndrome. In addition, if it is thought that the patient has developed a compartment syndrome in the setting of external compression, including splints or casts, these devices should be loosened or removed immediately. This can aid in the diagnosis of the cause of the patient's symptoms as well as provide some measure of relief from the compressive insult. Often, the removal or loosening of a cast can provide adequate treatment; but even if the patient does show resolution of symptoms, practitioners are encouraged to remain vigilant and continue to closely monitor the patient's extremity until total resolution of symptoms.

Consent for operation should include fasciotomies, debridement of soft tissue, and possible amputation. The patient and family should be counseled that the patient will likely require additional operations for debridement and reconstruction.

Other planning should include early notification of anesthesia and operating room staff and the availability of blood for transfusion if it is indicated during the surgical procedure. In some cases, coagulopathy can contribute to or be the sole cause of compartment syndrome. Excessive bleeding following fracture reduction or continued bleeding following surgery can lead to increased compartmental pressures. If a bleeding diathesis is suspected, appropriate steps should be taken to correct the deficiency before operative intervention.

SURGERY

Patient Positioning

Once anesthetized, the patient should be positioned in a way that affords adequate access to the entire affected upper extremity for both surgeon and assistant. This includes turning the operating table at a right angle to the anesthesia provider and placing the affected upper extremity on an arm board that is attached to the operating room table. Good lighting is essential, especially because the viability of the muscles in the forearm and hand needs to be assessed at the time of fasciotomy. To test viability of the muscle, a monopolar electrocautery can be utilized in addition to having bipolar cautery available. While pneumatic tourniquets are frequently used for upper extremity surgery, they should not be used for a forearm fasciotomy because, as stated previously, the perfusion of the affected forearm musculature must be assessed at the time of fasciotomy.

Technique for Fasciotomies of the Forearm

There are two volar compartments and one true dorsal compartment and a mobile wad that should be addressed when performing forearm fasciotomies (Figs. 13-3 and 13-4). The classic teaching of forearm fasciotomies includes two incisions—one on the volar aspect and one on the dorsal aspect of the forearm. In general, both volar forearm compartments (superficial and deep) are decompressed via the volar incision, while the dorsal compartment and the mobile wad can be adequately decompressed via the dorsal incision. A variety of incisions on the volar forearm have been proposed and studied in cadavers. Ulnar-sided incisions have been shown to be the safest approach to both superficial and deep volar forearm compartments, providing adequate visualization while avoiding injury to the radial artery and median nerve.

Incision of the Volar and Dorsal Forearm

Typically, the volar forearm incision extends from the antecubital fossa down to the wrist. The most common design is that of a sigmoid incision. The incision is marked beginning on the medial aspect

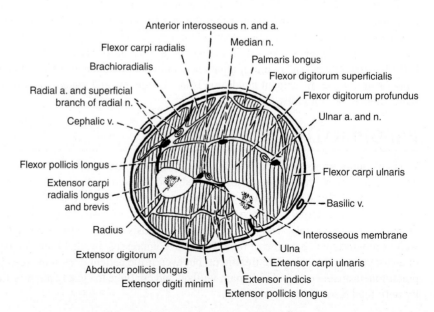

FIGURE 13-3

Cross-sectional anatomy of the midforearm. Note the deep position of the FPL and FDP adjacent to the radius, ulna, and interosseus membrane. This deep position against the rigid skeleton makes these muscles particularly vulnerable to damage due to compartment syndrome. (Used by permission of Mayo Foundation.)

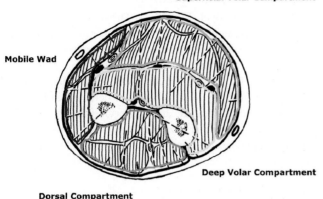

Superficial Volar Compartment

Mobile Wad

Deep Volar Compartment

Dorsal Compartment

FIGURE 13-4

Cross-sectional anatomy of the midforearm. Each compartment is labeled and outlined: superficial volar, deep volar, dorsal, and mobile wad.

of the elbow just anterior to the medial epicondyle, curving radially along the midforearm, curving back to the distal ulnar side of the forearm, and finally coming along the distal wrist crease to approximately the level of the carpal tunnel (Fig. 13-5).

An alternative incision design places the forearm incision on the volar ulnar aspect of the forearm (Fig. 13-6A, B). The purpose of this design is to, in theory, offer protection for the median nerve once decompression has been performed. The radially based flap in the distal forearm will provide this median nerve protection even with marked edema and gaping of the wound. Other surgeons have advocated leaving the carpal tunnel skin intact while releasing the transverse carpal tunnel ligament deep to the skin to protect the median nerve from exposure.

The incision of the dorsal forearm is designed in linear fashion over the midline of the forearm dorsum to allow access to the forearm extensors including the extensor muscle bellies, brachioradialis, and the radial wrist extensors (Fig. 13-6C).

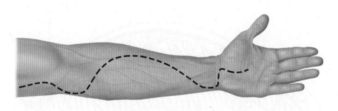

FIGURE 13-5

Incision pattern for fasciotomies of the forearm and carpal tunnel.

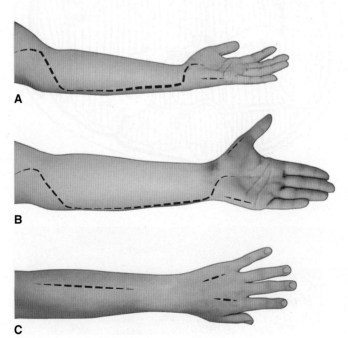

A

B

C

FIGURE 13-6

Alternative incision pattern for fasciotomies used by the authors. This incision varies in that entirety of the incision is along the very ulnar volar aspect of the arm. This approach ensures adequate coverage of the median nerve despite significant debridement and severe edema. **A:** Ulnar view of the forearm and hypothenar incision. **B:** Volar view of the forearm and hand incisions. **C:** Dorsal view of the forearm over the extensor muscle bellies and allowing access to the more radial mobile wad. The hand incisions are placed over the index and ring metacarpals to allow access to the first and second compartments and the third and fourth compartments, respectively.

Release of Superficial Compartments of the Volar Forearm

Once the skin incision is marked, it is incised with a scalpel (Fig. 13-7). The dissection is further carried down through the subcutaneous tissues with either electrocautery or scissor dissection. Once the antebrachial fascia of the volar forearm is visualized, the fascia is incised with curved tenotomy-type scissors. The fascial division should be extended proximally and distally until the entire superficial volar forearm compartment is decompressed (Fig. 13-8). Once the fascia is open, the viability of the musculature must to be assessed. If compartment syndrome has been detected early and a fasciotomy has been performed, myonecrosis can be avoided. If, after observing the musculature for several minutes, there is no reperfusion, or there is distinct myonecrosis of any of the forearm muscles, consideration should be given to immediate debridement of all dead tissue. At this point, only the superficial volar forearm compartment has been decompressed.

Release of Deep Compartments of the Volar Forearm

The deep volar compartment is approached through the interval between the flexor digitorum superficialis (FDS) and the flexor carpi ulnaris (FCU) (Fig. 13-9). The FDS muscle belly is retracted radially and the FCU muscle belly is retracted ulnarly; this allows visualization of the deep compartment and protects the median nerve and ulnar neurovascular bundle. The deep volar fascia is opened along the entire length of the flexor digitorum profundus (FDP) and flexor pollicis longus (FPL) muscle bellies. Once the fascia is incised, the muscles often appear edematous and will herniate from their respective compartments. The viability of these muscles must also be assessed. Consideration should be given to excision of any distinctly necrotic muscle at the time of fasciotomy, as this can become a nidus for infection if not removed.

Release of Compartments of the Dorsal Forearm

Some authors believe that decompression of the volar forearm compartments will secondarily lead to adequate decompression of the dorsal forearm compartment as well as the mobile wad (Fig. 13-10). However, if one is planning to take this approach, it is strongly advised that compartmental pressure

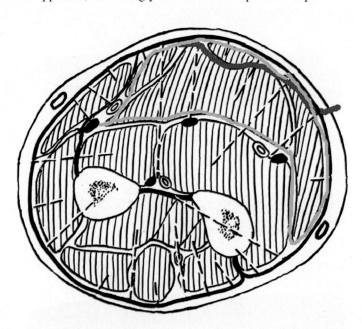

FIGURE 13-7

Cross-sectional anatomy of the volar aspect of the midforearm. The superficial volar compartment is highlighted. Incision and release indicated in *blue*.

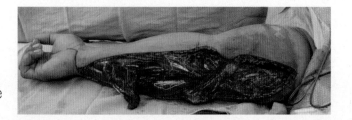

FIGURE 13-8

Intraoperative photo after superficial compartment release extending from the wrist crease to proximal to the elbow. The antebrachial fascia is released along the entirety of the incision ensuring complete release of the superficial compartment.

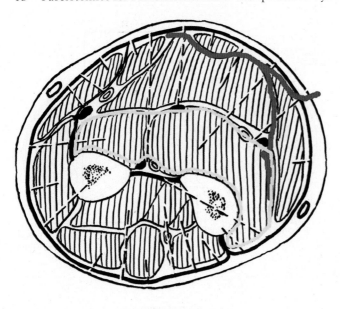

FIGURE 13-9

Cross-sectional anatomy of the volar aspect of the midforearm. The deep volar compartment is highlighted. Continued release indicated in *blue* between the FDS and the FCU.

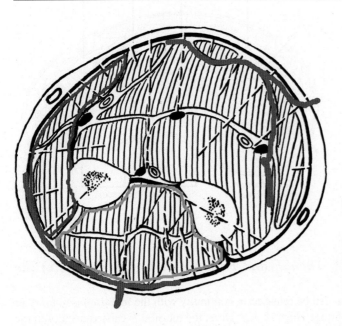

FIGURE 13-10

Cross-sectional anatomy of the dorsal aspect of the midforearm. Incision and release indicated in *blue* with release of the fascia overlying the dorsal extensor muscle bellies as well as a release of the radial mobile wad.

readings of the dorsal forearm compartment as well as the mobile wad be taken intraoperatively to confirm that decompression of the volar side of the forearm has indeed led to adequate decompression of the dorsal forearm.

Using the previously described markings, the skin is incised with a scalpel and carried down through the subcutaneous tissue with either electrocautery or scissor dissection. The dorsal forearm fascia is incised typically with tenotomy scissors along the length of the extensor muscle bellies both proximally and distally. Once the musculature of the dorsal forearm compartment has been assessed, one must then dissect in the subcutaneous plane in the radial direction to access the mobile wad. It is here that the fascia over the brachioradialis and the radial wrist extensors (extensor carpi radialis brevis and longus) are incised with scissors.

Technique for Fasciotomies of the Hand

The hand has seven compartments: the thenar, hypothenar, carpal tunnel, and four interosseus compartments (Fig. 13-11). All seven compartments can be decompressed with five small incisions (see Fig. 13-6B, C).

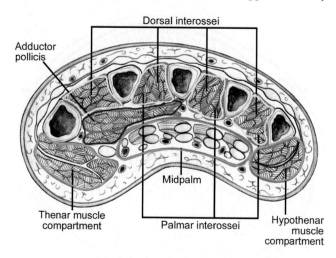

FIGURE 13-11

Cross-sectional anatomy of the hand. Each compartment is labeled and outlined. The volar compartments are the thenar, hypothenar, and carpal tunnel (midpalmar and adductor pollicis). The dorsal compartments consist of the four interossei compartments. (From Berger R, Weiss A-PC, eds. *Hand Surgery*. Philadelphia, PA: Lippincott Williams & Wilkins; 2003.)

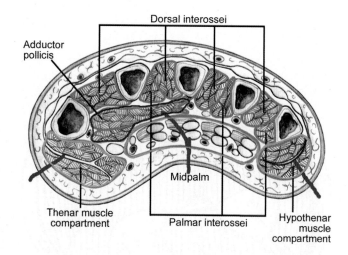

FIGURE 13-12

Cross-sectional anatomy of the hand. Two incisions along the far radial and ulnar aspects of the hand along the border between the glabrous and hair-bearing skin allow access to the thenar and hypothenar compartments of the hand. The carpal tunnel release gives way to the carpal tunnel, midpalmar space, and deep adductor pollicis space.

Release of the Carpal Tunnel, Thenar, and Hypothenar Compartments of the Volar Hand

The transverse carpal tunnel ligament can be released in continuity with the forearm fasciotomy or as described with an overlying skin bridge (Fig. 13-12). Here, the incision is carried distally to the distal point of the transverse carpal ligament (Fig. 13-13). After dividing the skin and subcutaneous tissues, the transverse carpal ligament is divided with scissors or a scalpel while the median nerve is protected.

The thenar and hypothenar compartments are decompressed next. These incisions are made at the border of the glabrous and hair-bearing skin of the thenar and hypothenar eminences, respectively, and are approximately 3 to 4 cm long (see Fig. 13-7B). Once the skin and fat is opened, the fascias of these compartments are also opened with spreading scissor dissection.

Release of the Four Interosseus Compartments of the Dorsal Hand

Finally, the four interosseus compartments can be opened with two incisions on the dorsum of the hand (see Figs. 13-7C and 13-14). These incisions are centered over the index and ring finger metacarpal bones and are 3 to 4 cm long. After making the index metacarpal incision, scissors are used to spread radially to open the first interosseus compartment and ulnarly to open the second interosseus space. Similarly, one enters the ring metacarpal incision to spread radially into the third interosseus compartment and ulnarly into the fourth interosseus compartment (see Fig. 13-15).

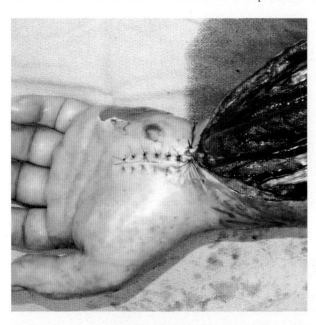

FIGURE 13-13

Intraoperative photo of patient with completed carpal tunnel incision for a volar fasciotomy release. After release of the carpal tunnel (midpalmar and adductor pollicis), the skin incision is closed to protect the underlying median nerve. Some advocate for subcutaneous release of the transverse carpal ligament leaving the skin bridge intact (not shown).

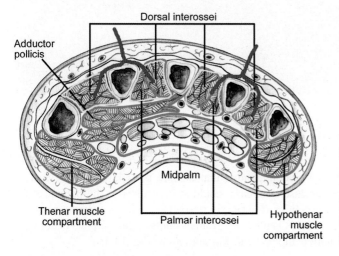

FIGURE 13-14

Cross-sectional anatomy of the hand. Two dorsal hand incisions placed over the index and ring metacarpals for decompression of the interosseous musculature of the hand.

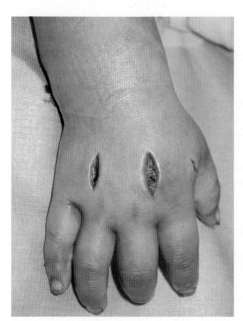

FIGURE 13-15

Intraoperative photo of pediatric patient with fasciotomy for hand compartment syndrome. These incisions are along the metacarpals and allow access to all four interosseous compartments.

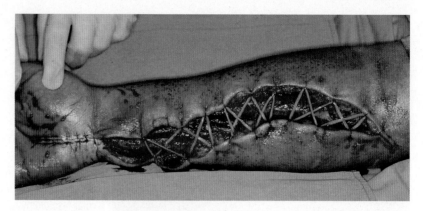

FIGURE 13-16

Partial coaptation of forearm fasciotomy wound edges using the "Roman sandal" method. Vessel loops or rubber bands are weaved across the wound to bring the skin edges closer while allowing for some expansion due to postoperative edema.

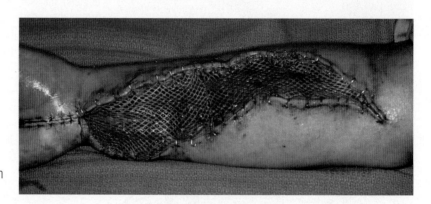

FIGURE 13-17

Forearm fasciotomy wound immediately following skin grafting.

Closure and Reconstruction

Temporary Closure

Once all compartments are released, it is recommended that closure be delayed for at least 24 to 48 hours. Closure of the skin, despite fascial release, could still predispose the patient to the redevelopment of increased interstitial pressures resulting in tissue ischemia. Temporary retention sutures or running elastic sutures (the "Jacob's ladder" or "Roman sandal") can be placed along the wound to provide some skin approximation and prevent skin retraction (Fig. 13-16).

Reconstruction

One should consider closure of the forearm and hand wounds following resolution of the patient's compartment syndrome, stabilization of vital signs, early resolution of edema, and assurance that there is further no underlying muscle necrosis or devitalized tissue within the wound bed. Skin closure can usually commence 1 to 7 days following a fasciotomy. Inflammation from compartment syndrome results in significant edema. If extremity edema has subsided, the skin may be closed with delayed closure or with skin grafting. Temporary retention mechanisms can be used to recruit overlying skin back to its original positions. This can be used in conjunction with a negative pressure dressings, which can help alleviate edema and prevent further skin edge retraction of the wound.

Delayed primary closure of both palmar and dorsal wounds may be impractical in cases where the antecedent trauma has been significant, or if swelling has not abated within approximately 1 week of fasciotomies. In such cases, skin grafting may be carried out over exposed muscle bellies to expedite wound coverage and patient rehabilitation (Fig. 13-17). Skin grafts can be later excised after the patient is healed and there is return of normal skin laxity.

POSTOPERATIVE MANAGEMENT

Immediately following fascial release, repeat wound exploration under anesthesia is recommended at 24 to 48 hours; this allows the surgeon to verify that all necrotic muscle has been removed. Between operative interventions, the patient should be well hydrated and the extremity should be kept elevated to reduce edema. Finger and hand therapy can be initiated to maintain joint range of motion. If the patient complains of increasing pain or numbness, one must be concerned for incomplete release of the compartments, and the patient should be immediately returned to the operating room.

For wound care, we most commonly use negative pressure dressings or gauze impregnated with either petroleum or antibiotics to prevent wound desiccation. Other options also include traditional frequent (daily or twice daily) wet-to-moist dressings and whirlpool and pulse lavage-type irrigation pending on the patient's clinical needs and pain tolerance.

Early involvement with our occupational therapy team is critical to functional outcomes for patients. This includes designing and manufacturing of custom removable thermoplast splints that allow for dressing changes and hold the hand in a functional position (intrinsic plus). It must be ensured that this splint does not induce external compression. They also provide instruction for hand motion exercises. The chief reason for these exercises is to ensure that the patient's range of motion remains relatively stable and that tendon gliding continues, especially with the flexor tendons at the wrist level. If the involvement is only of the forearm, a light compression glove can assist with edema control, range of motion, and pain.

COMPLICATIONS

As with any surgery, bleeding and hematoma are possible, especially in a forearm fasciotomy in which no tourniquet is used intraoperatively. Inadequate debridement can lead to infection. Finally, the most dreaded complication of forearm fasciotomy is continued muscle necrosis and eventual fibrosis despite forearm fasciotomies. In general, this does not occur with adequate decompression. As stated previously, the most likely reason for continued muscle necrosis following this operation is inadequate decompression of the forearm and hand compartments.

RESULTS

In general, adequate decompression of the compartments of the forearm and hand will allow resolution of the compartment syndrome and will lead to an outcome in which the patient has no or minimal residual dysfunction. The most frequent cause of muscle necrosis and subsequent fibrosis following forearm fasciotomy is due to delayed diagnosis or incomplete fasciotomy. Therefore, care must be taken intraoperatively to fully extend the fasciotomy proximally and distally, thereby decompressing the full length of all the affected muscle bellies. Following fasciotomy, patients require diligent wound care to ensure that the wounds remain clean so that they will be ready for either delayed primary closure or skin grafting.

PEARLS AND PITFALLS

- The surgeon must have a high suspicion for compartment syndrome in cases of fracture, crush, and ischemia.
- Swift, early, and complete fasciotomies are necessary to prevent muscle necrosis. Delayed or incomplete fasciotomies lead to unsatisfactory outcomes.
- If questionable muscle viability is encountered, plan for reexamination in the operating room in 24 to 48 hours.
- Reconstruction after fasciotomies can be approached with delayed primary closure, skin grafting, or healing by secondary intention.
- Adjuncts such as temporary tension mechanisms and negative pressure dressings can decrease the wound area needing coverage.
- Skin grafting for fasciotomies can shorten the healing period for patients, which can allow patients to more rapidly initiate hand rehabilitation. These skin grafts can be excised at a later date when edema and soft tissue suppleness has improved.

RECOMMENDED READING

Del Piñal F, Herrero F, Jado E, et al. Acute hand compartment syndromes after closed crush: a reappraisal. *Plast Reconstr Surg.* 2002;110(5):1232–1239.

Elliott KG, Johnstone AJ. Diagnosing acute compartment syndrome. *J Bone Joint Surg Br.* 2003;85(5):625–632.

Gelberman RH, Garfin SR, Hergenroeder PT, et al. Compartment syndromes of the forearm: diagnosis and treatment. *Clin Orthop Relat Res.* 1981;161:252–261.

Gulgonen A. Acute compartment syndrome. In: Green DP, Hotchkiss RN, Pederson WC, et al., eds. *Green's Operative Hand Surgery.* 5th ed. Philadelphia, PA: Elsevier; 2005:1986–1996.

McQueen MM, Gaston P, Court-Brown CM. Acute compartment syndrome: who is at risk? *J Bone Joint Surg Br.* 2000;82(2):200–203.

Naidu SH, Heppenstall RB. Compartment syndrome of the forearm and hand. *Hand Clin.* 1994;10(1):13–27.

Tsuge K. Treatment of established Volkmann's contracture. *J Bone Joint Surg Am.* 1975;57(7):925–929.

14 Soft Tissue Management of Delayed Compartment Syndrome

Milan Stevanovic and Frances Sharpe

The treatment of missed compartment syndrome of the upper extremity is a challenging problem for the reconstructive surgeon. The development of Volkmann's ischemic contracture produces flexor contractures of the wrist and fingers often crippling the hand and preventing useful function. In addition, the palmar skin may suffer from maceration and infection due to the difficulties of hygiene in a severely contracted palm. Several methods have been described for treating these contractures and include tendon lengthening, tendon transfers, and carpal fusion.

In 1923, Max Page described a forearm muscle sliding operation for the treatment of contracture of the muscles of the forearm. Since that time, there have been only a few case series describing various modifications of the technique typically for indications of Volkmann's ischemic contracture and for forearm muscle contracture of central neurologic origin. Surgical alternatives to a flexor origin slide include fractional muscle lengthening and superficialis to profundus transfer. In contrast to the other procedures, the flexor origin slide retains the muscle resting length of the contracted muscle and thus is capable of preserving muscle strength.

INDICATIONS/CONTRAINDICATIONS

The flexor origin muscle sliding procedure is used to treat wrist and finger flexion contractures resulting from scarred or fibrotic muscle of the forearm flexor muscle group seen in cases of Volkmann's or pseudo-Volkmann's contracture. Functional outcomes are better in pseudo-Volkmann's and mild and moderate cases of Volkmann's contracture. The better the remaining muscle function in the flexor muscle group, the better the ultimate grip strength. The procedure is also used to treat contractures of central neurological origin, including cerebral palsy, stroke, and neuromuscular disorders such as Parkinson's disease.

The requirements for using this technique include an intact soft tissue envelope and a stable neuromuscular examination, which usually occurs 6 to 12 months after the inciting event. The procedure can be performed in conjunction with other procedures such as wrist fusion, finger joint contracture release, and even tendon transfer.

Contraindications to the procedure include infection and fixed joint contractures. Further contraindications include thrombosis of the radial or ulnar arteries or damage to the common, anterior, or posterior interosseous arteries. Contractures at the wrist or finger joints may require correction prior to or simultaneously with the flexor origin slide. Relative contraindications include diabetes, peripheral vascular disease, or other autoimmune diseases.

Preoperative contracture can mask weakness of the wrist and finger flexors as well as weakness of the extensor compartment. Weakness and fibrosis of the muscle compartment will limit the final grip strength following this procedure; however, it is not a contraindication for this procedure and can be useful in correcting underlying contractures in anticipation of additional reconstructive procedures. Relative contraindications also include patients with athetoid cerebral palsy, cerebral palsy patients with a dynamic pattern of spasticity who experience frequent changes in tone and spasticity, and patients with progressive neurologic deterioration. The reason for the contraindications in this group of patients is primarily due to the fact that results are unpredictable and can deteriorate over time. Cerebral palsy is frequently associated with swan neck deformities of the fingers. This may appear worse after a flexor origin slide but is not a contraindication to this procedure.

PREOPERATIVE PLANNING

Preoperative planning includes a careful history, including the etiology of the contracture, the date of the injury, and a determination of whether the contracture is stable or worsening. A careful discussion of expected outcomes is necessary so that the patient has realistic expectations for the procedure. Clinical examination includes assessment of passive and active motion of the wrist and fingers and whether the finger contracture improves with passive flexion of the wrist (Fig. 14-1). It may be very difficult to assess wrist flexor and extensor strength due to the contracture. Hand intrinsic dysfunction may also be difficult to assess preoperatively. The rotational posture and or contracture of the forearm should be evaluated. If the patient has preoperative weakness of the pronator or a supination contracture, the surgical technique should be modified to preserve the origin of the pronator teres. Vascular and sensory examination should be performed and documented.

Special Evaluation

For patients with Volkmann's contracture, a preoperative MRI of the forearm can show the extent of muscle damage, including possible involvement of the extensor compartment as well as provide a more quantitative assessment of uninjured areas of the flexor compartment. Magnetic resonance angiography or arteriogram may be indicated for patients with a history of a previous vascular injury or an abnormal vascular exam.

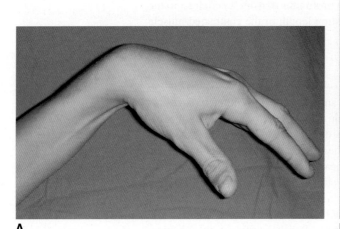

A

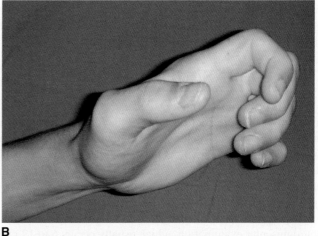

B

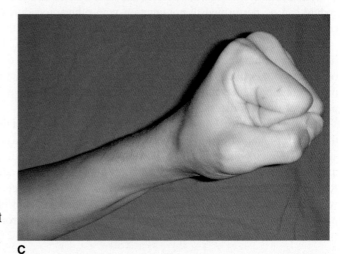

C

FIGURE 14-1

A: Preoperative evaluation of finger flexion, demonstrating full active extension of the fingers with the wrist in flexion. **B:** With the wrist in neutral, the fingers assume a position of flexion and cannot be passively extended. **C:** Preoperative finger flexion. (Copyright Milan Stevanovic and Frances Sharpe.)

For patients with spasticity, the preoperative use of Botox or selected nerve block may help in the preoperative evaluation to distinguish spasticity from joint contracture. This may also unmask extrinsic extensor weakness or intrinsic spasticity. This can help guide both surgeon and patient expectations for the procedure.

SURGERY

Patient Positioning

The patient is positioned supine with a hand table for the operative extremity. The procedure can be performed with a regional anesthetic, but we prefer general anesthesia with paralysis. A sterile tourniquet is used. No special equipment is required for the procedure; however, bipolar cautery and loupe magnification can be useful for the dissection.

Technique

Both volar and ulnar incisions have been described for the surgical approach for a flexor-pronator slide. We favor a modification of the extensile ulnar approach and technique initially described by Page. The surgical incision begins on the medial distal arm and continues along the ulnar border of the forearm all the way to the wrist. The ulnar nerve is identified and mobilized for several centimeters proximal and distal to the medial epicondyle, including proximal release at the arcade of Struthers (Fig. 14-2). Six centimeters of intermuscular septum between the brachialis and triceps is

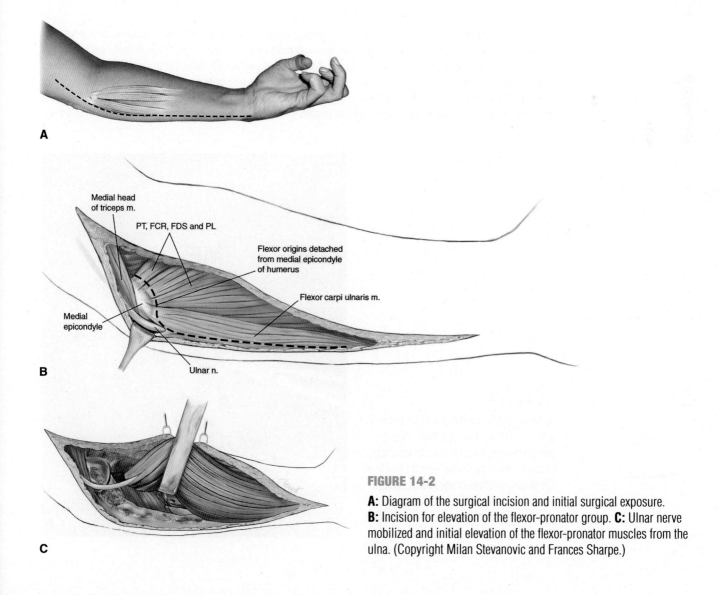

FIGURE 14-2

A: Diagram of the surgical incision and initial surgical exposure.
B: Incision for elevation of the flexor-pronator group. **C:** Ulnar nerve mobilized and initial elevation of the flexor-pronator muscles from the ulna. (Copyright Milan Stevanovic and Frances Sharpe.)

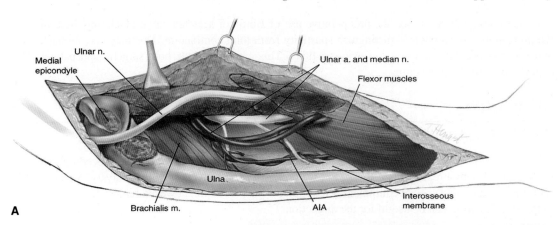

Ulnar n.
Medial
epicondyle
Ulnar a. and median n.
Flexor muscles
Ulna
Brachialis m.
AIA
Interosseous
membrane

A

FIGURE 14-3

A: Diagrammatic representation showing elevation of the flexor-pronator and common interosseous artery. (AIA, anterior interosseous artery.) **B:** Surgical dissection showing elevation of the flexor-pronator mass. (Copyright Milan Stevanovic and Frances Sharpe.)

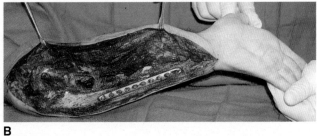

B

excised to prevent kinking of the ulnar nerve after transposition. The flexor-pronator mass is elevated off of the medial epicondyle. This includes the common origin of pronator teres, flexor carpi radialis, palmaris longus, the humeral origin of flexor digitorum superficialis, and the humeral origin of flexor carpi ulnaris (Fig. 14-3). Care is taken to preserve the medial collateral ligament and elbow joint capsule. Inadvertent disruption of the joint capsule is repaired with absorbable suture. In advertent disruption of the medial collateral ligament is repaired with a nonabsorbable no. 2 suture (Fig. 14-4).

FIGURE 14-4

Anatomy of the medial ulnar collateral ligament (MUCL) of the elbow. *Short arrow* showing the anterior oblique fibers of the ligament and *short arrow* showing the posterior fibers of the MUCL. (ME, medial epicondyle; OL, Olecranon.) (Copyright Milan Stevanovic and Frances Sharpe.)

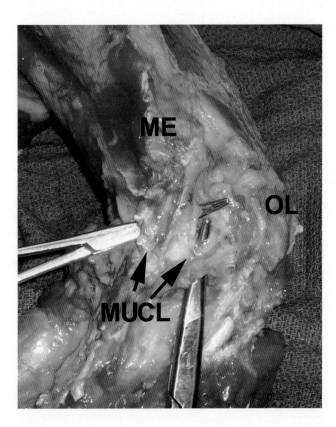

ME

OL

MUCL

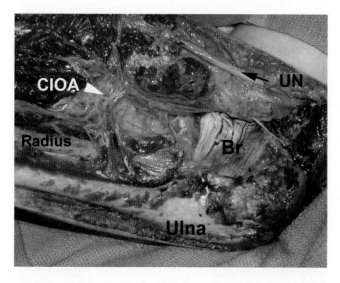

FIGURE 14-5

Proximal dissection. Insertion of the brachialis muscle (Br) on the coronoid in the proximal portion of the dissection. The common interosseous artery (CIOA) is seen dividing into the anterior interosseous artery and the posterior interosseous artery, which dives into the posterior compartment at the proximal edge of the interosseous membrane. This artery is the main blood supply to the extensor compartment and should be protected throughout the dissection. (UN, ulnar nerve.) (Copyright Milan Stevanovic and Frances Sharpe.)

The origins of the flexor carpi ulnaris, flexor digitorum profundus, and flexor digitorum superficialis are mobilized from the ulna and interosseous membrane (IOM). The dissection is carried out above the periosteum of the ulna and along the anterior surface of the interosseous membrane toward the radius. The tendinous insertion of the brachialis muscle onto the coronoid will be seen in the proximal portion of the dissection. The common interosseous artery arises as a branch of the ulnar artery about 4 cm distal to the origin of the ulnar artery. This artery crosses the flexor digitorum profundus, where it bifurcates into the anterior and posterior interosseous artery (Fig. 14-5). The posterior interosseous artery enters the posterior compartment at the proximal edge of the interosseous membrane. As the posterior interosseous artery is the dominant blood supply to the extensor compartment, protection of this branch is mandatory (see Pearls and Pitfalls). The dissection continues from proximal to distal and from medial to lateral over the interosseous membrane toward the radius. The origin of the flexor pollicis longus (FPL) is released. The FPL branches from the anterior interosseous nerve enter the muscle belly along its proximal medial and deep surface. Special attention is needed in this area to protect the anterior interosseous nerve and its FPL branches by keeping the dissection just above the intermuscular septum and the periosteum of the radius. If there is incomplete correction of the thumb after completely elevating the FPL from the IOM and radius, then additional correction can be achieved with a fractional lengthening of the FPL at the musculotendinous junction.

Throughout the procedure, the wrist and fingers are manipulated to check whether the contracture is improving and to help localize where there is still tightness within the muscle origin (Fig. 14-6). The dissection must often be carried down to the level of the wrist to release adhesions between the flexor tendons and pronator quadratus before full correction is achieved. If necessary, the carpal tunnel should be opened and tendon adhesions released in this area as well.

It has been our experience that the lacertus fibrosus and the superficial fascia around the antecubital fossa are often tight and contribute to residual elbow flexion contracture. The fascia can also tether the superficial flexors of the wrist and fingers, contributing to incomplete correction of the wrist and fingers with the muscle sliding only. Release of this fascia helps correct elbow flexion and finger contracture deformity. It can also prevent median nerve compression between the heads of the pronator teres. If the patient has a significant elbow flexion contracture, the brachialis insertion on the ulna can be released. Alternatively, a fractional lengthening of the brachialis at the musculotendinous junction can be performed slightly more proximally. We do not lengthen the biceps tendon, but the fascia around the biceps muscle and tendon can be released with some improvement in muscle excursion.

When a pronation contracture is present and not corrected by the release of the flexor-pronator origin, we release the pronator quadratus from the distal ulna. Even with a complete release of both pronators and volar distal radioulnar joint capsule, complete correction of the pronation deformity

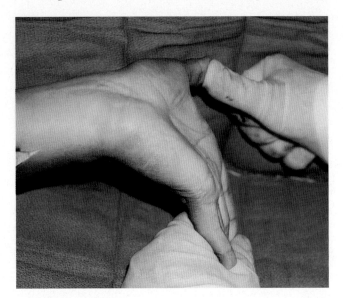

FIGURE 14-6

Frequent manipulation during the dissection is done to check for any areas still tight with passive manipulation. The slide is complete when the fingers and thumb can be fully extended with the wrist in full extension. (Copyright Milan Stevanovic and Frances Sharpe.)

may not be possible due to fibrosis and contracture of the interosseous membrane. We do not release the pronator teres at its insertion, as this could potentially lead to a supination deformity at the forearm.

At the completion of the muscle slide, the tourniquet is released and meticulous hemostasis is obtained. Thrombin is sprayed onto the exposed surfaces. A large drain is placed below the flexor muscles, and the ulnar nerve is transposed to an anterior subcutaneous position. There is no fascial layer closure. Only subcutaneous and skin layers are closed. The hand is casted in a position of neutral to relaxed forearm supination (Fig. 14-7). The wrist and fingers to the level of the distal phalanx are held in full extension. The thumb is positioned in extension and palmar abduction. Immobilization is continued for a period of 6 weeks to allow the flexor-pronator to heal adequately to its new origin.

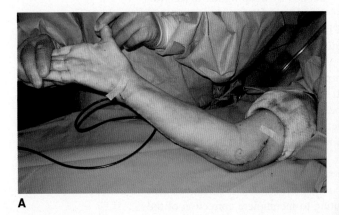

A

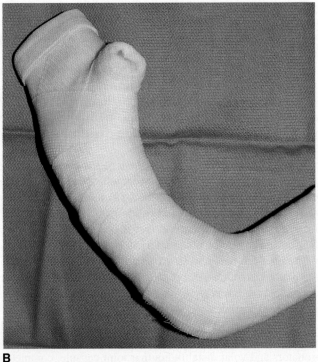

B

FIGURE 14-7

A: Wound closed over a large Hemovac drain. **B:** Application of cast with wrist and fingers in full extension and thumb in extension and palmar abduction. Care is taken to not allow thumb MCP hyperextension. (Copyright Milan Stevanovic and Frances Sharpe.)

POSTOPERATIVE MANAGEMENT

The patient is immobilized in a sugar-tong splint or long-arm cast immediately after surgery. If an elbow flexion contracture has been released, the elbow is positioned in maximum extension. The forearm is positioned in neutral to relaxed supination. The wrist and fingers are held in full extension, and the thumb is positioned in palmar abduction and extension. The initial cast should be bivalved. If a drain has been used, this is removed at 12 to 24 hours.

The patient is transitioned to a to short-arm cast still maintaining wrist and finger extension and thumb abduction-extension for an additional 2 to 3 weeks (full 6 weeks postoperatively). The patient is encouraged to work on elbow range of motion and nerve gliding during this period.

The cast is removed at 6 weeks postoperatively. Formal therapy begins, and the patient is to continue with elbow range of motion and nerve gliding. Finger and wrist range of motion are added to the therapy and continued for 6 to 12 weeks. A removable splint or custom thermoplast orthosis is applied to maintain wrist and finger extension and thumb abduction-extension. Daytime use is weaned as the patient tolerates this. However, nighttime use is recommended until the patient reaches skeletal maturity. Activities are increased as the patient regains strength and motion.

Additional reconstructive surgical procedures may be necessary 3 to 6 months postoperatively to improve the functional outcome. This will depend on the etiology of the flexion contracture. In the setting of Volkmann's ischemic contracture, this will depend on the extent and severity of the initial ischemic event. Subsequent procedures may include wrist fusion, tendon transfers, or free functional muscle transfers.

COMPLICATIONS

Early complications for any surgical procedure include bleeding, infection, and injury to nerves and blood vessels. A flexor origin muscle slide involves an extensive dissection of the forearm, which can lead to bleeding and hematoma formation. The most vulnerable neurovascular structures at risk include the ulnar nerve, which is transposed, the common interosseous artery, and the anterior interosseous nerve.

The most frequent intermediate and long-term complications or outcomes are incomplete correction of the contracture, limited grip strength, and hand deformity associated with unmasking underlying intrinsic dysfunction. There have been reports of supination contracture following flexor origin slide, and some authors recommend selective preservation of pronator teres origin in patients who do not have a preoperative pronated position of the forearm. The procedure has also been criticized for postoperative swan neck deformity of the fingers, which can be related to unmasking of intrinsic spasticity or weakening of the flexor digitorum superficialis.

RESULTS

Expectations following flexor origin slide are that of correction of the muscle component of the wrist and finger flexion contractures. The procedure cannot correct fixed joint contractures due to ligamentous or capsular contractures or restore normal function to fibrotic or spastic muscles. Functional outcomes depend on multiple factors, including etiology of the contracted muscle and remaining muscle function. Correction of the contraction of the external finger flexors may unmask an underlying intrinsic muscle dysfunction. In the clinical setting of a Volkmann's contracture, intrinsic dysfunction is a result of nerve ischemia and perineural fibrosis. In patients with spasticity, underlying spasticity of the intrinsics may be unmasked.

The broad spectrum of patient presentation and small numbers of patients requiring this procedure limit the outcome data available. Nevertheless, improvement in wrist and finger position can result in significant functional improvement. In our experience, patients with mild to moderate Volkmann's contracture can have significant functional improvement following flexor muscle slide. Corrected wrist and finger position and functional grasp can often be achieved (Fig. 14-8). Flexor origin slide for severe contractures can improve passive finger and wrist motion and is useful as a first stage of treatment before functional reconstruction with tendon transfer or functional free muscle transfer. Patients with contracture from central neurological origin have improvement in wrist and finger position with improvement in Zancolli and House functional scores. Outcomes are better in patients without intrinsic involvement.

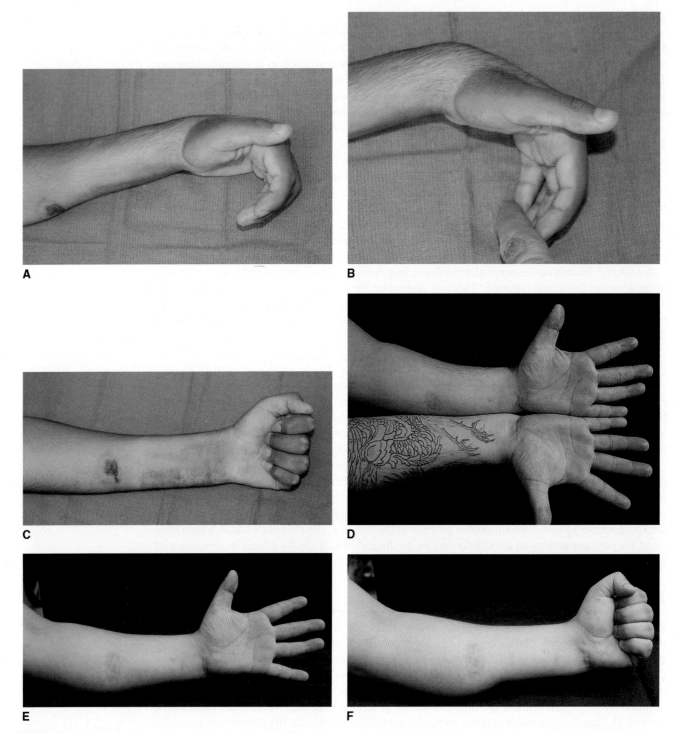

FIGURE 14-8

A 15-year-old high school football player sustained a minimally displaced both-bone forearm fracture that was minimally displaced but angulated. He was treated with a long-arm cast with extreme molding in the midforearm. On cast removal at 6 weeks, he was noted to have a flexion contracture of the thumb and fingers. The fingers could be extended, but only with maximal wrist flexion. He could actively flex his fingers into a full fist. At 9 months postinjury, the patient underwent a flexor origin slide. He was casted with the wrist, fingers, and thumb in maximum extension for 6 weeks after surgery. At 10-year follow-up, he is working in light construction and builds motorcycles. He reports that he is satisfied with his grip strength and notes occasional fatigue in the forearm with prolonged use. **A:** Preoperative finger position with wrist in neutral. **B:** Improved passive finger extension with wrist in flexion. **C:** Preoperative finger flexion. **D:** There is mild shortening of the affected left forearm. **E:** He has full finger extension with a slight thumb interphalangeal joint flexion contracture when the wrist is in full extension. **F:** He has full finger flexion with good grip strength. (Copyright Milan Stevanovic and Frances Sharpe.)

PEARLS AND PITFALLS

- The surgical incision is extensile. For a "mild-type" Volkmann's contracture or a pseudo-Volkmann's contracture, an incision at the proximal to midforearm may be sufficient to release the flexor digitorum profundus (FDP) from its ulnar and IOM origin and allow correction of a FDP contracture.
- Frequent passive extension of the wrist and fingers helps to identify structures that remain tight. The release is complete when full passive wrist and finger extension is achieved.
- Tenolysis of the flexor tendons at the pronator quadratus or at the carpal tunnel may be necessary if complete flexor origin slide fails to achieve full extension.
- Inaccurate preoperative assessment of flexor muscle strength may lead to suboptimal grip strength following correction of the contracture. *Prevention*: Finger flexion strength may be difficult to assess preoperatively. Careful clinical examination and preoperative MRI when indicated can help in identifying compromised flexor muscles. Even careful examination may not predict outcome. It is important to advise the patient and family that a possible outcome of surgery is that there may be correction of the wrist and finger position, but inadequate functional strength. The possible need for additional surgery such as tendon transfer or functional free muscle transfer helps to guide patient and family expectations.
- Inadequate wrist and finger extensor strength after contracture release. Wrist and finger extensor strength may be difficult to assess preoperatively because of the preoperative contracture. The extensor compartment may be compromised by the original injury, or further insult to the extensor compartment may be caused by surgical injury to the posterior interosseous artery. *Prevention*: Preoperative assessment and MRI where indicated may help identify extensor weakness. Preoperative discussion with the patient and family may help manage patient expectations and potential anticipation of additional surgeries.
- Postoperative hematoma or seroma. *Prevention*: This dissection involves an extensive release of muscle and can lead to postoperative hematoma formation. Careful hemostasis after tourniquet release and when the patient has been brought to a normotensive condition should be performed. Topical thrombin or tranexamic acid in appropriately selected patients as well as the liberal use of drains can reduce this risk.

RECOMMENDED READING

Deeney V, Kaye JJ, Geary SP, et al. Pseudo-Volkmann's contracture due to tethering of flexor digitorum profundus to fractures of the ulna in children. *J Pediatr Orthop.* 1998;18:437–440.

Eichler G, Lipscomb P. The changing treatment of Volkmann's ischemic contractures from 1955–1965 at the Mayo Clinic. *Clin Orthop Relat Res.* 1967;50:215–223.

Gosset J. Surgical desinsertion of the anterior long muscles of the forearm in the treatment of contractures and ischemic retraction. *J Chir.* 1956;72(5):487–494.

Guilleminet M, Blanchet A, Picault. Early results of the Page-Gosset operation for a one-year old Volkmann's contracture. *Lyon Chir.* 1956;51(4):464–467.

Inglis AE, Cooper W. Release of the flexor-pronator origin for flexion deformities of the hand and wrist in spastic paralysis: a study of eighteen cases. *J Bone Joint Surg Am.* 1966;48(5):847–857.

Keenan MA, Korchek JI, Botte MJ, et al. Results of transfer of the flexor digitorum superficialis tendons to the flexor digitorum profundus tendons in adults with acquired spasticity of the hand. *J Bone Joint Surg Am.* 1987;69(8):1127–1132.

Page C. An operation for the relief of flexion-contracture in the forearm. *J Bone Joint Surg Am.* 1923;3:233–234.

Sharma P, Swamy MK. Results of the Max Page muscle sliding operation for the treatment of Volkmann's ischemic contracture of the forearm. *J Orthop Traumatol.* 2012;13(4):189–196.

Stevanovic M, Sharpe F. Management of established Volkmann's contracture of the forearm in children. *Hand Clin.* 2006;22(1):99–111.

Thevenin-Lemoine C, Denormandie P, Schnitzler A, et al. Flexor origin slide for contracture of spastic finger flexor muscles: a retrospective study. *J Bone Joint Surg Am.* 2013;95(5):446–453.

White WF. Flexor muscle slide in the spastic hand: the Max Page operation. *J Bone Joint Surg Br.* 1972;54(3):453–459.

15 Soft Tissue Interposition Flaps in the Management of Heterotopic Ossification and Proximal Radioulnar Synostosis

M. Claire Manske, Douglas P. Hanel, and Seth D. Dodds

The elbow and forearm play a critical role in upper extremity function to position the hand in space. Loss of motion of the elbow or forearm following trauma is severely debilitating, impairing activities of daily living, occupational obligations, and recreational activities. Heterotopic ossification (HO) about the elbow can be one of the causes of poor joint motion following trauma. This complication of elbow trauma is poorly tolerated, rarely compensated for by adjacent joints, and often requires surgical intervention.

Proximal radioulnar synostosis is a specific type of heterotopic ossification consisting of the formation of a bony bridge between the radius and ulna limiting forearm rotation. It most commonly occurs following forearm fractures but can also occur secondary to crush injuries, burns, congenital anomalies and biceps tendon repair. The incidence of proximal radioulnar synostosis following forearm fractures is estimated at 1.2% to 6.6%, but the rate of synostosis is higher with certain risk factors. Concomitant closed head injury, soft tissue trauma (including crush or burn injuries), and interosseous membrane instability all predispose to radioulnar synostosis. The location of forearm fractures is also predictive, with proximal forearm fractures being at greater risk than distal forearm fractures, especially when the fractures of the radius and ulna occur at the same level or when the ulna fracture is proximal to the radius fracture. Finally, surgical technique during operative fixation of forearm fractures may contribute; iatrogenic disruption of the interosseous membrane, surgical implants extending into the interosseous space, and failure to clear bony fragments and reamings from of the surgical field are associated with increased risk of radioulnar synostosis.

INDICATIONS/CONTRAINDICATIONS

The indication for surgery in the setting of proximal radioulnar synostosis is a loss of forearm rotation causing functional limitations. Normal forearm rotation is 76 degrees of pronation and 82 degrees of supination; however, most tasks require a much smaller arc of motion, from 50 degrees of pronation to 50 degrees of supination. Any decrease in this 100 degrees of functional arc of motion should prompt consideration of surgical intervention. In addition, radioulnar synostosis may occur in association with heterotopic ossification and capsular contracture about the elbow, limiting elbow flexion and/or extension and further impairing upper extremity function. Concomitant pathology limiting elbow motion to less than a 30 to 130 degrees of arc of motion must also be addressed. If elbow contractures exist, we prefer to stage corrective procedures, with contracture release and excision of heterotopic ossification about the elbow being performed first, with radioulnar synostosis release 3 months later. It should be noted that physical therapy is rarely effective in improving limited range of motion in the setting of ectopic ossification and radioulnar synostosis. Consequently, we do not advocate for a prolonged course of therapy in patients with clear synostosis or heterotopic ossification limiting motion.

Surgery may be contraindicated in several situations including active infection and a compromised soft tissue envelope. Moreover, surgery should not occur until ossification is mature, as demonstrated by the presence of well-rounded cortical edges and cessation of progressive expansion on radiographs. Additional contraindications to surgery include the presence of degenerative joint changes that may be better managed with elbow arthroplasty, inability to participate in postoperative rehabilitation, comorbid medical conditions precluding surgery, and symptoms insufficiently bothersome to warrant surgery.

PREOPERATIVE PLANNING

As with any surgical procedure, preoperative evaluation begins by determining a patient's principle concern. Patients with radioulnar synostosis complain of stiffness and the inability to rotate the forearm. If the heterotopic ossifications involve the distal humerus or proximal ulna, limited elbow flexion and extension may be present as well. Pain is typically not the predominant symptom in radioulnar synostosis with or without heterotypic ossification about the elbow. The presence of pain, especially in the midarc of motion, should alert the clinician to look for another source of symptoms, including fracture nonunion, degenerative joint changes, elbow or forearm instability, or peripheral nerve compression, which are not addressed by procedures aimed at improving elbow and forearm motion. A thorough understanding of the original injury, associated injuries (especially closed head injuries), and subsequent treatments should be sought and often provide insight into the causes of impaired motion. Knowledge of previous treatments, including surgical procedures, allows surgeons to establish an appropriate treatment plan and anticipate intraoperative findings; operative reports are particularly helpful in determining the need to remove surgical implants, identify transposed neurovascular structures, and avoid complications. In addition, any history of neurologic deficit, both peripheral and central, is important to elucidate because they may influence surgical treatment or the ability to participate in postoperative rehabilitation. In particular, surgeons should inquire about parasthesias or motor deficits, which may indicate a compressive peripheral neuropathy. Finally, the patient's occupation, recreational activities, and postoperative goals should be discussed to determine their expectations and functional demands, as well as to establish realistic goals postoperatively.

On clinical exam, the clinician should assess the status of the soft tissue envelope and note the location of previous incisions in relation to palpable and radiographic landmarks. Areas of pain, swelling, and erythema suggest alternative causes that may need to be addressed in addition or prior to a surgery aimed at restoring elbow and forearm motion. Elbow stability, elbow flexion and extension, and forearm rotation should be documented and correlated with imaging findings. Wrist and hand function are also assessed. Finally, it is important to perform and document a thorough neurovascular exam to determine if there is involvement of these structures that needs to be addressed and to compare postoperative findings with the preoperative evaluation. Sensation should be objectively documented with 2-point discrimination or monofilament testing. Motor function should be quantified on a 5-point scale. If sensory or motor dysfunction is present on exam, electrodiagnostic studies should be obtained prior to surgery.

We routinely obtain AP, lateral, and oblique radiographs of the elbow and AP and lateral radiographs of the forearm to identify the extent of ectopic ossification or synostosis (Fig. 15-1). It is helpful to classify the extent of synostosis using the Jupiter and Ring modification of the Vince and Miller classification of proximal radioulnar synostosis, as this influences surgical management:

- Type I: distal third of forearm
- Type II: middle third of forearm
- Type IIIA: proximal third of forearm, distal to the bicipital tuberosity

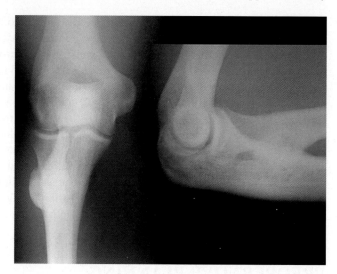

FIGURE 15-1

The anteroposterior and lateral elbow radiographs of a 42-year-old power lifter 8 weeks after a single incision repair of distal biceps tendon rupture. The forearm is ankylosed in mid pronation-supination.

- Type IIIB: synostosis of the radial head and proximal radioulnar joint
- Type IIIC: proximal forearm synostosis contiguous with heterotopic bone extending to the distal humerus

An axial CT scan of the elbow and forearm with coronal and sagittal reformatted images is useful to elucidate the location of heterotopic ossification and radioulnar synostoses (Fig. 15-2). A preoperative CT scan will also demonstrate the status of the articular surfaces, including degenerative changes or joint incongruity, which may require an alternative treatment strategy. For fracture malunions or complex deformity, three-dimensional reconstructions of CT imaging can be helpful. If there are concerns about the integrity of the blood supply to the soft tissue envelope or a pedicle interposition flap is being considered, a CT angiogram or formal vascular studies of the extremity can be obtained. Unless there is concern for infection, we do not routinely obtain tests to assess infection or inflammatory status (complete blood count [CBC], erythrocyte sedimentation rate [ESR], c-reactive protein [CRP], joint aspiration).

The timing of surgical intervention is controversial. There is insufficient evidence in the scientific literature to support the use of nuclear medicine scans or blood alkaline phosphatase levels to guide operative intervention, as both of these have been shown to be unreliable determinants of bony maturation or risk of recurrent ectopic ossification. Rather, we proceed when the heterotopic ossification is mature on x-rays, as indicated by stable-size and well-delineated borders. Typically, this occurs within 4 to 12 months of injury.

Excision of heterotopic ossification, synostosis resection, and soft tissue interposition requires little special equipment. The equipment we routinely have available is listed in Table 15-1.

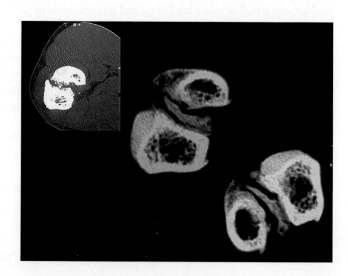

FIGURE 15-2

Coronal CT image reveals the extent of heterotopic bone involvement in the region of the bicipital tuberosity.

TABLE 15-1	Operative Equipment for Soft Tissue Interposition Flap Surgery	
Standard Equipment	**Optional Equipment**

Standard Equipment	Optional Equipment
• Sterile tourniquet	• Fluoroscopy
• Wide retractors	• Hardware removal instruments
• Lamina spreader	• Total elbow arthroplasty
• Vessel loops	• Lidocaine infusion pump
• Rongeurs (including Kerrison and pituitary osteotomes and curettes)	• Continuous passive motion machine
• Suture anchors	• Postoperative radiation therapy
• Hinged elbow distractor	• Static progressive splinting
• Tensor fascia lata allograft	
• Closed suction drain	

SURGERY

Anatomy

Operating on the elbow and proximal forearm requires a detailed understanding of the osseous, ligamentous, and neurovascular structures for efficient surgical dissection, to address all relevant pathology, and avoid iatrogenic injury. The relationships among these structures are described in further detail in the discussion of surgical technique; however, the following provides a brief overview.

The osseous structures of the forearm, the radius and ulna, articulate with the distal humerus proximally to form the radiocapitellar and ulnohumeral joints of the elbow, respectively. They articulate with the carpus distally to form the wrist joint and with each other both proximally and distally to form the proximal and distal radioulnar joints; it is these articulations between the radius and ulna that permit forearm rotation. Relative to the longitudinally straight ulna, the radius is bowed; maintaining the straight ulna and curved radius, especially during fracture fixation, is necessary for forearm rotation. Disruption of this relationship may also limit forearm rotation, even in the absence of ectopic ossification.

Between the radius and ulna is the interosseous membrane, a complex confluence of oblique fibers that forms a radioulnar syndesmosis. In addition to participating in force transmission from the radius to the ulna, the interosseous membrane provides stability between the radius and ulna and serves as the origin for forearm muscles that participate in forearm rotation. The width of the interosseous membrane is greatest in the distal and middle thirds of the forearm and narrower proximally where the radius and ulna are closer together. The small size of this space may explain the predisposition of proximal forearm fractures to limitations in forearm motion, as any ectopic ossification in this area interferes with the ability of the radius to rotate about the ulna.

The pertinent neurovascular structures in the anterior elbow include the median nerve, brachial artery, and radial nerve. Just proximal to the elbow joint, there is a constant relationship from medial to lateral of the median nerve, brachial artery, and biceps brachii tendon. The median nerve then enters the cubital fossa by passing deep to the lacertus fibrosus and anterior to the brachialis muscle. In the proximal forearm, the median nerve supplies the pronator teres, palmaris longus, and flexor carpi radialis. The median nerve enters the forearm between the deep and superficial heads of the pronator teres and then travels through an arch created by the two heads of the flexor digitorum sublimis. Approximately 5 cm distal to this arch, the anterior interosseous nerve branches from the median nerve proper, to supply the flexor digitorum profundus, flexor pollicis longus, and pronator teres.

The brachial artery lies just lateral to the median nerve in the distal arm and passes under the lacertus fibrosis with the median nerve to enter the forearm. Approximately 1 cm distal to the elbow joint, at the level of the radial neck, the brachial artery bifurcates into the radial and ulnar arteries, which both provide collateral branches to supply the elbow prior to continuing distally on their respective sides of the forearm. The radial recurrent branch of the radial artery deserves particular mention, as the first major branch, arising from the radial artery at the level of the radial neck and traveling proximally between branches of the radial nerve to supply the brachialis and brachioradialis. The radial artery then runs deep to the brachioradialis, where its branches supply the brachioradialis distally. Care must be taken when working on the lateral side of the elbow to protect the branches of both the radial nerve and artery.

The radial nerve also passes anterior to the elbow, in the interval between the brachialis and brachioradialis, and then continues into the forearm in the interval between the brachialis and extensor carpi radialis longus (ECRL). As it enters the forearm, it branches into superficial and deep branches at approximately the level of the radiocapitellar joint. The superficial branch continues as the sensory branch of the radial nerve, passing anterior to the supinator to run deep to the brachioradialis into the distal forearm. The deep branch continues as the posterior interosseous nerve (PIN), diving deep to the supinator muscle through a fibrous opening in the proximal edge of the superficial head (arcade of Frohse). The PIN passes obliquely through the supinator, crossing the neck of the radius to enter the dorsal extensor compartment of the forearm. When the supinator or neck of the radius is involved with heterotopic bone, the PIN is at risk of injury and must be protected throughout the dissection.

In the medial arm, ulnar nerve is located anterior to the medial intermuscular septum until it pierces through the septum approximately 8 to 10 cm proximal to the medial epicondyle and lies posterior to the septum as it courses distally, passing dorsal to the medial epicondyle of the elbow and entering the forearm between the two heads of the flexor carpi ulnaris. It is at risk with excision of heterotopic ossification of the medial elbow and forearm, as it may become encased in heterotopic bone. In addition, after release of chronic elbow contracture, improved elbow extension may result in neurapraxic injury to the ulnar nerve postoperatively.

The posterior aspect of the elbow is void of neurovascular structures, with the only exception being the radial nerve. The radial nerve crosses the posterior humerus from medial to lateral, at approximately 11 cm proximal to the lateral epicondyle.

Patient Positioning

The patient is positioned supine on a well-padded operating table. Either a general anesthetic or brachial plexus block may be used. Although the operative upper extremity may be positioned across the patient's chest, we prefer the limb abducted from the torso and placed on a hand table. If the shoulder is mobile, external rotation provides access to the medial and anterior elbow, while internal rotation allows access to the posterior and lateral elbow. This position also allows easy access to the forearm for intraoperative fluoroscopy.

The extremity is then prepped and draped from the fingertips proximally to the axilla and clavicle. We recommend having a sterile tourniquet available, but prefer not to use a tourniquet, as it limits tissue mobilization, causes venous engorgement during prolonged cases, obscures small vessel bleeding, and causes reactive hyperemia when the tourniquet is deflated. Rather, we inject the planned incision with local anesthetic mixed with 1/200,000 epinephrine after the limb is prepped, which provides excellent hemostasis when the injection is performed approximately 20 minutes prior to skin incision.

Technique

The goal of surgical intervention is to excise all impediments to forearm and elbow motion and minimize risk of recurrent synostosis. The specific surgical techniques vary based on the pathology to be addressed. Described below is our technique for excision of heterotopic bone limiting elbow flexion and extension, resection of radioulnar synostosis limiting forearm rotation, and soft tissue interposition to prevent recurrence.

Excision of Heterotopic Ossification at the Elbow

The essential components of heterotopic bone excision to improve elbow motion are:

- Remove all HO from the brachialis, triceps, and adjacent to collateral ligaments.
- Release the anterior and posterior joint capsules.
- Clear the coronoid and olecranon fossa of fat, synovium, and bony impediments to motion.
- Decompress and transpose the ulnar nerve.
- Assess elbow instability and repair/reconstruct collateral ligaments if necessary.

INCISION. We do not use a tourniquet for the reasons described above. After the limb is prepped and draped, the planned incision is injected with 0.25% bupivacaine with 1/200,000 epinephrine prior to skin incision. The choice of skin incision is influenced in part by location of heterotopic ossification and location of previous incisions. Ideally, existing incisions are incorporated into the surgical approach, but the safest approach to the ectopic ossification to be resected should be utilized. A posterior skin incision for elbow release surgery provides circumferential access to the medial, lateral, anterior, and posterior elbow, as well as avoiding injury to the medial and lateral antebrachial cutaneous nerves supplying the forearm. Separate medial and lateral incisions can be used, if preferred, using the same medial and lateral intermuscular intervals as in the posterior approach. An anterior approach to the elbow for heterotopic ossification excision is of little utility, indicated only for isolated flexion contractures with full flexion and no evidence of bony or soft tissue pathology posteriorly.

The posterior approach begins with a longitudinal skin incision along the posterior elbow with a 15 blade scalpel; ideally, the incision is just medial or lateral to the olecranon to avoid a scar, which may be painful if directly over the olecranon tip. The length of the incision depends on the extent of heterotopic ossification, but can extend from the proximal arm to the distal forearm. Sharp dissection is performed down to the triceps fascia proximally and to the extensor fascia along the subcutaneous border of the ulna distally. Full-thickness medial and lateral skin flaps are elevated, with care to identify and protect the ulnar nerve medially.

MEDIAL EXPOSURE. After full-thickness skin flaps are raised, the ulnar nerve is identified proximally in the arm where it crosses the medial intermuscular septum, approximately 8 to 10 cm proximal to the medial epicondyle, outside of the zone of dense scarring. The nerve is followed distally through the cubital tunnel and through the two heads of flexor carpi ulnaris, releasing all constricting structures, including heterotopic ossification that may be encasing the nerve; freer elevators, synovial and Kerrison rongeurs, and osteotomes are helpful for this task. The nerve is then mobilized from the cubital tunnel with a cuff of medial triceps to preserve the vascular supply; a latex-free Penrose drain can be looped around the nerve to atraumatically manipulate the nerve during exposure and transposition (Fig. 15-3). The medial intermuscular septum, supracondylar ridge of the humerus, and flexor-pronator origin are then identified. The medial intermuscular septum is exposed down to its insertion on the humerus and then excised completely, with care to identify and cauterize the crossing vessels. This facilitates exposure of the brachialis muscle. The brachialis muscle is elevated off the supracondylar ridge proximally and the flexor-pronator mass elevated off the medial epicondyle distally. The interval between the brachialis and the anterior elbow capsule with its associated ectopic ossification is developed, protecting the median nerve and brachial artery just anterior to the brachialis. As the flexor-pronator mass is elevated from the medial epicondyle and proximal ulna, care should be taken to preserve the medial collateral ligament if possible, especially the anterior band that lies deep the flexor carpi ulnaris, to

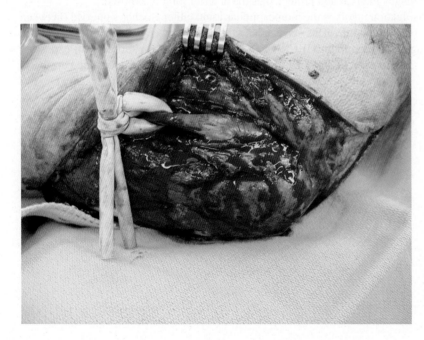

FIGURE 15-3

This previously "transposed ulnar nerve" sits directly on the medial epicondyle. It is essential to identify and protect the ulnar nerve before proceeding with capsular and heterotopic bone resection.

prevent elbow instability; in chronic severe contractures, release of the posterior band of the medial collateral ligament may be indicated.

Exposed ectopic ossification on the medial side is then excised with a combination of an oscillating saw, osteotomes, and rongeurs. Contracted anterior capsule should be excised with the heterotopic bone. When the coronoid fossa is encountered, it should be cleared of fat and synovium. As the excision proceeds radially, the radial nerve is at risk in the depth of the exposure; if lateral heterotopic ossification requires excision, a lateral approach should be used so that the radial nerve can be identified and protected during ectopic bone excision.

With any procedure that will result in increased elbow extension, we routinely perform an anterior submuscular ulnar nerve transposition at the conclusion of the procedure. Many patients present with ulnar nerve symptoms preoperatively, and even among patients without ulnar nerve symptoms, improvement in elbow range of motion postoperatively carries risk of increased traction on the ulnar nerve postoperatively. If a submuscular ulnar nerve transposition is performed, the median nerve must be exposed, which we find easiest to do just prior to excision of the medial intermuscular septum, by tracing the septum to its insertion on the humerus and identifying the nerve just anterior to the brachialis muscle; alternatively, the median nerve may be more easily identified distally, deep to the lacertus fibrosis.

LATERAL EXPOSURE. In a manner similar to the medial side, a full-thickness fasciocutaneous flap is elevated from the triceps to the lateral side of the elbow. A lateral column approach proximally and Kocher or Kaplan approach distally are used to expose the elbow joint. In the proximal aspect of the surgical field, the brachioradialis and extensor carpi radialis longus are identified and elevated from the supracondylar ridge and medial epicondyle to expose the underlying brachialis (Fig. 15-4). At this point in the procedure, we recommend identifying the radial nerve so it can be protected. The radial nerve exits the arm in the interval between the brachialis and brachioradialis and enters the forearm in the interval between the brachioradialis and extensor carpi radialis longus. In densely scarred tissue, the radial nerve may not be easily identified in these intervals. Several techniques can be used to locate the radial nerve in areas of dense scarring. One strategy is to locate the posterior antebrachial cutaneous branch of the radial nerve that can often be in the undersurface of the lateral skin flap (Fig. 15-5). The nerve is traced proximally to the lateral intermuscular septum at its branch point from the radial nerve proper. Alternatively, the insertion of the lateral intermuscular septum on the lateral epicondyle is identified and followed proximally by carefully releasing the triceps muscle off the septum. Branches of the radial nerve (lateral brachial cutaneous nerve, posterior antebrachial cutaneous nerve) are identified as they cross the septum, which can then be traced back to the radial nerve proper, where it pierces the septum between 6 and 10 cm proximal to the tip of the lateral epicondyle. After the radial nerve has been identified, it can be traced distal to the brachioradialis-extensor carpi radialis longus interval and protected as the anterior joint is exposed.

If the heterotopic ossification involves the radiocapitellar joint, either Kocher's interval (between extensor carpi ulnaris [ECU] and anconeus) or Kaplan's interval (between extensor carpi radialis brevis and extensor digitorum communis [ECRB-EDC]) may be used for more distal exposure. After either the ECU-anconeus or ECRB-EDC intermuscular plane is developed, the capsule is

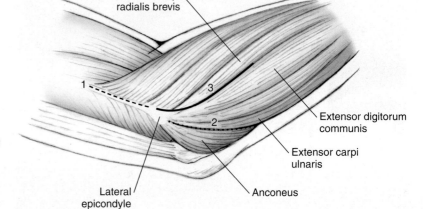

FIGURE 15-4

Three intervals to approach the anterior elbow. (*1*) Partial elevation of the muscles taking origin from the lateral epicondyle, the brachioradialis, and cephalad portion extensor carpi ulnaris. (*2*) Anconeus and extensor carpi ulnaris. (*3*) Extensor carpi radialis brevis and extensor digitorum communis.

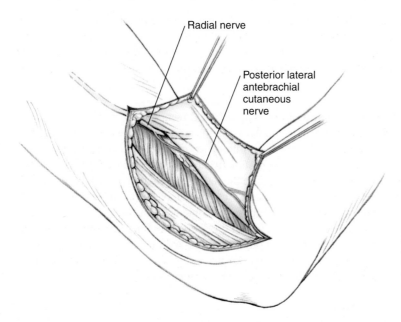

FIGURE 15-5

The posterior antebrachial cutaneous nerve is identified distally and followed proximally into the lateral intermuscular septum. This cutaneous nerve leads to the radial nerve proper.

incised along the anterior border of the lateral ulnar collateral ligament (Fig. 15-6). If needed, the proximal fibers of the supinator are elevated subperiosteally. As long as the dissection remains subperiosteal, the PIN is protected within the substance of the supinator as it crosses the radial neck 3 to 4 cm distal to the radiocapitellar joint.

As heterotopic bone is encountered, blunt elevators are used to dissect it free from the surrounding muscle but not the underlying joint capsule, so the capsule and heterotopic bone can be excised

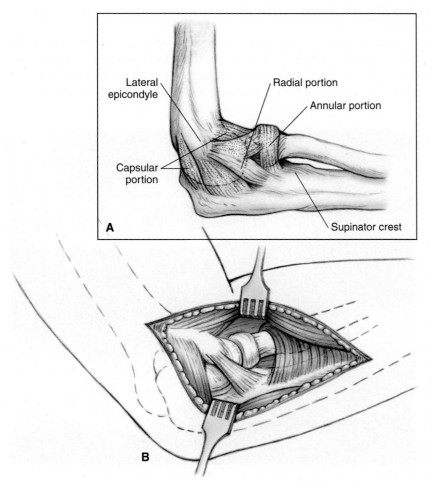

FIGURE 15-6

A: Lateral collateral ligament complex of the elbow consisting of the capsular, radial, and annular portions (*stippled*) removed to expose the lateral elbow articulations. **B:** The *stippled portion* of **(A)** has been removed, exposing the radial head and neck and the distal humerus. Preserving the ulnar portion of the lateral collateral ligament (*shaded area*), when possible, preserves elbow stability.

as a unit. Dissection proceeds medially until the coronoid is encountered or the ectopic ossification becomes confluent with the forearm bones. We find it helpful to place a blunt right-angled retractor in interval between the brachialis muscle and the underlying capsule to allow direct visualization during excision of the heterotopic ossification and contracted anterior capsule to minimize the risk of neurovascular injury.

POSTERIOR EXPOSURE. Lastly, the posterior elbow is approached from the lateral side by elevating the triceps from the lateral column and posterior humerus. With care to preserve the triceps insertion on the olecranon, the interval between the triceps and posterior joint capsule is developed with a blunt elevator. The radial nerve crosses the posterior humerus approximately 11 cm proximal to the lateral epicondyle, so care should be taken not to injure the radial nerve when using a blunt elevator to release the triceps off the distal humerus. The posterior capsule and associated heterotopic ossification are excised to improve elbow flexion and to expose the contents of the olecranon fossa. Using rongeurs and osteotomes, the olecranon fossa is cleared of fat, synovium, fracture callus, heterotopic ossification, and any other impediments to elbow motion. If necessary, the posteromedial elbow can be approached by working on the medial side of the triceps and incising the posterior band of the medial collateral ligament to access the medial side of the posterior elbow joint.

Proximal Radioulnar Synostosis Resection

For patients with isolated proximal radioulnar synostosis without heterotopic ossification affecting ulnohumeral joint motion (type IIIA and IIIB), a lateral approach to the elbow may be used (Fig. 15-7A, B). The lateral epicondyle, olecranon, and radial head are identified by palpation, and an oblique incision paralleling the interval between the anconeus and extensor carpi ulnaris is made from lateral supracondylar ridge of the humerus across the lateral epicondyle to the subcutaneous border of the ulna. Electrocautery is used to dissect through the subcutaneous tissue and scar down to the extensor fascia, which is incised from the lateral epicondyle along the interval of the anconeus and extensor carpi ulnaris. If proximal exposure is needed to improve visualization, the incision may be extended in line with the humeral shaft and a lateral column approach performed as described for elbow heterotopic bone excision.

The radioulnar synostosis is exposed from the lateral side by elevating the anconeus and extensor carpi ulnaris with electrocautery as a full-thickness flap from the posterior lateral aspect of the ulna. The flap is elevated from distal to proximal with care to preserve the proximal insertion of the anconeus to protect the recurrent posterior interosseous artery supplying the flap as well as

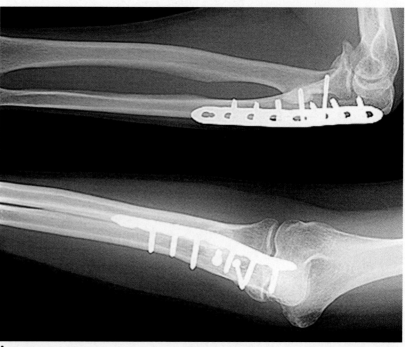

FIGURE 15-7

A: The patient developed radioulnar synostosis after treatment of a Monteggia fracture.   **A**

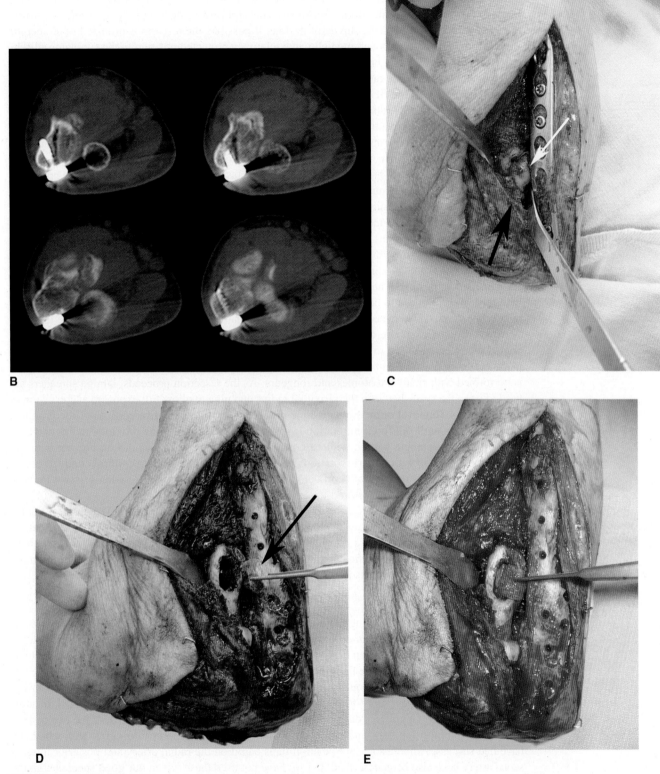

FIGURE 15-7 (*Continued*)

B: The CT scans demonstrate the location of the synostosis adjacent to the tuberosity. **C:** The entire anconeus and extensor carpi ulnaris complex have been elevated from the ulna (*black arrow*), exposing the bridge of heterotopic bone between the radius and ulna (*white arrow*). **D:** The synostosis encased the bicipital tuberosity and tendon. The ectopic bone was removed and the tendon left attached to a block of heterotopic bone (*arrow*). The resection exposed the medullary canal of the radius. The fixation plate was removed. **E:** The medullary canal is packed with allograft bone chips to minimize extrusion of marrow content. The biceps tendon and attached bone block are pushed into the medullary canal and secured with a stout nonabsorbable suture.

the lateral collateral ligament of the elbow. The dissection proceeds radially across the ulna to the interosseous space at the site of the synostosis. The supinator is elevated subperiosteally to protect the PIN in the substance of the supinator muscle. If possible, the forearm is pronated to protect the PIN by moving it anteriorly and medially, in a relatively protected position in the supinator muscle. Alternatively, the PIN may be identified via a separate anterior incision adjacent to the ulnar border of the brachioradialis. The radial nerve proper is identified in the interval between the brachioradialis and brachialis and traced distally until its bifurcation into the PIN and the superficial branch of the radial nerve. The PIN is then dissected distally into the supinator, where the arcade of Frohse and any additional compressive tissue or scar is excised (Fig. 15-7C–E).

Occasionally, an anterior approach is needed for complete radioulnar synostosis excision in addition to the lateral approach. An incision along the ulnar border of the brachioradialis from the elbow flexion crease to the distal forearm is made with a scalpel. The fascia along the ulnar border of the brachioradialis is identified and the muscle elevated to identify the superficial branch of the radial nerve along its undersurface. The superficial branch of the radial nerve is traced proximally into the antecubital fossa to its origin from the radial nerve. All branches of the radial nerve must be identified and protected, including its branches to the brachioradialis, extensor carpi radialis longus (ECRL), and most importantly, the PIN. The PIN is then dissected distally into the supinator where the arcade of Frohse (the stout fibers of the proximal edge of the supinator) is released to prevent nerve compression. In addition to identification of neurologic structures, the radial artery and the radial recurrent artery along with their branches need to be preserved. In the anterior dissection, the median and ulnar nerves are relatively protected by the medially retracted flexor-pronator mass on the ulnar aspect of the forearm.

After adequate exposure of the synostosis and protection of the PIN, broad Homan or right-angled retractors are used to maintain visualization; anecdotally, narrow retractors are thought to place excessive pressure on neurovascular structures, especially the PIN. Excision of the synostosis is performed with small osteotomes and rongeurs. As the resection proceeds, lamina spreaders are used to open the space between the proximal radius and ulna to allow full exposure and excision of the synostosis. Removal of heterotopic bone proceeds down to the native cortices of the proximal radius and ulna until full forearm rotation is restored. The cortices of the proximal radius and ulna are debrided to a smooth border, without bony prominences or sharp spicules, to prevent injury to the interposition flap with forearm rotation. Image intensification is used to confirm complete resection of the synostosis and smooth cortical edges. The resection is complete when passive forearm pronation and supination are restored.

Several precautions against recurrent synostosis are undertaken at this time. The surgical field is irrigated with 3 L of normal saline, followed by meticulous hemostasis with bipolar electrocautery. Exposed cancellous surfaces are covered with bone wax, and any exposure of the intramedullary canal due to a breach in the cortical surface is packed with cancellous allograft soaked in thrombin to prevent efflux of marrow cells into the excision bed.

Soft Tissue Interposition

Soft tissue interposition following radioulnar synostosis resection is recommended to prevent recurrent ectopic ossification and lessen pain with forearm rotation. Numerous synthetic and biologic interposition materials have been described, including bone wax, silicone sheets, free nonvascularized grafts, vascularized pedicle flaps, and vascularized free flaps.

Synthetic grafts have fallen out of favor, given that biologic grafts have been shown to have a superior ability to prevent scar formation compared to synthetic grafts in an animal model. In addition, the use of free fat grafts is discouraged given the risk of dislodgment. We describe two pedicle myofascial interposition flaps and one nonvascularized biologic interposition graft with which we have had success. Adipofascial interposition flaps based on the radial artery and posterior interosseous artery have also been described, but we have not used these, given our good success with the anconeus, brachioradialis, and tensor fascia lata grafts described below.

Pedicled Anconeus Myofascial Flap Interposition

The anconeus myofascial flap is a thin pedicled flap well suited for type III proximal radioulnar synostosis. Owing to its small side, it does not have the excursion to address type II or I synostoses. In addition, if previous trauma or surgery has injured the muscle, it may not be a viable interposition option.

The anconeus receives its blood supply proximally from the collateral circulation of the elbow, predominantly the medial collateral artery (MCA) branch of the profunda brachii artery. It also has

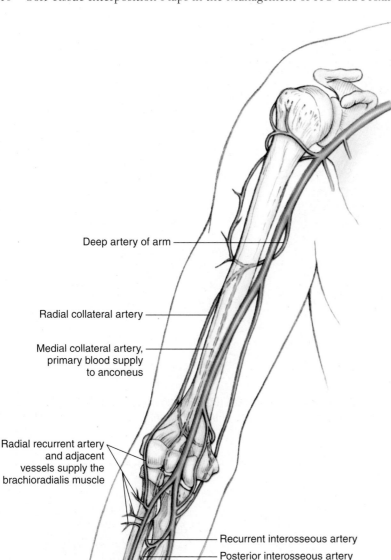

Deep artery of arm

Radial collateral artery

Medial collateral artery,
primary blood supply
to anconeus

Radial recurrent artery
and adjacent
vessels supply the
brachioradialis muscle

Recurrent interosseous artery
Posterior interosseous artery

FIGURE 15-8

The arterial anatomy of the distal arm. The medial collateral artery (MCA), a branch of the profunda brachii, is the primary blood supply to the anconeus. The radial recurrent artery (RRA), a branch of the radial artery, and small arterial branches within 3 cm of the RRA provide the primary blood supply to the brachioradialis muscle.

a distal vascular supply from the recurrent posterior interosseous artery, which is sacrificed during flap mobilization (Figs. 15-8 and 15-9). The anconeus is elevated by the posterior border of the ulna from distal to proximal, beginning at the junction of the proximal and middle one-third of the ulna. Elevation proceeds proximally until the flap is sufficiently mobile to reach the distal extent of the synostosis. Care must be taken to preserve the insertion of the anconeus on the lateral epicondyle and its attachment to the triceps to avoid disrupting its proximal vascular supply. With the forearm pronated, the anconeus is then rotated into the interosseous space and its distal edge secured to the ulnar aspect of the biceps tuberosity with sutures in the biceps tendon or suture anchors in the proximal radius. We use a stout nonabsorbable suture in a mattress or Bunnel locking fashion. With forearm supination, the flap advances into the interosseous space at the site of previous synostosis, creating an effective barrier against recurrent ectopic ossification (Fig. 15-10).

Additional applications of the proximally based anconeus myofascial flap have been described. This flap can be used for coverage of soft tissue defects around the elbow, including the lateral epicondyle, posterior olecranon, and the radial olecranon at the triceps insertion. The muscle is elevated, rotated into the defect, secured in position, and covered with a split-thickness skin graft. This flap has also been used as an interposition flap between the capitellum and proximal radius following radial head excision or failed radial head arthroplasty, as described by Morrey

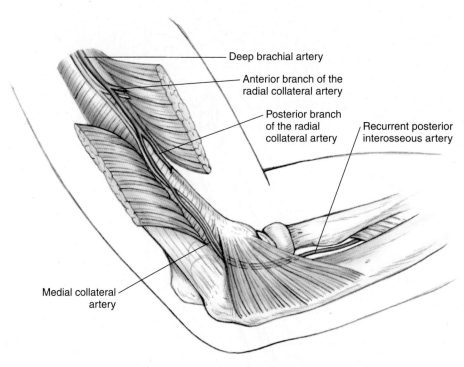

FIGURE 15-9

In addition to the medial collateral artery (MCA), the anconeus receives blood supply distally from the recurrent posterior interosseous artery (RPIA). The MCA and RPIA are frequently sacrificed in the process of elevating this flap.

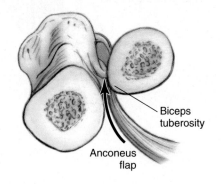

FIGURE 15-10

With the forearm placed in full pronation, the distal end of the anconeus flap is attached to the ulnar edge of the biceps tuberosity with a suture anchor or direct stitch into the biceps tuberosity. As the forearm is supinated (*arrow*), the anconeus will be drawn into the proximal radioulnar space.

and Schneeberger (Fig. 15-11). Three interposition options are described: type I, interposition into the radiocapitellar joint; type II, into the proximal radioulnar joint, posterior to the intact fibers of the lateral ulnar collateral ligament; and type III, as a proximal radioulnar wrap. After interposition, the flap is secured with stout nonabsorbable sutures placed through drill holes. Distally based anconeus flaps based on the recurrent posterior interosseous artery have also been described for management of soft tissue defects around the elbow resulting from burns or skin avulsion. Its use is discouraged in the setting of fractures or radioulnar synostosis, given that it is a small vessel that is easily injured during fracture fixation or synostosis resection.

Pedicled Brachioradialis Myofascial Flap Interposition

The brachioradialis interposition flap, based proximally on the radial recurrent artery, is useful when both anterior and posterior approaches are needed to excise the radioulnar synostosis. After the synostosis has been excised and the surgical field prepared, the brachioradialis tendon is released distally and the muscle elevated from distal to proximal with care to cauterize or ligate branches of the underlying radial artery as well as protect the underlying superficial branch of the radial nerve.

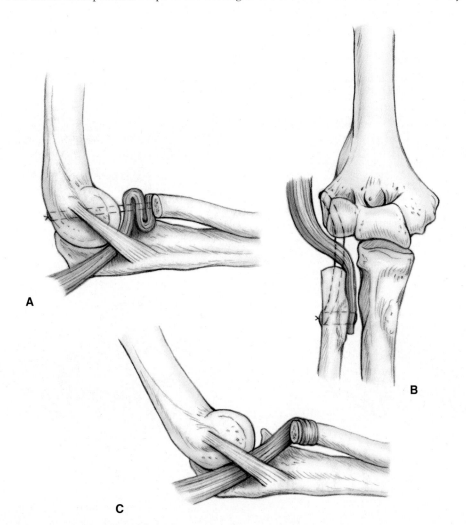

FIGURE 15-11

Three interposition options for the anconeus flap after radial head resection: type I, radiocapitellar joint; type II, radiocapitellar and proximal radioulnar joint; and type III, proximal radioulnar wrap.

Dissection proceeds until there is sufficient length to interpose between the proximal radius and ulna, with care to preserve the radial recurrent artery, which supplies the brachioradialis proximally. It is not necessary to release the brachioradialis from the lateral epicondyle or lateral intermuscular septum (Fig. 15-12).

The brachioradialis is then interposed between the radius and ulna from anterior to posterior and secured by one of two methods. One method is to secure the muscle flap to the posterior surface of the fully supinated radius with suture anchors or sutures passed through drill holes, which allows the muscle to pass/migrate into the interosseous space with pronation. The second method, described by Diego Fernandez, wraps the muscle around the proximal radius, deep to the superficial branch of the radial nerve, which is then secured to itself with locking sutures that pass through muscle fascia and tendon fibers.

Additional uses for the brachioradialis flap include coverage of medium-size soft tissue defects about the elbow, the antecubital fossa, the posterolateral elbow, or the volar forearm. Myofascial flaps and myofasciocutaneous flaps have both been described. A myofascial flap is elevated as described above, rotated into the defect and covered with a split-thickness skin graft. Alternatively, a myofasciocutaneous flap is designed with a skin paddle centered over the radial recurrent artery, extending 2 to 3 cm in width and 6 to 10 cm long from proximal to distal. The skin paddle, which can be used for flap monitoring, is rotated into the defect, and the donor defect is narrow enough to be closed primarily.

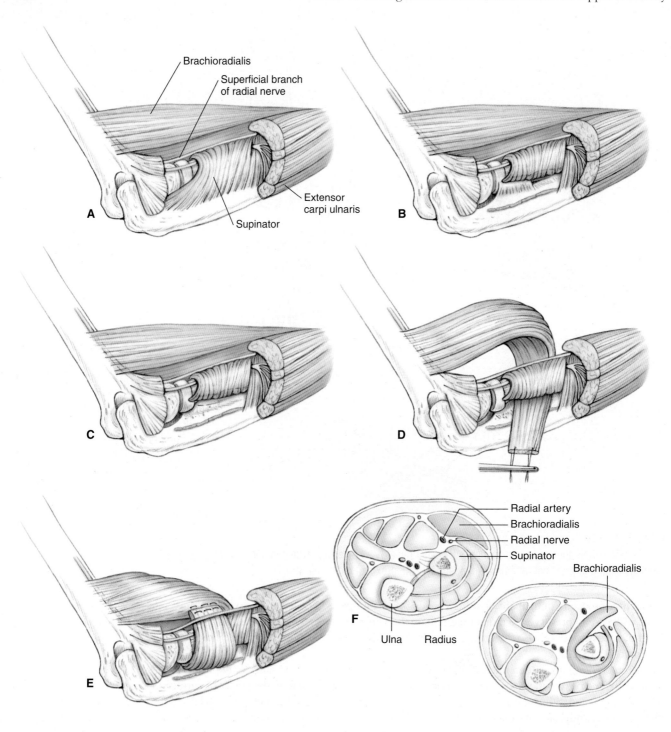

FIGURE 15-12

A: Posterior lateral approach (Kocher). Through a separate incision, the interval between the anconeus and extensor carpi ulnaris is developed. **B:** The supinator muscle is sharply elevated off the ulna, exposing the radioulnar synostosis. **C:** The synostosis is removed, and if necessary, the interosseous ligament membrane is excised. **D:** A separate anterior incision runs just ulnar to the brachioradialis muscle. The tendon is divided distally, the superficial branch of the radial nerve is separated from the under belly of the muscle, and the vascular bundles entering the muscle in the proximal forearm are preserved. The muscle is passed through the interosseous space created by the resection. **E:** The tail of the muscle is brought deep to the radial nerve and sutured to the proximal muscle belly. **F:** Cross section of the forearm. Note the muscle passes radial to the radial artery in the midforearm, distal to the biceps tendon and deep to the superficial branch of the radial nerve.

Tensor Fascia Lata Interposition

Revision surgery, extensive heterotopic ossification, or previous muscle or vascular disruption may render transposition of a local flap exceedingly difficult, if not impossible. In these situations, a tensor fascia lata graft is a desirable alternative. Both autograft and allograft tensor fascia lata grafts have been described. Although autograft has the advantage of biocompatibility, it causes significant donor site mobility, including superficial nerve injury, scaring, hematoma, and muscle herniation causing thigh asymmetry. Given the risk of complications and the recognition that neither allograft nor autograft is vascularized after harvest, we favor allograft.

We perform this procedure as described by Friedrich et al. (Fig. 15-13). After resection of the synostosis, a tensor fascia lata allograft approximately 4 to 5 cm wide and 10 to 12 cm long is obtained. The graft is then wrapped around either the radius or the ulna, whichever is more accessible, had the

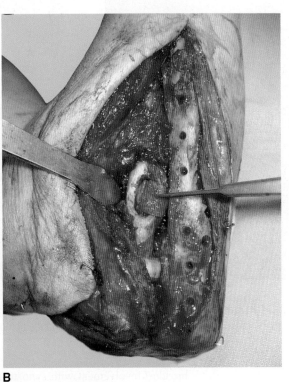

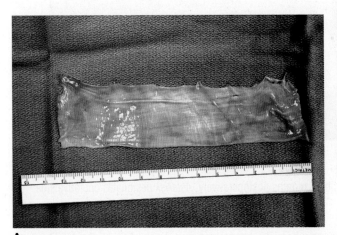

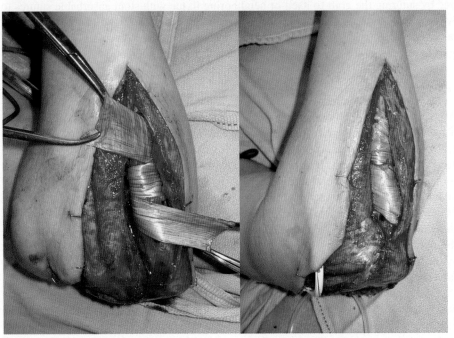

FIGURE 15-13

A: This 4 × 14–cm tensor fascia lata allograft is used as interposition material. **B:** This is the forearm of the patient shown in Figure 15-7. After synostosis resection, the rough surfaces of the radius and the ulna are prone to reformation of the synostosis. **C:** The tensor fascia lata allograft is wrapped around the ulnar and secured with stout absorbable sutures.

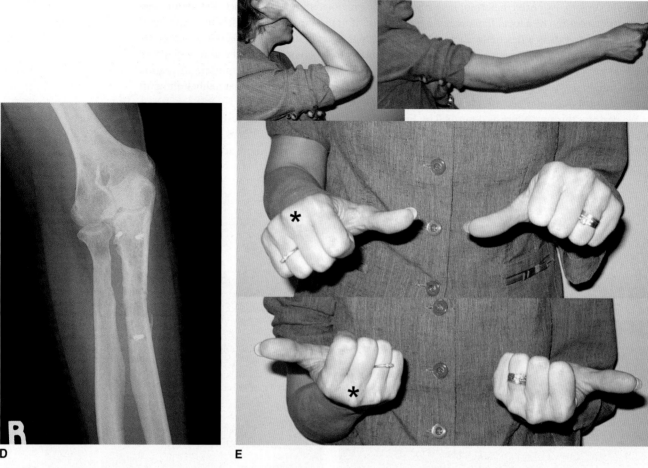

D   E

FIGURE 15-13 (Continued)
D: Radiographs of the elbow 6 months postoperatively. **E:** Range of motion 6 months postoperatively. *Asterisk* designates operative side.

broadest involvement with synostosis, or where the synostosis was deemed to originate. The graft is then secured by suturing the graft to itself or neighboring tissue with stout absorbable sutures to create a sleeve around the proximal forearm bone. Alternatively, the graft can be sutured to the ulna, interposed in the interosseous space, and secured to the pronated radius with suture anchors, which allows the graft to be drawn into the interosseous space with forearm supination.

Closure

Prior to wound closure, we recommend assessing elbow stability. If either the medial or lateral collateral ligaments were intentionally or unintentionally released during the procedure, they should be reconstructed with tendon allograft (palmaris or plantaris) and secured with suture anchors or bone tunnels. Of particular importance are the anterior band of the medial collateral ligament and the ulnar lateral collateral ligament. If stability cannot be restored with ligament reconstruction, a dynamic external fixator should be considered.

After thorough irrigation, closed suction drains are placed anteriorly and posteriorly, deep to the fascia. In addition, continuous infusion pumps delivering lidocaine or bupivacaine may be placed to augment postoperative pain control. Muscle attachments to the humerus, radius, and ulna are then repaired with suture or suture anchors. If the flexor-pronator mass was elevated for medial exposure of the elbow, the ulnar nerve may be transposed anteriorly adjacent to the median nerve prior to repair of the flexor-pronator mass; alternatively, the flexor-pronator mass can be repaired and the nerve transposed to a subcutaneous position secured with a cuff of flexor-pronator fascia. The deep fascia is closed with absorbable suture in a running or interrupted fashion, followed by subcutaneous and skin closure. Care should be taken to ensure that the skin is not under tension. A sterile soft dressing is applied to the wound to allow immediate postoperative motion.

A single-shot or "continuous catheter" brachial plexus block is placed by the anesthesia team, which provides pain relief that facilitates immediate passive range of motion postoperatively. Our patients are routinely admitted to the hospital postoperatively for initiation of continuous passive motion for flexion and extension while the block or pump is in place. After the nerve block has lapsed, transition to active and passive range-of-motion exercises, demonstrated by hand therapists, is initiated.

POSTOPERATIVE MANAGEMENT

Range-of-motion exercises are initiated on postoperative day 1. Patients with an axillary block or infusion pump are provided with continuous passive motion machines. When the block has worn off or the catheter discontinued, active and active-assisted range-of-motion exercises are initiated. With the elbow flexed to 90 degrees and an object grasped in the hand to minimize radiocarpal pronation-supination, the patient actively pronates and supinates the forearm. When not performing exercises, static progressive splints are utilized, including at night, alternating nightly between supination splints and pronation splints. We do not use dynamic splints. After 2 weeks, nighttime splinting in the position of the greatest loss of motion replaces alternating splints nightly. We recommend splinting and forearm exercises for 6 months postoperatively, after which there does not appear to be any improvement in range of motion with exercises and splints. Strengthening exercises are initiated at 6 weeks postoperatively. Anecdotally, however, patients often report that even though their range of motion does not quantitatively improve beyond 6 months, their strength and ease of motion continue for up to 2 years.

Both pharmacologic and radiologic treatments have been described to decrease the risk of recurrent ectopic ossification. Patients without a history of gastrointestinal ulcers or renal disease are prescribed ketorolac 30 mg IV as an inpatient, but we do not prescribe oral nonsteroidal anti-inflammatory medications, such as indomethacin, postoperatively, given their high potential for gastrointestinal and renal complications and low rate of patient compliance.

We do recommend perioperative radiation therapy in select patients with a high risk of recurrence, including those with recurrent ankylosis or synostosis of the radioulnar joint that extends proximal to the biceps tuberosity. After a discussion of the risk and benefits of perioperative radiation therapy, including wound breakdown, neuritis, lymphedema, and remote risk of postradiation sarcoma, in this patient population, we use a single 700-cGy dose of external beam radiation within 36 hours of surgery.

RESULTS

The ideal operative technique to treat proximal radioulnar synostosis remains unknown, with variable results reported in the scientific literature, all based on the outcomes of small groups of patients.

Early studies of patients treated with posttraumatic proximal radioulnar synostosis resection suggested a guarded prognosis. Among the first to publish their results, Vince and Miller described three patients with proximal synostosis, two of whom experienced recurrent ankylosis. Similarly, Failla et al. reported their outcomes in 20 patients treated with synostosis excision and soft tissue interposition with various materials (including silicone, polyethylene sheets, fascia, fat, and muscle). Although intraoperative passive arc of motion improved to 121 degrees (pronation 78 degrees, supination 55 degrees), the mean final active arc of motion at 40 months decreased to 55 degrees. In addition, 7 of 20 patients (35%) experience recurrent synostosis. More recent studies are more encouraging. Jupiter and Ring presented their results of proximal forearm synostosis excision in 18 forearms, 8 of which had free fat interposition, and the remaining had no interposition material. The arc of motion at final follow-up in their patient population was 139 degrees with only one patient (who had a closed head injury) experiencing recurrent synostosis.

Anconeus Interposition Flap

Daluiski et al. treated 23 patients with radioulnar synostosis with resection and anconeus interposition. They report a mean improvement in forearm rotation from 21 to 132 degrees (pronation improved from 12 to 70 degrees; supination improved from 9 to 62 degrees) at nearly 5 years postoperatively. Notably, in their series, patients with a radioulnar synostosis secondary to forearm fracture had less improvement than those with radioulnar synostosis following biceps tendon disruption and repair, which is consistent with other reports.

Bell and Berger published their small series of patients treated with forearm synostosis excision and anconeus interposition and report improvement in forearm rotation of 100, 140, and 150 degrees in each of their three patients. Morrey and Schneeberger also treated three patients with anconeus interposition for proximal forearm synostosis and found forearm arc of motion improved by a mean of 105 degrees.

Brachioradialis Interposition Flap

Fernandez and Joneschild evaluated the outcome of three patients with recurrent radioulnar synostosis treated a "wrap-around" brachioradialis flap, combining their results with those of two patients with recurrent middiaphyseal forearm synostosis treated with a "wrap-around" flexor carpi ulnaris flap. All patients were prescribed indomethacin for 3 weeks postoperatively. At a mean of 8 years of follow-up, patients had a mean of 60 degrees pronation and 54 degrees supination; no patient experienced recurrence.

Tensor Fascia Lata Interposition Graft

The outcomes of tensor fascia lata interposition following synostosis excision are also promising. Friedrich and colleagues reported their results of radioulnar synostosis excision in 13 patients treated with tensor fascia lata autograft (3 patients) or allograft (10 patients) and followed for a mean of 30 months postoperatively. The mean arch of forearm rotation improved from 9 degrees preoperatively to 124 degrees at final follow-up. Pronation improved from 14 to 62 degrees, and supination improved from −4 degrees (4 degrees of pronation) to 62 degrees.

Other Pedicled Adipofascial Flaps

Jones and colleagues reported his outcomes in one patient with a type II radioulnar synostosis treated with resection and interposition of a radial forearm adipofascial flap; preoperative, this patient's forearm was locked in a neutral position with no forearm rotation. Postoperatively, he achieved 90 degrees of pronation and 90 degrees of supination at 3 years after surgery, without radiologic evidence of recurrent synostosis. Another report by Sonderegger et al. reviewed their six patients (five with proximal radioulnar synostosis and one with distal radioulnar synostosis) treated with a pedicle adipofascial flap based on either the radial or posterior interosseous artery. They demonstrated improved forearm rotation to 76 degrees of pronation and 78 degrees of supination intraoperatively, which decreased only slightly to 70 degrees of pronation and 71 degrees of supination at a mean of 32 months postoperatively. No patients had radiographic recurrence of synostosis.

The varied outcomes in the literature with various interposition materials and adjunctive treatment suggest there is much that remains unknown with regard to proximal radioulnar synostosis. As with any reconstructive procedure, treatment must be individualized to the patient, taking into account their specific mechanism of injury, associated trauma, overall health, and expectations. Although this chapter focuses on surgical intervention, compliance with postoperative rehabilitation is paramount.

COMPLICATIONS

The most common complications of proximal forearm synostosis excision are nerve injury, wound healing difficulties, and recurrent ankylosis. Most commonly, postoperative nerve complications are neurapraxic injuries resulting from overzealous retraction. Sonderegger reported on one PIN palsy that resolved spontaneously after 4 weeks. Although complete nerve disruption is rare, they can happen in the distorted anatomy of dense scar tissue and when nerves are encased in heterotopic bone. Thorough understanding of elbow and forearm anatomy, frequent assessment of nerve location, avoiding rigorous retraction, using broad, rather than narrow retractors, and limiting the duration of retraction, can reduce nerve injuries.

Wound complications have also been reported. In his series of 13 patients, Friedrich described one postoperative wound dehiscence that required wound debridement and revision closure. Daluski reported three postoperative hematomas, including one that required surgical evacuation. Avoiding the use of a tourniquet, meticulous hemostasis with electrocautery and ligation, and the use of drains can minimize wound healing difficulties. Migration of interposition material can occur, but this risk is minimized with the use of stout sutures securely placed in muscle, fascia, or bone.

Although not truly a complication, one of the most dreaded outcomes of synostosis excision is recurrent ankylosis. In many cases, there may be evidence of recurrent calcification on radiographs, but often these are not associated with significant loss of motion. As long as the physical exam demonstrates maintained motion, these calcifications are insignificant and do not require monitoring. Some loss of motion from the gains obtained intraoperatively is common; however, the majority of patients who are diligent with postoperative exercises maintain a functional arc of motion and achieve an optimal outcome.

PEARLS AND PITFALLS

- Preoperative planning is essential. All causes of limited motion should be identified, and surgical treatment should address all pathologic structures.
- A through appreciation of the patient's anatomy is essential.
- Careful discussion with patients preoperatively is important to establish postoperative expectations and emphasize the importance of postoperative rehabilitation.
- Meticulous hemostasis decreases the risk of recurrence.
- Avoid aggressive retraction of soft tissues, especially in proximal forearm to avoid injury to the PIN.
- Careful dissection and soft tissue handling to avoid iatrogenic injury.
- Copious irrigation prior to soft tissue interposition to remove any bone fragments to prevent recurrent HO/synostosis.
- Compliance with postoperative rehabilitation exercises is the most important element to maintaining range of motion.

RECOMMENDED READING

Beingessner DM, Patterson SD, King GJ. Early excision of heterotopic bone in the forearm. *J Hand Surg Am.* 2000;25(3):483–488.

Bell SN, Benger D. Management of radioulnar synostosis with mobilization, anconeus interposition, and a forearm rotation assist splint. *J Shoulder Elbow Surg.* 1999;8(6):621–624.

Cullen JP, Pellegrini VD Jr, Miller RJ, et al. Treatment of traumatic radioulnar synostosis by excision and postoperative low-dose irradiation. *J Hand Surg Am.* 1994;19(3):394–401.

Daluiski A, Schreiber JJ, Paul S, et al. Outcomes of anconeus interposition for proximal radioulnar synostosis. *J Shoulder Elbow Surg.* 2014;23(12):1882–1887.

Failla JM, Amadio PC, Morrey BF. Post traumatic proximal radio-ulnar synostosis: results of surgical treatment. *J Bone Joint Surg Am.* 1989;71(8):1208–1213.

Fernandez DL, Joneschild E. "Wrap around" pedicle muscle flaps for the treatment of recurrent forearm synostosis. *Tech Hand Up Extrem Surg.* 2004;8(2):102–109.

Friedrich JB, Hanel DP, Chilcote H, et al. The use of tensor fascia lata interposition grafts for the treatment of posttraumatic radioulnar synostosis. *J Hand Surg Am.* 2006;31(5):785–793.

Garland, DE, Hanscom DA, Keenan MA, et al. Resection of heterotopic ossification in the adult with head trauma. *J Bone Joint Surg Am.* 1985;67(8):1261–1269.

Hanel DP, Pfaeffle HJ, Ayalla A. Management of posttraumatic metadiaphyseal radioulnar synostosis. *Hand Clin.* 2007;23(2):227–234.

Hastings H, Graham TJ. The classification and treatment of heterotopic ossification about the elbow and forearm. *Hand Clin.* 1994;10(3):417–437.

Henket M, van Duijn PN, Doornberg JN, et al. A comparison of proximal radioulnar synostosis after trauma and distal biceps reattachment. *J Shoulder Elbow Surg.* 2007;16(5):626–630.

Jones NF, Esmail A, Shin EK. Treatment of radio-ulnar synostosis by radical excision and interposition of a radial forearm adipofascial flap. *J Hand Surg Am.* 2004;29(6):1143–1147.

Jupiter JB, Ring D. Operative treatment of post-traumatic proximal radio-ulnar synostosis. *J Bone Joint Surg Am.* 1998;80(2):248–257.

Lindenhovius ALC, Jupiter JB. The posttraumatic stiff elbow: a review of the literature. *J Hand Surg Am.* 2007;32(10):1605–1623.

McAuiffe JA, Wolfson AH. Early excision of heterotypic ossification about the elbow followed by radiation therapy. *J Bone Joint Surg Am.* 1997;79(5):749–755.

Morrey BF, Schneeberger AG. Anconeus arthroplasty: a new technique for reconstruction of the radiocapitellar joint and/or proximal radioulnar joint. *J Bone Joint Surg Am.* 2002;84(11):1960–1969.

Sonderegger J, Gidwani S, Ross ML. Preventing recurrence of radioulnar synostosis with pedicled adipofascial flaps. *J Hand Surg Eur.* 2012;37(3):244–250.

Tubbs RS, Apaydin N, Uz A, et al. Anatomy of the lateral inter muscular septum of the arm and its relationship to the radial nerve and its proximal branches: laboratory investigation. *J Neurosurg.* 2009;111(2):336–339.

Vince KG, Miller JE. Cross-union complicating fracture of the forearm. Part I: adults. *J Bone Joint Surg Am.* 1987;69(5):640–653.

Viola RW, Hanel DP. Early "simple" release of posttraumatic elbow contracture associated with heterotopic ossification. *J Hand Surg Am.* 1999;24(2):370–380.

16 Principles of Hand Incisions

Laura W. Lewallen and Marco Rizzo

INDICATIONS/CONTRAINDICATIONS

Because of the intricate balance of function in the hand and wrist, incisions in this area are unique. In an effort to ensure healing and maintain function, it is important to plan the incisions appropriately. Surgical exposure in the fingers has been well established over time to allow for good visualization of deeper structures without compromising skin healing or long-term motion. The hand and wrist are exposed using similar principles that allow for preservation of skin vascularity and avoid contracture over time. Poorly placed incisions result in restrictive scaring (Fig. 16-1), which may lead to diminished motion and function. In addition, the limited skin redundancy on the palmar surface of the hand may make primary closure difficult in edematous hands, resulting in the exposure of vital structures. Sound planning of incisions about the hand and wrist will help to avoid some of these difficulties. The purpose of this chapter is to review the principles and technique of skin incisions used for surgical exposure of the hand and wrist.

PREOPERATIVE PLANNING

Volar Approach to the Fingers

There are several commonly used approaches to the volar aspect of the fingers and thumb; however, the traditional Bruner incision is the most commonly used. The Bruner incision is a zigzag incision that angles at the flexion creases of the metacarpophalangeal, proximal interphalangeal, and distal interphalangeal joints (Fig. 16-2). As the incision is carried more proximally into the hand, the flexion creases of the palm are points of incisional direction change. The principle behind this technique is that longitudinal incisions axial to the lines of skin tension can generate excessive scarring that can limit extension. Oblique incisions are less likely to result in hypertrophic scaring and are less likely to restrict motion after undergoing longitudinal contraction during the scar maturation process. For optimal healing of the flaps, it is best to keep the angles close to 90 degrees. Angles more acute than 60 degrees carry a higher incidence of skin necrosis.

An alternative to the Bruner incision in the finger is the midlateral approach (Fig. 16-3A). It has the advantage of being cosmetically less conspicuous. The incision is based about the lateral (or medial) side of the finger, and the skin is elevated to provide exposure of the underlying tissues. A good way to ensure that the surgeon is not directly over the neurovascular bundles is to connect the incisions at the apex of the flexion creases (Fig. 16-3B). This is also a preferred

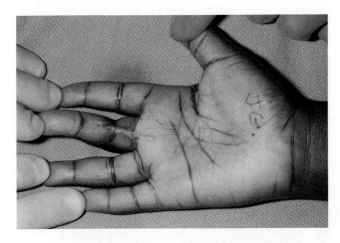

FIGURE 16-1

Example of restrictive scar resulting from straight line incision placed over the flexor surface of the finger.

approach in cases of replantation surgery. Although cosmetically appealing, this technique requires care in elevating the skin to ensure its viability, as it is perfused by the contralateral arterial digital artery.

In cases of flexion deformity of the fingers, seen in condition such as Dupuytren disease and prior scar contracture, a straight midline incision with Z-plasties is an alternative approach to the traditional Bruner incision (Fig. 16-4). This will allow for the elongation of the incision as the flexion deformity is corrected. Z-plasty angles of 60 degrees help preserve viability at the apex of the skin flap.

Incisions over the distal pulp of the finger, such as is necessary in felons, are best made directly over the area of swelling and induration. Whenever possible, it is better to position the incision in fingers away from the thumb pulp diminishing the impact of any scar sensitivity. These wounds can

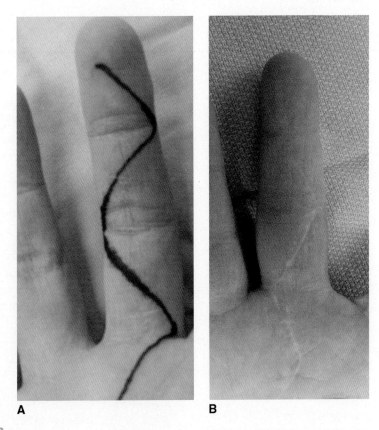

A **B**

FIGURE 16-2

Bruner incision approach to the volar aspect of the fingers. **A:** The most commonly preferred method of crossing flexion creases is with these undulating angled incisions. **B:** A nicely healed incision following a Bruner incision.

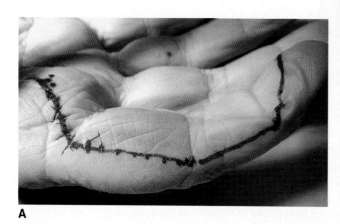

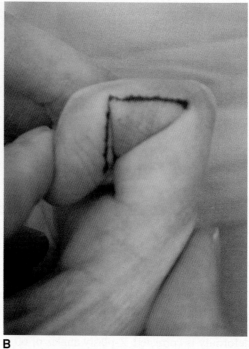

A   **B**

FIGURE 16-3

A: The midaxial or lateral approach to the fingers. This technique can be a more cosmetically appearing alternative to the Bruner incision.
B: Care must be taken to connect the incision at the apex of the flexion creases so as to avoid direct dissection over the underlying neurovascular structures and prevent excessive volar scarring.

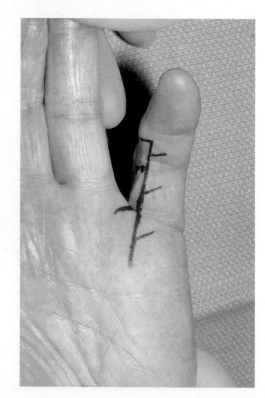

FIGURE 16-4

A longitudinal Z-plasty approach to the volar aspect of the finger can be useful in cases of preexisting flexion contracture, such as in Dupuytren contracture.

be loosely closed or allowed to heal via secondary intention. If it appears that the incision may need to be extended proximal to the distal interphalangeal joint, a Bruner incision can be preferred for better exposure.

Dorsal Incisions about the Fingers

The dorsal skin of the hand has more redundancy and lacks glabrous skin; this is due to the requirements of joint flexion. This skin redundancy allows one to use longitudinal incisions with little risk of creating joint contractures. A longitudinal incision (Fig. 16-5) allows for protection of the venous and lymphatic drainage, while giving good visualization of the extensor mechanism. One should remember that majority of venous and lymphatic drainage from the fingers runs dorsal through the web spaces and into the metacarpal valleys. Lazy S or curvilinear incisions may also be designed to avoid crossing extension creases (see Fig. 16-5). Incisions over the distal interphalangeal joint can be longitudinal as well, but dissection can be limited due to the nail bed and fold distally. An alternative is the T- or H-shaped (Fig. 16-6) incision that allows for visualization of the extensor mechanism and distal interphalangeal joint.

Volar Incisions about the Hand

Transverse incisions or incisions that parallel the palmar flexion creases offer the best cosmetic results. However, these incisions are perpendicular to the underlying vessels, nerves, and tendons. Therefore, care must be taken when performing these approaches. Incisions for trigger finger releases are a good example (Fig. 16-7). In addition, transverse incisions (similar to those along the distal palm flexion crease) in the metacarpophalangeal joint flexion crease at the base of the thumb for A1 pulley release have been found to produce better aesthetic results and result in less restrictive scarring. In cases where more exposure is necessary, as seen in patients with concomitant retinacular cysts, traditional longitudinal Bruner-type incisions may be used. Again you want to follow the basic premise of changing directions at the creases to minimize scarring. Wounds or scars in the web spaces are at risk of developing functionally limiting scars. Depending on the patient, these can sometimes necessitate revision Z-plasties and web space deepening.

In exposing the carpal tunnel, a longitudinal incision, preferably in or parallel to the palmar crease, is commonly used. If the incision needs to be extended proximally, Bruner-type zigzag

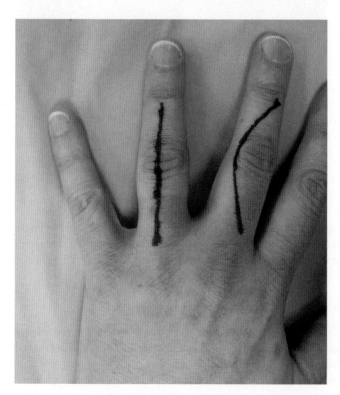

FIGURE 16-5

Two common approaches to the dorsum of the fingers: a straight longitudinal and a more curved longitudinal that avoids the extension creases.

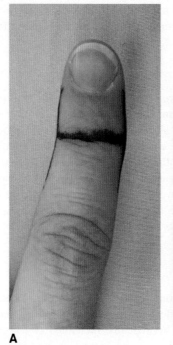
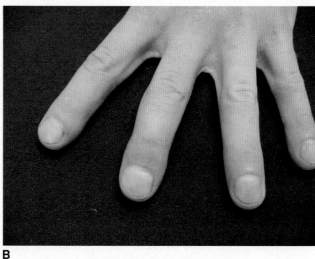

A   **B**

FIGURE 16-6

A: An H-shaped incision over the dorsal aspect of the distal interphalangeal joint in a patient who underwent distal interphalangeal arthrodesis. **B:** The wound went on to heal very nicely.

FIGURE 16-7

An incision to trigger finger approach utilizing the palm flexion crease. These can result in cosmetically appealing scars with little/no residual deficit. In cases where greater exposure is necessary, a longitudinal Bruner-type incision is preferred.

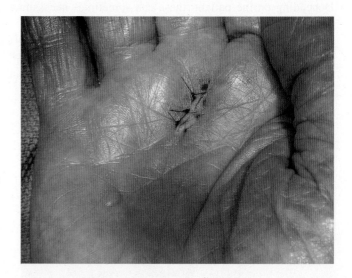

incisions can be made between the distal and proximal wrist flexion creases (Fig. 16-8). These angled incisions are the most common and useful method of crossing flexion creases in the hand and wrist. Care should be taken to stay ulnar to the palmaris longus tendon to avoid injury to the palmar sensory branch of the median nerve.

Dorsal Incisions about the Hand and Base of Thumb

Longitudinal incision can be successfully used over the dorsum of the hand without the risk of significant restrictive scarring. Transverse and curvilinear incisions can also be used over the dorsum of the hand if desired. The skin over the dorsum of the hand is mobile, and scarring is generally less of a functional problem. Approaches to the carpometacarpal joint can be made longitudinally between

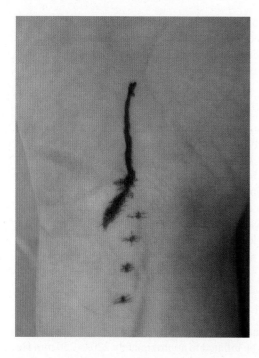

FIGURE 16-8

An extensile carpal tunnel incision. Angulation at the wrist flexion crease will minimize scarring of the wound. By keeping incision ulnar to the palmaris longus tendon (*dotted line*), injury to the palmar sensory branch of the median nerve can be avoided.

the abductor pollicis longus and extensor pollicis brevis tendons or they can be more radial (along the plane of the intersection of the dorsal and volar skin) and extended proximally transversely along the wrist flexion crease, forming a "hockey-stick" appearance as described by Eaton and Littler.

Incisions about the Wrist

Volar incisions to the wrist can be along flexion creases or longitudinal provided the incision changes direction at the flexion creases in a modified Bruner fashion. Dorsal approaches to the wrist can be longitudinal, transverse, or curvilinear. The tissues on the dorsal aspect of the wrist are redundant, and dorsal scarring is not typically a problem. These can include incisions to expose the base of the thumb. Radial and ulnar incisions may be performed longitudinally, curvilinearly, or transversely.

Incisions about the Forearm

As we extend proximally, more traditional incisions can be utilized. If it is a fairly short incision, such as in open treatment of distal radius fractures, a longitudinal incision will suffice (Fig. 16-9).

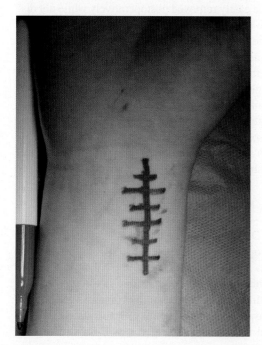

FIGURE 16-9

A longitudinal approach to the distal radius in a case of open reduction and internal fixation of a distal radius fracture. Angulation of the incision can be performed if the incision needs to be extended distally.

If the incision is extended distally, a Bruner angulation is made at the wrist flexion crease. In cases where extensive exposure is necessary, such as is required in compartment syndrome release, an undulating longitudinal incision works well. If the elbow must be crossed, this is usually done in a lazy S fashion passing to the medial aspect of the antecubital fossa.

Healing by Secondary Intention

In cases such as infection and Dupuytren contracture, it may be advantageous to leave the wounds at least partially open. These wounds can heal nicely by secondary intention. Modalities such as whirlpool and wound vacuum–assisted closure can be helpful in accelerating wound healing as well as minimizing risk of infection. Disadvantages include time to healing and the fact that some patients find the healing process cosmetically unappealing. Unfortunately, functional limitations such as joint contractures can result as rehabilitation is delayed during the wound healing process. However, with good postoperative wound care, this can be an effective way to manage some of the more difficult cases or cases where it is necessary to leave the wounds open.

SURGERY

Patient Positioning

Typically, the patient is in a supine position, and a hand table is used. A tourniquet is placed in the proximal portion of the arm. We prefer the pressure to be inflated to approximately 220 to 250 mm Hg for adults and 200 to 225 mm Hg for children (generally 70 to 100 mm Hg above the patient's systolic pressure). If the surgery is isolated to the distal aspect of the finger, a finger tourniquet can be placed. In these cases, we routinely also place the upper arm tourniquet, which can be utilized if need be. Tourniquets are generally not necessary in cases where lidocaine with epinephrine is utilized, as in wide awake local anesthesia technique (WALANT) is utilized. The entire extremity is prepped. Perioperative antibiotics are administered when indicated.

Technique

Loupe magnification should be utilized and will help avoid injury to important underlying structures. The incision is typically made with a no. 15 blade knife, taking care to keep the blade perpendicular to the skin and not skiving. The knife can be used to cut the dermis and epidermis. Generally speaking, dissection should proceed from known to unknown or normal to abnormal tissues. Electrocautery, with needle-point cautery, can be used for small veins or vessels. We prefer the use of bipolar cautery. Drains should be liberally used, especially in contaminated wounds or wounds with compromised hemostasis. Options include a small silastic, Penrose or Hemovac drain. The drain can be placed without suture so that it can be easily removed postoperatively while not disturbing the overlying dressing. Otherwise, drains can be sutured for added protection if the surgeon wants to secure it in place for a longer period of time. It is our preference to deflate the tourniquet prior to wound closure to evaluate hand perfusion and achieve hemostasis prior to wound closure. After ensuring adequate hemostasis and viability of the hand, the tourniquet may be reinflated during wound closure. Incisions can be closed in a single layer with a nonabsorbable interrupted 4-0 or 5-0 suture such as nylon or Prolene. Either horizontal or vertical mattress sutures can be utilized. Vertical mattresses are better for everting the skin edges, while horizontal mattress sutures will allow for less overall sutures. Increased ischemia of the soft tissues can occur with horizontal mattress closure. In young children, an absorbable suture such as catgut or chromic is preferred as it obviates the need for suture removal and will help minimize stress to the child postoperatively.

POSTOPERATIVE MANAGEMENT

A thoughtfully applied hand dressing is imperative. Depending on the injury or surgery performed, some period of immobilization may be necessary. Proper immobilization will allow for the skin and soft tissues to heal with minimal stretch and tension. However, this needs to be balanced with the risk of developing joint contractures. In cases of fracture care, immobilization is often prolonged compared with the soft tissue–only procedures. The dressing should be mildly compressive and supportive (Fig. 16-10). Surgeries involving the distal aspects of the digits may be adequately dressed with a tube-gauze type of dressing. More proximal reconstructive surgeries will require varying

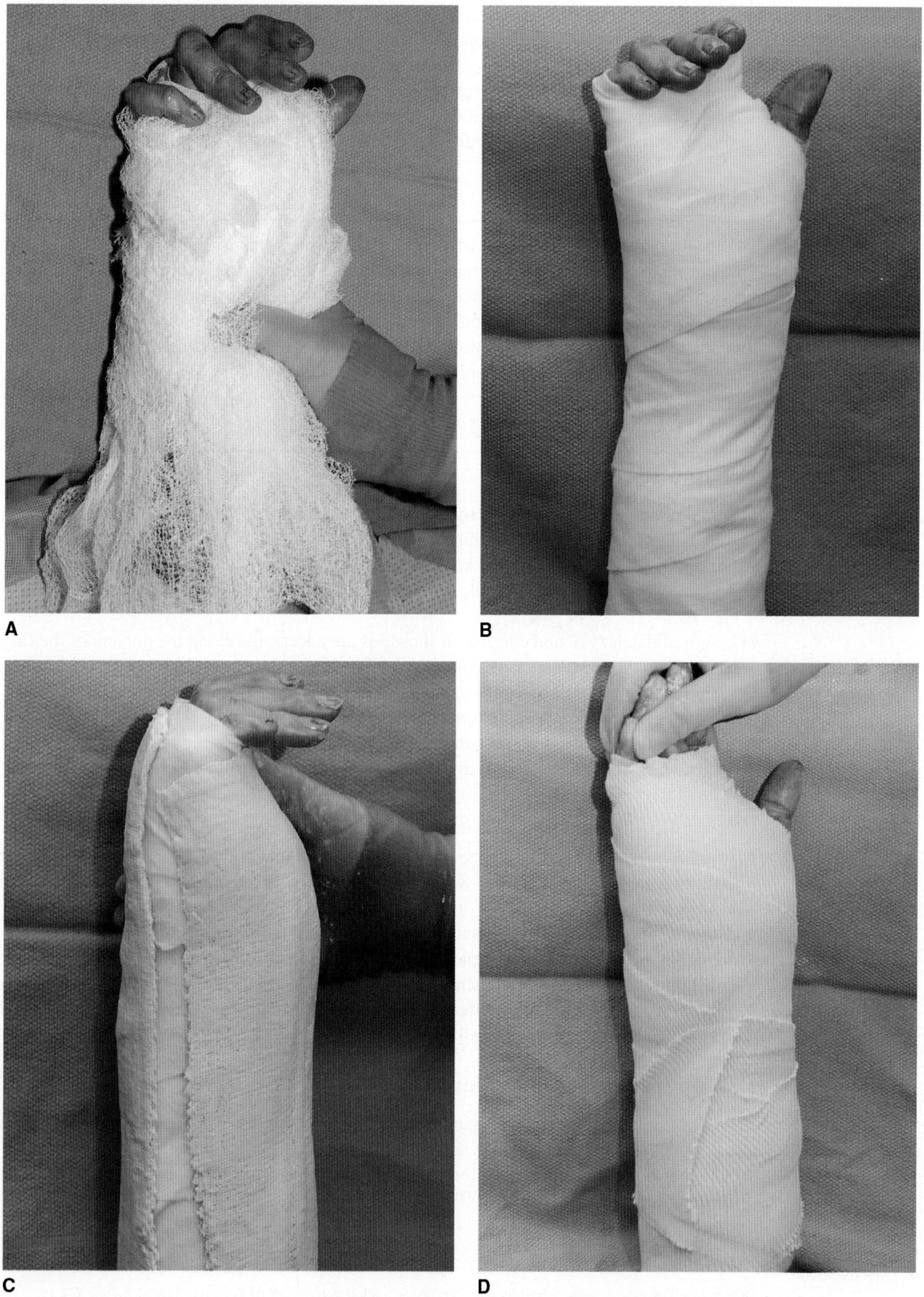

FIGURE 16-10

Example of a compressive dressing in a patient with rheumatoid arthritis who underwent metacarpophalangeal joint arthroplasty.
A: Following application of xeroform on the incision, fluffs are placed on the volar, dorsal, radial, and ulnar aspects of the wrist and hand. Gauze is lightly placed within the web spaces of the digits. **B:** Cast padding is applied over the gauze. **C:** Plaster is then applied over the cast padding. **D:** A bias wrap completes the dressing. In this example, the MP joints need to be immobilized in extension and neutral deviation. If finger motion is not contraindicated, care should be taken not to have the dressing restrict finger motion.

periods of immobilization of the wrist and hand in the position of function. Specifically, with the wrist in mild extension, metacarpophalangeal joints are flexed and interphalangeal joints extended (intrinsic plus position). Elective soft tissue procedures such as carpal tunnel releases can be immobilized with the wrist in mild extension and the fingers free to move immediately. Although this is our preference, we acknowledge these can be successfully treated with simply a soft dressing. Drains are discontinued when output is acceptable.

COMPLICATIONS

The most common adverse result of poorly planned incisions is scar contracture (see Fig. 16-1). This can lead to cosmetic and/or functional deficits. A more difficult problem is skin necrosis and subsequent wound healing problems. These can lead to problems such as infection, excessive scar formation, and diminished function. Other less common complications related to inadequate or suboptimal incisions include injury to nerves, arteries, or tendons. However, with good preoperative planning and technique, these complications are usually avoidable.

PEARLS AND PITFALLS

Preoperative Planning

- Sound planning of incisions is crucial, in order to minimize scarring and other complications, as well as to optimize motion and function.
- For optimal flap healing, aim to keep angles close to 90 degrees in the Bruner incision.
- To avoid the neurovascular bundle during the midlateral approach, connect the apex of the flexion creases.
- Longitudinal, lazy S, and curvilinear incisions are acceptable along the dorsum of the fingers and hand, given the redundancy and mobility of the skin in this area.
- Transverse incisions or incisions that parallel the palmar flexion creases are effective and cosmetically appealing for cases such as trigger finger release.
- A longitudinal incision, in or parallel to the palmar crease, is recommended for carpal tunnel release. Bruner-type incisions may be used if proximal exposure is necessary.

Surgery

- A tourniquet is inflated to 220 to 250 mm Hg for adults and 200 to 225 mm Hg for children. Deflating the tourniquet prior to wound closure allows for adequate hemostasis and evaluation of hand perfusion.
- A finger tourniquet is placed if surgery is isolated to the distal aspect of the finger.
- 4-0 or 5-0 nylon or Prolene is typically used for wound closure in adults. Absorbable suture, such as catgut or chromic, is recommended in children to avoid the need of suture removal.
- Vertical mattress technique is effective for everting the skin edges, while the horizontal mattress technique allows for fewer overall sutures.

Postoperative Management

- Proper immobilization is necessary to allow for healing. It is important to also bear in mind the risk of developing joint stiffness secondary to prolonged immobilization.
- A longer period of immobilization is required for fracture healing, compared with isolated soft tissue procedures.

RECOMMENDED READING

Bruner JM. The zigzag volar digital incision for flexor tendon surgery. *Plast Reconstr Surg.* 1967;40:571.
Eaton RE, Littler JW. Ligament reconstruction for the painful thumb carpometacarpal joint. *J Bone Joint Surg.* 1973; 55A:1655.
Graham WP. Incisions, amputations, and skin grafting in the hand. *Orthop Clin North Am.* 1970;1:227.
McCash CR. The open palm technique in Dupuytren's contracture. *Br J Plast Surg.* 1964;17:271.

17 Lateral Arm Flap for Hand and Wrist Coverage

Ryan P. Ter Louw and James P. Higgins

The lateral arm flap was originally described by Song et al. in 1982 as a thin and pliable fascio-cutaneous flap for head and neck reconstruction. Subsequent publications have described the great versatility of this flap as it may be harvested with other elements of the lateral brachium including vascularized fascia, bone, and nerve for reconstruction of composite defects. The donor site may often be closed primarily and produces minimal morbidity. For upper extremity injuries, it may be harvested from the ipsilateral arm localizing all trauma to one extremity. The vascular pedicle is constant in its anatomy, and harvest of the pedicle does not require sacrifice of any of the major vessels supplying the upper extremity. The main drawbacks of the conventionally designed lateral arm flap included its relative thickness and short pedicle length.

Here, we provide a description of the "extended" lateral arm flap (ELAF). The "conventional lateral arm flap" utilized a vertical ellipse of skin based over the distal half of the lateral brachium. The "extended" lateral arm modification repositions the ellipse distally, such that the skin segment includes the tissue over the lateral epicondyle and proximal dorsal forearm. This modification provides three main advantages (Table 17-1). First, the skin segment harvested is thinner in the distal design. Second, the distal positioning of the skin provides a functionally longer vascular pedicle for improved ease of insetting. Finally, the more distal position of the skin paddle allows the surgeon to better visualize the radial nerve during pedicle dissection protecting it from any iatrogenic injury.

INDICATIONS/CONTRAINDICATIONS

The indications for this flap are summarized in Table 17-2.

If the flap is going to be used as a free flap, it is important to remember that free tissue transfer requires significant time under general anesthesia, and the flap will require postoperative monitoring to ensure vessel patency. Patients with significant comorbidities should be medically optimized and carefully selected prior to lengthy surgical procedures. Patients who have suffered previous elbow fractures that required surgical dissection of lateral column of the humerus are at high risk of flap failure, and some alternative means of reconstruction should be chosen in these patients. Though the donor site of the lateral arm flap is typically closed primarily, the scar can be at risk for hypertrophy and may extend distal to the elbow. In addition, flaps larger than 6 to 8 cm in width usually cannot be closed primarily and will require split-thickness skin grafting for donor site closure. This possibility should be discussed with the patient preoperatively. The diameter of the pedicle can be 1.5 mm, which is considerably smaller than other fasciocutaneous flaps. We would recommend that the surgical anastomosis be performed with the operating room microscope.

ANATOMY

The lateral arm flap receives its blood supply from arterial perforators of the lateral intermuscular septum (Fig. 17-1). The radial collateral artery originates from the profunda brachii and travels from the posterior brachium to the lateral humerus along the spiral groove. At the spiral groove, it branches into anterior and posterior divisions. The posterior radial collateral artery (PRCA) provides

TABLE 17-1   Advantages and Disadvantages of the Lateral Forearm Flap

Advantages
- Thin/pliable skin paddle
- Harvest from ipsilateral arm limiting surgical sites to one extremity
- Reliable arterial anatomy
- No position change
- Rapid harvest under tourniquet
- Multiple composite tissue options
- Similar pigmentation and hair bearing status to hand/wrist

Disadvantages
- Smaller pedicle size
- Shorter pedicle length
- Visible scar when extended beyond elbow
- Sensory deficit in posterior cutaneous nerve of forearm

TABLE 17-2   Indications for a Lateral Forearm Flap

Small- to medium-sized defects within the hand and wrist
    Dorsal/volar wounds requiring tendon gliding surface
    First webspace resurfacing after radical contracture release
    Vascularized bone graft
    Scar resurfacing
    Vascularized nerve graft/sensate flap
Wounds requiring free tissue transfer
    Head and neck wounds: intraoral resurfacing, tongue reconstruction, segmental bony defects
    Lower extremity wounds requiring reconstruction over gliding surfaces, one-stage Achilles tendon reconstruction
    Burn scar resurfacing
Small- to medium-sized defects within the hand and wrist
    Olecranon wounds (as a reversed flap)
    Antecubital contractures (as a reversed flap)

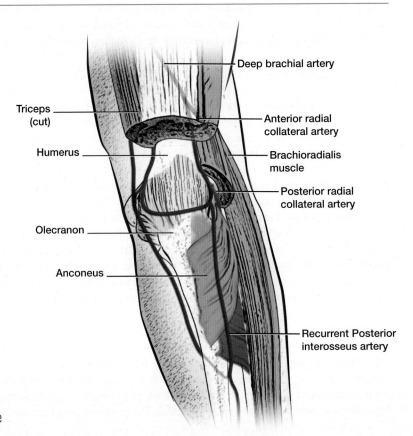

FIGURE 17-1

The arterial anatomy of the lateral arm demonstrating the rich vascular plexus. Note the connection between the PRCA and the recurrent posterior interosseous artery. The PRCA is the pedicle for the free lateral arm flap. The recurrent posterior interosseous artery is the basis for the pedicled reverse lateral arm flap for olecranon coverage.

TABLE 17-3 Lateral Forearm Flap Anatomy	
Artery	Posterior radial collateral
Vein	Venae comitantes (deep system)
Nerve	Posterior brachial cutaneous nerve
Maximum size	25 × 6 cm
Pedicle length	8 cm (13 cm with extended lateral arm flap)
Pedicle size	1.5–2.5 mm
Average flap thickness	6.3 cm
Composite tissue	Skin, vascularized humerus, vascularized nerve graft, fascia only, triceps tendon

the primary blood supply to the lateral arm flap. The PRCA is located within the lateral intermuscular septum and is intimately associated with the periosteum of the humerus. It serves as a reliable 6- to 8-cm pedicle for the proximally based free lateral arm flap (Table 17-3).

Venous drainage of the flap is provided by the venae comitantes of the PRCA system. Additional superficial veins are not required for harvest. The posterior brachial cutaneous nerve courses with the vascular pedicle and may be used if a sensate flap is desired.

The lateral intermuscular septum is found between the lateral head of the triceps and the brachioradialis. The radial nerve can be found emerging from the spiral groove and entering interval between the brachioradialis and brachialis muscles. Identifying the nerve early in dissection allows for more rapid flap elevation.

The PRCA arborizes into a filigree of smaller branches distal to the elbow. In an anatomic injection study of the ELAF, the PRCA extended an average 8 cm beyond the lateral epicondyle. The radial recurrent artery and recurrent posterior interosseous artery anastomose with the PRCA. These connections allow for design of a distally based pedicled flap, which is particularly useful in elbow coverage.

PREOPERATIVE PLANNING

When selecting a reconstructive donor site for the hand and wrist, a thin and pliable flap is essential. A recent study comparing parascapular, lateral thigh, and lateral arm flaps found that the lateral arm flap was consistently the thinnest fasciocutaneous flap, at an average of 6.3 cm. Though the pedicle is shorter and smaller in diameter than other fasciocutaneous flaps, the hand and wrist are a privileged microsurgical site with ample recipient vessels.

The lateral arm flap requires no preoperative workup in an atraumatic donor brachium due to the predictability of the PRCA.

SURGERY

Patient Positioning

The patient is positioned supine under general anesthesia with the donor extremity on a hand table. The arm is prepped and draped up to and including the axilla. A sterile tourniquet is placed as proximally as possible but may require removal to complete pedicle dissection.

Technique

Flap design should be determined after the wound has been thoroughly debrided. The defect is assessed for the need of any vascularized bone or fascial requirements. The defect is then measured. The flap design is transposed along the longitudinal axis of the lateral arm and forearm. The use of Doppler for skin paddle perforator identification is possible, but not routinely performed by the senior author because of the flap's reliability. The traditional marking for the lateral arm flap extends from the deltoid insertion on the humerus to the lateral epicondyle, overlying the lateral intermuscular septum (Fig. 17-2). The ELAF is designed to incorporate the thinner skin on the posterior lateral forearm and increase the length of the vascular pedicle. The longitudinal ellipse is designed such that the long axis is aligned with the lateral intermuscular septum of the brachium and continues in this trajectory over the dorsal forearm with the elbow in full extension. The lateral epicondyle is placed in the center of the flap. The distal limits of the ELAF angiosome have not been determined.

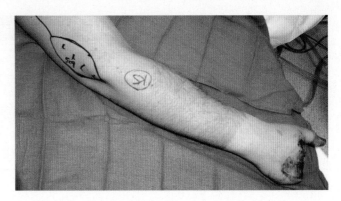

FIGURE 17-2

Traditional lateral arm flap skin paddle extending to lateral epicondyle.

The authors routinely harvest the flap to the junction of the middle and proximal thirds of the forearm (Fig. 17-3).

The extremity is fully exsanguinated, then a sterile tourniquet is inflated. The senior author prefers to start with the anterior approach; this allows for immediate identification of the radial nerve, which is the only structure that requires caution during harvest of the flap.

The entire anterior margin of skin paddle is carried through the muscular fascia of the anterior compartment muscles. Several muscle groups will come into view. These contain obliquely oriented fibers making specific muscles difficult to identify. From distal to proximal, these muscle groups are the extensor carpi ulnaris, extensor digiti quinti, extensor digitorum communis, extensor carpi radialis brevis, extensor carpi radialis longus, brachioradialis, and brachialis muscles. The radial nerve courses in the interval between the brachialis and brachioradialis. The brachioradialis origin is more proximal than one might expect given its anatomic position in the forearm. Its most proximal fibers originate at the midpoint of the humerus and mark the location where the radial nerve will lie adjacent to the vascular pedicle. Distal to this point, the radial nerve will course anteriorly and outside of the zone of flap dissection. In the typical ELAF design, this point of divergence will exist proximal to the location of the skin paddle. Identifying the radial nerve prior to the flap elevation and confirming that it is proximal to the skin paddle will enable the surgeon to expediently elevate the flap without concern for radial nerve injury.

The flap is then elevated by continuing the anterior compartment subfascial dissection until the anterior surface of the humerus is visible. Attention is then directed to the posterior margin of the flap, and a similar rapid subfascial dissection is performed until the posterior surface of the humerus is visible. The flap should now be adherent to the lateral column of the humerus only by a narrow (2- to 3-mm) strip of periosteum.

Attention is then turned to the portion of the flap overlying the forearm musculature. Here, the extensor fascia is less distinct. The flap is elevated from distal to proximal immediately above the common tendon of the forearm extensors. Once the lateral epicondyle is encountered, the dissection is converted to a sharply subperiosteal plane. This continues proximal to the lateral epicondyle elevating the narrow strip of remaining periosteal attachments to the lateral column of the humerus. Maintaining a strictly subperiosteal plane protects the PRCA from injury. As dissection proceeds more proximally, the pedicle becomes more superficial within the septum (Fig. 17-4).

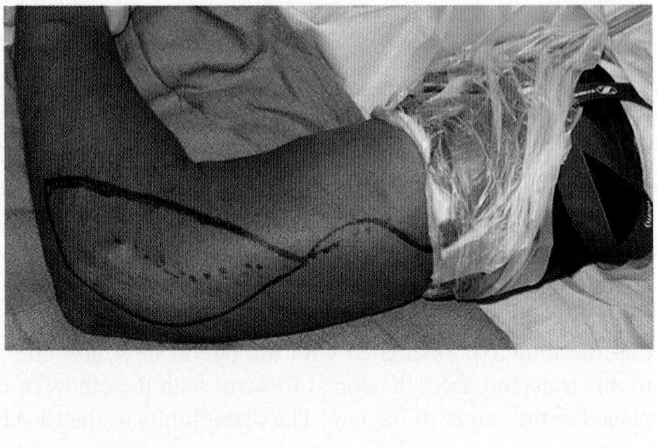

FIGURE 17-3

Distal design of lateral arm flap allowing increased pedicle length and sterile tourniquet placement.

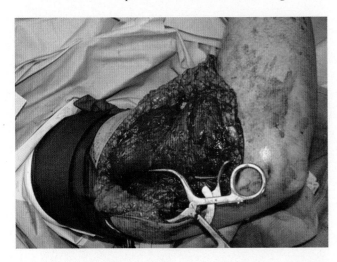

Proximal exposure of the PRCA within
the lateral intermuscular septum.

When the pedicle dissection reaches the spiral groove, the anterior branch of the radial collateral
artery (ARCA) is encountered heading distally with the radial nerve in the brachioradialis/brachialis
interval. The ARCA is ligated, and the radial nerve is gently retracted anteriorly enabling the continued elevation of the radial collateral artery pedicle (Fig. 17-5).

There are several techniques described to lengthen the lateral arm flap pedicle. By splitting the
lateral and long heads of the triceps, the PRCA can be traced to the profunda brachii, yielding an
additional 1 to 2 cm of pedicle length. However, the motor innervation of the triceps becomes intri-
cately associated with the pedicle, increasing likelihood of injury. This technique is rarely necessary
with distal design of the ELAF.

Figures 17-6 to 17-8 document three cases managed with conventional lateral forearm
flaps.

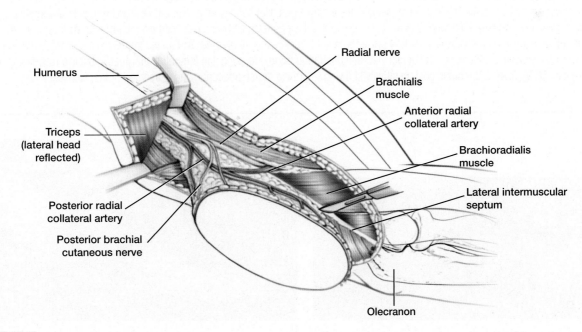

FIGURE 17-5

Anatomy of conventional lateral arm flap harvest. Elevation of flap is demonstrated in subperiosteal plane of lateral column of humerus. The
flexor compartment is reflected anteriorly and extensor compartment posteriorly. The ARCA travels with the radial nerve. As the flap is raised
on the PRCA, the anterior branch is ligated to permit continued proximal dissection and increase pedicle length.

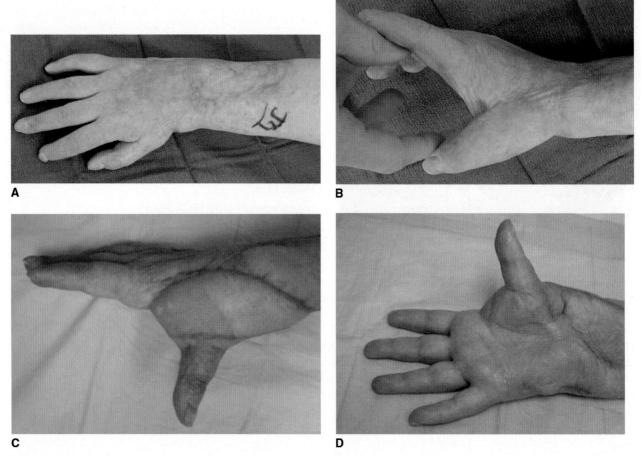

FIGURE 17-6

A 36-year-old woman presented with septic shock following postoperative C-section infection. She developed ischemic wounds to bilateral upper and lower extremities, resulting in bilateral below-knee amputations. Her hand wound required skin grafting and subsequently developed contracture. Webspace contracture was resurfaced with EIP opponensplasty and extended lateral arm flap. **A:** Posttraumatic scarring of dorsal hand and first webspace initially closed with split-thickness skin grafting. **B:** Limited thumb extension and abduction secondary to first webspace contracture. **C:** Dorsal view demonstrating improved extension 3 months after first webspace resurfacing with lateral arm flap. **D:** Volar view 3 months postoperatively showing improved thumb abduction and deepening of first webspace.

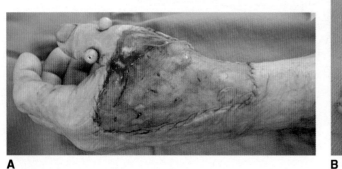
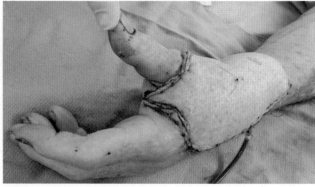

FIGURE 17-7

This traumatic hand injury resulted in significant soft tissue loss of the dorsal hand and first webspace. There were no fractures or other injuries sustained. Without vascularized fascial coverage, this injury would likely result in first webspace contracture and limited finger extension. **A:** Dorsal view of skin avulsion and intra-articular metacarpal phalangeal fracture, initially treated with skin grafting. **B:** Immediate postoperative view of dorsal hand resurfacing and first webspace deepening with extended lateral arm flap.

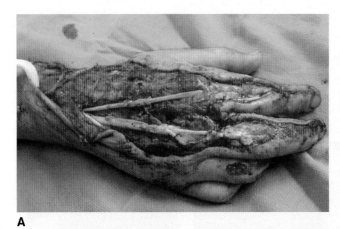

A

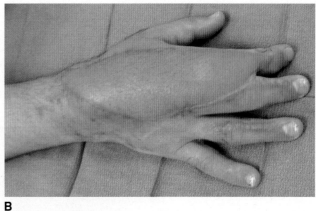

B

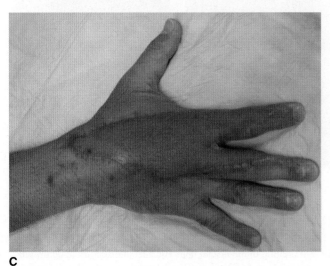

C

FIGURE 17-8

This partial dorsal hand defect extended distal to the metacarpal phalangeal joints and involved the dorsal skin of several fingers. Reconstruction with an extended lateral arm flap was performed with intentional incomplete syndactyly. The webspace was recreated, and the flap was debulked at a second stage to improve contour and hand function. **A:** Dorsal view of traumatic avulsion and extensor tendon lacerations extending to proximal phalanges. **B:** Three months postoperatively from extended lateral arm flap with intentional syndactylization. **C:** Three months after syndactyly release, adequate finger abduction is demonstrated.

Variations

Lateral Arm Fascia Flap

Conventionally, the lateral arm flap harvest width is limited by the desire to close the donor site primarily. The amount of skin capable of excision while still permitting primary closure is approximately 6 to 8 cm. When hand or wrist defects are wider, a fascia-only flap provides a good option. The flap is then covered with full- or split-thickness skin grafting (Fig. 17-9). Fascial perforators are found 1 to 15 cm proximal to the lateral epicondyle and will support any axial fascial flap of up to 12 × 9 cm.

Skin Flap with Tendon

A slip of triceps tendon may also be incorporated within the lateral arm flap and has been described in one-stage Achilles reconstruction. Though the skin paddle of the lateral arm flap is thin and pliable, it remains durable enough for total palmar or plantar skin resurfacing and has been described with 13-year follow-up in patients with refractory Dupuytren and Ledderhose disease.

Osteocutaneous Flap

The PRCA also provides periosteal branches to the humerus. This allows for design osteocutaneous flaps in both free and pedicled fashion. Vascularized bone segments of 10 to 15 cm can be safely taken immediately above the lateral epicondyle provided it does not include more than 25% of the circumference of the humeral cortical circumference. The osseous component requires harvest of a small slip of triceps tendon and brachioradialis to ensure perforator inclusion to the periosteum. This provides the option of inclusion of bone within a skin flap harvested; the bone segment is primarily cortical, and it's quite narrow in anteroposterior dimensions.

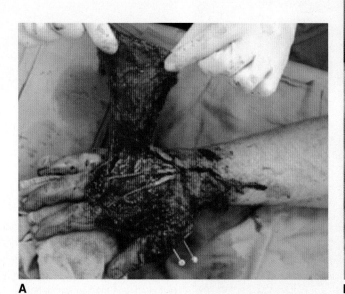
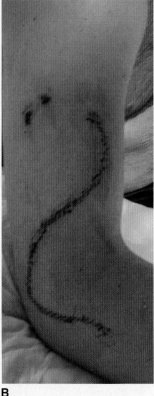

A   **B**

FIGURE 17-9

This large dorsal hand wound presented with exposed extensor tendons. The soft tissue deficit was too large for coverage with the skin paddle of the lateral arm flap with primary closure. A free fascial lateral arm flap was harvested followed by split-thickness skin grafting of the fascial flap. The vascularized fascia below the skin graft allowed for improved extensor tendon gliding. **A:** Significant dorsal hand wound with extensor tendon laceration. A free fascial flap was harvested from the lateral arm to provide a gliding surface for tendon excursion. **B:** Donor site closure 1 week after surgery following drain removal.

Nerve-Sparing Dissection

The lateral arm flap may be made sensate via the posterior brachial cutaneous nerve. A second nerve, the posterior cutaneous nerve of the forearm, may be observed passing through the territory of harvest. This nerve is often sacrificed resulting in loss of sensation in the dorsal proximal forearm. Preservation of the posterior cutaneous nerve of the forearm has been described by Fogdestam et al. Although this technique limits the donor site morbidity, it also requires additional dissection around the pedicle, which may result in pedicle injury.

Reversed Lateral Arm Flap

The distally based "reverse lateral arm flap" is used primarily for coverage of wounds over the olecranon. The flap is designed using a longitudinal ellipse over the brachium. Dissection begins at the proximal margin of the flap. At the level of the spiral groove, the profunda brachial artery is ligated while protecting the radial nerve. The anterior and posterior dissection is performed in the subfascial plane as described above, while elevating the pedicle subperiosteally along the lateral edge of the humerus. The distally based flap is adequately mobilized to permit coverage of the olecranon wound when transposed. The surgeon may then elect to maintain the proximal skin pedicle in order to protect the small vascular connections between the PRCA and the posterior interosseous system. This rotation and inset will leave a prominent skin fold ("dog-ear") at the posterior-distal flap margin. This may be revised to improve contour at a second surgery if desired (Fig. 17-10A, B). Alternatively, the surgeon may elect to complete the proximal skin incision

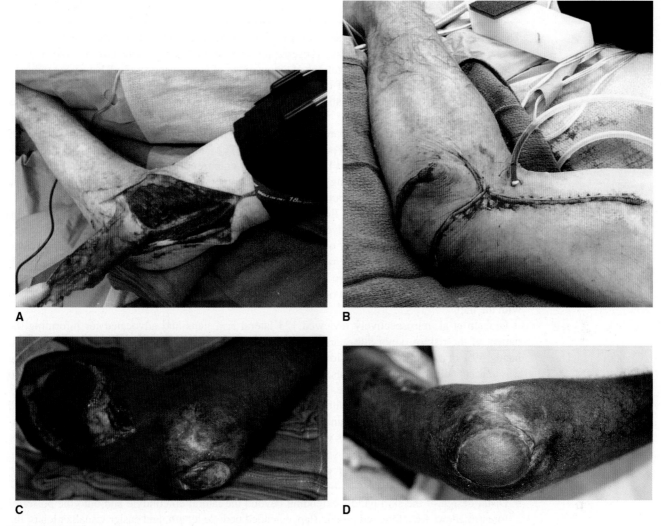

FIGURE 17-10

These recalcitrant elbow wounds shown have failed prior attempts at primary closure and splinting. Distally based "reversed" lateral arm flap for elbow coverage may be elevated as a transposition skin flap **(A, B)** or as an island flap **(C, D)**. **A:** Recalcitrant olecranon wound from infected olecranon bursitis with reverse lateral arm flap harvest. **B:** A distally based lateral arm transposition flap. **C:** Another olecranon wound complicated by ulnar osteomyelitis. After adequate debridement and antibiotic therapy, a reverse lateral arm island flap harvest. **D:** Three months after a distally based lateral arm island flap.

through the level of the dermis while protecting the fibrofatty subcutaneous plane of tissue. The surrounding skin is mobilized in the subdermal plane, and the flap is rotated ninety degrees into the olecranon wound as an island flap (Fig. 17-10C, D). In both techniques (transposition or island flap), the flap is positioned so that suture lines are not positioned on that the apex of the olecranon and the flap is inset without tension.

POSTOPERATIVE MANAGEMENT

Primary closure of the donor site can be achieved with appropriate flap design. As a large segment of fascia has been removed with the flap, fascial closure at the donor site should not be attempted. A closed suction drain should be placed in the donor site prior to closure. A posterior elbow splint aids in protecting tight donor site closures, but should be removed early to allow for range of motion. With appropriate physical therapy and patient education, elbow contractures and weakness are easily avoided.

COMPLICATIONS

The most common complications associated with the lateral arm flap include infection, hematoma, wound dehiscence, and paresthesias. These represent routine complications encountered with all microvascular reconstruction. Limitations of elbow range of motion and strength have been reported in the literature, but are unlikely if early postoperative range of motion is initiated. Radial nerve injury is the most feared complication. However, with proper flap elevation, the radial nerve is identified and protected.

Klinkenberg et al. recently compared the donor site morbidity, aesthetic and functional outcomes of the lateral arm, lateral thigh, and parascapular flaps. The authors found no significant differences between flaps with regard to patient DASH scores, lower extremity functional scale, and the Short-Form 36. All 20 patients undergoing lateral arm flaps reported numbness in the distribution of the posterior cutaneous nerve of arm, but 85% stated they would agree to the same flap again.

Akinci reviewed 72 lateral arm flaps for upper extremity reconstruction and found that in the setting of electrical injury, early coverage led to higher rates of venous thrombosis and advocated for delay. The donor site morbidity of 17 ELAFs was investigated by Hamdi et al., which revealed no significant differences in elbow range of motion or strength when compared to the unoperated arm. They reported on postoperative hypoesthesia over the lateral brachium averaging 45 cm^2; this corresponds to the distribution area of posterior cutaneous nerve of the forearm, which is harvested with the flap.

Graham et al. retrospectively reviewed 123 lateral arm flaps and advocated for informing the patient of the risk of donor site scarring and lateral arm hypoesthesia following surgery. In their hands, 59% of patients reported residual posterior forearm numbness at 3 years. Donor site scarring was unacceptable in 27 % of patients, and twice as likely in female patients. Some patients required skin grafting to close the donor site. Depner et al. reviewed the donor site morbidity of 22 ELAFs with primary closure of the donor site. They found patient satisfaction to be high in both males and females when assessed on a visual analogue scale, with an average score of 8.2 out of 10. Mild postoperative donor site sensory deficits were not a cause of patient dissatisfaction.

PEARLS AND PITFALLS

- Distal design of the skin paddle extending beyond the lateral epicondyle and onto the posterior forearm allows for a thin and pliable flap, extended pedicle length, and easier visualization of the radial nerve during harvest.
- In obese patients, the lateral arm flap may be too thick for hand and wrist coverage. A more distally designed flap and subsequent flap debulking may be required.
- The radial artery provides an excellent recipient vessel for all traumatic defects of the hand and wrist. The senior author prefers end-to-side anastomosis in the radial artery at the anatomic snuffbox if possible.
- Early identification and protection of the radial nerve in the brachioradialis/brachialis interval allow for expedient flap elevation without concern for injury to the nerve.
- Skin paddle width should be limited 6 to 8 cm to allow for primary closure of the donor site. Placement of posterior splint may be helpful in preventing dehiscence if donor site closure is tight.
- Early postoperative mobilization of elbow is recommended to prevent decreased range of motion.

RECOMMENDED READING

Akinci M, Ay S, Kamiloglu S, et al. Lateral arm free flaps in the defects of the upper extremity: a review of 72 cases. *Hand Surg.* 2005;10(2–3):177–185.

Berthe JV, Toussaint D, Coessens BC. One-stage reconstruction of an infected skin and Achilles tendon defect with a composite distally planned lateral arm flap. *Plast Reconstr Surg.* 1998;102(5):1618–1622.

Busnardo FF, Coltro PS, Olivan MV, et al. Anatomical comparison among the anterolateral thigh, the parascapular, and the lateral arm flaps. *Microsurgery.* 2015;35(5):387–392.

Coessens B, Vico P, De MA. Clinical experience with the reverse lateral arm flap in soft-tissue coverage of the elbow. *Plast Reconstr Surg.* 1993;92(6):1133–1136.

Depner C, Erba P, Rieger UM, et al. Donor-site morbidity of the sensate extended lateral arm flap. *J Reconstr Microsurg.* 2012;28(2):133–138.

Fogdestam I, Tarnow P, Kalaaji A. Extended free lateral arm flap with preservation of the posterior cutaneous nerve of the forearm. *Scand J Plast Reconstr Surg Hand Surg.* 1996;30(1):49–55.

Graham B, Adkins P, Scheker LR. Complications and morbidity of the donor and recipient sites in 123 lateral arm flaps. *J Hand Surg Br.* 1992;17(2):189–192.

Haas F, Rappl T, Koch H, et al. Free osteocutaneous lateral arm flap: anatomy and clinical applications. *Microsurgery.* 2003;23(2):87–95.

Hamdi M, Coessens BC. Distally planned lateral arm flap. *Microsurgery.* 1996;17(7):375–379.

Hamdi M, Coessens BC. Evaluation of the donor site morbidity after lateral arm flap with skin paddle extending over the elbow joint. *Br J Plast Surg.* 2000;53(3):215–219.

Kan HJ, Hovius SE. Long-term follow-up of flaps for extensive Dupuytren's and Ledderhose disease in one family. *J Plast Reconstr Aesthet Surg.* 2012;65(12):1741–1745.

Katsaros J, Schustermann M, Beppu M, et al. The lateral upper arm flap: anatomy and clinical applications. *Ann Plast Surg.* 1984;12:489–500.

Klinkenberg M, Fischer S, Kremer T, et al. Comparison of anterolateral thigh, lateral arm, and parascapular free flaps with regard to donor-site morbidity and aesthetic and functional outcomes. *Plast Reconstr Surg.* 2013;131(2):293–302.

Kuek LB, Chuan TL. The extended lateral arm flap: a new modification. *J Reconstr Microsurg.* 1991;7(3):167–173.

Moffett TR, Madison SA, Derr JW Jr, et al. An extended approach for the vascular pedicle of the lateral arm free flap. *Plast Reconstr Surg.* 1992;89(2):259–267.

Ng SW, Teoh LC, Lee YL, et al. Contralateral pedicled lateral arm flap for hand reconstruction. *Ann Plast Surg.* 2010;64(2):159–163.

Okada M, Takamatsu K, Oebisu N, et al. Reversed lateral upper arm flap with a vascularised fragment of the humerus for reconstruction of ulna shaft fracture after resection of malignant tumour: a case report. *J Plast Reconstr Aesthet Surg.* 2011;64(10):1373–1376.

Patel KM, Higgins JP. Posterior elbow wounds: soft tissue coverage options and techniques. *Orthop Clin North Am.* 2013;44(3):409–417.

Prantl L, Schreml S, Schwarze H, et al. A safe and simple technique using the distal pedicled reversed upper arm flap to cover large elbow defects. *J Plast Reconstr Aesthet Surg.* 2008;61(5):546–551.

Sauerbier M, Germann G, Giessler GA, et al. The free lateral arm flap: a reliable option for reconstruction of the forearm and hand. *Hand (NY).* 2012;7(2):163–171.

Song R, Song Y, Yu Y, et al. The upper arm free flap. *Clin Plast Surg.* 1982;9(1):27–35.

Wong M, Tay SC, Teoh LC. Versatility of the turn-around technique of the lateral arm flap for hand reconstruction. *Ann Plast Surg.* 2012;69(3):265–270.

Yousif NJ, Warren R, Matloub HS, et al. The lateral arm fascial free flap: its anatomy and use in reconstruction. *Plast Reconstr Surg.* 1990;86(6):1138–1145.

18 Radial Forearm and Radial Forearm Fascial Flap for Coverage of the Dorsum of the Hand and Wrist

Yoo Joon Sur, Mohamed Morsy, and Michel Saint-Cyr

INDICATIONS/CONTRAINDICATIONS

The skin and soft tissues of the dorsum of the hand are thin and pliable while providing an efficient gliding surface for the extensor tendons. The tissue is also durable and sensate to withstand continuous external insults. Due to the specialized nature of this tissue, reconstruction of soft tissue defects on the dorsum of the hand is a challenge as the surgeon must find tissue of similar quality to bring to the site of the defect. Small defects on the dorsum of the hand can be treated with wound care alone and be left to heal through secondary intention or treated with skin grafting; however, in cases where there are exposed nerves, vessels, joints, bones, or tendon without paratenon, flap coverage must be considered.

Although there are numerous methods of providing vascularized coverage for such situations, the reverse radial forearm flap has been the workhorse flap for soft tissue coverage of the dorsum of the hand. The reverse radial forearm flap is reliable and versatile. It can be harvested as a fasciocutaneous, adipofascial/fascial flap, or as a composite flap with addition of adjacent flexor carpi radialis muscle belly, tendon (e.g., palmaris longus), partial bone from the radius or cutaneous nerves. Although the radial forearm flap can be designed as a proximally based or distally based pedicled flap, or a free flap, a distally based pedicled flap is the most commonly used application for soft tissue reconstruction of the hand. Its advantages include consistent anatomy, long pedicle length, large-vessel caliber, thinness of the flap, and low technical demand without the need for microsurgery.

The traditional radial forearm flap, which was described by Yang and Yuzhi in 1978, is a fasciocutaneous flap. This simple one-stage procedure is indicated for coverage of the first web space, the palm, and the dorsum of the hand. This flap also can be used for coverage of the thumb and proximal parts of other fingers. The donor site is usually covered with a skin graft at the time of flap harvest.

There are two major downsides of the traditional radial forearm flap: the unsightly donor site and sacrifice of the radial artery (Fig. 18-1). Surgical techniques have been refined to limit these shortcomings. The more recent use of the radial forearm adipofascial/fascial flap can decrease morbidity at the donor site remarkably by harvesting only the adipofascial component of the flap. This leaves the overlying skin intact, allowing one to close the donor site with a linear scar. The flap does require skin grafting once transferred to the hand, but this can be a better option when a super-thin coverage is needed. More recent advances have also allowed for preservation of the radial artery by elevating the radial forearm fasciocutaneous or adipofascial/fascial flap based on perforators of the radial artery.

216

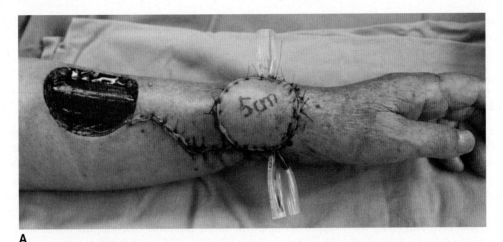

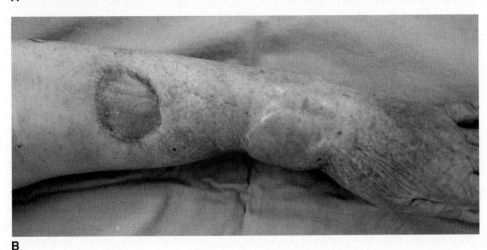

FIGURE 18-1

A 68-year-old woman with a soft tissue defect of the left wrist. **A:** The soft tissue defect was reconstructed with a distally based pedicled radial forearm flap following appropriate debridement. **B:** Subfascial flap harvest and split-thickness skin graft resulted in an unsightly dented scar on the donor site.

Contraindications to use of the flap include cases where the radial artery has been damaged or is missing (as may be seen in patients following cardiac bypass or radial artery catheterization). An Allen test should be performed to verify that the patient has an intact carpal arch, as flow to the reverse radial forearm flap is dependent on intact arterial flow through the ulnar artery into the carpal arterial arch and then retrograde into the radial artery. If the Allen test is abnormal, the traditional reverse radial forearm flap is contraindicated. On the other hand, the radial artery perforator pedicled flap can be safely elevated even if the palmar arch is not competent or the radial artery is the only inflow to the hand as the perforator-based flap will not sacrifice the radial artery. If there is any question about the blood flow to the hand, a vascular ultrasound or formal angiogram may be obtained prior to proceeding with flap coverage.

While not an absolute contraindication to flap use, a history of peripheral vascular disease, smoking, and diabetes may compromise the blood flow through smaller perforators making a perforator-only flap less reliable in these patients.

PREOPERATIVE PLANNING

Soft tissue coverage of the hand should be attempted as early as possible to maximize its functional recovery. Early coverage is predicated on radical debridement of all nonviable tissue and skeletal stabilization. When considering a radial forearm flap, circulation of the radial and ulnar artery should be checked to verify the patency of the carpal arch. To identify major perforators for a perforator-based flap, intraoperative exploration still remains the gold standard to determine the exact location of the radial artery perforators; but CT angiogram and MRA may also allow one to see the location of the major skin perforators.

SURGERY

Anatomy

The route of the radial artery is represented by a line connecting the midpoint of the cubital fossa to the point just medial to the radial styloid process. The radial artery runs within the lateral intermuscular septum, which connects the periosteum of the anterior border of the radius and the deep fascia surrounding the limb and separates the anterior and posterior compartments of the forearm. The radial artery originates from the brachial artery at approximately the neck of the radius and passes between the supinator and pronator teres. The division of the radial artery from the brachial artery can be found under the bicipital aponeurosis. In the proximal forearm, the radial artery is just deep to the brachioradialis, lying between the brachioradialis and the pronator teres. If the brachioradialis is pulled laterally, the entire length of the radial artery can be seen. As the radial artery runs distally, it lies between the tendons of the brachioradialis and the flexor carpi radialis. More distally, the radial artery is covered by only skin and fascia and lies just lateral to the tendon of the flexor carpi radialis. After reaching the radial styloid process, the radial artery turns posteriorly, passing underneath the tendons of the abductor pollicis longus and the extensor pollicis brevis, and enters the anatomical snuff box. It then passes between the first two metacarpal bones and forms the deep palmar arch by joining the deep branch of the ulnar artery. The radial artery is accompanied by two venae comitantes. The venae comitantes are connected to each other by multiple communicating branches, which make reverse flow possible by crossover and bypass patterns. The diameter of the radial artery is approximately 2.5 mm, and that of the venae comitantes is 1.3 to 2.5 mm.

The radial artery provides an average of 24.6 cutaneous perforators per arm, and among them, 9.2 cutaneous perforators are clinically relevant major cutaneous perforators (a caliber of 0.5 mm or greater) (Fig. 18-2). The radial artery major perforators are clustered to the proximal third and distal fifth of the forearm (Fig. 18-3). *At least two major perforators can be found within 2 cm proximal to the radial styloid process without exception.* The perforators of the proximal third of the forearm are usually larger but less frequent, whereas those of the distal fifth are smaller and grouped densely. There are few perforators in the midportion of the forearm. Perforators coming off the radial artery travel to the dermis and form a network by means of linking vessels (Fig. 18-4). These linking vessels connect adjacent perforators and usually run parallel to the radial artery, thus following the longitudinal axis of the forearm. Linking vessels help maintain flow between adjacent perforators and explain why flaps

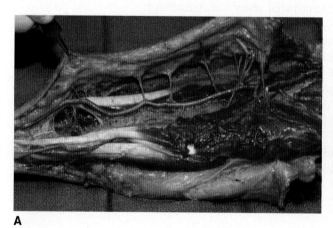
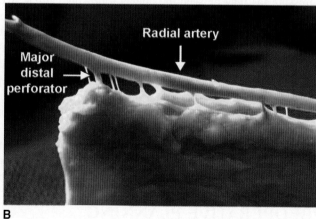

A   **B**

FIGURE 18-2

A: Dissection of a red Microfil-injected cadaveric specimen showed multiple cutaneous perforators of the radial artery. **B:** Those with a caliber of 0.5 mm or more were clinically relevant major cutaneous perforators. (Reprinted from Saint-Cyr M, Mujadizic M, Wong C, Hatef D, et al. The radial artery pedicle perforator flap: vascular analysis and clinical implications. *Plast Reconstr Surg.* 2010;125:1469–1478, with permission.)

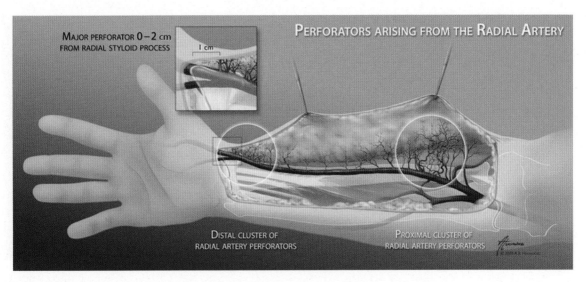

FIGURE 18-3

Illustration of proximal and distal clusters of clinically relevant, major cutaneous perforators of the radial artery. There are always at least two major cutaneous perforators within 2 cm proximal to the radial styloid process. (Reprinted from Saint-Cyr M, Mujadizic M, Wong C, Hatef D, et al. The radial artery pedicle perforator flap: vascular analysis and clinical implications. *Plast Reconstr Surg.* 2010;125:1469–1478, with permission.)

can survive based on a single dominant perforator. Because the vascular network of linking vessels lies between the fascia and the dermis, the radial forearm flap can be harvested suprafascially (Fig. 18-5). Suprafascial dissection does not compromise blood supply to the radial forearm flap (Fig. 18-6).

Patient Positioning

In most cases, the radial forearm flap is harvested from the same upper extremity. The patient is placed in supine position on the operating table equipped with a hand table. A pneumatic tourniquet is applied to arm and the entire upper extremity is scrubbed and draped in standard surgical fashion.

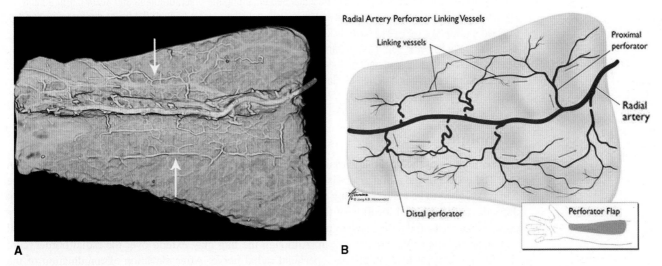

FIGURE 18-4

A: A 3D reconstruction coronal CT angiographic image of a radial forearm flap after suprafascial harvest. The linking vessels (*white arrows*) run parallel to the radial artery. (Reprinted from Schaverien M, Saint-Cyr M. Suprafascial compared with subfascial harvest of the radial forearm flap: an anatomic study. *J Hand Surg Am.* 2008;33:97–101, with permission.) **B:** The radial artery perforator linking vessels. *Blue arrows* indicate the direction of blood flow. Linking vessels can maintain blood flow between adjacent cutaneous perforators (interperforator flow) even after they are ligated. (Reprinted from Saint-Cyr M, Mujadizic M, Wong C, et al. The radial artery pedicle perforator flap: vascular analysis and clinical implications. *Plast Reconstr Surg.* 2010;125:1469–1478, with permission.)

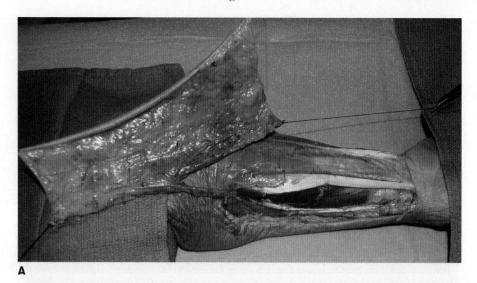

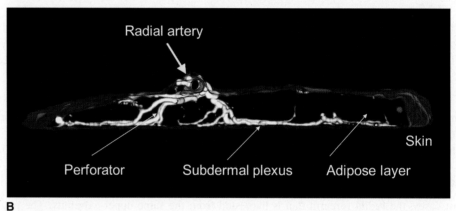

FIGURE 18-5

A: Suprafascial harvest of a radial forearm flap from a cadaveric specimen. The deep fascia was preserved up to a few millimeters from the lateral intermuscular septum along the brachioradialis and flexor carpi radialis. The flexor tendons remain covered by deep fascia, with only the muscle belly of the flexor digitorum profundus exposed, providing a well-vascularized skin graft bed. **B:** A 3D reconstruction axial CT angiographic image of a radial forearm flap after suprafascial harvest. The subdermal plexus is well protected by adipose tissue, and flap perfusion is dependent mainly on the cutaneous perforators that course obliquely down to the subdermal plexus. (Reprinted from Schaverien M, Saint-Cyr M. Suprafascial compared with subfascial harvest of the radial forearm flap: an anatomic study. *J Hand Surg Am.* 2008;33:97–101, with permission.)

Technique

Before inflation of the pneumatic tourniquet, patency of the palmar arch is confirmed with an Allen test. The course of the radial artery is marked out on the forearm using a handheld Doppler and the flap is designed to be centered along the path of the radial artery (Fig. 18-7). The design of the flap depends on the size and location of the soft tissue defect. The flap size should be equal or slightly greater than measured defect size to prevent closing tension. The limit of the flap width is the radial and ulnar borders of the volar forearm. Although the flap may extend over the radial border, care should be taken not to damage the superficial radial nerve. After elevation exsanguination of the upper extremity, dissection proceeds under tourniquet control and loupe magnification. At first, a curvilinear or straight skin incision is made along the path of the radial artery from the planned pivot point to the distal margin of the flap. The pivot point of the pedicle is usually about 2 to 4 cm proximal to the radial styloid process. The radial artery and venae comitantes are identified between the tendons of the flexor carpi radialis and the brachioradialis, and the skin incision is continued proximally to the ulnar side of the flap. The incision is deepened to the deep fascia along the ulnar margin of the flap. In the original flap description, flap harvest was performed in the subfascial plane. However, authors prefer a suprafascial dissection in order to minimize donor site morbidity. The potential

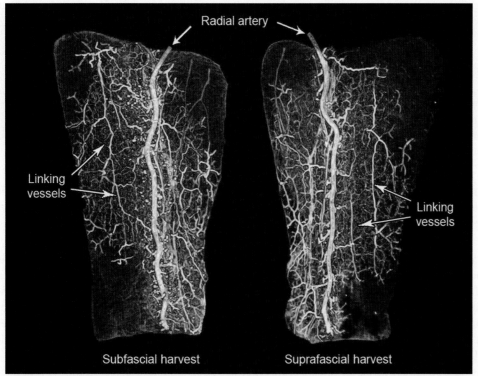

A

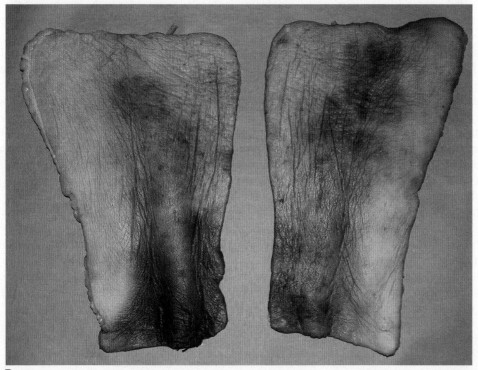

B

FIGURE 18-6

A: Three-dimensional reconstruction with anteroposterior CT angiographic scans of paired radial forearm flaps after injection of the radial arteries with barium sulfate/gelatin mixture (subfascial flap harvest on the left and suprafascial flap harvest on the right). Note that the suprafascial plexus and longitudinal linking branches are preserved during suprafascial harvest and that the vascular filling pattern and cutaneous territory are virtually identical for both flaps. **B:** Same flaps after injection with methylene blue dye showing identical patterns of vascular territory surface areas between both subfascial (left) and suprafascial (right) harvested radial forearm flaps. (Reprinted from Schaverien M, Saint-Cyr M. Suprafascial compared with subfascial harvest of the radial forearm flap: an anatomic study. *J Hand Surg Am.* 2008;33:97–101, with permission.)

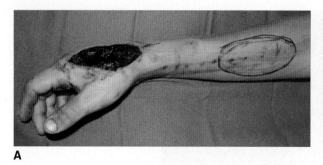
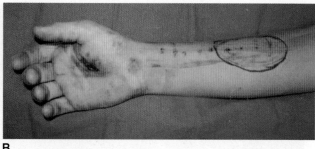

FIGURE 18-7

A: A 26-year-old man with a skin and soft tissue defect of the dorsum of the right hand. **B:** The course of the radial artery was marked using a handheld Doppler. A distally based pedicled radial forearm flap was designed to be centered along the course of the radial artery. The flap was intentionally designed slightly larger than the measured defect size to prevent closing tension. (Courtesy Sean Bidic MD.)

advantages of preservation of the deep fascia include prevention of tendon exposure or the formation of adhesions with the overlying skin graft, improved functional outcome, and a superior bed for skin graft. The suprafascial dissection plane also facilitates visualization and protection of the superficial radial and antebrachial cutaneous nerves. The suprafascial dissection is carried out radially up to the radial border of the flexor carpi radialis, and the dissection proceeds deep into the subfascial layer so that a cuff of fascia surrounding the radial artery and venae comitantes is maintained. This technique enables preservation of cutaneous perforators as they pass through the deep fascia. Next, the skin incision is continued along the radial border of the flap and the suprafascial dissection is continued to the ulnar border of the brachioradialis. Then, the dissection deepens to the subfascial plane. Distally, the radial artery and associated venae comitantes are located more volar to the brachioradialis tendon; therefore, careful attention must be made to retract the brachioradialis tendon radially to expose the vascular pedicle and not injure the septum and radial artery perforators. The radial artery and venae comitantes are ligated at the proximal margin of the flap, and the flap and the vascular pedicle are lifted from proximal to the pivot point (Fig. 18-8). When a sensate flap is needed, the medial or lateral antebrachial cutaneous nerve can be used for neurotization, but superficial veins are mostly ligated. One of the proximal superficial veins should be ligated with enough length to allow for additional venous outflow anastomosis in case of venous congestion after flap harvest. Skeletonization of the vascular pedicle should be avoided to ensure sufficient retrograde venous flow. The tourniquet is deflated, and the perfusion of the flap is checked. Before the flap is transposed, a time interval is helpful to enhance proper perfusion of the flap and to prevent vasospasm of the pedicle. Finally, the flap is inset to the defect and suction drains are placed beneath the flap (Fig. 18-9). Although the flap can be transposed through a subcutaneous tunnel, the threshold for skin incision from the pivot point to the defect should be low to secure robust flap perfusion. Transposing the flap pedicle underneath a tight skin envelop is fraught with complications, and the dorsal skin with its increased laxity should be favored in the majority of cases. Keeping a small skin island over the pedicle can allow skin incision and pedicle coverage with minimal tension. The donor site can be closed primarily when the width of the flap is less than 4 cm. A larger donor site is covered with unmeshed split-thickness or full-thickness skin grafts. A clinical case of a distally based pedicled radial forearm flap for soft tissue reconstruction of the thumb is illustrated in Figure 18-10.

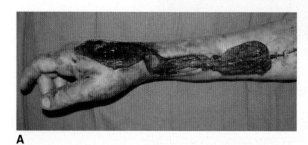
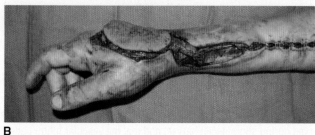

FIGURE 18-8

A: The distally based pedicled radial forearm flap was harvested. The vascular pedicle was not skeletonized to prevent venous congestion. **B:** The flap was rotated to reach the defect, and its perfusion was checked after tourniquet deflation.

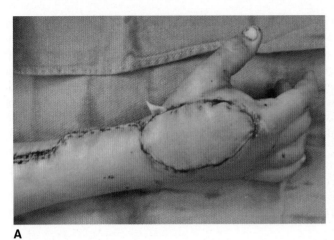
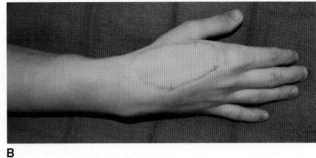

FIGURE 18-9

A: Skin incision was made between the pivot point and the defect, and the flap was inset to the defect. Although a distally based pedicled radial forearm flap can be transferred though a subcutaneous tunnel, skin incision should be made when compression of the pedicle is doubted. In this case, the donor site was closed primarily. **B:** Lipoaspiration of the radial forearm flap was performed 8 weeks after the initial surgery for improved contouring.

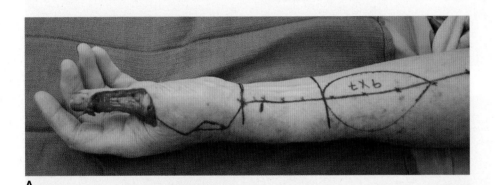
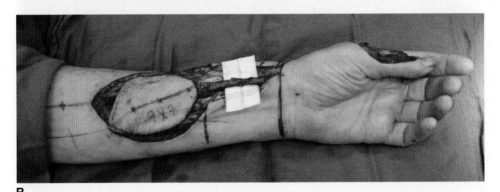
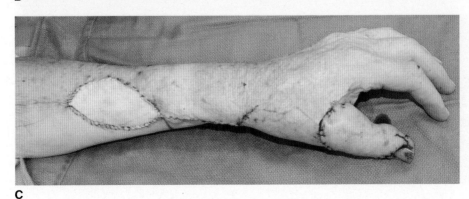

FIGURE 18-10

A 46-year-old man with left thumb soft tissue defect. **A:** After appropriate debridement and wound care, a distally based pedicled radial forearm flap was planned. **B:** A 9 × 7 cm flap was harvested suprafascially. **C:** The flap was inset through a subcutaneous tunnel, and the donor site was covered by full-thickness skin graft.

When the radial forearm flap is harvested as an adipofascial/fascial flap (without the skin), the only difference from the previous surgical technique is in the initial dissection. A curvilinear or straight skin incision is made along the path of the radial artery from the pivot point to the proximal margin of the flap. In the adipofascial/fascial flap, the skin is lifted off the subcutaneous tissue, leaving a thin layer of fat on the skin to avoid damaging the subdermal vascular plexus. After exposing proper width of subcutaneous tissue, the suprafascial dissection proceeds to the space between the flexor carpi radialis and the brachioradialis. The suprafascial dissection itself does not jeopardize flap perfusion as long as a portion of fascia surrounding the vascular pedicle is preserved. Next steps are identical to the previously described techniques. The adipofascial/fascial flap is usually covered with unmeshed split-thickness skin grafts. Meshing of skin grafts is discouraged not only due to the poor cosmesis but also due to the increased risk of contractures, especially over the web spaces and crease folds.

The radial forearm fasciocutaneous or adipofascial/fascial flap also can be harvested without sacrifice of the radial artery (Fig. 18-11). The distal cluster of the radial artery cutaneous perforators, which

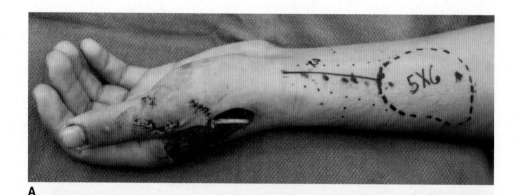

A

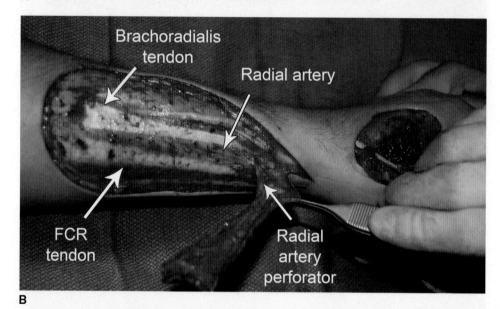

B

FIGURE 18-11

A 21-year-old man with left hand degloving injury. After debridement and repair of extensor pollicis longus, the soft tissue defect was covered with a distally based radial artery perforator flap. **A, B:** A flap based on a major cutaneous perforator within 2 cm proximal to the radial styloid process was harvested suprafascially.
C: The flap was transferred through a subcutaneous tunnel and the donor site was closed with full-thickness skin graft from the groin.

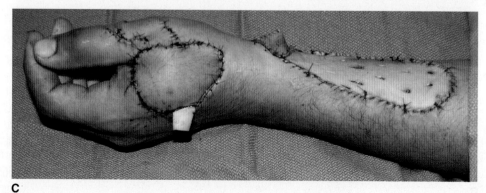

C

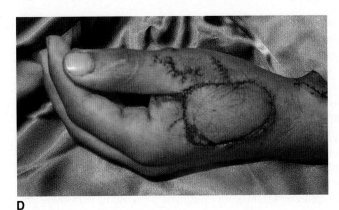

D

is located at the distal fifth of the forearm, is used to supply the distally based radial artery perforator flap. There are always at least two major perforators (a caliber of 0.5 mm or greater) within 2 cm of the radial styloid process (see Fig. 18-3). The flap is dissected with a wide (greater than 3 cm) subcutaneous pedicle, which rises through the intertendinous septum between the flexor carpi radialis and the brachioradialis. Dissection can be performed along the subfascial plane or the suprafascial plane. Because cutaneous perforators of the radial artery travel directly to the skin and communicate with each other in the subcutaneous tissue by means of multiple linking vessels (see Fig. 18-5), the suprafascial dissection does not compromise blood supply to the radial artery perforator pedicled flap (see Fig. 18-6). The pivot point is about 2 to 4 cm proximal to the radial styloid process, the base of pedicle is preserved as widely as possible, and the individual perforators should not be skeletonized. This is to guarantee inclusion of as many of the cutaneous perforators and linking vessels as possible and thus maximizing flap vascularity. After the flap is elevated, the tourniquet is deflated, and perfusion of the flap is checked. Because this flap is nourished by wide subcutaneous pedicle with small cutaneous perforators, arterial perfusion pressure is low, and it sometimes takes time to recover physiologic perfusion after tourniquet deflation. By the same token, caution is required to prevent kinking or compression of the pedicle when the flap is transposed. In case of an adipofascial/fascial flap, it can be flipped over to reach the defect.

POSTOPERATIVE MANAGEMENT

Routine postoperative protocols for flap reconstruction, such as maintaining warm environment, adequate hydration, and pain control, also apply to the radial forearm flap. The upper extremity is initially immobilized with a long arm splint for the first week and then with a short arm splint for another week. A suction drain is usually removed after 24 hours, and the upper extremity is elevated to decrease edema for the first week. Sequential clinical examinations of the flap circulation are performed for the first 3 days. Venous congestion occasionally happens in early postoperative period but usually subsides spontaneously. When a skin graft is used for the donor site or for the coverage of adipofascial/fascial flap, the fingers and wrist should be immobilized to allow the skin graft to adhere to the recipient bed. Gentle range of motion exercise can be initiated when the flap is stable and the skin graft is taken, approximately 1 week after the reconstruction.

RESULTS

After the first description of the distally based pedicled radial forearm flap by Lu in 1982, the distally based pedicled radial forearm flap has been the workhorse flap in the field of hand surgery for over three decades. The robust vascularity of this flap provides excellent wound healing, and cases of partial or total flap loss are rare. Most of the unsatisfactory results are related to poor cosmesis of the donor site. Efforts have been developed to improve the cosmesis of the donor site. The suprafascial radial forearm flap can reduce donor site morbidity by allowing a smoother skin graft recipient site. The radial forearm adipofascial/fascial flap provides even better cosmesis for both of the donor and recipient sites.

COMPLICATIONS

One of possible major complication is flap failure. The most common reason for failure of the radial forearm flap is technical error. Partial or total flap loss is usually related to venous congestion rather than arterial insufficiency. The best solution is to detect the problem as soon as possible. Early signs of venous congestion may be addressed with loosening overlying dressings or removing a couple of stitches. However, if not improving, a rapid return to the operating room is mandatory. Surgical exploration is needed to find kinking, stretching, or compression of the vascular pedicle.

At the donor site, partial or total loss of the skin graft sometimes occurs due to hematoma, seroma, infection, or poor immobilization. However, it is avoidable with strict short-term immobilization and careful compression dressing. The superficial radial nerve can be hurt during flap elevation. This injury induces loss of sensation and a painful neuroma. For such cases, nerve repair may be required.

The most detrimental complication, although rare, is the problem induced by sacrifice of the radial artery. There have been case reports of total hand ischemia, digital ischemia, and chronic vascular insufficiency, as well as some case reports of cold intolerance following sacrifice of the radial artery. A thorough physical examination and supplemental imaging examination should be performed preoperatively to verify flow in the ulnar artery and carpal arch thus preventing this complication.

Although the adipofascial/fascial flap and the radial artery perforator flap can provide more favorable cosmesis and can save the radial artery, they are more technically demanding, and they may have higher rates of marginal necrosis and partial and total loss than the traditional radial forearm flap. The safe dimension of the radial artery perforator flap that can be transferred reliably is smaller than the traditional radial forearm flap. The wide subcutaneous pedicle of the radial artery perforator flap is also cumbersome and occasionally needs to be skin grafted.

PEARLS AND PITFALLS

- Always obtain an Allen test prior to performing this flap. If there is any question about the patency of the ulnar or radial artery, obtain a vascular ultrasound or CT angiogram.
- At least two major perforators from the radial artery can be found within 2 cm proximal to the radial styloid process without exception.
- Do not completely exsanguinate the arm prior to inflating the tourniquet. This will aid in identifying the perforators to the skin.
- Maintain the peritenon over the tendons during flap harvest to maximize skin graft take.
- Although a distally based pedicled radial forearm flap can be transferred though a subcutaneous tunnel, a skin incision should be made when compression of the pedicle is suspected.
- Consider placing a nonmeshed skin graft over the donor site.
- The flap can be performed under regional anesthesia.
- Venous congestion can occur in rare cases; if this occurs, consider delaying flap inset by 48 hours. Return the flap to its native bed, and cover the wound with a moist dressing or a negative pressure dressing (VAC). Alternatively, a cutaneous vein contained within the flap can be anastomosed to a dorsal hand vein to facilitate venous drainage from the flap.
- If the flap appears ischemic after elevation and release of the tourniquet, one can consider converting the pedicled flap to a free flap for flap salvage.
- To improve skin graft adherence at the donor site, always use a bolster or VAC and some form of wrist immobilization.
- To avoid an unsightly donor site, do not use this flap for defects larger than 12 × 12 cm.

RECOMMENDED READING

Chang SM, Hou CL, Zhang F, et al. Distally based radial forearm flap with preservation of the radial artery: anatomic, experimental, and clinical studies. *Microsurgery.* 2003;23(4):328–337.

Ho AM, Chang J. Radial artery perforator flap. *J Hand Surg Am.* 2010;35(2):308–311.

Jeng SF, Wei FC. The distally based forearm island flap in hand reconstruction. *Plast Reconstr Surg.* 1998;102(2):400–406.

Kaufman MR, Jones NF. The reverse radial forearm flap for soft tissue reconstruction of the wrist and hand. *Tech Hand Up Extrem Surg.* 2005;9(1):47–51.

Saint-Cyr M, Muajdzic M, Wong C, et al. The radial artery pedicle perforator flap: vascular analysis and clinical implications. *Plast Reconstr Surg.* 2010;125(5):1469–1478.

Schaverien M, Saint-Cyr M. Suprafascial compared with subfascial harvest of the radial forearm flap: an anatomic study. *J Hand Surg Am.* 2008;33(1):97–101.

Taghinia AH, Carty M, Upton J. Fascial flaps for hand reconstruction. *J Hand Surg Am.* 2010;35(8):1351–1355.

Weinzweig N, Chen L, Chen ZW. The distally based radial forearm fasciosubcutaneous flap with preservation of the radial artery: an anatomic and clinical approach. *Plast Reconstr Surg.* 1994;94(5):675–684.

Yang D, Morris SF, Tang M, et al. Reversed forearm island flap supplied by the septocutaneous perforator of the radial artery: anatomical basis and clinical applications. *Plast Reconstr Surg.* 2003;112(4):1012–1016.

19 Posterior Interosseous Artery Island Flap for Dorsal Hand Coverage

Eduardo A. Zancolli

The posterior interosseous flap is an island pedicled fasciocutaneous flap from the dorsal aspect of the forearm supplied by the cutaneous branches of the posterior interosseous artery. The posterior interosseous artery is located in the septum between the extensor carpi ulnaris and the extensor indicis proprius. This flap has proven to be an excellent coverage option for the dorsum of the hand and the first interdigital web. The dorsal cutaneous area of the forearm supplied by the posterior interosseous artery was initially described by Manchot in 1889 and later by Salmon in 1936.

INDICATIONS/CONTRAINDICATIONS

The posterior interosseous artery island flap is capable of transporting the skin of the distal two-thirds of the forearm. The flap's pedicle length determines its distal coverage possibilities. Buchler et al. were the first to note that the flap could reach the dorsum of the proximal interphalangeal joints. It is particularly useful for covering extensive defects on the back of the hand as far distally as the dorsal aspect of the proximal phalanges of the fingers and for obtaining coverage of the first web space after the release of severe adduction contractures of the thumb. It can be indicated in different types of pathologies such as burn sequelae, wounds on the dorsum of the hand, tumors, and congenital deformities.

Contraindications for flap use include any injury to the posterior interosseous artery or deep laceration or crush wounds to the posterior forearm in the area of the flap pedicle. The flap is not recommended in patients with diabetes, in whom small vessels may be diseased. The flap has been used successfully in smokers, but smoking certainly carries a higher risk of flap complications.

Patients need to be informed that a skin graft may be necessary to close the donor site. And the donor site may be prone to the development of heavy scaring in some individuals.

PREOPERATIVE PLANNING

Successful flap harvest is predicated on a thorough knowledge of the flap anatomy. Normally, the anterior and posterior interosseous arteries in their course through the forearm are united through two main anastomoses: one proximal at the level of the distal border of the supinator muscle and one distal at the most distal part of the interosseous space (2 cm proximally of the distal radioulnar joint; Fig. 19-1). The posterior interosseous island flap is supplied by the reverse arterial blood flow through the distal anastomosis once the proximal anastomosis has been ligated. Venous drainage is produced by the venae comitantes of the posterior interosseous artery.

The angiosomal territory of the posterior interosseous artery was studied in a series of 80 cadaveric forearms in 1993. Ink injections performed through catheter placed in the distal part of the anterior interosseous artery stained the distal two-thirds of the posterior forearm skin through the reverse flow through the distal anastomosis. The proximal third of the forearm skin remained unstained even

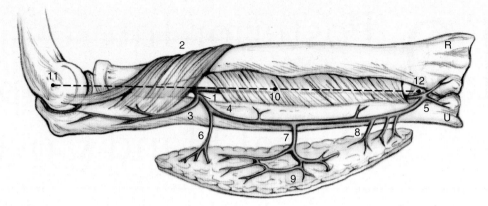

FIGURE 19-1

Anatomy of the posterior interosseous artery. (*1*) Proximal end of the posterior interosseous artery at the distal border of the supinator muscle. (*2*) The artery is emerging as a division of the common interosseous artery. (*3*) Recurrent interosseous artery. (*4*) Posterior interosseous artery following the longitudinal line X-X', between the lateral epicondyle (*11*) and the distal radioulnar joint (*12*). (*5*) Distal anastomosis between both interosseous arteries (2 cm proximal to the distal radioulnar joint). Cutaneous branches from the posterior interosseous artery that irrigate the two distal thirds of the posterior skin of the forearm. Proximal (*9*), middle (*7*), and distal (*8*) branches. (*10*) Middle of the forearm where the middle cutaneous branch is located 1 to 2 cm distal to this point.

when larger amounts of ink were injected (Fig. 19-2). Ink injections through the catheter placed in the proximal part of the posterior interosseous artery stained the proximal two-thirds of the posterior forearm through the direct flow through the proximal cutaneous branch.

Other anatomic conclusions from this study can be summarized as follows: the posterior interosseous artery usually branches from the common interosseous artery in the proximal third of the forearm in 90% of cases; it can however be a direct branch of the ulnar artery in 10% of cases. It pierces the interosseous membrane about 6 cm distal to the lateral epicondyle of the humerus, forming its origin or proximal anastomosis between the anterior and posterior interosseous arteries. It enters into the posterior compartment of the forearm below the distal edge of the supinator muscle, located at the junction of the proximal one-third and distal two-thirds of the dorsal aspect of the forearm (60 mm distal to the lateral epicondyle). At its entrance into the posterior compartment of the forearm, the posterior interosseous artery gives off branches to the recurrent interosseous artery that anastomoses at the elbow with the medial (also called middle) collateral artery. The medial collateral artery will anastomose with the posterior radial collateral artery and posterior ulnar recurrent artery at the dorsum of the distal humerus through the anastomotica magna. In its ascending course, the recurrent interosseous artery runs between the lateral condyle and the olecranon (Fig. 19-3).

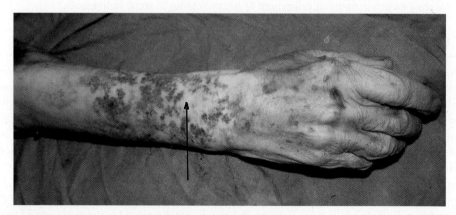

FIGURE 19-2

Fresh cadaver injected with 20 mL of black ink through a catheter placed in the distal anterior interosseous artery. The distal and middle thirds of the dorsal forearm are stained.

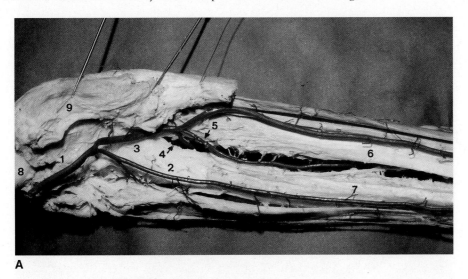

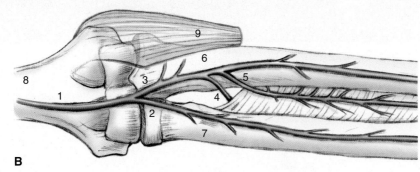

FIGURE 19-3

A: Cadaver specimen dissected to show the proximal origin of the posterior interosseous artery. **B:** Volar view of the proximal part of the forearm and the elbow. (*1*) Brachial artery. (*2*) Radial artery. (*3*) Ulnar artery showing the separated origin of the posterior interosseous artery (*4*) and the anterior interosseous artery (*5*). (*6*) Ulna. (*7*) Radius. (*8*) Humerus. (*9*) Medial epicondyle muscles.

From the proximal anastomosis, the posterior interosseous artery follows a line between the lateral epicondyle and the distal radioulnar joint. In its course, it can be divided into three parts: proximal, middle, and distal.

In the proximal part, the artery runs deep to the abductor pollicis longus muscle and is covered by the extensor digiti minimi and the extensor carpi ulnaris muscles and in close relation with the posterior interosseous nerve and a large venous plexus. In the middle part, it becomes superficial, just beneath the superficial antebrachial fascia in the middle third of the forearm, running between the extensor digiti minimi and the extensor carpi ulnaris muscles. In this part, the artery reduces its diameter in 90% of the cases and is usually found to be between 0.3 and 0.6 mm in diameter (Fig. 19-4).

In the distal part, the posterior interosseous artery joins with the distal end of the anterior interosseous artery, forming the distal anastomosis between the two vessels. This anastomosis is located 2 cm proximal to the distal radioulnar joint and very close to the periosteum of the ulnar metaphysis (Fig. 19-5). This anastomosis has been present in all our cadaver specimens and operative cases and represents the point of rotation of the vascular pedicle of the posterior interosseous flap. At the distal anastomosis, the posterior interosseous artery enlarges between 0.9 and 1.1 mm.

During its course, the posterior interosseous artery gives four to six cutaneous branches, which run through the septum between the extensor digiti minimi and the extensor carpi ulnaris muscles to reach the dorsal skin of the forearm; *of these, the principal cutaneous branches are the proximal and middle branches.* The proximal cutaneous branch emerges from the proximal part of the artery, forming a large branch that irrigates the skin over the upper third of the dorsal aspect of the forearm. It is consistently present but it has a variable origin. Of our 80 specimens, it was found

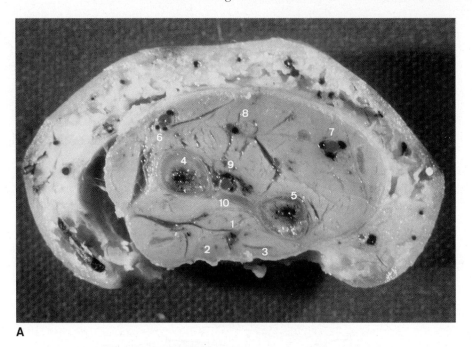

A

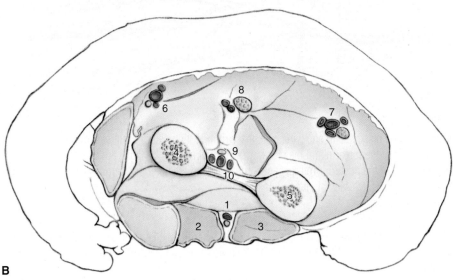

B

FIGURE 19-4

Transverse section of the forearm at its middle third. (*1*) Posterior interosseous artery—in its proximal course—running deep between the extensor digiti quinti (*2*) and the extensor carpi ulnaris (*3*) muscles. (*4*) Radius. (*5*) Ulna. Radial artery (*6*) and ulnar artery (*7*) both with their venae. Median nerve and median nerve artery (*8*). Anterior interosseous artery and its venae (*9*). Interosseous membrane (*10*).

as a branch of the recurrent interosseous artery in 28 (35%), as a branch of the common interosseous artery in 22 (27.5%), and as a branch of the posterior interosseous artery in 30 (37.5%). This variation indicates that the proximal cutaneous branch cannot be preserved to supply the flap in all cases.

The middle cutaneous branch originates in the middle third of the forearm where the posterior interosseous artery becomes superficial. It represents a large branch located at 1 to 2 cm distal to the middle of the forearm. It was consistently present in our cadaveric investigations and clinical cases.

No cutaneous branches were found between the described proximal and middle branches. In our cadaveric observations, one or two large interconnecting venous perforators were consistently found

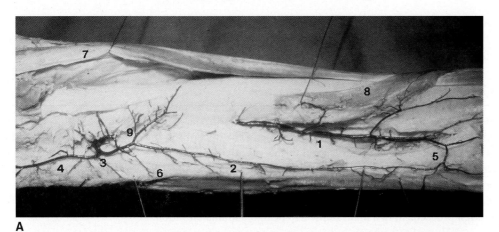

A

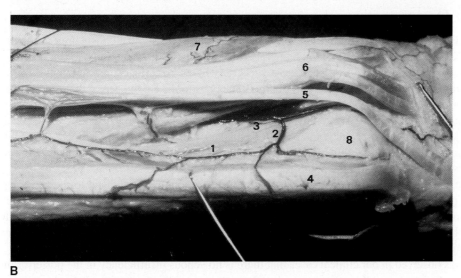

B

FIGURE 19-5

A: Cadaver specimen injected with latex (right forearm). Dissection of both interosseous arteries. (*1*) Anterior interosseous artery. (*2*) Posterior interosseous artery piercing the interosseous membrane (*3*) and showing the emergence of the recurrent interosseous artery (*4*). The cutaneous branches have been eliminated. (*7*) Distal anastomosis between both interosseous arteries located very close to the periosteum of the distal metaphysis of the ulna. (*8*) Extensor carpi ulnaris. (*9*) Extensor carpi radialis brevis muscle. (*10*) Extensor pollicis brevis and abductor pollicis longus muscles. (*11*) Large branch of the posterior interosseous artery to irrigate common extensor muscle. **B:** Posterior interosseous artery showing its proximal anastomosis (*2*) with the anterior interosseous artery (*3*). Right forearm. Several branches to the dorsal muscles of the forearm are seen. (*4*) Extensor carpi ulnaris tendon. (*5*) Extensor digiti quinti tendon. (*6*) Extensor communis digitorum tendons. (*7*) Extensor pollicis brevis and abductor pollicis longus muscles. (*8*) Distal head of the ulna.

running together with the middle cutaneous arterial branch, uniting the superficial to the deep venous system (the venae comitantes of the posterior interosseous artery). At the distal third of the posterior forearm, the posterior interosseous artery may also contribute six to eight cutaneous branches to the skin of variable diameter. The posterior interosseous artery also gives several branches to the muscles of the posterior compartment of the forearm and contributes some blood supply to the periosteum of the radius and ulna.

In our studies, there were only two cases where the continuity of the posterior interosseous artery was absent at the level of the middle of the forearm: one occurred in an anatomic specimen and one in a clinical case. This uncommon anatomic finding is in accordance with other reports in the medical literature. Thus, Penteado et al. found absence of the posterior interosseous artery in the forearm in 4 of 70 specimens. In their same series, the distal anastomosis was absent in only one case. Buchler and Frey found the posterior interosseous artery missing at the middle of the forearm in 2 of 36 cases. Despite this, angiograms and Doppler examination are not part of our standard preoperative protocol.

SURGERY

The surgical procedure is performed under general anesthesia. A pneumatic tourniquet is employed. Exsanguination is obtained by simple elevation of the upper limb for 30 seconds. Loop magnification (4×) permits a better identification of the vascular pedicles and their cutaneous branches. The patient is placed in the supine position with the forearm placed in pronation over the inferior-lateral thoracic wall with the elbow flexed in 90 degrees (Fig. 19-6). This position facilitates flap preparation and dissection. The tourniquet is insufflated (250 mm Hg) after the flap has been designed. The operation proceeds in two main steps: flap design and flap elevation.

Flap Design

Flap design (Fig. 19-7A) is strictly related to the shape and size of the recipient area. A longitudinal line (X-X′) is drawn from the lateral humeral epicondyle to the distal radioulnar joint. This line represents the course of the posterior interosseous artery in the posterior forearm. A point *A* is marked 1 cm distal to the middle of line. This point corresponds to the emergence of the middle cutaneous branch of the posterior interosseous artery and to the medial interconnecting venous perforator. The flap is planned to be irrigated by this middle cutaneous pedicle, so the point A must be always included in the flap. A second point, point *B*, is marked at the distal end of the line X-X′ and is 2 cm proximal to the distal radioulnar joint. Point *B* corresponds to the distal anastomosis between both interosseous arteries and is the point of rotation of the pedicle flap.

   The proximal limit of the flap can be safely placed to a point 6 cm distal to the lateral epicondyle (point *C*). The flap may be extended distally up to the wrist joint. In this case, distal cutaneous branches can be included. It should be remarked that the medial vascular cutaneous pedicle is capable of irrigating a flap as large as the complete width of the posterior forearm. The center of the flap always corresponds to the line X-X′.

   It was observed in our clinical cases that there is no venous insufficiency in the posterior interosseous reverse forearm flap if it is raised with the large middle venous interconnecting perforator. It ensures sufficient drainage of the subcutaneous tissue and skin into the venae comitantes of the posterior interosseous artery.

   A flap approximately 3 to 4 cm wide will allow for direct closure of the donor area of the forearm leaving an inconspicuous scar (Figs. 19-8 and 19-9). Wider flaps will require a skin graft to cover the dorsum of the forearm and may lead to a poorer aesthetic result (Fig. 19-10).

Flap Elevation

Flap elevation (see Fig. 19-7B) begins at its radial side. The dissection is carried out between the subcutaneous tissue and the superficial fascia. The incision is continued in the direction of the wrist, and the proximal and medial cutaneous branches are easily identified. The interconnecting venous

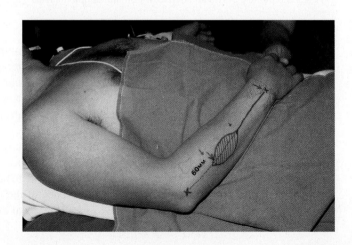

FIGURE 19-6

Position of the upper limb during surgery. In this patient, a posterior interosseous artery island flap 4 cm wide has been designed to cover the first interdigital web. The flap is located at the level of the middle cutaneous branch of the posterior interosseous artery. Details on the flap design are completed in Figure 19-7.

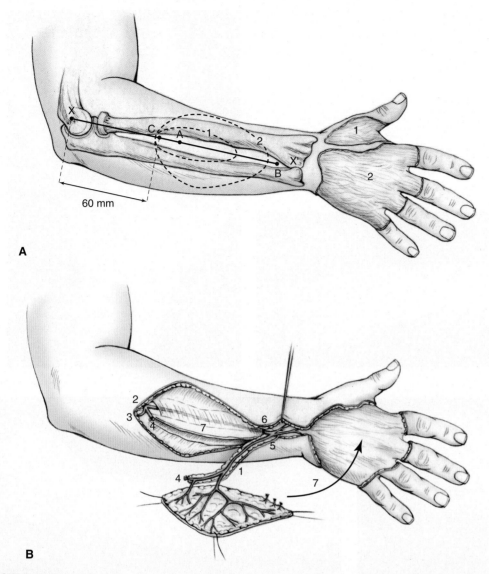

FIGURE 19-7

A: Design of the flap. The location of the island flap is in the line X-X′, between the lateral epicondyle (X) and the distal radioulnar joint (X′). Three points are marked in the skin. Point *A* corresponds to the location of the middle cutaneous branch of the posterior interosseous artery. Point *B* is located 2 cm proximal to the distal radioulnar point and corresponds with the location of the distal anastomosis; and point *C* is located at the distal edge of the supinator muscle where the posterior interosseous artery pierces the interosseous membrane. This point is 60 mm distal to the lateral epicondyle. The width, length, and shape of the island flap are in accordance with the defect to be covered: *1* is representing the shape, size, and location of a flap to cover the first interdigital web and *2* represents a flap to cover the dorsal aspect of the hand. **B:** Raising of the island flap. The flap has been raised with the posterior interosseous artery and its venae comitantes (*1*). In this case, the middle and the proximal cutaneous branches are irrigating the flap. The intermuscular septum and a strip of fascia are raised with the posterior interosseous artery. (*2*) Common interosseous artery. (*3*) Recurrent interosseous artery. (*4*) The posterior interosseous artery has been ligated at its emergence (proximal anastomosis between both interosseous arteries). (*5*) Distal anastomosis is preserved (point of rotation of the flap). (*6*) Anterior interosseous artery. (*7*) In this case, the flap is rotated to cover the dorsum of the hand. The donor area is covered with a free skin graft (see Figs. 19-8 and 19-9).

perforator that accompanies the medial cutaneous branch is clearly visualized. The proximal cutaneous branch can be coagulated. Our clinical cases have shown that the flap can be safely raised with the middle cutaneous branch. The posterior interosseous artery is sectioned at its proximal origin proximal to the medial cutaneous branch. The posterior interosseous artery with its venae comitantes is raised with the intermuscular septum located between the extensor carpi ulnaris and

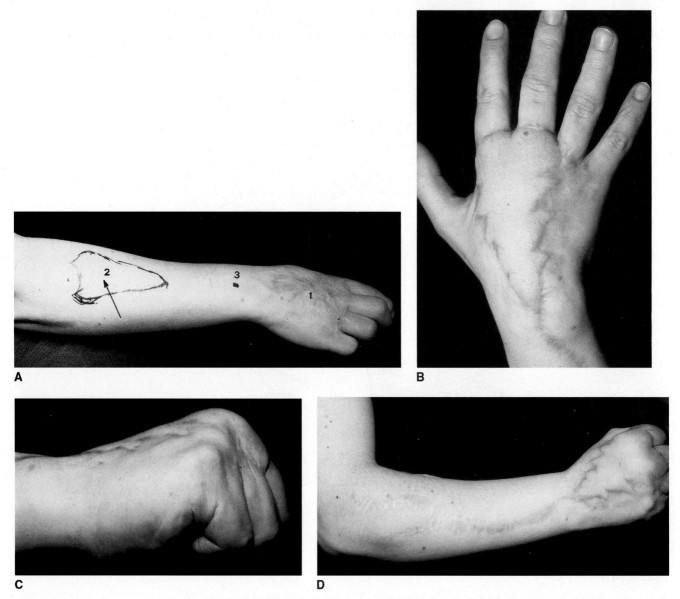

FIGURE 19-8

A: Sequela of an injury in a 19-year-old girl on the dorsum of the hand (*1*) with laceration of the long extensor tendons of the index and middle fingers and stiffness of their metacarpophalangeal joints. A posterior interosseous artery island flap was designed (*2*) with the shape of the area to be covered on the hand. Middle and proximal pedicles were preserved to irrigate the flap. Excision of the injured extensor tendons and metacarpophalangeal capsulectomies were indicated simultaneously with the island flap. The fingers were immobilized in flexion during the postoperative period. Location of the distal anastomosis (*3*). **B:** Finger extension obtained after a secondary surgical stage with Z-plasties at the borders of the flap and tendon transfer from the flexor superficialis tendon of the ring finger, divided into two strips, to the base of the middle and index fingers proximal phalanges. The interdigital webs were reconstructed with the flap. **C:** Digital flexion obtained. **D:** The donor area of the forearm was initially closed.

the extensor indicis proprius and a very thin strip of fascia covering the muscles. Elevation is completed after sectioning the skin at the ulnar side of the flap. Finally, the flap is turned through 180 degrees to cover the recipient area: to the dorsum of the hand, or to a released first web space, or to both. Now, the pneumatic tourniquet is released to observe flap circulation.

At the end of the procedure, the hand is immobilized in a neutral position of the wrist or with some dorsiflexion. In the case of coverage of the back of the hand, where the extensor tendons have been excised and a metacarpophalangeal capsulotomy has been performed, the fingers are immobilized in flexion to prevent the recurrence of metacarpophalangeal stiffness in extension. In these cases, tendon grafts can be indicated during a second surgical stage (see Figs. 19-8 and 19-9).

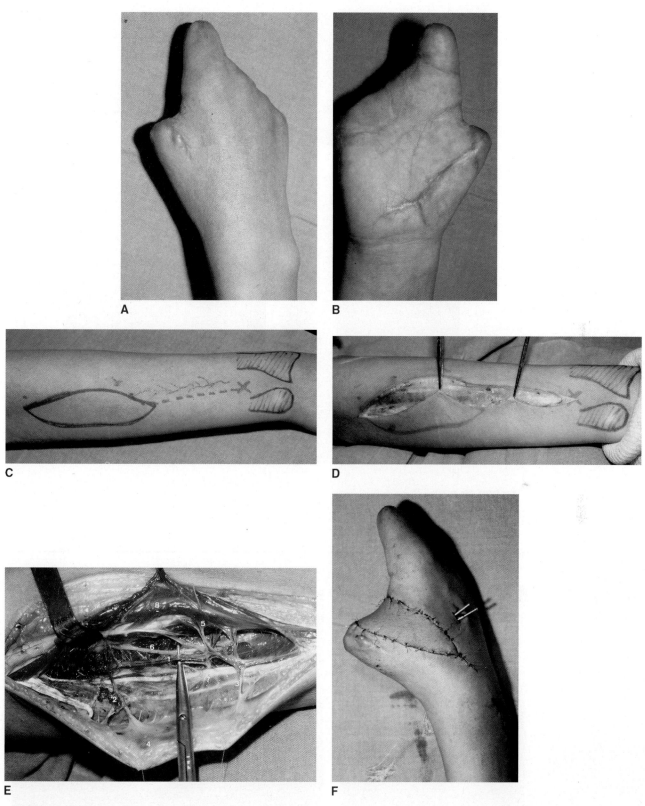

FIGURE 19-9

A, B: Sequela of a trauma with amputation of the digits and adduction contracture of the first intermetacarpal space in an 18-year-old man. **C:** Design of the posterior interosseous artery island flap of 3 cm width. The middle cutaneous branch was preserved to nourish the island flap. **D:** The initial skin incision is shown. The radial side of the flap is initially elevated from its radial side. **E:** Anatomy of the dissected posterior interosseous artery (*1*) with its middle (*2*) and distal (*3*) cutaneous branches to the dorsal skin of the forearm (*4*). Several arterial branches to the dorsal muscles of the forearm (*5*) and the posterior interosseous nerve (*6*) are shown. The extensor carpi ulnaris muscle (*7*) and the extensor muscles to the fingers (*8*) are separated. The hand is at the right of the picture. **F:** A few days after the release of the first intermetacarpal space and the transport of the island flap. Two KW are maintaining the separation of the first two metacarpals.

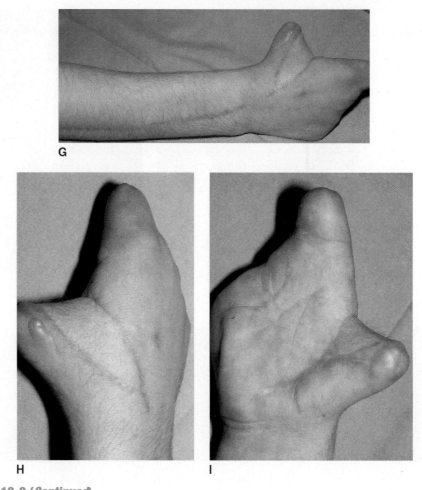

FIGURE 19-9 (*Continued*)

G: Direct closure of the donor area. **H, I:** Result obtained.

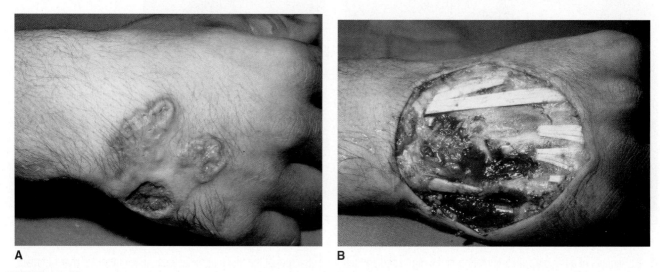

FIGURE 19-10

A: An epithelioid sarcoma with invasion of skin on the dorsal aspect of the forearm in a 20-year-old man. **B:** An ample excision of the affected skin, including the extensor tendons of the two last fingers, was indicated.

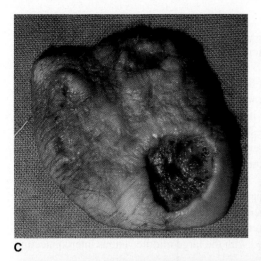

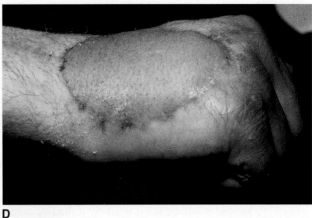

C

D

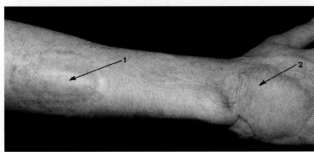

E

FIGURE 19-10 (*Continued*)

C: Piece of the lesion. **D:** Immediate postoperative period after a posterior interosseous artery island flap. In a secondary surgical stage, the extensor tendons were reconstructed. **E:** Result after 2 years following the initial operation showing the free skin graft in the donor area (*1*) and the posterior interosseous artery island flap in the recipient area (*2*). Complete function of the fingers was obtained.

POSTOPERATIVE MANAGEMENT

The hand and wrist are immobilized in a long plaster splint for 2 weeks after the surgery. A large window is left in the dressing to monitor the flap for signs of ischemia or venous congestion. No blood thinning agents are used during the postoperative period. Following removal of the splint, the sutures are removed and the patient may begin postoperative therapy.

RESULTS

Our series of 80 cases (47 men and 33 women) was published in 1993. In this series, 22 flaps were indicated for the coverage of skin defects in the dorsum of the hand, 37 for the reconstruction of the first interdigital web, 5 to cover the dorsum of the hand and first web space, 15 for the volar wrist, and 4 for the palm of the hand. In three cases, extensor tendon grafts to extend the fingers were indicated in a second surgical stage. Seventy-six flaps were successful and four were lost. Two of these were clearly due to twisting of the pedicle. The flap provides a large amount of skin for hand reconstruction without interfering with lymphatic drainage, venous drainage, or the integrity of the principal vessels of the volar side of the forearm. It furnishes good quality skin to permit secondary surgical reconstructions of tendons or the skeleton of the hand.

COMPLICATIONS

As mentioned previously, flap loss is the most serious complication; this is most commonly due to inadvertent twisting of the pedicle or injury to the veins during dissection resulting in flap congestion. Injury to the radial nerve has also been reported with temporary paralysis to the extensor carpi ulnaris and extensor digiti minimi muscles following flap harvest. Such occurrences are rare but can be avoided by meticulous dissection with the aid of the tourniquet during the case.

PEARLS AND PITFALLS

- Knowledge of the route of the posterior interosseous artery is critical to ensure safe elevation of the flap.
- The posterior interosseous artery follows a line between the lateral epicondyle and the distal radioulnar joint and gives four to six cutaneous branches, which run through the septum between the extensor digiti minimi and the extensor carpi ulnaris muscles to reach the dorsal skin of the forearm; of these, the principal cutaneous branches are the proximal and middle branches.
- When designing the flap, a longitudinal line is drawn from the lateral humeral epicondyle to the distal radioulnar joint. This line represents the course of the posterior interosseous artery in the posterior forearm
- A point is marked 1 cm distal to the middle of the line marking the route of the posterior interosseous artery. This point corresponds to the emergence of the middle cutaneous branch of the posterior interosseous artery and to the medial interconnecting venous perforator.
- Venous insufficiency is unlikely if the flap is raised with the large middle venous interconnecting perforator.
- Flaps wider than 4 cm will require skin grafting for closure of the donor site.

RECOMMENDED READING

Angrigiani C, Grilli D, Dominikow D, et al. Posterior interosseous reverse forearm flap: experience with 80 consecutive cases. *Plast Reconstr Surg.* 1993;92(2):285–293.

Buchler U, Frey HP. Retrograde posterior interosseous flap. *J Hand Surg.* 1991;16A(2):283–292.

Costa H, Soutar DS. The distally based island posterior interosseous flap. *Br J Plast Surg.* 1988;41:221–227.

Costa H, Smith R, McGrouther DA. Thumb reconstruction by the posterior interosseous flap. *Br J Plast Surg.* 1988;41:228–233.

Dap F, Dantel G, Voche P, et al. The posterior interosseous flap in primary repair of hand injuries. *J Hand Surg.* 1993;18-B(4):437–445.

Goubier JN, Romaña C, Masquelet AC. Le Lambeaux interosseoux posterieur chez l'enfant. *Chir Main.* 2002;21:102–106.

Gilbert A, Masquelet AC, Hentz VR. Pedicle flaps of the upper limb. In: Dunitz M, ed. *Vascular Anatomy: Surgical Technique and Current Indications.* Philadelphia, PA: Lippincott Williams & Wilkins; 1992.

Manchot C. *The Cutaneous Arteries of the Human Body. (Translation of Hautarterien des menslischen Korpers. 1889.)* New York: Springer; 1983.

Masquelet AC, Penteado CV. Le Iambeau interosseoux posterieur. *Ann Chir Main.* 1987;6:131–139.

Mazzer N, Barbieri CH, Cortez M. The posterior interosseous forearm island flap for skin defects in the hand and elbow: a prospective study of 51 cases. *J Hand Surg.* 1996;21B:237–243.

Penteado CV, Masquelet AC, Chevrel JP. The anatomic basis of the fascio-cutaneous flap of the posterior interosseous artery. *Surg Radiol Anat.* 1986;8:209–215.

Zancolli EA, Angrigiani C. Colgajo dorsal del antebrazo (en "isla) (Pedículo de vasos interoseos posteriores). *Rev Asoc Arg OrtopTraumatol.* 1986;51(2):161–168.

Zancolli EA, Angrigiani C. Dorsal forearm island flap. *Posterior interosseous vessels pedicle. 3rd Congress of the International Federation of Societies for Surgery of the Hand*, Tokyo, 1986 (abst).

Zancolli EA, Angrigiani C. Posterior interosseous island flap. *J Hand Surg.* 1988;13-B(2):130–135.

Zancolli EA, Cozzi E. *Atlas de Anatomía Quirúrgica de la Mano.* Ed Medica Panamericana Madrid; 1993:93.

20 Fillet Flaps in Cases of Mutilating Trauma

Ryan W. Schmucker and Michael W. Neumeister

Fillet flaps take advantage of tissue that would otherwise be discarded in order to cover vital structures and preserve limb length in the setting of amputations. Fillet flaps are, by definition, axial flaps that may provide skin, muscle, fascia and bone. They can be harvested either as a pedicled or as a free flap. Careful planning and execution of these flaps can allow for reconstruction of local defects with a flap of a similar tissue type. By taking advantage of the spare parts that would otherwise be disposed of, the morbidity of a separate flap harvest can be avoided. For these reasons, fillet flaps are an essential tool in the armamentarium of the reconstructive surgeon.

Fillet flaps are most commonly employed after mutilating trauma to the hand. Frequently the traumatized area is left without soft tissue coverage of vital structures such as bone, joint, tendon, or neurovascular bundles. Vascularized coverage of these structures can be obtained by using attached parts of the mangled hand that otherwise are rendered dysfunctional or from amputated parts that still contain a preserved vascular pedicle. The concept of spare parts surgery can be broadly applied to include any tissue that would otherwise be discarded; these flaps may include bone, nerve, tendon, joints, or an entire digit. Segments of the injured part can be harvested with their blood supply intact and thereby be used as a vascularized tissue graft or flap.

The key component to the safe harvest of a fillet flap is an understanding of the vascular supply to the tissue. Since the entire upper extremity and lower extremity can both be used in a fillet fashion, the blood supply to the arm and leg must be understood. In the upper extremity, the axillary artery terminates at the lateral border of the pectoralis minor muscle becoming the brachial artery to a point just distal to the antecubital fossa. The brachial artery runs in the medial upper arm in relative proximity to the ulnar and median nerves. At the level of the elbow, the brachial artery is lateral to the median nerve. The brachial artery bifurcates into the radial and ulnar arteries, respectively, under the superficial flexor muscles of the forearm. The radial artery travels under the flexor carpi radialis muscle exiting more superficial in the forearm just lateral to the tendon of the flexor carpi radialis. The ulnar artery travels with the ulnar nerve under the muscle belly of the flexor carpi ulnaris becoming more superficial in the distal forearm. The ulnar artery travels through Guyon canal and bifurcates into a superficial and deep branch, each of which communicates with the radial artery component of the superficial and deep palmar arches. The radial artery bifurcates at the wrist into a superficial palmar and deep dorsal branch. The superficial palmar branch courses around the base of the thenar eminence, while the larger deep branch travels under the abductor pollicis longus, extensor pollicis brevis, and the extensor pollicis longus, through the anatomical snuffbox. It then courses between the first and second metacarpals, through the adductor space to form the radial component of the superficial and deep palmar arches. The common digital vessels arise from the superficial palmar arch and travel to the level of the metacarpophalangeal joint, where the vessels bifurcate to become the digital vessels proper (Fig. 20-1).

In the lower extremity, the superficial femoral and the profunda femoral vessels may be used as arterial inflow for fillet flaps of the thigh. The superficial femoral vessels continue distally to form the popliteal artery, which bifurcates in the popliteal fossa to form the anterior tibial and posterior tibial arteries. The posterior tibial artery subsequently bifurcates to become the posterior tibial artery and the peroneal artery. The anterior tibial artery travels in the anterior compartment above the interosseous membrane, becoming more superficial as it approaches the extensor retinaculum

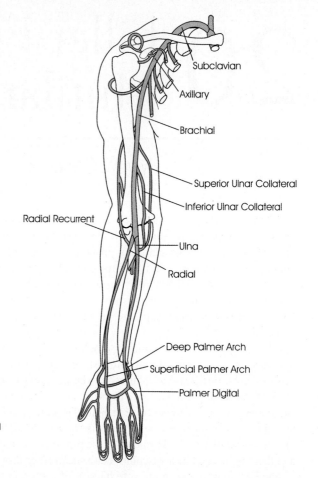

FIGURE 20-1

Upper extremity vascular anatomy. Axial pattern flaps can be designed from known vasculature and their smaller branches.

of the ankle. At this point, the vessel becomes the dorsalis pedis artery, which travels between the first and second metatarsal of the foot. The superficial arcuate branch provides arterial inflow to the dorsum of the foot, while the deep branch pierces between the first and second metatarsal to form the plantar vascular arch. The common digital vessels arise from this arch and bifurcate at the metatarsal-phalangeal joints to become the digital vessels to the toes. The peroneal artery travels near the medial aspect of the fibula and terminates as the lateral calcaneal artery behind the lateral malleolus. The posterior tibial artery travels in the posterior compartment of the lower leg and exits superficial behind the medial malleolus and subsequently bifurcates into the medial and lateral plantar vessels (Fig. 20-2).

INDICATIONS/CONTRAINDICATIONS

Before harvesting a fillet flap for soft tissue coverage, the surgeon should identify the ultimate goal of the immediate and delayed reconstructive procedures. Decisions may be less complex for some lower extremity trauma, where discarding the mutilated limb may be in the best interest of the patient from a functional point of view. Prostheses may be much more functional than attempts at salvage where stability and sensation are compromised. Conversely, mangled hands can have significant function if pinch and grasp can be restored. Reconstructive efforts in these cases may be turned toward salvaging fingers and the thumb, rather than using their tissue as spare parts for soft tissue coverage for the remaining injured hand. Restoring some sensate function to the hand allows it to continue to play a key role in the patient's activities of daily living. This separates the overall treatment protocols and goals for upper extremity reconstruction from that of the lower extremity (Fig. 20-3). Nerve regeneration, revascularization, tendon and bone reconstruction, and secondary toe-to-hand procedures are alternatives to amputation of digits or hands and permit acceptable restoration of function. However, in both the upper and lower extremities, there arise opportunities to use tissue that would otherwise be discarded for definitive soft tissue closure.

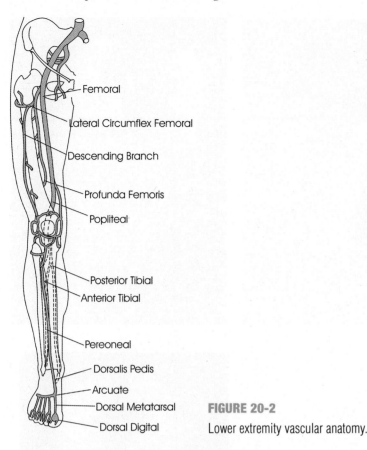

FIGURE 20-2

Lower extremity vascular anatomy.

The availability of adequate tissue often depends on the mechanism of injury to a limb. Clean guillotine-type lacerations or amputations offer the best results and restoration of function because there is minimal tissue loss. These injuries rarely necessitate the need of spare parts or fillet flaps due to the lack of soft tissue deficits. More traumatic injuries such as with crush or avulsion mechanisms or electrical burns require greater debridement and have more tissue loss. Consequently, these injuries frequently take advantage of spare parts and fillet flap surgery for coverage.

Pedicled or free tissue fillet flaps can be used for proximal amputations that require stable coverage to better preserve functions such as elbow flexion or knee mobility. This technique is usually indicated for amputations with significant proximal soft tissue loss and in situations where replantation is contraindicated. The remaining distal tissue is filleted and, based on one neurovascular bundle, transferred to cover the proximal exposed structures as a free tissue transfer. If there is an intact and reliable neurovascular bundle, but with segmental intervening tissue loss, the fillet flap of distal tissue can be harvested as a pedicled flap, leaving the vessels and nerves intact. Indications for fillet flaps are included in Table 20-1.

PREOPERATIVE PLANNING

The preoperative planning should take into consideration patient stability, premorbid health, a history of smoking, possibility of limb function (i.e., preservation of elbow function), available local tissue, prosthesis application, and patient occupation. Patient selection is vital when contemplating the use of fillet flaps for soft tissue coverage of limb or trunk defects. In acute, mutilating trauma, the patient must be stabilized initially as survival is always the first goal. Following the full advanced trauma life support (ATLS) workup with primary and secondary surveys, limb salvage is planned to optimize function.

The initial surgery should entail an aggressive irrigation and debridement to make sure all tissue is viable. Many times, second and third surgeries are required to allow tissue to demarcate and to avoid infection. When planning a fillet flap, the surgeon should identify the blood supply to the spare tissue and ensure that this is intact and undamaged. Fillet flaps can be transferred as a free flap or a pedicled flap. Digital fillet flaps are neurovascular flaps usually based on the digital arterial and

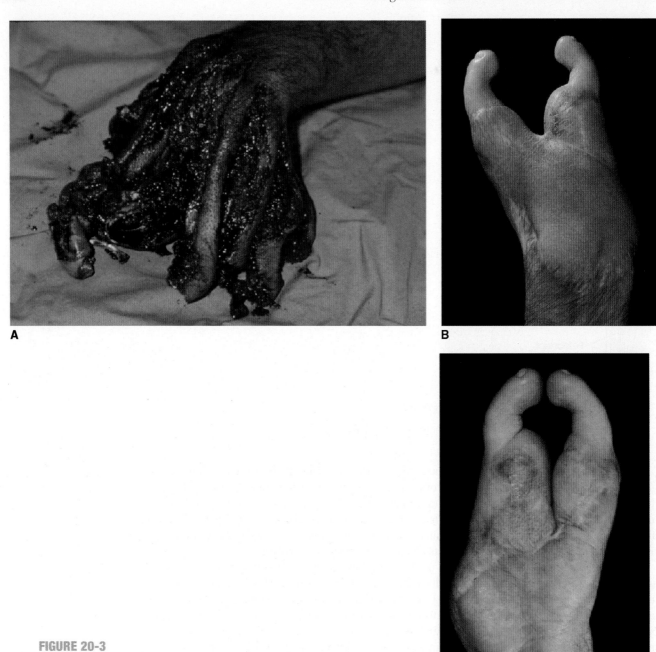

FIGURE 20-3

A: Mutilated hand from corn picker injury with complete loss of all fingers. **B, C:** Restoration of pinch from two toe-to-hand transfers.

nerve supply to the finger (Fig. 20-4). The surgeon can use these digital flaps in cases where a finger has one intact neurovascular bundle and is viable distally but has been, in part, rendered otherwise dysfunctional as a result of proximal trauma. In elective cases, angiography may help identify intact vascular anatomy before transfer. However, angiography is rarely indicated in the acute traumatic case as the surgeon can directly visualize the vessels and observe the vascularity (bleeding) of the distal tissues.

TABLE 20-1   Indications for Fillet Flap
Nonreplantable extremity with adjacent tissue loss from trauma
Nonsalvageable digit with proximal or adjacent digit/hand defect
Availability of tissue from discarded, amputated, or nonfunctioning limb or digit
Segmental loss tumor extirpation or trauma

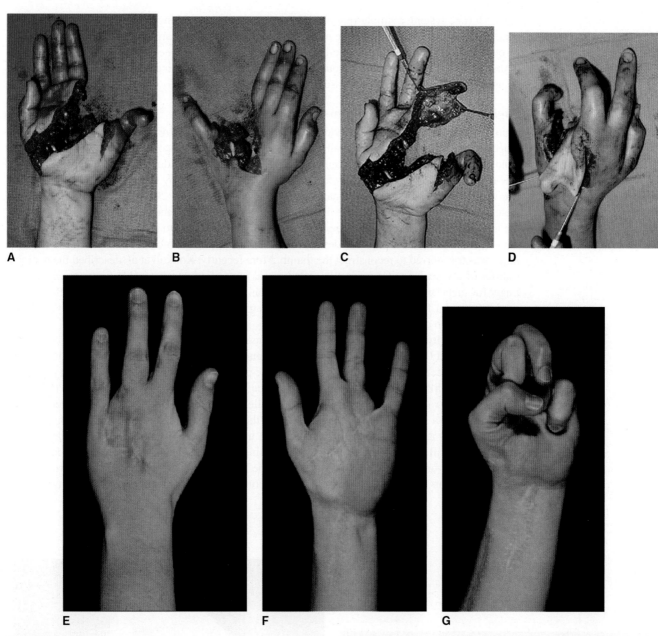

FIGURE 20-4

A–G: Table saw to the right hand with intrusion through the web space between the small and ring finger in an ulnar to radial direction. Complex repair of flexor/extensor tendons, along with neurovascular repair of the arch and common digital vessels was undertaken. The ring finger is filleted based on its radial neurovascular bundle. Resection of the head of the fourth metacarpal was performed secondary to the level of comminution. Long-term follow-up reveals good prehension.

SURGERY

Patient Positioning

The patient should be positioned appropriately to allow dissection of the digit, arm, or leg based on the blood supply of that part. Most upper and lower extremity flaps can be dissected from the supine position. An exception to this is the use of an entire leg fillet flap for recurrent, recalcitrant pressure sores on the ischial and parasacral areas, for which the patient will need to be in the prone position for inset of the flap.

Technique

Before inflation of the tourniquet, vascular integrity should be assessed by observing bleeding skin edges and use of a handheld Doppler when needed. Smaller particulate debris can be removed using a pulse lavage system, a simple spray bottle, or even cystoscopy tubing hooked to a 3-L bag of saline (Fig. 20-5). Larger debris should be mechanically debrided with sharp dissection. The preservation of questionable tissue is acceptable if further debridement is planned in the subsequent 24 to 48 hours. In these cases, temporary wound coverage with moist dressings, allograft, or xenograft can be used to prevent desiccation of tissues in the interim (Fig. 20-6).

Digital Fillet Flaps of the Hand

Mutilating injuries of the hand provide an ideal setting for the use of fillet flaps for soft tissue coverage. A single finger can provide all the components required for composite reconstruction of the hand. Digital fillet flaps can be designed to cover both palmar and dorsal hand defects (Fig. 20-7). The use of adjacent digits that have been rendered dysfunctional by the injury can provide coverage with glabrous skin and maintenance of normal sensation (Fig. 20-8). Similarly, microsurgical techniques can be used to move the filleted digit to an area of the hand not immediately adjacent to the flap. Idler et al. describe the use of a filleted digit as a free flap to cover proximal hand wounds. An osteocutaneous fillet flap was described by Gainor et al. in which the index finger with bone intact was transferred to reconstruct the thumb. More recently, Kokkoli et al. described the pedicled transfer of a vascularized proximal interphalangeal joint of an unsalvageable finger to an adjacent finger for metacarpophalangeal joint reconstruction. A composite neurovascular island flap can be used in a similar fashion incorporating distal phalanx, nail bed, and skin for sensate reconstruction of a hemi-thumb defect (Fig. 20-9).

The vascularity of the digit to be used in fillet fashion is determined by gross inspection and the use of handheld Doppler. The arc of rotation depends on the fillet flap's vascular pedicle. The fillet flap must reach the primary defect based on the pivot point of the pedicle. Al-Qattan described lengthening a fillet of finger flap by incising the skin longitudinally and unfurling the finger based on either radial or ulnar neurovascular bundle to increase its functional length. Preoperative planning using a surgical lap sponge to measure the arc of rotation and subsequent length of the flap required is a helpful tool in determining the utility of the proposed flap. Incomplete filling of the defect will result in the need for skin grafting or some other form of additional soft tissue coverage. Split or full-thickness skin grafts can be harvested from remaining spare parts. Excess tissue within the fillet flap can be used to fill in contour defects. In such cases, the distal portion

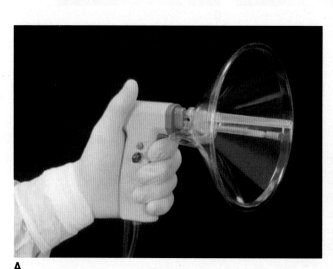

A

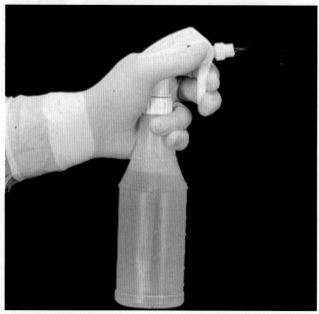

B

FIGURE 20-5
A: Pulse lavage system. **B:** Simple spray bottle.

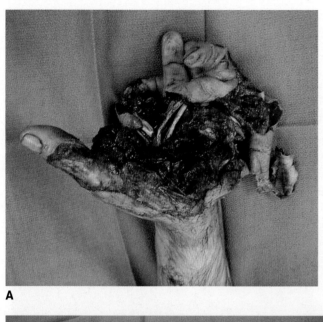

A

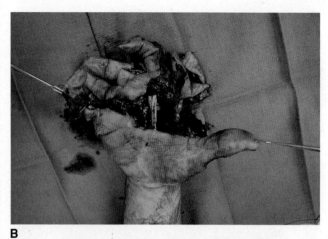

B

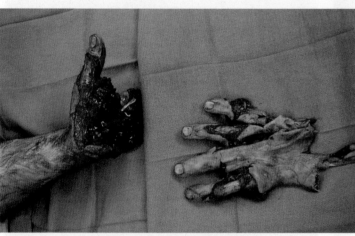

C

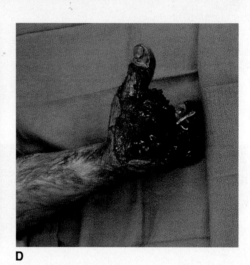

D

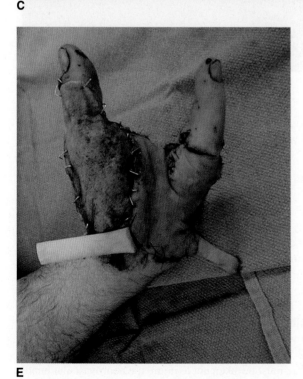

E

FIGURE 20-6

A–E: Mutilating injury necessitating temporary coverage with allograft secondary to the size of the wound, and possible need for further debridement.

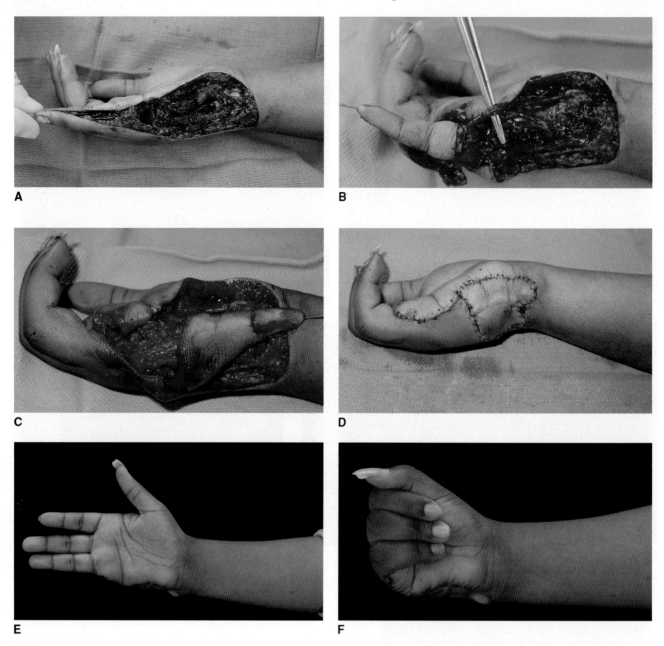

FIGURE 20-7

A 14-year-old patient with hypothenar defect. **A–D:** The small finger is filleted based on its radial neurovascular bundle for coverage. This technique provides stable, sensate closure of the defect. **E, F:** Three-month follow-up reveals stable coverage and good hand function.

of the fillet flap can be deepithelialized and folded beneath the remaining flap to augment soft tissue bulk.

Fillet Flaps of the Arms and Legs

Fillet flaps of the arms and legs are used to cover proximal amputation stumps to prevent further shortening of the limb or to add length around the elbow or shoulder. In upper extremity trauma, these axial fillet flaps are based on the radial or ulnar arteries. The flap is usually a free tissue transfer because there is often an intervening defect in the vessels. The brachial artery and venae comitantes act as the recipient vessels around the elbow. In lower extremity trauma, the fillet flap can be based on either the anterior tibial or the posterior tibial vessels. Incisions in the distal amputated part are made on the opposite side of the limb from where the blood supply is located. This preserves the blood supply to the skin, subcutaneous tissue, and muscles based axially, with the medial and lateral tissues at equal distances from the pedicle. Care must be taken not to injure the neurovascular bundle

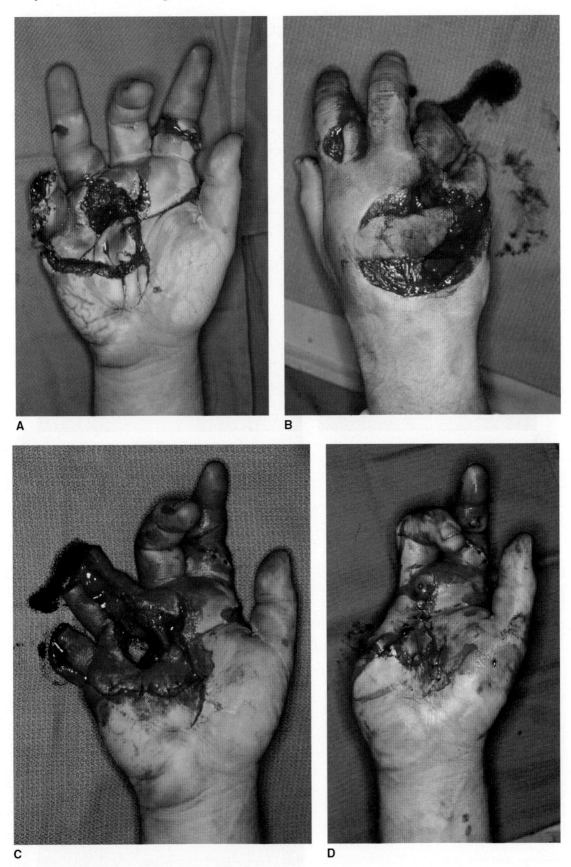

FIGURE 20-8

A–G: Punch press injury to the ulnar aspect of the left hand. Ring and small fingers filleted for coverage. A small skin graft is placed dorsally beyond the reach of the tip of the flap. Long-term postoperative follow-up reveals stable coverage.

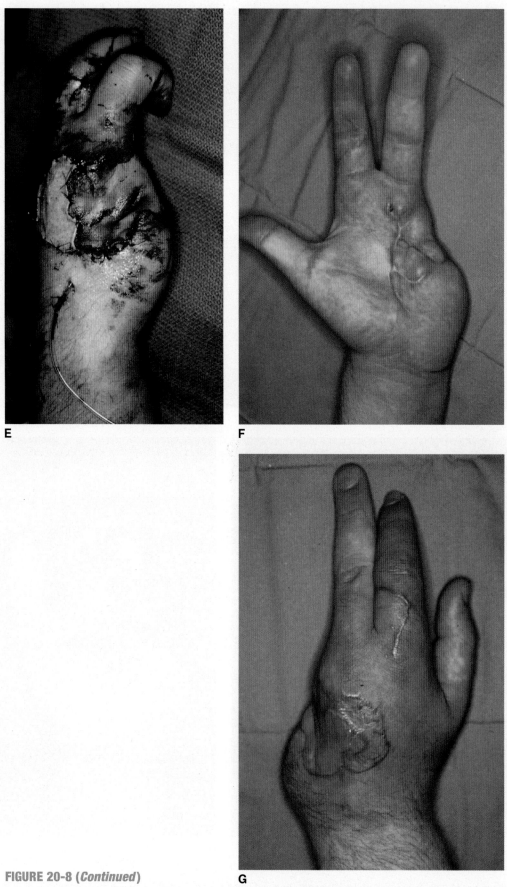

FIGURE 20-8 (*Continued*)

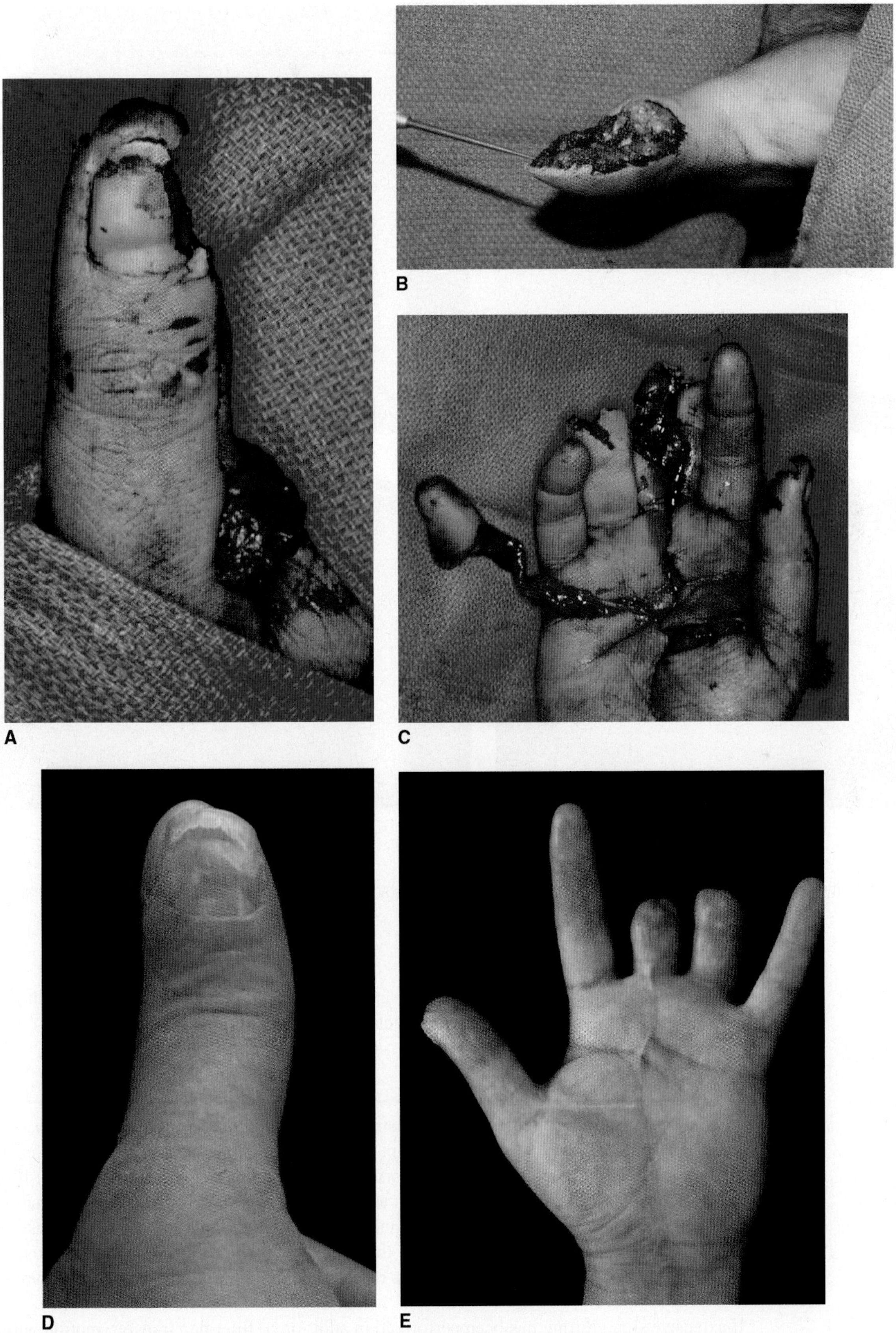

FIGURE 20-9

A, B: Table saw injury to the ulnar aspect of a thumb. **C–E:** Additional injury to the middle and ring fingers. Neurovascular island flap harvested from the middle finger transferred for composite coverage of the thumb.

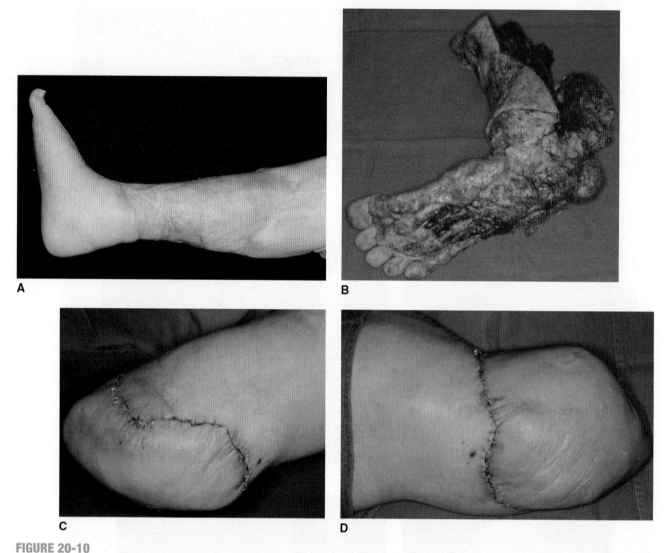

FIGURE 20-10

A–D: Lower extremity reconstruction after amputation. The sole of the foot is filleted and transferred proximally to cover the proximal stump after amputation.

or its branches during the removal of the bony and muscular components of the flap. The flap is then trimmed appropriately to fit the recipient defect (Fig. 20-10).

POSTOPERATIVE CARE

Postoperative care depends on the area reconstructed. For upper extremity defects, bulky noncompressive dressings are used to protect the flap, and elevation is encouraged to decrease edema. A window is left within the dressing for monitoring of the vascular status of the fillet flap. If microvascular reconstruction with the spare part as a free flap has been performed, then flap monitoring is performed hourly with clinical assessment and Doppler for the first 24 to 48 hours to ensure there are no signs of venous or arterial compromise that would necessitate an emergent return to the operating room. In cases where flap compromise is detected, rapid re-exploration of the anastomosis can prevent flap failure.

If extensive skin grafting has been performed in addition to fillet flap transfer, motion within the digit or extremity is usually delayed for 5 to 7 days to allow for skin graft take. If a bolster dressing has been placed or the skin graft secured with vacuum-assisted closure (VAC), motion may be initiated earlier.

RESULTS AND COMPLICATIONS

Flap loss is obviously the most devastating complication follow fillet flap reconstruction. In such cases, alternative means of wound coverage will be necessary to cover resultant defects. Küntscher et al. presented their results from pedicle fillet flaps of fingers for dorsal, palmar, and adjacent digital defects secondary to trauma, burns, Dupuytrens disease, malignant tumor resection, and diabetic gangrene. In their series of 30 patients, the fillet flap provided a stable coverage option with normal sensibility compared to the unaffected digits. The overall complication rate was 18%, with a flap loss, revision surgery, and infection rate of 7.5%. Oliveira et al. had a series of seven patients with total upper extremity avulsions treated with free fillet flaps to preserve amputation site length. They had two major complications including one total flap loss secondary to infection and one patient death on postoperative day 3 secondary to acute respiratory distress syndrome (ARDS). The postoperative course in the other five patients was uneventful.

In conclusion, free and pedicled fillet flaps offer an option for tissue coverage and preservation of length in the setting of amputations that does not require a second donor site and makes use of "spare parts" tissue that would otherwise be discarded. In the setting of mutilating extremity trauma, it is important to consider the overall stability of the patient before embarking on reconstruction. However, in the right situation with a stable patient, fillet flaps can be utilized effectively and should be an essential tool in the armamentarium of all reconstructive surgeons.

PEARLS AND PITFALLS

- Do not discard anything until the completion of the case. Amputated parts can be a valuable source of skin, bone, nerve, and vascular graft.
- A reliable source vessel in an amputated part can allow that piece of tissue to serve as a pedicled or free fillet flap.
- In cases of crush or avulsion, careful examination of the source vessel must be performed prior to elevation of the fillet flap to rule out thrombosis. A handheld Doppler can be used to assess the reliability of the pedicle prior to flap preparation.

RECOMMENDED READING

Al-Qattan MM. Lengthening of the finger fillet flap to cover dorsal wrist defects. *J Hand Surg Am.* 1997;22:550–551.
Chan SW, LaStayo P. Hand therapy management following mutilating hand injuries. *Hand Clin.* 2003;9(1):133–148.
Gainor BJ. Osteocutaneous digital fillet flap: a technical modification. *J Hand Surg Br.* 1985;10:79–82.
Ghali S, Harris PA, Khan U, et al. Leg length preservation with pedicled fillet of foot flaps after traumatic amputations. *Plast Reconstr Surg.* 2005;115(2):498–505.
Idler RS, Mih AD. Soft tissue coverage of the hand with a free digital fillet flap. *Microsurgery.* 1990;11:215–216.
Kokkoli E, Spyropoulou GA, Shi HS, et al. Heterotopic procedures in mutilating hand injuries: a synopsis of essential reconstructive tools. *Plast Reconstr Surg.* 2015;136(5):1015–1026.
Küntscher, MV, Erdmann D, Homann HH, et al. The concept of fillet flaps: classification, indications, and analysis of their clinical value. *Plast Reconstr Surg.* 2001;108:885–896.
Lin CH, Webb K, Neumeister MW. Immediate tissue transplantation in upper limb trauma: spare parts reconstruction. *Clin Plast Surg.* 2014;41(3):397–406.
Oliveira IC, Barbosa RF, Ferreira PC, et al. The use of forearm free fillet flap in traumatic upper extremity amputations. *Microsurgery.* 2009;29(1):8–15
Russell RC, Neumeister MW, Ostric SA, et al. Extremity reconstruction using nonreplantable tissue ("spare parts"). *Clin Plast Surg.* 2007;34(2):211–222.

21 Free Flaps for Upper Extremity Reconstruction and the Anterolateral Thigh Flap

Samir Mardini, Harvey Chim, Steven L. Moran, and Chih-Hung Lin

INDICATIONS/CONTRAINDICATIONS

Soft tissue deficiencies within the upper extremity are common following trauma, burns, infection, and tumor extirpation. The coverage of such defects can usually be accomplished with the use of pedicled flaps or local rotational flaps. However, when local and regional donor sites are limited or when defects are very large or encompass multiple structures including nerve, bone, or muscle, the use of composite free tissue transfer provides a reliable and single-stage means of reconstructing complex defects.

The benefits of free tissue transfer within the upper extremity include the transfer of additional vascularized tissue to the injured area; the ability to carry vascularized nerve, bone, skin, and muscle to the injured area in one procedure; and the avoidance of any additional functional deficits to the injured limb, which may be incurred with the use of a local or pedicled flap. Free flaps are not tethered at one end, as is the cases for pedicled flaps, and this allows for more freedom in flap positioning and insetting. More recent axial fasciocutaneous flaps as well as perforator flaps also allow for primary closure of donor sites without the need to sacrifice muscle. With current microsurgical techniques, free flap reexploration rates are between 1% and 20%, with flap failure rates between 1% and 4% for cases requiring elective free tissue transfer. Finally, the upper extremity is particularly suited for free tissue transfer as the majority of recipient vessels used for anastomosis are located close to the skin and are of a variety of sizes. This allows a wider range of donor sites including free-style flaps that can be transferred with a short pedicle to reconstruct various defects in the upper extremity.

Major indications for free tissue transfer are (a) primary coverage of large traumatic wounds with exposed bone, joint, and tendons or hardware; (b) coverage of complex composite defects requiring bone and soft tissue replacement; (c) coverage of soft tissue deficits resulting from release of contractures or scarring from previous trauma; and (d) significant burns.

There are few absolute contraindications for free flap transfer, and in many cases, free tissue transfer may be the only option for upper limb salvage following significant soft tissue loss. Further workup and evaluation must be performed for patients with a history of a hypercoagulable state, history of recent upper extremity DVT, and evidence of ongoing infection with the traumatic defect. Most of these issues can be resolved with proper evaluation and treatment. To have success in any free flap surgery, recipient vessels must be available for microvascular anastomosis. In single-vessel extremities, end-to-side anastomosis of the artery or flow-through flaps must be performed. Disregarding technical error, the status of the recipient vessel used for flap anastomosis may play the greatest role in flap failure. Recipient vessels should ideally be located out of the zone of injury, radiation, or infection as vessels in these zones are highly prone to thrombosis, in both the intraoperative period and the postoperative period. When nearby healthy recipient vessels are not present, flaps with long pedicles are chosen for transfer. The design of the anterolateral thigh flap can be modified to provide a longer effective pedicle length. The most distal perforator is chosen, and the skin island is designed placing the perforator in the most proximal aspect of the flap. When needed, arteriovenous fistulas may be created proximally within the upper extremity or axilla using the cephalic or saphenous vein. These fistulas can be brought into the zone of injury and divided to provide adequate inflow and outflow for free tissue transfer.

Specific Indication for the Anterolateral Thigh Flap

There are many choices for free flap coverage of the upper extremity. The scapular, parascapular, lateral arm, and latissimus dorsi myocutaneous flap have long been favorites of surgeons for reconstruction of traumatic upper extremity injuries. If joints are to be crossed, fasciocutaneous flaps are much preferred as muscle flaps can undergo atrophy and fibrosis and restrict flexion and extension across joints or fingers (Fig. 21-1).

Classic cutaneous free flaps, such as the radial forearm flap, lateral arm flap, and scapular flap, have limitations in size, donor site morbidity, and bulkiness. The advantage of the anterolateral thigh flap is that it allows for a two-team harvest, an 8-cm wide flap with primary closure of the donor site, a long pedicle, inclusion of multiple tissue types, the ability to thin the flap, and the potential to harvest a large skin island measuring up to 25 cm × 25 cm on a single perforator. Musculocutaneous flaps such as the latissimus dorsi and rectus abdominis flaps result in functional loss and donor site morbidity including, particularly in the abdomen, potential hernia formation. In addition, in coverage of joint surfaces, muscle flaps tend to undergo fibrosis and atrophy over time, which may limit muscle excursion, particularly when placed over the elbow or dorsum of the hand. Muscle flaps continue to be used for coverage of defects involving osteomyelitis or significant soft tissue

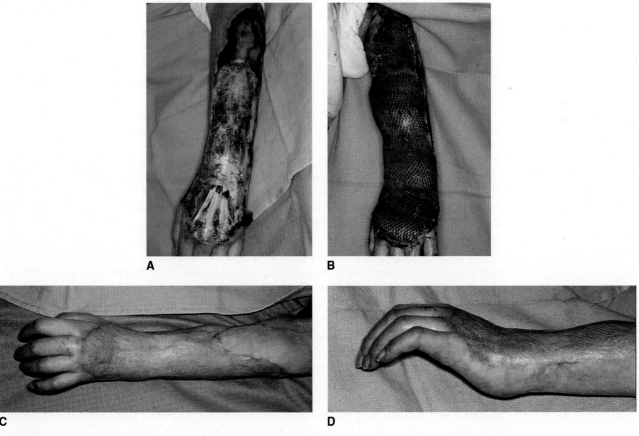

FIGURE 21-1

A: An extensive IV infiltrate to back of hand and forearm resulted in full-thickness skin loss over the majority of the hand and forearm in this 56-year-old woman. **B:** Soft tissue coverage was obtained with the use of a rectus abdominis free flap. **C, D:** Despite successful soft tissue coverage, atrophy and fibrosis within the muscle over time have lead to limitations in wrist motion resulting in decreased wrist flexion.

contamination, despite lack of strong evidence supporting this practice. Chimeric anterolateral thigh flaps including skin and other tissues such as muscle and fascia and nerve have been used with excellent outcomes for the reconstruction of complex defects.

The anterolateral thigh flap has become a commonly used flap in reconstructive microsurgery for a variety of defects around the body, including the upper extremity. The skin overlying the anterior thigh region has a relatively constant anatomy with the descending branch of the lateral femoral circumflex artery (LFCA), giving rise to either musculocutaneous or septocutaneous perforators that supply the area. Based on their experience with over 1,500 anterolateral thigh flaps for various anatomic defects including the upper extremity, Chen et al. determined that 12% were based on direct septocutaneous perforators and 88% were based on musculocutaneous perforators. Variations in perforator anatomy can exist, which include absence of skin perforators, perforators that are too small for elevation, and perforator arteries that have no accompanying vein. These anatomical variations are rare, accounting for 2% of cases; however, they need to be noted by the surgeon. As proposed by Chen, an algorithm for managing anatomical variations begins with attempting to identify a more proximal perforator in the upper thigh, usually arising from the transverse branch of the LFCA and harvesting the flap based on this perforator. Alternatively, an anteromedial thigh flap may be raised or the vastus lateralis may be taken as a musculocutaneous or muscle-only flap with a skin graft. Finally, exploration can be performed on the contralateral side as the anatomy may be different.

Yu et al. studied the perforator pattern in the anterolateral thigh flap and found a predictable anatomy of the perforators and a way to localize the perforators in a simple and effective manner. They found that there are usually one to three cutaneous perforators in the anterolateral thigh flap region that they term perforator A, B, and C. They found that perforator B is the most consistent perforator and is located near the midpoint of the line connecting the anterior superior iliac spine (ASIS) and the superolateral corner of the patella. After finding perforator B, they found that approximately 5 cm proximally and distally, they were able to find perforator A and C, respectively. In 11% of the patients, perforator B was not found, and in those cases, perforator A and perforator C were each found in 73% of the patients. They found that the overall probability of finding another cutaneous perforator (A or C or both) on which to base the flap was 100%. Outside of this group of patients, they had an overall incidence of not being able to raise the flap in both thighs of 0.7%.

The anterolateral thigh flap serves as the ideal flap, particularly in upper extremity reconstruction. The flap provides a pedicle length of 12 cm (range 8 to 16 cm) with suitable vessel diameters; the arterial diameter measures 2.1 mm (range 2 to 2.5 mm). The artery is accompanied by two venae comitantes measuring 12 cm in length (range 8 to 16 cm) and with a diameter of 2.3 mm (range 1.8 to 3.3 mm). The anterolateral thigh flap is also a versatile flap with the ability to incorporate different tissue components with large amounts of skin, as the flap can be harvested as a cutaneous, fasciocutaneous, or musculocutaneous flap with vastus lateralis. In addition, based on the supply of the LFCA system, a chimeric flap incorporating the rectus femoris or tensor fascia lata can be raised to cover extensive, complex defects. The flap may be harvested as a sensate flap by including the lateral femoral cutaneous nerve or as a flow-through flap in cases of significant arterial trauma. Inclusion of thigh fascia with the flap allows its use as an interposition graft for tendon reconstruction. The flap may be debulked primarily, optimizing the match of donor tissue for the upper extremity. Ordinary skin flaps can sometimes produce bulkiness with poor aesthetics. Thick skin paddles, such as with parascapular flaps, may interfere with motor function and flexion of the metacarpophalangeal joints or interphalangeal joints. The anterolateral thigh flap can be thinned to 3 to 5 mm and used for resurfacing of the hand and forearm. The donor site of the anterolateral thigh flap results in minimal morbidity with most sites able to be closed primarily, resulting in a linear scar and absence of any long-term leg dysfunction. Hanasono et al. evaluated the outcomes at the donor site of the anterolateral thigh flap in 220 patients and concluded that the anterolateral thigh flap is associated with a low rate of complications and functional morbidity. Even when the motor nerve to the vastus lateralis is divided, or substantial amounts of thigh fascia or vastus lateralis muscle are included in the flap design, all patients return to their preoperative level of function. Sensory issues such as tingling were found in some patients following anterolateral thigh flap harvest. Lastly, its anatomic location allows for a two-team approach for flap elevation and recipient site preparation, saving considerable operative time.

ANTEROLATERAL THIGH FLAP FOR UPPER EXTREMITY RECONSTRUCTION

Preoperative Planning

Preoperative requirements for flap consideration begin with the preparation of a clean wound bed. Radical debridement of all necrotic tissue is the most important component of a successful reconstruction. Tissue considered to be of marginal viability should be debrided early rather than performing multiple dressing changes or utilizing vacuum-assisted therapy in the hopes of rescuing traumatized tissue; such measures can lead to delayed definitive surgical reconstruction, perpetuate the inflammatory component of wound healing, perpetuate distal edema, and result in hand and limb stiffness. If the surgeon can guarantee a clean wound bed, free of any necrotic material, immediate flap coverage may be attempted in cases of acute trauma. Most high-energy traumatic injuries and agricultural accidents require at least one to two surgical debridements prior to definitive wound closure. Wound cultures for bacteria and fungal species are obtained. The ideal timing for upper limb free tissue reconstruction has been debated within the literature but should be within 72 to 96 hours of injury.

The upper extremity is evaluated for any evidence of concomitant bony or neurovascular injury. A careful vascular evaluation is also performed and if there is any question as to the status of the inflow vessels, an angiogram or a CT angiogram may be obtained to verify inflow. Our preference is to perform the majority of arterial anastomoses in an end-to-side fashion while the veins are anastomosed in an end-to-end fashion. If consideration is being given to performing an arterial anastomosis in an end-to-end fashion to either the radial or ulnar artery, the surgeon must verify a patent palmar arch with an Allen's test or Doppler examination prior to surgery. The donor leg for the anterolateral thigh flap should be free of concomitant soft tissue trauma. If the patient has a history of lower extremity arterial atherosclerotic disease or diabetes, examination of the lower extremity is warranted, to verify that there is an intact profundus femoral artery, which gives rise to the lateral femoral circumflex system.

Patient Positioning

The patient is positioned in the supine position for harvest of the anterolateral thigh flap. The injured arm is positioned on a standard hand table. Recipient site preparation is aided with the use of an upper extremity tourniquet.

Flap harvest is performed under general anesthesia, though spinal/epidural block for flap elevation and axillary block of the affected extremity can be undertaken when general anesthesia is contraindicated. This would be a rare situation that we have not encountered.

Flap Elevation Surgery

General principles and steps in elevation for perforator flap include the following:

1. Doppler mapping of the perforators
2. Design of the flap
3. Exploration and identification of the perforators leading to the main pedicle
4. Intramuscular or intermuscular dissection of the perforators with preservation of the motor nerve to the vastus lateralis
5. Harvest of the flap
6. Thinning of the flap
7. Transfer of the flap to cover the defect

The anterolateral thigh flap is based on the descending branch of the lateral femoral circumflex vessel, which courses inferiorly along the intermuscular septum giving rise to subcutaneous and/or intramuscular perforators that penetrate the fascia to supply the skin and subcutaneous tissue overlying the anterolateral thigh. A preoperative Doppler examination of the lower leg is performed to identify these perforators. A line is drawn from the ASIS to the lateral margin of the patella. At the midpoint of this line is a reliable perforator identifiable in most cases (Fig. 21-2). Two additional perforators are identified around 5 cm proximal and 5 cm distal to the midpoint perforator in the majority of cases. The skin paddle, incorporating more than one perforator when possible, is designed in an elliptical fashion based on the dimensions of the defect in the upper extremity.

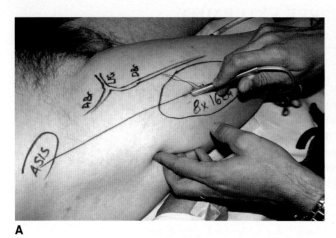

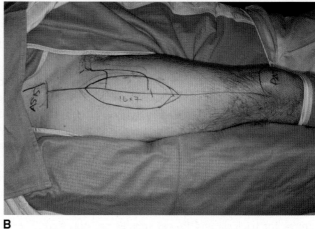

A   **B**

FIGURE 21-2

Prior to flap elevation, the arterial perforators to the ALT flap are identified on the leg. A line is drawn from the anterior superior iliac spine (ASIS) to the lateral margin of the patella. In 90% of cases, a major perforator can be identified within 3 cm of the middle portion of this line. A second major perforator is usually identified at the upper third of this line. **A:** The sites for the perforators are confirmed with a handheld Doppler probe and marked with a skin scribe. **B:** The flap is then designed around the perforators in an elliptical fashion.

Subfascial Dissection

Dissection begins medially by dissecting down to the fascia lata overlying the rectus femoris muscle. The fascia is incised and dissection proceeds in a lateral direction until the intermuscular septum separating the rectus femoris and vastus lateralis muscles is encountered. Medial retraction of the rectus femoris muscle exposes the entire septum, allowing for visualization of the descending branch of the LFCA in addition to its branch going to the rectus femoris itself (Fig. 21-3). At this point, there may be one to three major perforators exiting from the descending branch and passing through the muscle of the vastus lateralis as musculocutaneous perforators or passing directly through the septum as septocutaneous perforators to the skin. Usually, one large perforator is sufficient to supply a large skin island and allows for easy thinning of the flap. However, more perforators may be included if the skin island is very large. If septocutaneous perforators are present, the dissection proceeds proximally until adequate pedicle length is obtained. If the perforator is an intramuscular one, it is carefully dissected free from the surrounding muscle. A cuff of muscle may be included in

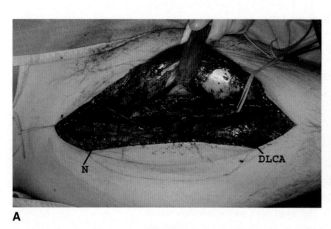

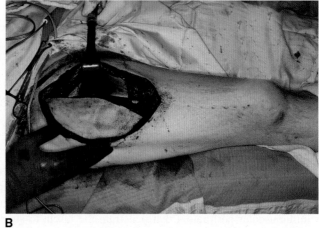

A   **B**

FIGURE 21-3

A: After the flap has been marked, the medial incision is made first and the rectus femoris muscle is identified. The rectus femoris (RF) muscle is retracted medially to reveal the descending branch of the lateral femoral circumflex vessels (DCLA). A branch of the lateral femoral cutaneous nerve (n) can usually be identified running superior to the vastus lateralis muscle. **B:** Once the flap perforators are identified, dissection may begin at the lateral margin of the flap.

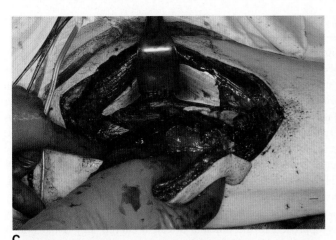

C

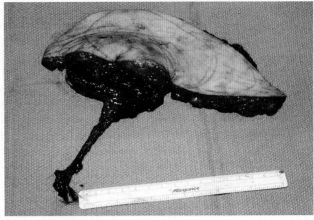

D

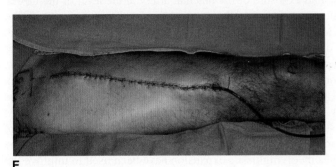

E

FIGURE 21-3 (*Continued*)
C: Two perforators of the lateral femoral circumflex vessels are seen passing into the vastus lateralis. These vessels may be dissected through the muscle into the fascia of the overlying skin flap or a small cuff of muscle may be preserved around the vessels. **D:** The flap is now ready for transfer to the arm. The muscle cuff can be seen beneath the skin paddle. The pedicle length and large diameter allow for easy insetting and microvascular anastomosis. **E:** The donor site may be closed primarily over a closed suction drain.

the flap should the upper extremity wound require additional bulk or if the wound contains exposed bone or significant dead space (see Fig. 21-3D).

Dissection proceeds along the descending branch of the LFCA separating venae comitantes from the artery. The pedicle can be dissected back to the main trunk of the LFCA or divided at the descending branch. If one traces the vessels back to the origin, the motor nerve to the vastus lateralis will need to be dissected free from the arterial pedicle. This may be a tedious dissection as the nerve may pass through and around the venous pedicle. Dissection of the vessels back to the origin results in very large caliber vessels of up to 3 mm in some cases.

Suprafascial Dissection

The medial margin of the flap incision is made through the skin and subcutaneous tissue. Dissection then proceeds above the fascia in a medial to lateral direction until the previously dopplered skin vessels are reached. Strict hemostasis allows for less blood staining of the surrounding tissues and easier visualization of the skin vessels. Cutaneous nerves overlying the fascia are preserved at the donor site whenever possible. After identifying a suitable skin vessel and confirming its course piercing through the fascia and entering the subcutaneous tissue, the lateral skin flap incision is made down to the same suprafascial plane and dissection proceeds in a lateral to medial direction until the same skin vessel is visualized. A fascial incision is made in the direction of the skin vessel (usually caudad) and the vessel is traced in a retrograde fashion until adequate vessel length and caliber are achieved. Inclusion of a cuff of fascia can avoid damage and twisting of the skin vessel. Dissection then proceeds in a retrograde fashion with all small branches carefully ligated or cauterized. Minimal and gentle manipulation of the skin vessel avoids vessel spasm. Traction on the pedicle is always avoided, keeping in mind that traction can occur due to the weight of the flap itself.

When added bulk is required to cover a complex wound, the anterolateral thigh flap can be harvested as a chimeric flap along with the vastus lateralis or rectus femoris muscles, the tensor fascia lata, or other skin flaps in the thigh based on the supply of lateral femoral circumflex system. The flap can also be split into different skin paddles based on individual perforators for coverage of complex defects. This may allow coverage of separate defects in the hand and fingers with the same flap.

ADIPOFASCIAL AND FASCIA-ONLY FLAP

When a thin flap that does not require skin is desired, an adipofascial flap can be elevated by using techniques as described earlier. Once the fascia is exposed and incised, a subfascial dissection is performed until the perforator is located (Fig. 21-5). A minimum of 3 mm of fat should be preserved over the fascia to avoid problems with the vascularity of the flap. The vascular network runs over the fascia. Alternatively, the anterolateral thigh flap can be harvested as a fascia-only flap. This has the advantage of providing extremely thin tissue for coverage in the hand, which can be contoured to the dimensions of the defect and covered with a skin graft.

Sensory reinnervation of the flap can be achieved by including the lateral femoral cutaneous nerve in the proximal portion of the flap. The nerve arises from the deep fascia approximately 10 cm caudad to the ASIS and divides into two or three branches.

Preparation of the recipient vessels is performed. If the radial artery is to be used, a Henry approach is usually carried out. For approach to the brachial artery, a curved lazy-S incision is performed over the antecubital fossa and exposure of the brachial artery at the level of the medial forearm is performed. The flap is then transferred to the upper extremity. The tourniquet is then released in order to verify adequate arterial inflow. Once adequate arterial inflow has been verified, the anterolateral thigh flap may be divided from the lower extremity and transferred to the upper extremity. The anastomosis is then performed in an end-to-side fashion using 9-0 or 10-0 nylon. Venous coupling is used for the venous anastomosis unless there is a reason not to use it (Fig. 21-4).

The donor site is approximated primarily over closed suction drainage when flap width is less than 8 cm, or a skin graft may be used for larger width flaps. If the width of the flap does not allow for primary closure, the skin edges are brought close to each other using sutures from the deep tissue of the skin margin to the underlying muscle in order to prevent retraction of the tissues (Fig. 21-5I). Other techniques involving tissue expansion have been used to improve the donor site morbidity, pretransfer, concurrent transfer, or posttransfer.

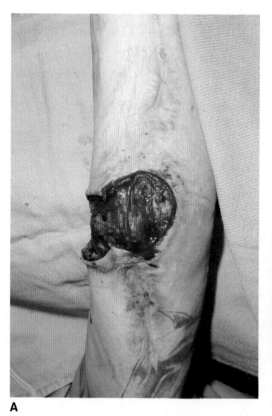

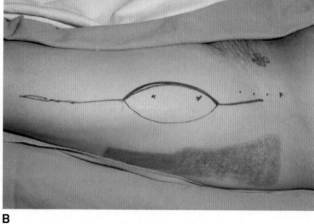

A   B

FIGURE 21-4

A: A 34-year-old man, status post liver transplantation, with a chronic left posterior elbow wound. The multiple posterior scars are evidence of previous attempts to close this defect. **B:** The skin incision for an ipsilateral ALT flap is marked on the thigh after identification of the underlying perforators.

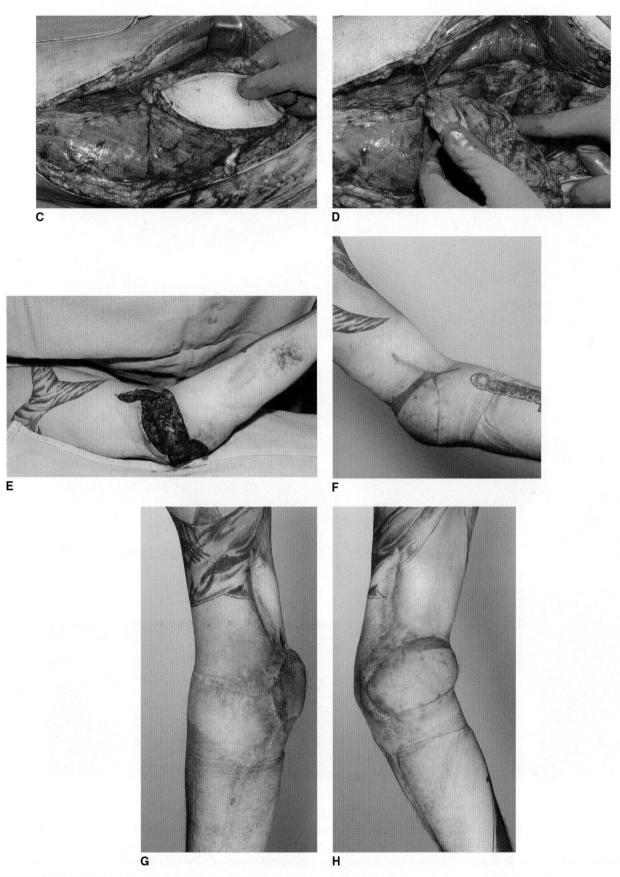

FIGURE 21-4 (*Continued*)

C: The flap is separated from surrounding tissue. **D:** The lateral femoral circumflex vessels can be seen above the surgeon's index finger entering the flap. **E:** In preparation for flap transfer, the brachial artery is exposed at the level of the elbow. **F–H:** The result at 3 months postoperatively with well-healed wound, with good contour and no signs of infection.

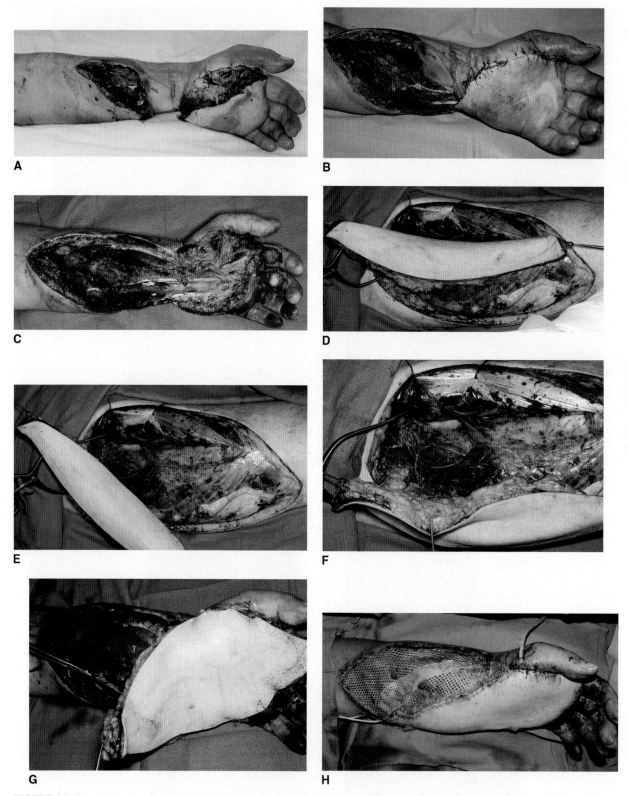

FIGURE 21-5

A 43-year-old man was baling hay when his left hand was caught in between the wheel and the belt of the baling mechanism, and he sustained severe degloving injury of his hand and left forearm. He was reconstructed with a free anterolateral thigh perforator flap. **A:** Hand and forearm on presentation. **B:** Hand and forearm following debridement and partial closure. **C:** The patient was taken back to the operating room and required debridement of the palmar tissue of the hand. **D:** An anterolateral thigh flap measuring 13 cm wide was harvested from the right thigh. **E, F:** Right thigh showing the rectus femoris muscle retracted medially and the intramuscular dissection of the perforator through the vastus lateralis muscle. **G:** Partial inset of the anterolateral thigh flap into the hand showing the pedicle directed proximally toward the recipient vessels, the ulnar artery and cephalic vein. **H:** Inset of the anterolateral thigh flap and skin grafting of the remaining defect.

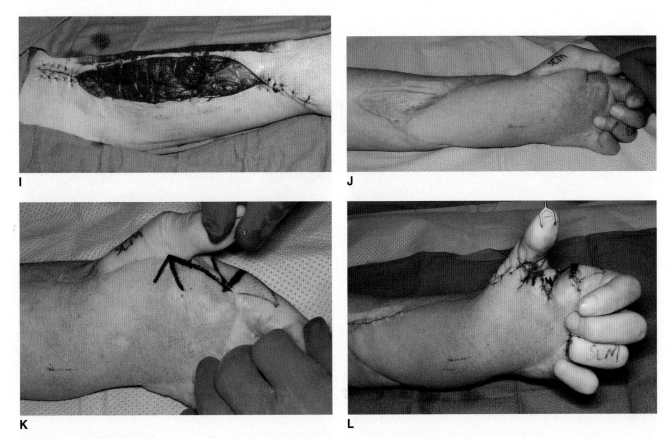

FIGURE 21-5 (*Continued*)
I: The donor site required skin grafting from the adjacent skin of the thigh. The flap was wide and primary closure was not possible. Therefore, approximation of the thigh skin was performed using horizontal mattress sutures prior to skin grafting. **J–L:** Postoperative result showing healing of the flap and the skin graft, in addition to a contracture in the first web space requiring Z-plasties.

Thinning of the Flap

When a thick flap is required, either the flap can be elevated in a suprafascial plane to reduce the thickness of the flap and preserve the fascia at the donor site or it can be raised in the subfascial plane and then thinned. After the flap is isolated on its pedicle, further defatting of the flap can be undertaken. The flap is usually thinned by excising the deep fat consisting of wide, flat fat lobules up to the junction of the superficial fat, made up of smaller, round lobules. Defatting before ligation of the pedicle allows for monitoring of flap perfusion during the thinning process. Individual perforators can be dissected following their course from deep to superficial. A cuff of adipose tissue should be preserved around the perforator but the fat lobules at other areas may be thinned more aggressively. The flap may be thinned up to 3 mm without compromise to the blood supply. A more conservative approach toward primary flap thinning should be undertaken until adequate experience is gained as flap debulking can be performed safely and easily as a secondary procedure (Fig. 21-6).

The microdissection procedure is another method of thinning the flap. This involves the dissection of blood vessels within the adipose layer under operative microscopic magnification and visualization, also identifying the vessel distribution in the adipose layer. In this fashion, the flap is elevated in a one-step procedure without damaging any perfusing blood vessels. Fat lobules are bluntly removed from the perforator and its branches until the insertion of these vessels into the subdermal vascular network.

Another case is shown in Figure 21-7.

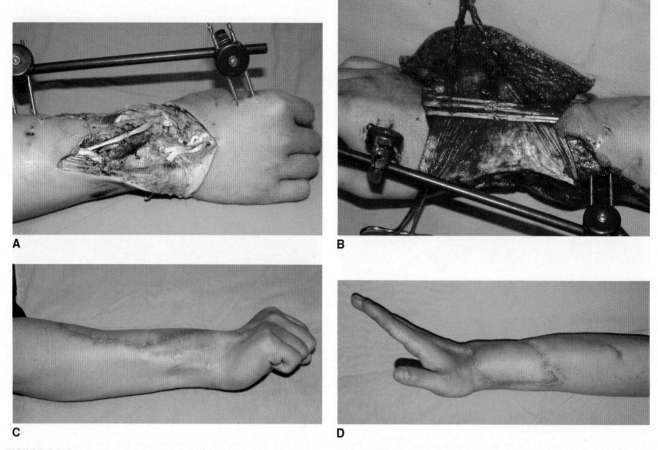

FIGURE 21-6

A 31-year-old man sustained an open fracture of the right forearm with disruption of the extensor muscles and tendons. **A:** Dorsal view of the hand and wrist showing disruption of the extensor tendons. **B:** A free anterolateral thigh flap with vascularized fascia lata was used to reconstruct the dorsal hand and wrist defect and provide a smooth gliding surface. **C, D:** Postoperative photographs at 14 months showing good flexion and extension of the wrist and digits.

POSTOPERATIVE MANAGEMENT

Monitoring

Flap monitoring is of paramount importance following microvascular surgery. Postoperative thrombosis of either the artery or vein can be salvaged in greater than 50% of patients if detected early. Intraoperatively, a stitch is placed over the perforator on the skin paddle to facilitate postoperative monitoring with a Doppler probe. Alternatively, an implantable Doppler probe can be placed around the vein or artery intraoperatively to allow for continuous monitoring of the anastomosis. The Doppler signal over the marked skin paddle is checked hourly with the use of a handheld Doppler while the patient remains in the intensive care unit. The highest incidence of postoperative arterial thrombosis is within the first 24 hours, with the incidence of venous thrombosis occurring most frequently within the first 3 days. Donor site drain output is recorded and drains are kept in place until daily output is less than 30 mL. The patient is allowed to ambulate on postoperative day 2. Postoperative complications include partial to total flap loss, temporary weakness in the lower extremity that usually resolves within the first 2 weeks, and sensory deficit at the donor site if there has been any stretching or injury to the lateral femoral cutaneous nerve. In cases of venous congestion, exploration of the anastomosis is necessary. If prolonged venous thrombosis is experienced, the use of either TPA or leeches can sometimes be used to salvage the flap.

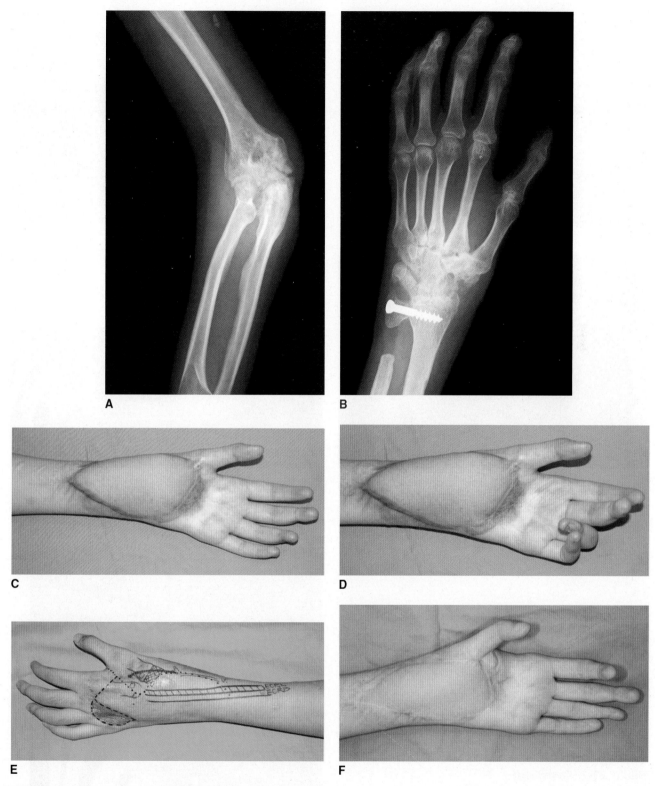

FIGURE 21-7

A 19-year-old woman sustained an open fracture of the right elbow and a crush injury of the left hand. At another institution, she underwent tendon release for the hand, a free groin flap, and a Kapandji procedure. She presented with complaints of a stiff right elbow due to posttraumatic elbow fusion and limitation in finger flexion. **A:** Radiograph showing fusion of the right elbow. **B:** Radiograph demonstrating fusion of the left wrist and thumb basal joint. **C:** Volar view of the hand and forearm showing the fingers in extension. **D:** Volar view showing the limitation of thumb and finger flexion and opposition. **E:** View of the hand and forearm prior to scar release, first web space release, tenolysis, tendon transfer, and a free anterolateral thigh flap for web space creation and suspension interpositional arthroplasty for thumb basal joint. **F:** The hand in extension 1 year after surgery.

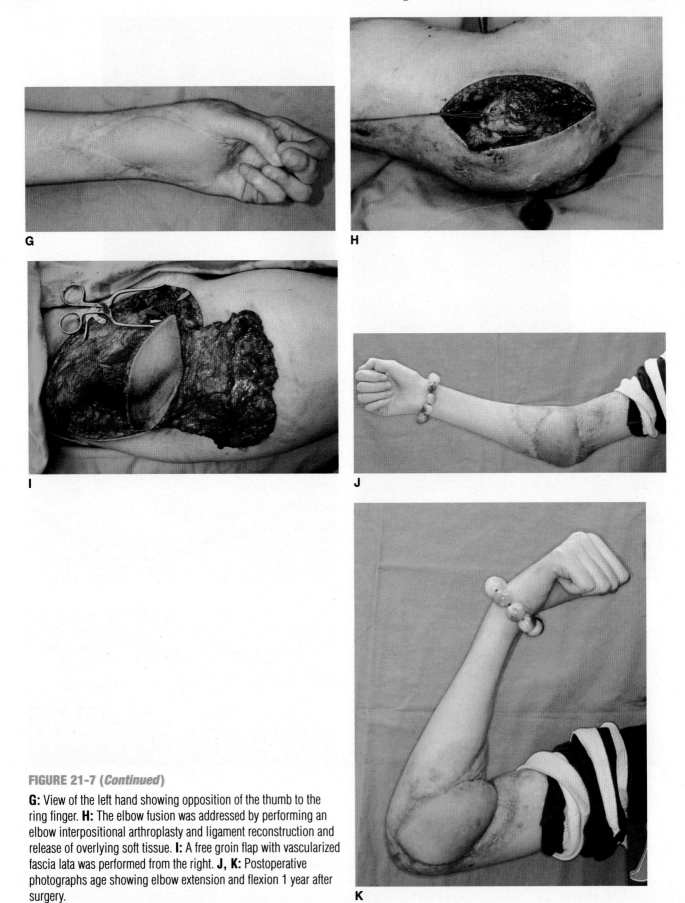

FIGURE 21-7 (*Continued*)

G: View of the left hand showing opposition of the thumb to the ring finger. **H:** The elbow fusion was addressed by performing an elbow interpositional arthroplasty and ligament reconstruction and release of overlying soft tissue. **I:** A free groin flap with vascularized fascia lata was performed from the right. **J, K:** Postoperative photographs age showing elbow extension and flexion 1 year after surgery.

The use of postoperative anticoagulation is debated. Our patients are given one baby aspirin per day and are continued on subcutaneous heparin while they are in the hospital. Formal anticoagulation with heparin is discouraged and has been linked to an increase risk of hematoma formation and flap loss. For those situations where arterial inflow has been difficult to establish, dextran at 25 mL/hour may be used in adults.

Rehabilitation

Underlying injuries usually dictate when motion may begin. We usually wait 5 days for the anastomosis to mature and for the postoperative swelling to subside. At this point, if the underlying bone injury is stabilized, early mobilization is initiated. A light Ace wrap is applied to the flap beginning on day 5 to help aid in resolution of postoperative swelling. Reelevation of the flap for additional bone grafting or tendon grafting can be done as soon as 4 to 6 weeks. Defatting or thinning of the flap is usually delayed for 6 to 9 months after the original surgery.

RESULTS

Good success has been reported with the use of anterolateral thigh flaps in the upper extremity. Flap failure rates have been noted to be as low as 2%. Additional thinning procedures may be required in patients with continued bulk. Microvascular surgery and free tissue transfer within the upper extremity are facilitated by large recipient vessels and a relatively shallow operating field.

COMPLICATIONS

The greatest complication of free flap surgery is flap loss due to arterial or venous thrombosis. The best means of preventing these problems is adequate preoperative planning. Repairs within the zone of injury, technical errors including inadequate visualization of vessels, and tension or kinking at the anastomosis site can all lead to flap failure. Ongoing infection can also result in partial flap loss. For the anterolateral thigh flap, twisting of the pedicle can occur easily due to the absence of muscle to keep its proper orientation. Marking the anterior wall of the pedicle and lifting of the flap in the air to allow the pedicle to lie in its natural orientation prior to final inset may prevent pedicle twisting. It is also important to avoid compression of the flap.

CONCLUSION

With proper planning, the anterolateral thigh flap is capable of managing many complex injuries within the upper extremity. It is now often our first choice for coverage of upper extremity defects. The advantages of the ALT flap are relatively consistent anatomy; ease in dissection; long pedicle length; ability to achieve a thin, pliable flap; ability to provide sensate coverage through the lateral femoral cutaneous nerve; no sacrifice of major artery of the lower limb; and versatility in flap construct, which allows one to harvest not only muscle but also functional muscle such as the rectus femoris. The donor site can be closed primarily.

PEARLS AND PITFALLS

- The anterolateral thigh flap is a good fasciocutaneous flap for upper extremity coverage.
- A cuff of vastus lateralis can be included with the ALT flap if there is dead space to be filled.
- A chimeric ALT flap with multiple skin paddles based on different perforators may be used to resurface complex defects.
- The ALT flap may be thinned by harvesting it in a suprafascial plane followed by thinning of the deep fat, preserving a cuff of tissue around the perforators.
- A fascia-only ALT flap may be used when a very thin, supple flap is desired.
- The ALT flap can be made sensate by including the lateral femoral cutaneous nerve in the flap harvest.
- The ALT flap donor site may be closed primarily when flap width is less than 8 cm.

RECOMMENDED READING

Aggarwal A, Singh H, Mahendru S, et al. Pedicle streaking: a novel and simple aid in pedicle positioning in free tissue transfer. *Indian J Plast Surg.* 2015;48:274–277.

Attinger CE, Janis JE, Steinberg J, et al. Clinical approach to wounds: débridement and wound bed preparation including the use of dressings and wound-healing adjuvants. *Plast Reconstr Surg.* 2006;117(7 Suppl):72S–109S.

Bhadkamkar MA, Wolfswinkel EM, Hatef DA, et al. The ultra-thin, fascia-only anterolateral thigh flap. *J Reconstr Microsurg.* 2014;30:599–606.

Brandt K, Khouri RK, Upton J. Free flaps as flow-through vascular conduits for simultaneous coverage and revascularization of the hand or digit. *Plast Reconstr Surg.* 1996;98:321–327.

Cavadas PC. Arteriovenous vascular loops in free flap reconstruction of the extremities. *Plast Reconstr Surg.* 2008;121:514–520.

Chen HC, Tang YB, Mardini S, et al. Reconstruction of the hand and upper limb with free flaps based on musculocutaneous perforators. *Microsurgery.* 2004;24:270–280.

Chen KT, Mardini S, Chuang DC, et al. Timing of presentation of the first signs of vascular compromise dictates the salvage outcome of free flap transfers. *Plast Reconstr Surg.* 2007;120:187–195.

Chim H, Ng ZY, Carlsen BT, et al. Soft tissue coverage of the upper extremity: an overview. *Hand Clin.* 2014;30:459–473.

Fan KL, Patel KM, Mardini S, et al. Evidence to support controversy in microsurgery. *Plast Reconstr Surg.* 2015;135:595e–608e.

Gharb BB, Salgado CJ, Moran SL, et al. Free anterolateral thigh flap in pediatric patients. *Ann Plast Surg.* 2011;66:143–147.

Goh TL, Park SW, Cho JY, et al. The search for the ideal thin skin flap: superficial circumflex iliac artery perforator flap: a review of 210 cases. *Plast Reconstr Surg.* 2015;135:592–601.

Gutwein LG, Merrell GA, Knox KR. Paraumbilical perforator flap for soft tissue reconstruction of the forearm. *J Hand Surg Am.* 2015;40:586–592.

Hallock GG. Preservation of hand function using muscle perforator flaps. *Hand (NY).* 2009;4:38–43.

Hallock GG. Tissue expansion techniques to minimize morbidity of the anterolateral thigh perforator flap donor site. *J Reconstr Microsurg.* 2013;29:565–570.

Hanasono MM, Skoracki RJ, Yu P. A prospective study of donor-site morbidity after anterolateral thigh fasciocutaneous and myocutaneous free flap harvest in 220 patients. *Plast Reconstr Surg.* 2010;125:209–214.

Kimura N, Satoh K. Consideration of a thin flap as an entity and clinical applications of the thin anterolateral thigh flap. *Plast Reconstr Surg.* 1996;97:985–992.

Kimura N. Thinning and tailoring. In: Wei F-C, Mardini S, eds. *Flaps and Reconstructive Surgery.* 2nd ed. Philadelphia, PA: Elsevier; 2016.

King EA, Ozer K. Free skin flap coverage of the upper extremity. *Hand Clin.* 2014;30:201–209.

Koshima I, Nanba Y, Tsutsui T, et al. New anterolateral thigh perforator flap with a short pedicle for reconstruction of defects in the upper extremities. *Ann Plast Surg.* 2003;51:30–36.

Koshima I, Yamamoto T, Narushima M, et al. Perforator flaps and supermicrosurgery. *Clin Plast Surg.* 2010;37:683–689.

Luenam S, Prugsawan K, Kosiyatrakul A, et al. Neural anatomy of the anterolateral thigh flap. *J Hand Microsurg.* 2015;7:49–54.

Mardini S, Chim H, Wei FC. Anterolateral and anteromedial thigh flap. In: Wei F-C, Mardini S, eds. *Flaps and Reconstructive Surgery.* 2nd ed. Philadelphia, PA: Elsevier; 2016.

Peng F, Chen L, Han D, et al. Reconstruction of two separate defects in the upper extremity using anterolateral thigh chimeric flap. *Microsurgery.* 2013;33:631–637.

Qing L, Wu P, Liang J, et al. Use of flow-through anterolateral thigh perforator flaps in reconstruction of complex extremity defects. *J Reconstr Microsurg.* 2015;31:571–578.

Salgado CJ, Mardini S, Jamali AA, et al. Muscle versus nonmuscle flaps in the reconstruction of chronic osteomyelitis defects. *Plast Reconstr Surg.* 2006;118:1401–1411.

Scheker LR, Ahmed O. Radical debridement, free flap coverage, and immediate reconstruction of the upper extremity. *Hand Clin.* 2007;23:23–36.

Schiaverien MV, Hart AM. Free muscle flaps for reconstruction of upper limb defects. *Hand Clin.* 2014;30:165–183.

Senchenkov A, Agag RL, Lee J, et al. Management of anterolateral thigh free flap donor site defects with a continuous external tissue expander. *Microsurgery.* 2015;35:290–294.

Torres-Ortíz Zermeño CA, López MJ. Aesthetic and functional outcomes of the innervated and thinned anterolateral thigh flap in reconstruction of upper limb defects. *Plast Surg Int.* 2014;2014:489012.

Townley WA, Royston EC, Karmiris N, et al. Critical assessment of the anterolateral thigh flap donor site. *J Plast Reconstr Aesthet Surg.* 2011;64:1621–1626.

Tsai FC, Yang JY, Mardini S, et al. Free split-cutaneous perforator flaps procured using a three-dimensional harvest technique for the reconstruction of postburn contracture defects. *Plast Reconstr Surg.* 2004;113:185–193

Wang HT, Fletcher JW, Erdmann D, et al. Use of the anterolateral thigh free flap for upper-extremity reconstruction. *J Hand Surg Am.* 2005;30:859–864.

Wei FC, Jain V, Celik N, et al. Have we found an ideal soft tissue flap? An experience with 672 anterolateral thigh flaps. *Plast Reconstr Surg.* 2002;109:2019–2226.

Wei FC, Jeng SF, Mardini S. Free style flaps. In: Wei F-C, Mardini S, eds. *Flaps and Resconstructive Surgery.* 2nd ed. Philadelphia, PA: Elsevier; 2016.

Wei FC, Mardini S. Free-style free flaps. *Plast Reconstr Surg.* 2004;114:910–916.

Yamamoto T, Narushima M, Yoshimatsu H, et al. Free anterolateral thigh flap with vascularized lateral femoral cutaneous nerve for the treatment of neuroma-in-continuity and recurrent carpal tunnel syndrome after carpal tunnel release. *Microsurgery.* 2014;34:145–148.

Yang LC, Wang XC, Bentz ML, et al. Clinical application of the thoracodorsal artery perforator flaps. *J Plast Reconstr Aesthet Surg.* 2013;66:193–200.

Yu P, Youssef A. Efficacy of the handheld Doppler in preoperative identification of the cutaneous perforators in the anterolateral thigh flap. *Plast Reconstr Surg.* 2006;118:928–933.

Zheng X, Zheng C, Wang B, et al. Reconstruction of complex soft-tissue defects in the extremities with chimeric anterolateral thigh perforator flap. *Int J Surg.* 2016;26:25–31.

22 Pedicled Flaps from the Groin and Lower Abdomen for Upper Extremity Coverage

S. Raja Sabapathy

The pedicled groin flap, first described by McGregor and Jackson in 1972, marked a milestone in upper extremity reconstruction. The flap, with its favorable length-to-width ratio, was seen as a great advance over the then-existing techniques. With the advent of microsurgery and free tissue transfers, the enthusiasm for this flap was reduced, but in spite of this, the groin flap still holds a useful place in the armamentarium of the reconstructive surgeon nearly half a century after its original introduction. The groin flap has become a must-know flap for the upper extremity surgeon due to its reliability, ease of elevation, and versatility of usage. This chapter covers the techniques required for successful use of the groin flap. By combining the groin flap with flaps based on vessels in the adjoining areas of the abdomen, a large number of defects can be covered.

INDICATIONS/CONTRAINDICATIONS

The groin flap is an example of a distant pedicled flap. The flap maintains its blood supply through its primary pedicle, while new blood vessels are established at the recipient defect site. Maturation of the flap usually requires 2 to 3 weeks before one can divide the groin flap pedicle and inset the flap. This is the major drawback to using the flap. During the maturation process, the hand must be kept close to the groin, which can promote edema, stiffness, and infection.

The indications for the use of the groin flap are broad, and the flap can be used to cover most defects on the hand and distal forearm. It is easiest to use for dorsal defects of the hand and fingers. Nevertheless, it can be used to cover the palm, volar aspect of the fingers, or any defect in the hand. When combined with flaps from the adjacent abdominal territories, even circumferential defects and large defects extending from the fingers to the elbow can safely be covered.

The use of the groin flap has been most commonly used for hand soft tissue coverage in preparation for free toe transfer for thumb or digital reconstruction. Use of the groin flap allows one to avoid the use of a microvascular anastomosis, thus sparing arteries and veins, which can be used for the subsequent toe transfer. In multiple finger amputations, if the bases of the proximal phalanges are present, it is worth to preserve the metacarpophalangeal joints with the groin flap for the subsequent toe transfer.

The groin flap can also be used as a free flap. The superficial circumflex iliac perforator flap (SCIP flap) based on the superficial blood supply to the groin flap allows for rapid elevation of a thin cutaneous flap with a favorable donor site.

Extremes of age are not a contraindication for the groin flap. We have used it in a 5-month-old child as well as in an 80-year-old man. It has been believed that children do not tolerate the period of immobilization required prior to flap separation; however, we have found that children tolerate this well. Pain caused by pull against the flap acts as a restraint for children not to disturb the flap. In comparison to the young patient, we do need to exercise care when performing the flap in older individuals. In older adults, there is a concern that edema and stiffness can develop within the hand. We usually start physiotherapy within the hand while the flap is still pedicled to the groin to avoid the development of edema.

Prior history of appendectomy, inguinal hernia repair, and Pfannenstiel incision are not contraindications for the use of the groin flap, though one may need to be careful if the flap needs to capture the skin of the adjacent territories. Inguinal node dissection or radiation to the groin is our only absolute contraindications to the use of the groin flap as these procedures often result in the disruption of the cutaneous perforating vessels.

ANATOMY

For the purpose of upper extremity reconstruction, we need to be familiar with the blood supply of the lower part of the abdomen (Fig. 22-1).

The femoral artery gives off the superficial circumflex iliac artery (SCIA) 2 cm below the inguinal ligament. It may arise as a common trunk with the superficial inferior epigastric artery (SIEA). SCIA is the vessel supplying the groin flap. It runs parallel to the inguinal ligament and at the medial border of the sartorius muscle gives off a deep branch and the superficial branch on which the groin flap is based. The course of the vessel is two fingerbreadths inferior to the anterior superior iliac spine (ASIS) and parallel to the inguinal ligament. Any portion of the skin flap that is designed distal to the anterosuperior iliac spine is considered to be a random flap and should be raised at 1:1.5 breadth-to-length ratio. In practice, we have consistently found that longer flaps can safely be raised up to the posterior axillary fold.

The SIEA arises from the femoral artery 1 cm distal to the inguinal ligament or as a common trunk with the SCIA and then passes upward superficial to the inguinal ligament. The course almost corresponds to the line of the femoral artery. It soon becomes superficial to the Scarpa fascia, and the final branches can be traced up to the level of the umbilicus.

The other vessel that arises from the femoral artery is the superficial external pudendal artery. It arises close to the origin of the SCIA and SIEA and runs medially beneath the great saphenous vein, becomes superficial near the pubic tubercle, and supplies up to the level of the umbilicus. No specific flap is usually planned on this vessel, but its territory can be combined with the adjacent territories when a large flap is required.

Superiorly, paraumbilical perforators arise from the deep inferior epigastric artery and then fan out from the umbilicus. Anatomic knowledge helps us to design flaps to cover any defect in the hand and forearm in a comfortable position.

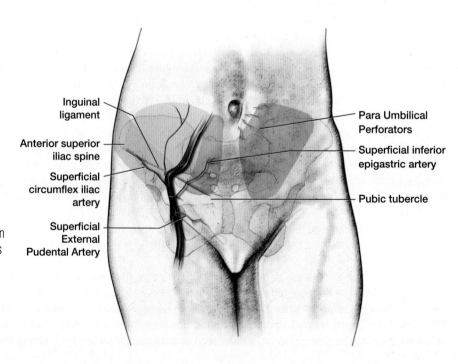

FIGURE 22-1

A schematic diagram showing the commonly used flaps from the lower part of the abdomen for upper limb reconstruction and the vessels on which they are based. (ASIS, anterior superior iliac spine; SCIA, superficial circumflex iliac artery; SIEA, superficial inferior epigastric artery; SEPA, superficial external pudendal artery; PT, pubic tubercle; PUP, paraumbilical perforators.)

SURGERY

Anesthesia

General anesthesia can be used, but in our center, the preference is for a combination of brachial block and spinal anesthesia. This combination cuts down on cost, gives prolonged pain relief, and most importantly in the immediate postoperative period, the patient cannot pull against the flap inset. Whichever anesthetic technique is chosen, temporary restraining tapes will be used to safeguard the position of the flap in the immediate postoperative period.

Patient Positioning

The patient is placed supine with the involved hand stretched out on a hand table. An arm tourniquet is tied to the upper limb. A small soft pillow can be placed under the gluteal region of the side of the flap harvest to elevate the iliac crest. The whole abdomen, from the lower margin of the chest wall to the thigh, is prepared, and the infraumbilical part of the abdomen and the upper thigh are kept open. If a large flap is planned, a thigh is made available for the harvest of skin graft.

Technique

Preparing the Hand for Flap Cover

The wound on the hand is thoroughly debrided. Adequate debridement is the key to success, and the quality of debridement is the same as what one would do when a free flap is used. Inadequate debridement causes infection under the flap, and even subclinical infection causes long-lasting edema of the flap. If fractures are present, they are stabilized. If K-wires are used, they *must not* be left protruding through the ulnar border of the hand, since it will be injuring the skin of the abdomen while the flap is pedicled. It is easier to plan the flap for a fully supinated hand than a fully pronated hand.

Planning and Raising the Groin Flap

Flaps can be raised with the guidance of anatomical landmarks, and we have found that preoperative Doppler study is not necessary. Whichever flap is raised from the lower abdomen, the following standard markings are done to design the ideal flap (Fig. 22-2):

Step 1. Mark the ASIS. This is the most important bony landmark to be marked. Since the course of the SCIA is marked in relation to the ASIS, mistake in this step in obese individuals can lead to flap problems. The finger is passed laterally along the inguinal ligament, and the first bony point felt is the ASIS. In obese individuals, mistakes can be made by marking it higher than it truly is.

Step 2. Mark the pubic tubercle and connect the ASIS and the point of the pubic tubercle, which will be the line of the inguinal ligament.

Step 3: At the midinguinal point (not the middle of the inguinal ligament), which is the midpoint between the ASIS and the midline along the inguinal ligament, palpate the pulsations of the femoral artery and mark the course for a few centimeters.

Step 4: Mark the outline of the sartorius muscle from the ASIS for a few centimeters.

Step 5: Mark the course of the SCIA. A point two fingerbreadths below the ASIS is marked on the lateral border of the sartorius. This would correspond to the point where the SCIA becomes superficial and flows into the territory of the groin flap. The course of the vessel is drawn parallel to the line of the inguinal ligament from the femoral artery passing along this point.

Step 6: Mark the course of the SIEA; it runs vertically along the line of the femoral artery.

With these markings, flaps could be planned with the axial vessels in the base. Since the arterial anatomy is reliable, pedicled flaps can be raised without specifically looking for the source vessel. It is also noted that at the site of entry of the source vessels into their respective flap territories, both SCIA and SIEA are only at a distance of 5 to 7 cm. We have found this constant, irrespective of the obesity status of the individual. So if we include both the vessels in the base of a flap, large flaps could be raised with a base of as narrow as 5 to 7 cm.

Step 7: A mental image of the available territory is envisioned at this stage. For elevation of the groin flap, the territory would be up to a line extended along the posterior axillary fold and for the SIEA (hypogastric flap); it would be the level of the umbilicus.

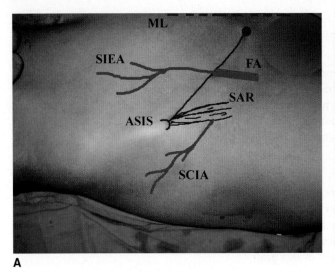

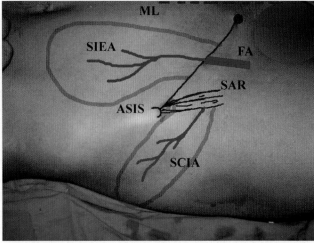

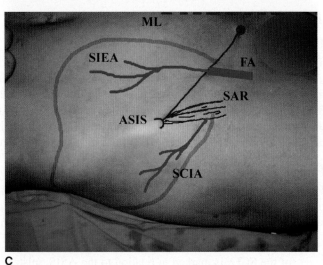

FIGURE 22-2

A: Basic marking for the planning of the groin flap. (ASIS, anterior superior iliac spine; SCIA, superficial circumflex iliac artery; SIEA, superficial inferior epigastric artery; FA, femoral artery; SAR, sartorius; ML, midline.) **B:** The standard safe territory of supply of groin flap and the hypogastric flap. **C:** Planning for a large flap by including both the vessels. Note the point of entry of both the vessels is usually only 5 to 7 cm. By keeping the base narrow, a large flap can be raised.

Designing the Flap

The flap is designed by planning in reverse (Fig. 22-3). We use an autoclaved cloth to plan the flap. We have found that linen templates are better than paper templates as they contour well over the defect. The hand after debridement is placed in the groin region in a comfortable position. The arm tourniquet if it has been applied is removed. Placing the hand in a comfortable position is the key to success. With the hand in the chosen position, the pattern that is cut with the pedicle is placed as it would be after the inset. Holding the pedicle in place, the hand is removed, and the pattern is allowed to fall into the zone of the flap territory. The flap outline is marked and once again the maneuver is repeated so that we ensure that the flap fits in the defect.

THE LENGTH OF THE PEDICLE. Conventionally and in the earlier publications, it has been stressed to keep the length of the pedicle long and tube the pedicle in order not to have a raw area and to be able to mobilize the hand in the postoperative period. We found that it had the disadvantage that the ultimate flap that covered the defect was too far away from the source vessel and the flap necrosis complications were higher. In our experience, we have found that narrowing the base and increasing the inset are the two primary determinants for postoperative comfort. So we do not raise long flaps, the pedicle is just long enough to promote pronation and supination of the hand. There is a small raw area at the base of the flap, but it has not posed any significant disadvantage. The drainage from this open area reduces in a few days and is easily manageable with dressing changes.

Raising the Flap

The flap is raised at the level of the fascia over the muscle in the lateral side and over the external oblique over the abdomen. It is better to raise the flap at the level of the muscle than fat, particularly

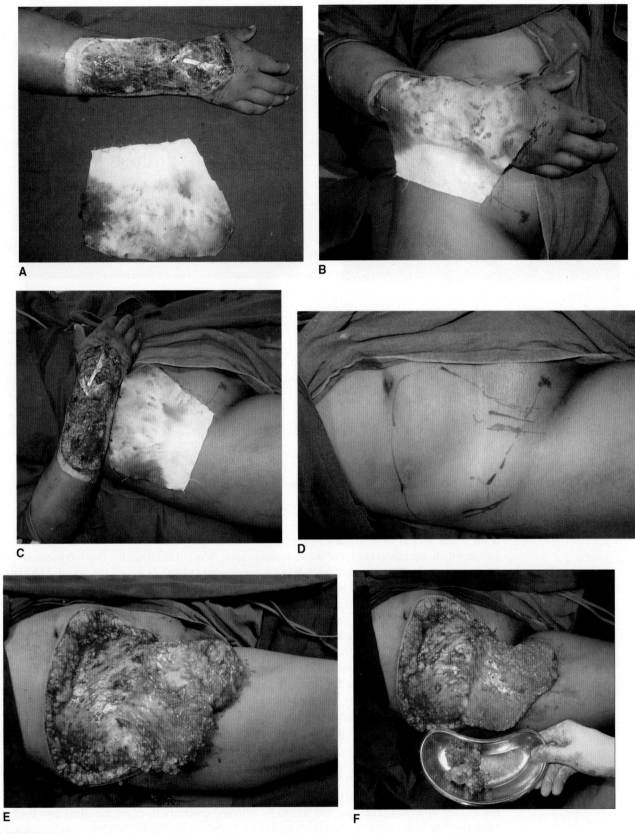

FIGURE 22-3

A: The posttraumatic defect of the dorsum of the hand and the distal forearm. The pattern of the defect is made in the cloth piece with an extension for the proposed pedicle. **B:** With the pattern on the defect, the hand is placed in the region of the flap in a comfortable position in such a way that the pedicle includes the source vessels. **C:** Holding the pattern in the location of the pedicle, the hand is removed and the outline of the flap marked. Adjustment can be done to narrow the pedicle or tilt the pattern so that the whole flap lies in the safe territory. **D:** The final design of the flap. **E:** The flap after raising from the bed. **F:** The part of the fat deeper to Scarpa fascia excised primarily to thin the flap, and the fat in the edges are trimmed to obtain a thinner flap.

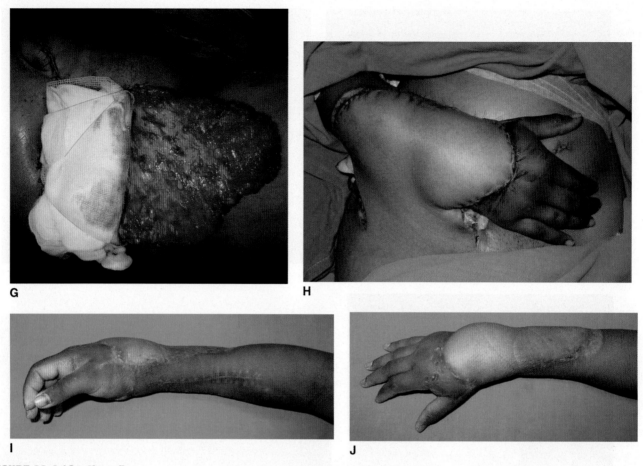

FIGURE 22-3 (Continued)
G: The donor area is narrowed, and the raw area is split skin grafted and covered with a tie over dressing. **H:** The flap after inset.
I, J: Postoperative result.

if the donor area is to be grafted as skin grafts take better on the muscle than on fat. The flap is elevated up to the lateral border of the sartorius muscle. Most of the time, the flap requirement can be met by raising the flap up to this point. It is not necessary to visualize the source vessel. The viability of the flap can be checked by bleeding in the flap at the subdermal plane.

The donor area is closed. If the breadth of the flap is 6 to 8 cm, the donor area can be primarily closed. The hip and the knee can be flexed by 30 degrees to reduce the tension at the suture line. If the flap raised is broader, then the raw area is narrowed and covered with split skin graft taken from the thigh. A tie over dressing is given to immobilize the graft.

The flap is then inset into the defect. To ease the inset of the flap, the flap can be thinned. The part of the fat deeper to the Scarpa fascia can be primarily excised. Further, the fat in the margin can be beveled so that suturing is easy, and there is less tension at the suture line. The distal part of the flap, which usually is used to cover the defect, is random in nature, and it depends upon the subdermal plexus for its viability. So this part can be thinned without jeopardizing the blood supply of the flap. Even in obese individuals, it is possible to obtain reasonably thin flaps to cover the hand defect.

Tips to Orient the Groin Flap for Hand Defects

To cover a dorsal defect, the flap has to face superiorly (Fig. 22-4). To cover a volar defect, the flap has to face inferiorly. The flap also has to be oriented correctly to cover the ulnar and the radial borders of the hand. After the required flap is raised, if the defect to be covered is on the dorsum of hand, the superior incision is prolonged roughly to the distance of the breadth of the flap. Then, if the lower margin is sutured to the original edge of the flap at the superior incision, the flap will point superiorly. To the cover the volar defect (Fig. 22-5), the inferior incision is prolonged. For radial (Fig. 22-6) and ulnar (Fig. 22-7) side defects, the superior and inferior incisions are prolonged but to half the extent as one would do for a dorsal or a volar defect.

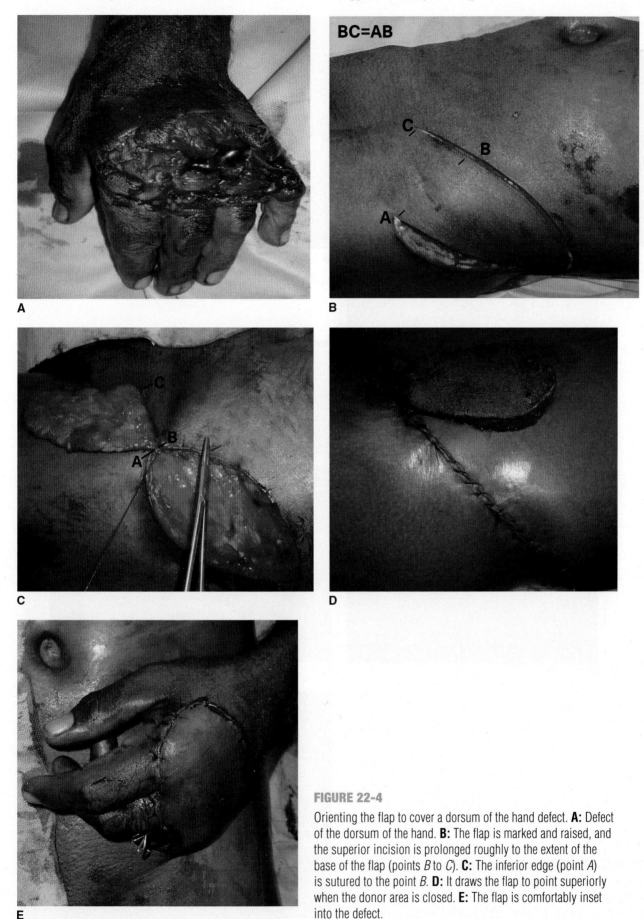

FIGURE 22-4

Orienting the flap to cover a dorsum of the hand defect. **A:** Defect of the dorsum of the hand. **B:** The flap is marked and raised, and the superior incision is prolonged roughly to the extent of the base of the flap (points *B* to *C*). **C:** The inferior edge (point *A*) is sutured to the point *B*. **D:** It draws the flap to point superiorly when the donor area is closed. **E:** The flap is comfortably inset into the defect.

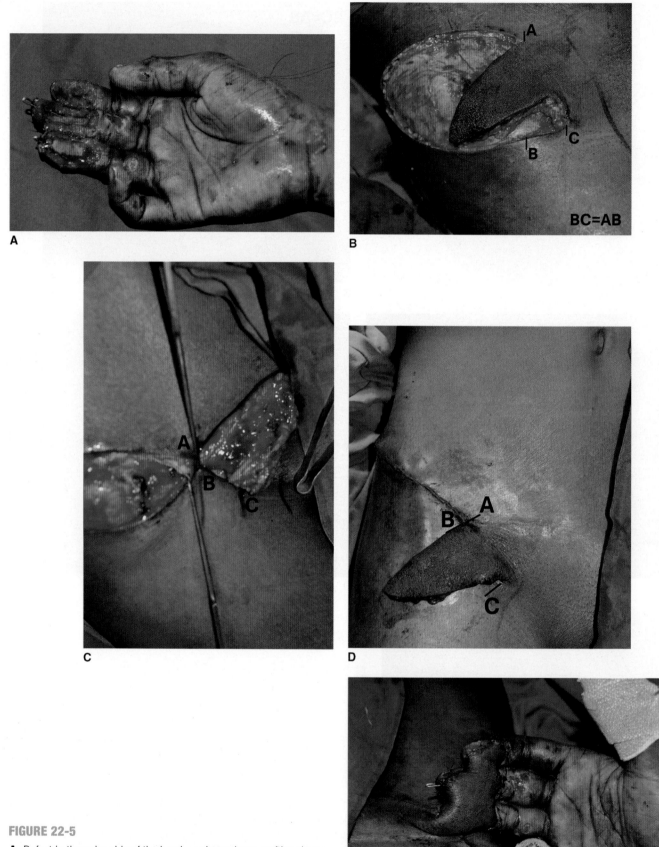

FIGURE 22-5

A: Defect in the volar side of the hand—primary bone grafting done and surgical syndactyly has been done. **B:** Groin flap has been raised, and for flaps to the volar side, the inferior incision is extended (points *B* to *C*). Point *A* is sutured to point *B* **(C)**, and making the flap point inferiorly **(D)**, and the flap is comfortably inset into the volar side **(E)**.

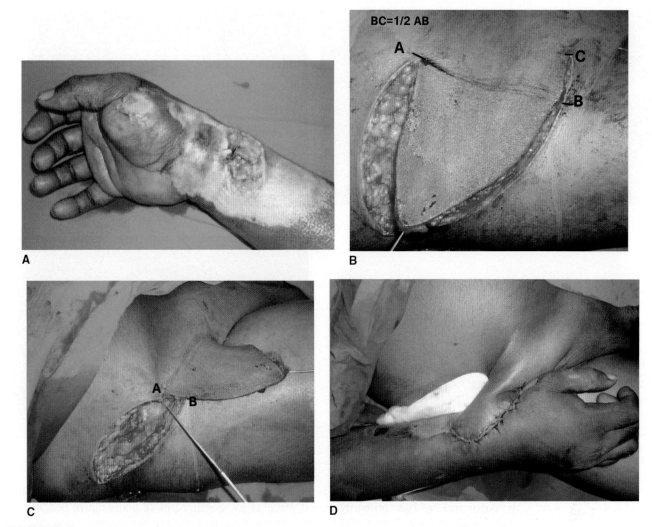

FIGURE 22-6

A: Defect in the radial side of the wrist. **B:** The flap is raised, and an extension of the incision is made on the inferior side, roughly matching to half the distance of the base of the flap (points *B* to *C*). **C:** When the points *A* to *B* are sutured, the flap turns obliquely downwards. **D:** The flap is easily inset into the radial defect without any kinking.

The flap is then inset. Good edge-to-edge opposition of skin is obtained since the flap survival depends upon good healing at the skin edges. When more than 80% of the margin is inset into the flap, with the hand in a position of ease, the patient will be comfortable in the postoperative period. If there is a potential dead space in the base or the wound covered was infected, a corrugated drain is placed beneath the flap and brought out through the open side.

POSTOPERATIVE MANAGEMENT

When the flap inset is complete, we use tapes to restrain the patient from making unwanted movement and pull off the flap. Broad tapes are used (Fig. 22-8). If surgery has been done under regional anesthesia, the flail upper limb has to be supported. One tape supports the arm, one supports the forearm, and one keeps the hand in such a way to prevent kinking of the pedicle. If the surgery has been performed under general anesthesia, similar tapes are used, and one has to stand guard till he recovers well and the position explained to the patient. These restraints are no longer required after 48 hours.

With the hand in the most desired position, three lines are drawn on the forearm or hand, and it is continued on the abdomen (Fig. 22-9). The patient and the nurse are instructed to just monitor that the lines stay aligned with one another. In this way, we ensure that the hand is in the correct position.

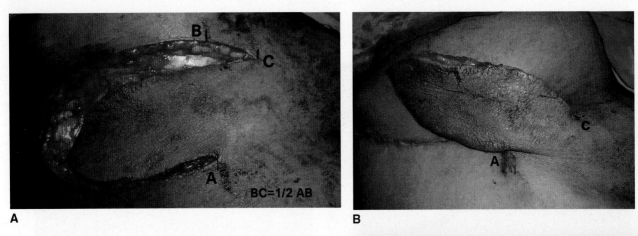

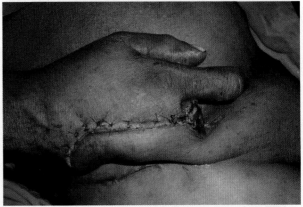

FIGURE 22-7

A: Flap for the ulnar border of the hand. After the flap has been raised, the superior incision is extended for half the distance of the base of the flap to point C. **B:** When points A to B are sutured, the flap points obliquely upward. **C:** In this way, the flap is comfortably inset into the ulnar side of the hand.

Postoperatively, a pillow is placed beneath the knee to reduce the tension at the suture line when the donor area has been primarily closed. Patients are mobilized in 48 hours out of bed and are ready for discharge in 3 days. The patients are encouraged to perform finger, elbow, and shoulder therapy.

Dividing the Flap

Flap pedicles are divided at 3 weeks. The flap can be divided in one sitting if one was able to inset 70% to 80% of the flap during the initial operation. A delay procedure is recommended when we do a tubed flap for reconstruction of a thumb or when a flap is used to cover circumferential raw area in an avulsed finger. In the delay procedure, a small skin incision is made in the pedicle of the flap in line with the source vessel. Ideally, the artery is identified and divided during the delay procedure. Delay procedures are done at 3 weeks. Complete flap division can then be performed 7 to 10 days following the delay procedure.

Thinning the Flap

Groin flaps from the lower abdomen can be bulky following transfer. Late flap thinning can be done safely 3 months after flap division. The prime advantage the pedicled flaps possess over free flaps is that during secondary thinning of the flap, the flap can be thinned aggressively as there is no worry of disrupting a microvascular anastomosis. The whole of the flap could be thinned in one sitting. We follow the technique of making a series of incisions of about 3 to 4 cm along the margin of the flap. Through these incisions, the whole flap can be thinned radically leaving only the subdermal layer intact. Most of the blood supply of the flap appears to be from the margins than from the bed, and so when less than one third of the flap margin is incised, we have never had any problem with flap necrosis. The undersurface of the flap is drained by corrugated drains, and the flap is then covered with a loose compression dressing.

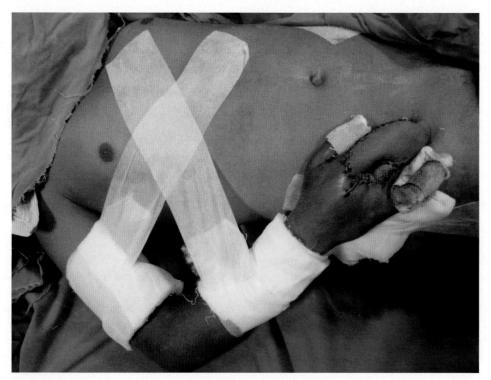

FIGURE 22-8

Basic support technique for protection of the flap in the immediate postoperative phase. The arm and the forearm need to be supported.

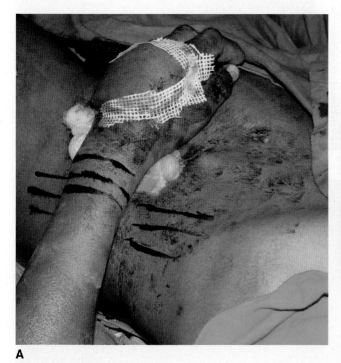

A

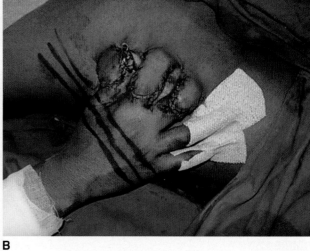

B

FIGURE 22-9

A: Three lines are drawn on the forearm and continued on to abdomen and thigh matching during the postoperative period. If the flap is big, the lines could be drawn on the flap with a marking pen. **B:** If some fingers are free and the flap is attached to the fingers or the thumb, then the fingers are restrained by tapes in the immediate postoperative period.

REFINEMENTS IN PEDICLED FLAPS FOR UPPER EXTREMITY COVER AND FLAPS IN SPECIAL SITUATIONS

Simultaneous Coverage of Dorsum and Volar Aspect of the Hand

On occasions when both the dorsum and palm need cover, bilobed flaps can be raised from the lower abdomen. The groin flap easily fits in the dorsum, and the hypogastric flap based on the SIEA can be used to cover the palm. The hand is sandwiched between the flaps. Since the anatomy of the vessels is very reliable, the base of the flaps can be made narrow, and it helps in increasing the arc of rotation of the flap, facilitates inset, and enhances the comfort of the patient in the postoperative period (Fig. 22-10).

Coverage of Large Defects

Groin flap can be combined with territories of the SIEA and the superficial inferior prudent artery to cover even large defects extending from the elbow to the metacarpophalangeal joints. The particular advantage of the pedicle flap is that a uniformly wide flap is available to cover the entire defect. This is in contrast to the free flap where when a large free flap is raised, the viability of the distal end of the flap may be precarious.

Most of the time, it is enough if the territories of the groin flap is combined with the hypogastric flap supplied by the SIEA. Both the vessels take origin from the femoral artery. At the site of entry of both of these vessels into the flap, they are only at a distance of 5 to 7 cm in any individual. So a large

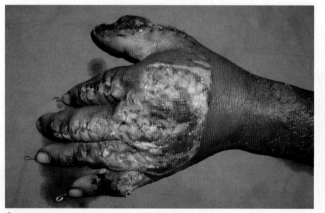

A

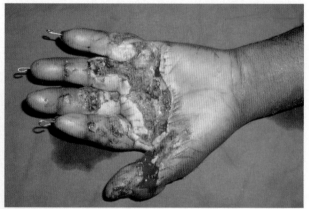

B

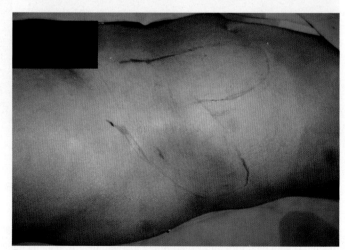

C

FIGURE 22-10

A, B: A 10-day-old hand injury requiring flap cover both on the dorsum and the palmar aspect of the hand. **C:** A bilobed flap marked, one a groin flap and the other the hypogastric flap on a common pedicle.

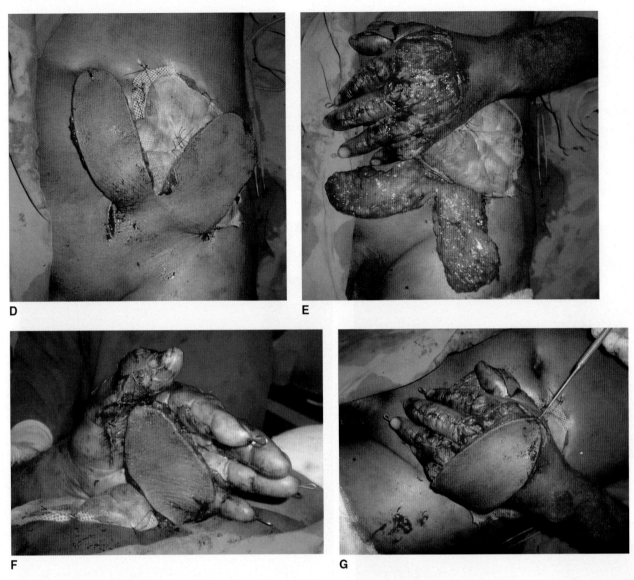

FIGURE 22-10 (*Continued*)
D, E: The raised flap, the donor area skin grafted, and the hand in preparation of inset. **F:** The hypogastric flap is used to cover the palm.
G: The groin flap covers the dorsum of the hand.

flap can be raised with the base of the pedicle just enough to include both these vessels. Narrowing the base of the flap helps us to design the flap to fit the defect (Fig. 22-11).

Flaps for Multiple Defects

Sometimes pedicle flaps might have to be done for nonadjacent defects on the same side or on volar and dorsal side or for multiple nonadjacent fingers (Fig. 22-12). The hand is first placed in the position of comfort in the flap area. The flap for the biggest defect is planned first. Most often, the groin flap is used for this. The donor area is closed or narrowed as much as possible, and a single suture is used to anchor the flap to the defect. With the hand in that position, the second flap is planned and raised. For small defects, more than trying to make it axial and based on a named particular vessel, a flap that will sit comfortably over the defect is chosen and designed. Now the anchoring suture is removed and the second flap is raised. In this way, the flaps sit well in the defect. If all the flaps are done initially, the orientation of the flaps may be altered when the donor areas are closed. To obviate it, the biggest flap is done first, donor area is closed, the flap temporarily attached, and the next flap is planned.

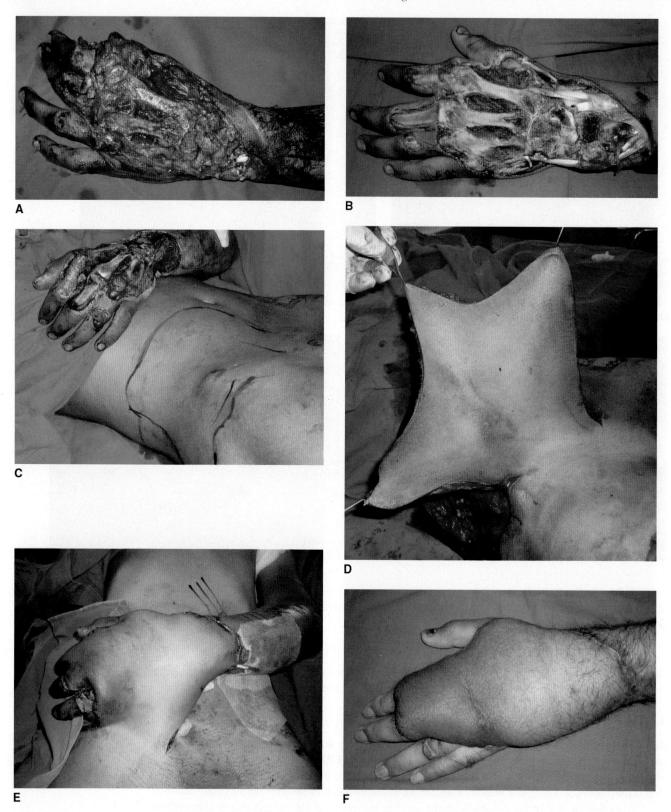

FIGURE 22-11

A: A dorsal composite loss of the hand and distal forearm in a road traffic accident. **B:** Postdebridement. **C:** Flap planned, including the territories of the groin and the hypogastric flaps. Note the lateral extent of the flap that is possible to be raised. **D:** The flap after being raised. **E:** The flap after being inset. **F:** After division.

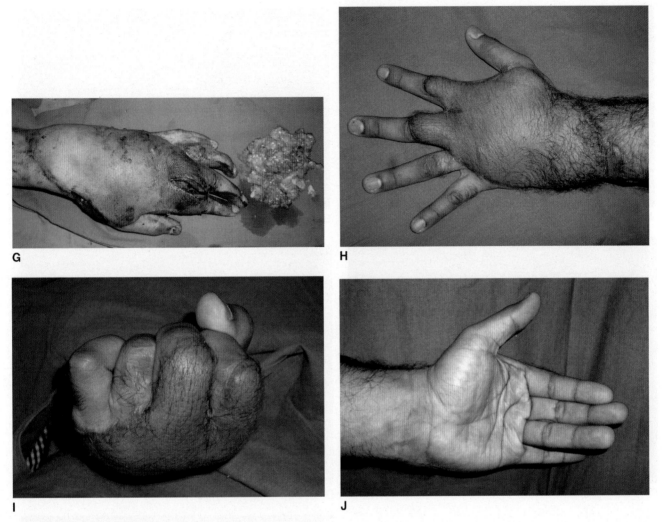

FIGURE 22-11 (*Continued*)
G: Thinning of the flap and division of the syndactyly between fingers after 3 months. **H–J:** Final functional result. Patient has extensor lag in the index, middle, and ring fingers but is doing well functionally.

Flaps in Children

Groin flaps and flaps from the lower abdomen can be performed in children safely (Fig. 22-13). Children have less postoperative stiffness. Contrary to popular opinion, there is no increased incidence of flap dehiscence in children. They also do not need any additional restraints. We have done flaps in children as young as 5 months of age and with no extra precaution and have obtained good results.

COMPLICATIONS

Groin flaps like any other flaps in trauma can develop a postoperative wound infection. We have found that these are most likely due to the poor initial debridement.

It is extremely rare to have total flap necrosis. Partial flap necrosis is due to poor planning of the flap and missing to include the axial vessel in the base of the flap. Since the anatomy is so consistent if the landmarks are followed, it is virtually impossible to miss including the vessels in the flap. Partial flap necrosis after division sometimes occurs. This indicates that the inset has been inadequate or the base is infected. If the inset is less than 70% of the perimeter of the defect or it is a tubed flap, then a prior surgical delay of the flap before division is indicated.

Physiotherapy is important for all patients undergoing pedicled flap. Shoulder and elbow therapy are instituted from the first postoperative day. When the groin flap is divided, under anesthesia, the shoulder and the elbow are mobilized fully so that joint stiffness complications are reduced.

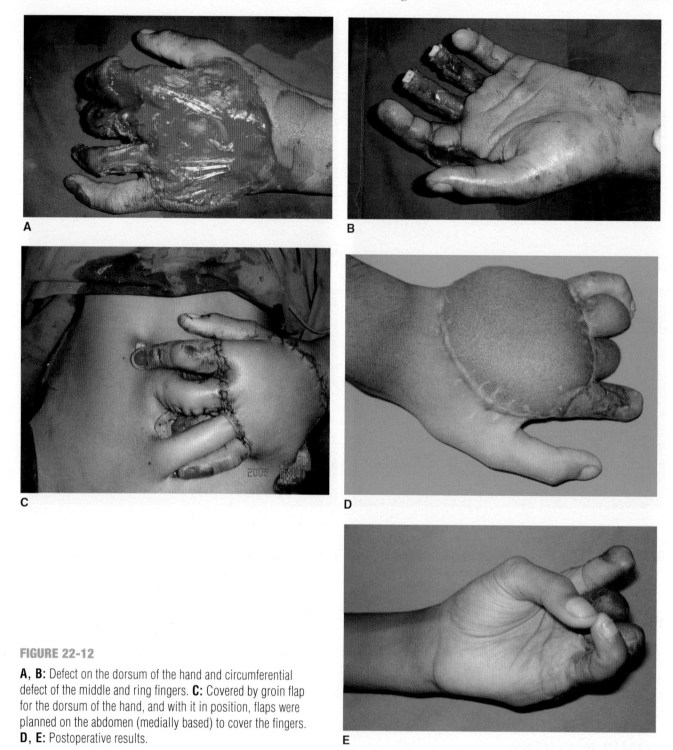

FIGURE 22-12

A, B: Defect on the dorsum of the hand and circumferential defect of the middle and ring fingers. **C:** Covered by groin flap for the dorsum of the hand, and with it in position, flaps were planned on the abdomen (medially based) to cover the fingers. **D, E:** Postoperative results.

PEARLS AND PITFALLS

- The anatomy of the axial arteries supplying the groin flap and the lower abdominal flaps is reliable. One must be careful in marking the ASIS (particularly in the obese), since the markings of the flap are based on this bony landmark.
- Design the flap according to the defect so that the inset will be increased.
- The pedicle needs to be just adequate to allow pronation and supination of the hand after inset. The pedicle need not be unduly long and tubed, which would compromise the blood supply of the critical area of the flap.

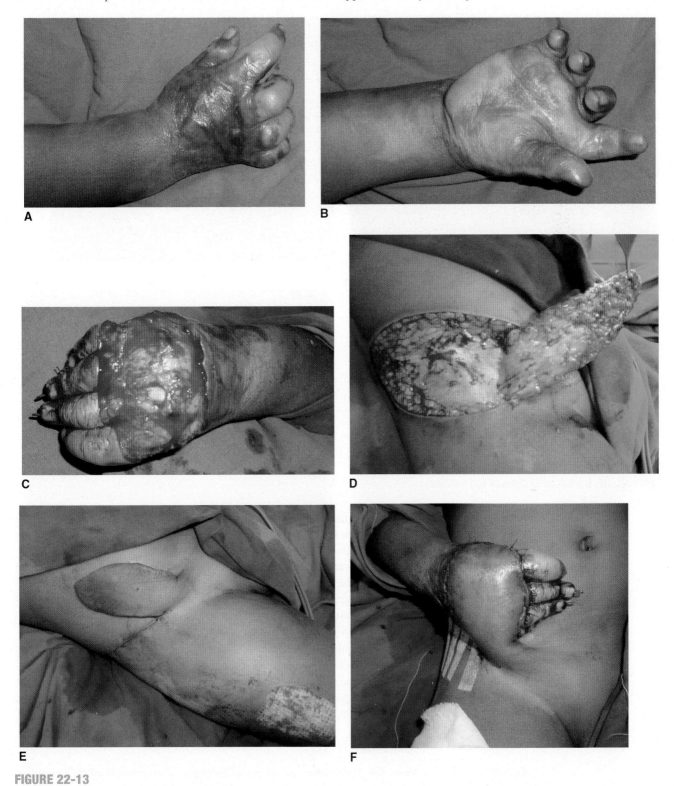

FIGURE 22-13

A, B: Postburn contracture of the hand and fingers of a 1-year-old child. **C:** After release of contracture and temporary pinning of the joints. **D:** Groin flap planned for the defect. **E:** Donor area sutured in a way so that the flap points superiorly. **F:** The flap inset into the defect.

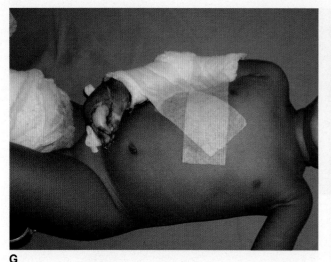

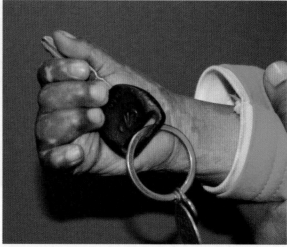

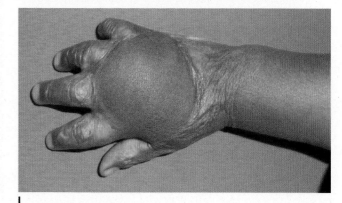

FIGURE 22-13 (*Continued*)
G: The child comfortable in the postoperative period with minimal restraints. **H, I:** Postoperative result and function.

- By combining the territories of the groin flap with that of the hypogastric flap, large flaps can be raised without delay. Since the site of entry of SCIA and SIEA into the flap is only about 5 to 7 cm, the base could be narrow and the flap large.
- The blood supply of the business end of the flap is usually random in nature, and it depends upon the subdermal plexus. So it can be thinned radically, making thin flaps possible.
- Bevel the fat obliquely in the edges so that the inset is easy to obtain without tension.
- If the inset is over 80%, there is no need to delay the flap before division at 3 weeks. Tubed flaps for thumb or degloving injuries of the digits must be delayed before division.
- Secondary thinning of the flap could be radical, and it could be done at 3 months after flap division.
- Debridement has to be radical as one would do prior to an emergency free flap to prevent infection.
- Primary reconstruction with bone grafts and tendon grafts is possible with pedicled flaps if the area of inset is more than 80% preventing exposure of the graft. Infection is dependent on the quality of debridement prior to flap cover than the flap itself.

RECOMMENDED READING

Bajantri B, Latheef L, Sabapathy SR. Tips to orient pedicled groin flap for hand defects. *Tech Hand Up Extrem Surg.* 2013;17:68–71.

Boyd JB, Taylor GI, Corlett R. The vascular territories of the superior epigastric and the deep inferior epigastric systems. *Plast Reconstr Surg.* 1984;73:1–16.

Chuang DC, Colony LH, Chen HC, et al. Groin flap design and versatility. *Plast Reconstr Surg.* 1989;84:100–107.

Friedrich JB, Katolik LI, Vedder NB. Soft tissue reconstruction of the hand. *J Hand Surg Am.* 2009;34:1148–1155.

McGregor IA, Jackson IT. The groin flap. *Br J Plast Surg.* 1972;25:3–16.

Sabapathy SR, Bajantri B. Indications, selection, and use of distant pedicled flap for upper limb reconstruction. *Hand Clin.* 2014;30:185–199.

Sabapathy SR, Venkatramani H, Giesen T, et al. Primary bone grafting with pedicled flap cover for dorsal combined injuries of the digits. *J Hand Eur Surg Eur Vol.* 2008;33:65–70.

Venkatramani H, Sabapathy SR. A useful technique to maintain the position of the hand following abdominal flap. *Indian J Plast Surg.* 2008;41:100–101.

Yilmaz S, Saydam M, Seven E, et al. Paraumbilical perforator based pedicled abdominal flap for extensive soft-tissue deficiencies of the forearm and hand. *Ann Plast Surg.* 2005;4:365–368.

PART IV
SOFT TISSUE COVERAGE OF THE FINGERS FOLLOWING TRAUMA

23 Cross-Finger Flaps for Digital Soft Tissue Reconstruction

Nicholas Pulos and Alexander Y. Shin

S oft tissue loss to the digits and fingertips is common following hand trauma. Treatment goals following such injuries include immediate coverage with well-vascularized tissue, restoration of sensation, and a durable thin reconstruction. The cross-finger flap can meet these goals.

Cross-finger flaps have been used for over 70 years to repair wounds and deformities requiring both skin and subcutaneous tissue. They provide durable skin coverage, preservation of adequate sensation, maintenance of finger length, and restoration of cosmesis. The purpose of this chapter is to describe the anatomy, indications and contraindications, technique, and results of treatment with the cross-finger and reverse cross-finger flaps.

INDICATIONS/CONTRAINDICATIONS

The cross-finger flap is indicated in the repair of wounds or deformities to the volar or flexor surfaces of the finger requiring the use of both skin and soft tissue. Specifically, this flap is used for soft tissue reconstruction of wounds not amenable to skin grafting alone. The main indication for the cross-finger flap is a volar fingertip wound with a major loss of skin and subcutaneous tissue with exposed bone, tendon, or distal interphalangeal joint. It is also commonly used for volar defects of the middle phalanx. A technique for restoration of the thumb pulp using the cross-finger flap has also been described.

A cross-finger flap can be used in any age group. In the pediatric patient, its use has been reported as early as the first year of life. It has been used in children for the treatment of congenital constricting bands, as well as burn contractures and ring avulsion injuries. Some authors have suggested caution in using this flap in patients older than 50 years of age due to the risk of persistent postoperative stiffness of the donor digit.

The reverse cross-finger flap is indicated in adults with defects on the dorsum of the finger or nail bed with major loss of skin and subcutaneous tissue and exposed bone, tendon, or joint that cannot be covered by other techniques. This flap consists of the same tissue used for the standard cross-finger flap but without the dermis and epidermis of the overlying skin. For this reason, it has also been referred to as a deepithelialized cross-finger flap or adipofascial flap.

Contraindications for the standard and reverse cross-finger flap include multiple injuries to the hand involving the potential donor digit; diseases affecting vascularity of the digit such as diabetes mellitus, Raynaud's disease, or Berger disease; or a preexisting disabling disease such as Dupuytren's contracture. Advanced age, osteoarthritis, and rheumatoid arthritis may be relative contraindications.

PREOPERATIVE PLANNING

Preoperative radiographs of the injured hand should be evaluated for concomitant injuries, which should be treated prior to the commencement of the cross-finger flap. The donor finger is adjacent to the injured finger. For defects of the index finger, the long finger is used. However, for all other defects, the radial digit is used as the donor site.

As a random flap, the base of the cross-finger flap is longer than the transverse limbs, and the entire dorsal skin of the finger can be raised. However, if the flap includes skin from the dorsal creases of the interphalangeal joints, the resultant scar may lead to stiffness and contracture. Additionally, the subcutaneous tissue over the distal interphalangeal and proximal interphalangeal joints is thin. To decrease the risk of contracture and provide adequate bulk, it is recommended that the flap be raised between the interphalangeal creases. Thus, the potential flap size will vary from patient to patient and depends on the size of the donor finger. Larger defects may require other methods of soft tissue reconstruction such as vascularized island flaps or partial toe transfers.

SURGERY

Anatomy

The cross-finger flap and reverse cross-finger flap are random pattern regional flaps, which are usually raised from the dorsum of the donor finger at the level of the proximal or middle phalanx. The small blood vessels of the subdermal and subcutaneous plexus provide the blood supply for these flaps. The palmar digital arteries and dorsal metacarpal arteries supply the collaterals to this flap. The dorsal carpal arch gives rise to the metacarpal arteries, which bifurcate to form the dorsal digital arteries. The dorsal digital arteries largely vascularize the skin and subcutaneous tissues of the dorsum of the proximal phalanx. Distally, the proper palmar digital arteries provide branches that feed the plexus of vessels covering the skin and subcutaneous tissues of the dorsum of the middle and distal phalanges.

Similarly, the innervation of the cross-finger flap may be derived from the sensory innervation of the dorsum of the hand and/or the proper digital nerves themselves. Up to the level of the proximal interphalangeal joint, the superficial branch of the radial nerve and dorsal sensory branch of the ulnar nerve innervates the dorsum of the hand. Distally over the middle phalanx, innervation is derived from dorsal sensory branches of the proper digital nerves. These dorsal sensory branches arise from each digital nerve at the level of the base of the proximal phalanx. At the level of the middle phalanx, the dorsal sensory branches arborize to innervate the dorsal skin. The proper digital nerves continue distally, trifurcating at or just past the distal interphalangeal joint, sending a dorsal branch to innervate the nail fold and nail bed (Fig. 23-1).

Patient Positioning

The majority of these flaps can be performed as outpatient surgery under regional anesthesia. The patient is positioned supine on the operating room table with the affected extremity placed on a radiolucent hand table. Hemostasis is facilitated with the use of either a brachial or digital tourniquet. Prophylactic antibiotic is given per the discretion of the surgeon.

Technique

The first step of the procedure involves adequate debridement and irrigation of the injured digit. All skin edges are freshened and trimmed to fit the dimensions of the flap (Fig. 23-2). Before planning the location and shape of the flap, the donor and recipient fingers are placed in a position of comfort. We recommend patterning the size of the defect on a piece of glove paper, allowing 20% excess of the flap pedicle to ensure adequate soft tissue coverage and a tension-free flap. The pattern is then transferred to the dorsum of the adjacent donor digit (Fig. 23-3).

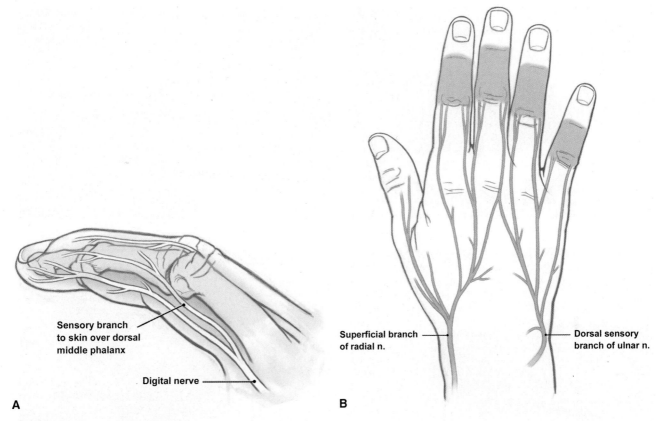

FIGURE 23-1

A: Innervation to the dorsum of the middle and distal phalanges from the proper digital nerves through dorsal and distal branches.
B: Innervation to the dorsum of the hand and dorsum of the proximal fingers from branches of the radial and ulnar nerves. (Reproduced with permission of the Mayo Foundation, 2015.)

The three sides of the flap are raised as a full-thickness graft including the subdermal fat on the donor finger down to the plane between the paratenon and the subcutaneous flap (Fig. 23-4A). The flap is hinged on the side closest to the injured digit. Fashioning the proximal transverse incision so that it extends more palmarly than the distal incision will allow the flap to face proximally, which may be preferable for coverage of an amputation stump. It is essential that the paratenon layer not be violated to ensure that a full-thickness skin graft will adhere to the donor site. Meticulous hemostasis is obtained with the use of bipolar cautery. The flap is assessed to ensure adequate mobility, without kinking, when the recipient site is covered (Fig. 23-4B). If further mobility of the flap is needed, the proximal or distal transverse incisions may be extended. Cleland's ligament may be incised taking care to protect the volar neurovascular bundle. Once the flap is reflected, the tourniquet is deflated and the vascularity of the flap and the paratenon are evaluated (Fig. 23-4C).

The free margins of the flap are sutured in placed on the finger defect with nonabsorbable 4-0 sutures in adults or absorbable sutures of adequate size in children (Fig. 23-5). The donor defect is covered with a full-thickness skin graft harvested from the antecubital fossa, upper brachium, or groin according to surgeon preference (Figs. 23-6 and 23-7). A compressive dressing of the surgeon's choice is applied over the skin graft, followed by a bulky hand dressing with appropriate splints. We prefer a petroleum bismuth dressing with mineral oil–soaked cotton balls that are bolstered.

Reverse Cross-Finger Flap

Preparations for the reverse cross-finger flap are similar to those of the standard cross-finger flap. However, this flap differs in two major ways: the placement of the flap hinge and the thickness of the donor tissue.

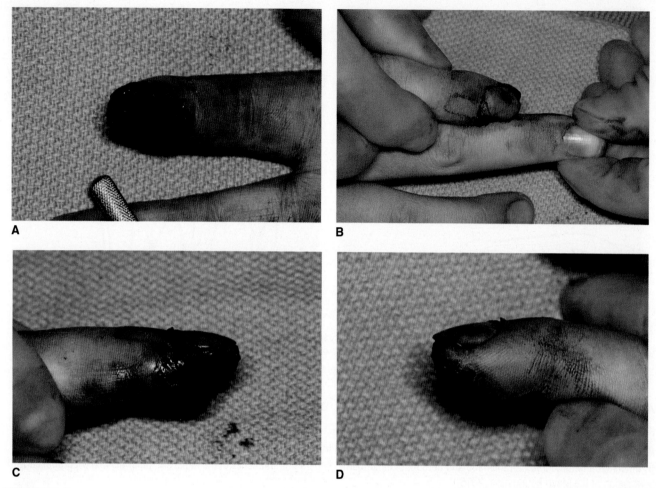

FIGURE 23-2

Volar **(A)**, dorsal **(B)**, and side views **(C, D)** of an oblique volar fingertip amputation. (Reproduced with permission of the Mayo Foundation, 2015.)

FIGURE 23-3

The injured finger is placed at the level of the planned flap from the dorsum of the middle finger at the level of the middle phalanx. The flap should be 20% larger than the actual defect to minimize tension at the time of closure. (Reproduced with permission of the Mayo Foundation, 2015.)

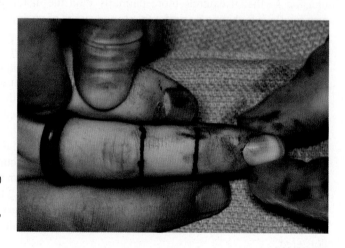

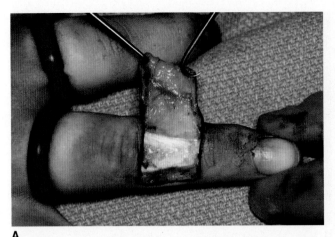

A

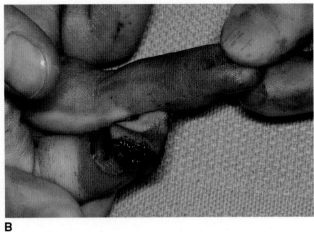

B

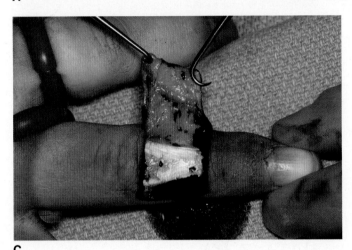

C

FIGURE 23-4

A: Elevation of the cross-finger flap, keeping the paratenon intact. **B:** Assessment of flap mobility and coverage.
C: Evaluation of the vascularity of the flap and the paratenon after release of the tourniquet. (Reproduced with permission of the Mayo Foundation, 2015.)

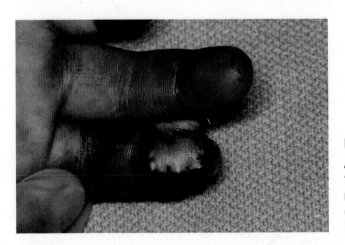

FIGURE 23-5

A clinical example of a cross-finger flap taken from the dorsum of the middle finger to cover the ring finger. (Reproduced with permission of the Mayo Foundation, 2015.)

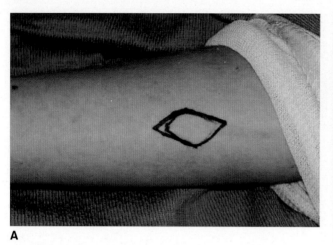

A

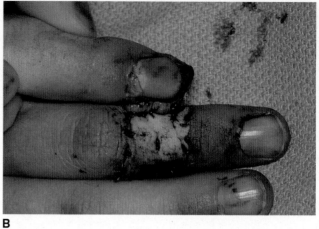

B

FIGURE 23-6

A full-thickness graft from the forearm **(A)** is used to cover the defect over the donor site **(B)**. (Reproduced with permission of the Mayo Foundation, 2015.)

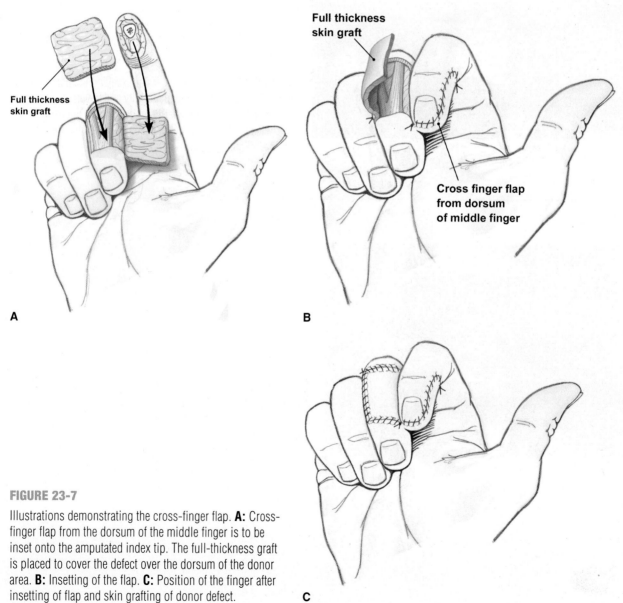

A

B

C

FIGURE 23-7

Illustrations demonstrating the cross-finger flap. **A:** Cross-finger flap from the dorsum of the middle finger is to be inset onto the amputated index tip. The full-thickness graft is placed to cover the defect over the dorsum of the donor area. **B:** Insetting of the flap. **C:** Position of the finger after insetting of flap and skin grafting of donor defect.

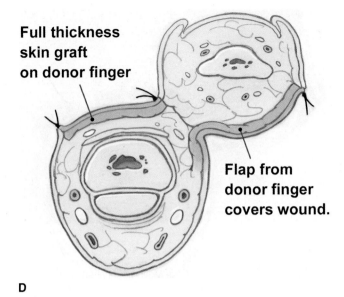

Full thickness skin graft on donor finger

Flap from donor finger covers wound.

D

FIGURE 23-7 (*Continued*)
D: Cross-section through donor and recipient sites. (Reproduced with permission of the Mayo Foundation, 2015.)

The hinge of the skin flap is opposite to the primary defect. This is in contradistinction to the standard cross-finger flap, where the hinge is adjacent to the site of the defect. Attention should be paid to raise a thin full-thickness skin graft, which does not include the subdermal fat layer from the dorsum of the donor finger at the level of the middle phalanx, below the hair follicles, and above the layer of subcutaneous veins. A flap of subcutaneous tissue is then raised, keeping the paratenon intact, with the hinge of subcutaneous tissue adjacent to the defect. The subcutaneous flap is then inset into the defect and the skin is placed back over the donor site. A full-thickness skin graft is harvested and set on the flap. The flap is secured and dressed in a manner similar to the standard cross-finger flap (Figs. 23-8 and 23-9).

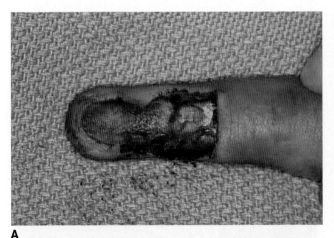

A

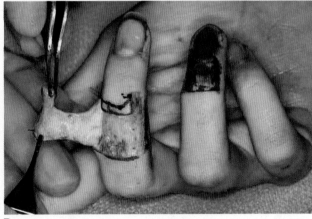

B

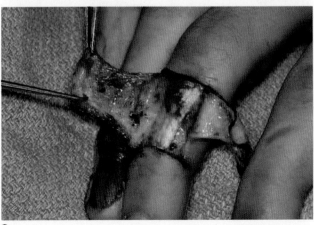

C

FIGURE 23-8

Clinical example of a reverse cross-finger flap. **A:** Surgical defect on the dorsum of the ring finger at the level of the distal phalanx and nail bed. **B:** Elevation of a full-thickness skin flap keeping the subcutaneous fat flap intact. **C:** Elevation of the subcutaneous flap, preserving the paratenon, with the hinge of subcutaneous tissue adjacent to the defect.

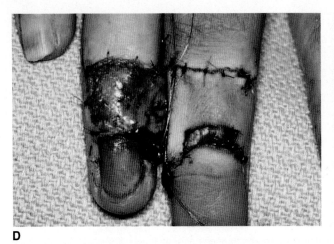

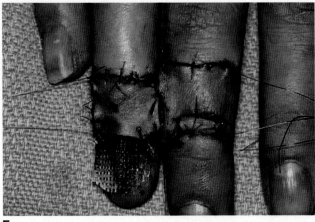

D

E

FIGURE 23-8 (*Continued*)

D: The flap is secured. **E:** A full-thickness skin graft is set on the flap. (Reproduced with permission of the Mayo Foundation, 2015.)

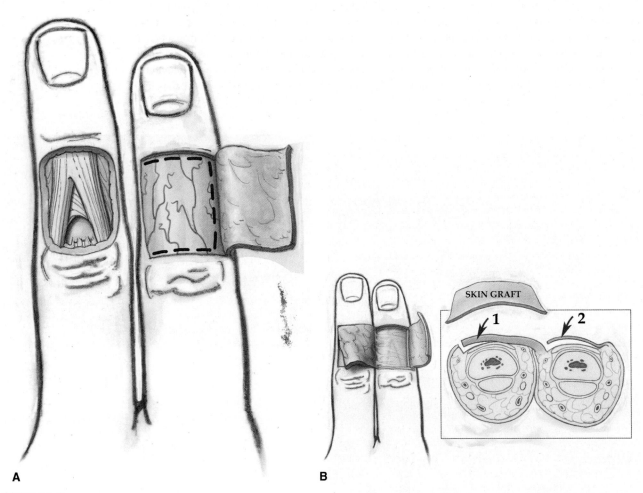

A

B

FIGURE 23-9

Illustrations demonstrating the reverse cross-finger flap. **A:** A thin-thickness skin flap is raised from the dorsum of the donor finger at the level of the middle phalanx, keeping the subcutaneous fat flap intact. The *dotted dashed lines* indicate the site of the planned reverse cross-finger flap, which is divided to the level of the paratenon. **B:** The reversed fat flap covers the dorsal finger skin defect (*arrow 1*). The raised thin-thickness skin graft is replaced again into its native site (*arrow 2*). A thin-thickness skin graft is placed over the reversed cross-finger flap.

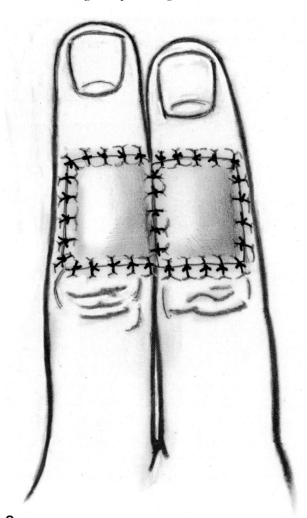

C

POSTOPERATIVE MANAGEMENT

Postoperatively, the wound is kept elevated and the patient is encouraged to move the uninjured digits. At 1 week, the postoperative dressings and splints are removed and a soft dressing is replaced. Nonabsorbable sutures are removed between 10 and 14 days postoperatively.

The flap is divided, contoured, and inset at approximately 3 weeks postoperatively. The timing of flap division can occur as early as 2 weeks (Figs. 23-10 and 23-11); however, it is our preference to wait until 3 weeks to allow for more complete integration. In our practice, this is done in the operating room under local or regional anesthesia on an outpatient basis to allow for adequate hemostasis and trimming if necessary.

Early active motion and passive stretching are initiated in a supervised therapy program shortly after flap division. This helps to eliminate stiffness and regain motion lost while the flap was maturing.

RESULTS

Kleinert et al. demonstrated high rates of patient satisfaction with only 2 of 56 patients stating that they would have preferred a more proximal amputation to cross-finger flap reconstruction. In another series, all patients were able to return to their former occupations and some were able to resume hobbies including playing piano and guitar. In a series of 54 patients treated with cross-finger flaps, 92% of patients were satisfied with the results and all patients recovered protective sensation. However, 53% suffered cold sensitivity and all of the flaps had diminished sweating and decreased sensory discrimination.

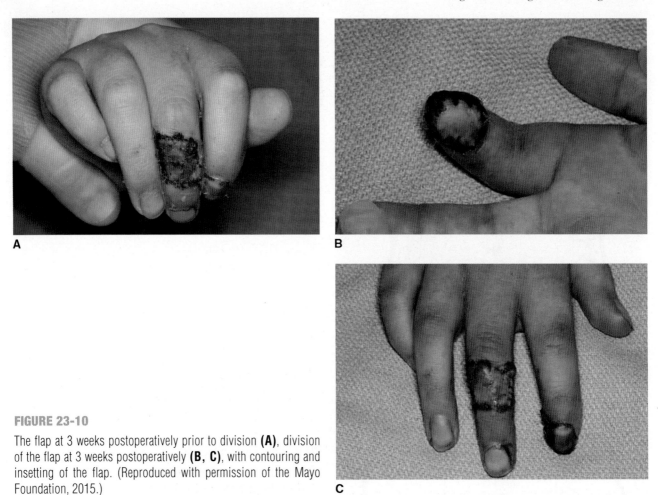

FIGURE 23-10

The flap at 3 weeks postoperatively prior to division **(A)**, division of the flap at 3 weeks postoperatively **(B, C)**, with contouring and insetting of the flap. (Reproduced with permission of the Mayo Foundation, 2015.)

An innervated cross-finger flap, whereby the dorsal sensory branch of the proper digital nerve of the donor digit is joined to the proper digital nerve of the injured digit, has been described in both the thumb and fingers. However, Kleinert et al. reported two-point discrimination of less than 8 mm in 70% of patients without neurorrhaphy. Additionally, two-point discrimination better than that

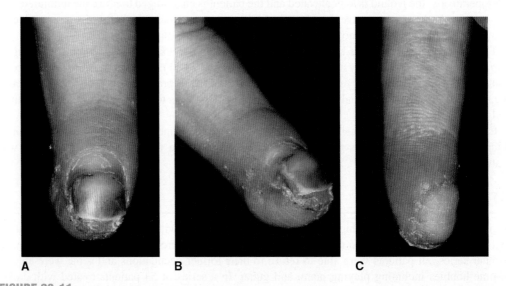

FIGURE 23-11

The appearance of the finger 3 months after surgery **(A–C)**. (Reproduced with permission of the Mayo Foundation, 2015.)

of the equivalent donor area on the unaffected hand has been reported. Sensation may continue to improve even after 3 months postoperatively. Thus, it appears that functional reinnervation of the cross-finger flap usually does occur. For these reasons, we do not routinely perform a neurorrhaphy with a cross-finger flap.

Atasoy reported on four patients satisfactorily treated with reverse cross-finger flap. In addition to coverage of the defect, nail growth and extensor tendon function were observed. Al-Qattan compared the results of reverse cross-finger flap reconstruction to adipofascial turnover flaps. All flaps survived with no infection or hematoma. However, patients who underwent reverse cross-finger flap reconstruction had more postoperative stiffness. Therefore, he recommended using the adipofascial turnover flap in older patients to avoid stiffness as well as pediatric patients to avoid the use of general anesthesia during flap division.

COMPLICATIONS

Postoperative infection and wound healing problems are unusual complications and may be associated with poor patient selection. Flap necrosis is a rare complication owing to the vigorous blood supply of the cross-finger flap. Color mismatch between the dorsum of the fingers and the pulp is minimal but may be more noticeable in patients with darker skin. Patients may also complain of hair growth depending on the site of the donor tissue. Other reported complications include development of a vascular malformation and epidermal inclusion cysts in reverse cross-finger flaps.

Altered sensation is the most common complication of this procedure with cold intolerance reportedly affecting as many as half of all patients. This cold intolerance may be more related to the injury than type of repair. The altered sensory recovery varies by age. More than 90% of patients younger than 12 years of age had 6 mm or less two-point discrimination, compared to 40% of patients older than 40 years of age. Similarly, cold intolerance, hyperesthesia, and joint stiffness were all less common in a pediatric population.

The major disadvantage of the cross-finger flap is that a normal finger, serving as the source of the flap, may have some residual scaring and stiffness as a result. The use of a thin cross-finger flap, which preserves the dorsal subcutaneous tissue, has been described to reconstruct volar defects that do not require bulk. Decreased grip strength of the donor digit has been reported. Donor site cosmesis may be improved with the use of full-thickness skin grafts, but color mismatch is common. Anesthesia at the tip of the donor finger, which took several months to resolve, has been reported. This highlights the caution necessary in elevating flaps to avoid damage to the digital nerves.

PEARLS AND PITFALLS

- The cross-finger flap allows for soft tissue reconstruction of fingertip and volar finger soft tissue injuries. The reverse cross-finger flap is used to reconstruct dorsal injuries.
- To decrease the risk of contracture and provide adequate bulk, it is recommended that the flap be raised between the interphalangeal creases.
- Pattern the size of the defect on a piece of glove paper, allowing 20% excess of the flap pedicle to ensure adequate soft tissue coverage and a tension-free flap.
- A full-thickness skin graft harvested away from the ipsilateral arm may provide a more cosmetically appealing result.
- Early active motion and passive stretching are initiated in a supervised therapy program shortly after flap division, which takes place at around 3 weeks.

RECOMMENDED READING

Al-Qattan MM. De-epithelialized cross-finger flaps versus adipofascial turnover flaps for the reconstruction of small complex dorsal digital defects: a comparative analysis. *J Hand Surg.* 2005;30(3):549–557.

Atasoy E. Reversed cross-finger subcutaneous flap. *J Hand Surg Am.* 1982;7(5):481–483.

Cohen BE, Cronin ED. An innervated cross-finger flap for fingertip reconstruction. *Rev Plast Reconstr Surg.* 1983;72(5):688–697.

Cronin TD. The cross finger flap: a new method of repair. *Am Surg.* 1951;17:419–425.

Gokrem S, Tuncali D, Terzioglu A, et al. The thin cross finger skin flap. *J Hand Surg Eur.* 2007;32(4):417–420.

Groenevelt F, Schoorl R. Cross-finger flaps from scarred skin in burned hands. *Br J Plast Surg.* 1985;38(2):187–189.

Hasting H II. Dual innervated index to thumb cross finger or island flap reconstruction. *Microsurgery.* 1987;8(3):168–172.

Horn JS. The use of full thickness hand skin flaps in the reconstruction of injured fingers. *J Plast Reconstr Surg.* 1951;78:463.

Jebson PJL, Louis DS, Bagg M. Amputations. In: Wolfe SW, Hotchkiss RN, Pederson WC, et al., eds. *Green's Operative Hand Surgery*, 6th ed. Philadelphia, PA: Elsevier Churchill Livingstone; 2011:1885–1927.

Kappel DA, Burech JG. The cross-finger flap: an established reconstructive procedure. *Hand Clin.* 1985;1(4):677–683.

Kleinert HE, McAlister CG, MacDonald CJ, et al. A critical evaluation of cross-finger flaps. *J Trauma* 1974;14:756–763.

Koshima I, Inagawa K, Urushibara K, et al. Fingertip reconstructions using partial-toe transfers. *Plast Reconstr Surg.* 2000;105(5):1666–1674.

Lee NH, Pae WS, Roh SG, et al. Innervated cross-finger pulp flap for reconstruction of the fingertip. *Arch Plast Surg.* 2012;39(6):637–642.

Ma GF, Cheng CJ, Chan KT, et al. Finger tip injuries: a prospective study on seven methods of treatment on 200 cases. *Ann Acad Med Singapore.* 1982;11(2):207–213.

Martin DL, Kaplan IB, Kleinert JM. Use of a reverse cross-finger flap as a vascularized vein graft carrier in ring avulsion injuries. *J Hand Surg Am.* 1990;15(1):155–159.

Nishikawa H, Smith PJ. The recovery of sensation and function after cross-finger flaps for fingertip injury. *J Hand Surg Br.* 1992;17(1):102–107.

Paterson P, Titley OG, Nancarrow JD. Donor finger morbidity in cross-finger flaps. *Injury.* 2000;31(4):215–218.

Warwick DJ, Milling MA. Growth of a vascular malformation into a cross-finger flap. *Br J Clin Pract.* 1993;47(1):48.

24 Heterodigital Arterialized Flap

Shian Chao Tay and Lam Chuan Teoh

INDICATIONS/CONTRAINDICATIONS

Indications

Hand trauma that results in exposed bone, tendon, joint, or neurovascular structures that are not suitable for skin grafting requires flap coverage. Skin defects across joints and in web spaces also require flap coverage to avoid contractures that could occur following split-thickness grafting. The location and size of these defects can often preclude the use of small rotation or advancement flaps. Free flap coverage is an option, but the presence of surrounding infection or a wide zone of trauma may make the recipient vessels' dissection difficult. In such situations, a heterodigital arterialized (HTA) flap may be an option to be considered.

The HTA flap is raised from the lateral side of a donor finger together with the digital artery and a dorsal digital vein. Unlike Littler's neurovascular island flap, or Hueston's extended neurovascular island flap, the HTA flap's main function is to provide nonsensory reconstruction of skin defects in the hand or fingers. Thus, this flap is never harvested with the finger pulp or the digital nerve of the donor finger. This is an important feature that serves to reduce morbidity to the donor finger. The inclusion of the digital dorsal vein into the flap improves venous drainage of the flap and reduces the incidence of venous congestion, which is a well-documented complication of the classic Littler's flap.

The HTA flap is a thin flap. In this aspect, it is ideal for reconstruction in the hand and fingers as it provides near like-to-like reconstruction for digital and palmar defects. The other advantage of this flap is that it is a regional pedicled flap. This allows one to avoid microsurgery and also allows for almost immediate motion of the reconstructed finger. One final benefit is that this flap allows for reconstruction to be performed as a single-stage procedure and avoids a second procedure as is required with a cross-finger flap or groin flap.

In our experience, the HTA flap has been used to reconstruct volar, lateral, or dorsal defects in the fingers proximal to the distal interphalangeal joint, web spaces, palm, dorsum of the hand, and the thumb. The average flap dimensions are 4.1 cm (range 1.5 to 5.5 cm) in the longitudinal axis and 2.1 cm (range 1.0 to 3.5 cm) in the transverse axis. The HTA flap is thus a useful option to consider when faced with the problem of a relatively large defect in the hand or finger that requires nonsensory flap reconstruction. The HTA flap has been used for reconstruction of defects following infection, trauma, replantation of digits, electrical burns, chemical burns, and high-pressure injection injuries.

In terms of flap mobility, the reach of the HTA flap is limited to coverage of defects in the adjacent fingers or thumb, or adjacent parts of the hand. This is principally due to the combined limitations in the reach of the dorsal vein and the digital artery of the flap. In situations where a greater reach is required, it is possible to divide the dorsal vein of the flap over the dorsum of the hand and reanastomose it in a region of healthy tissue after flap transfer. With this maneuver, the flap should have the ability to reach defects two to three fingers away, much like the traditional reach of Littler's neurovascular island flap, when pivoting at the common digital artery's takeoff at the superficial palmar arterial arch.

Contraindications

The HTA flap is absolutely contraindicated if there is only one functioning digital artery in the donor finger and when the vascular viability of any other adjacent fingers is threatened by flap harvesting. It is also relatively contraindicated if the functional prognosis of the finger to be reconstructed is judged to be so poor that it might be better to amputate it. However, we recognize that social or cultural practices may still dictate reconstruction for the purpose of cosmesis or the maintenance of the "whole" self. Conversely, if there is a rare situation wherein a need to perform a digital amputation exists in a hand containing a defect requiring flap reconstruction, the HTA flap can be used as a fillet flap from the amputated finger for defect reconstruction. In such a situation, the HTA flap is very useful in spare parts surgery as there is no concern for donor finger morbidity. If the defect occurs beyond the reach of the flap or in the contralateral hand, a free fillet HTA flap can be created from the finger to be amputated provided the conditions at the recipient finger allows for a free flap.

PREOPERATIVE PLANNING

All practical options available for reconstruction should be considered by the surgeon before deciding on the HTA flap. Risks of heterodigital donor finger morbidity should be carefully weighed against benefits of reconstruction. Often, the location, size, and nature of the defect will preclude other reconstructive options, leaving the HTA flap as the most viable option with the highest flap survival rate.

The choice of donor finger is often dictated by the location of the defect and is often an adjacent finger. The outside borders of the index and little fingers are not used as donor sites to preserve hand cosmesis and to maintain native skin for protection and sensation. This requirement is not absolute; however, we prefer the use of the middle finger, ring finger, and the ulnar border of the index finger. Theoretically, the radial border of the little finger can be used as a donor site, but this is rare as the little finger is small, providing little skin, and the remaining ulnar digital artery is often absent or vestigial.

A digital Allen's test must be performed on the intended donor finger to ensure that both digital arteries are sufficiently patent. In addition, the Allen's test should also be performed on the finger that is adjacent to the donor site as this would dictate if the digital artery mobilization can proceed proximal to the point of bifurcation of the common digital artery in order to create an arterial pedicle of sufficient length.

If the donor site is just next to the defect in the adjacent finger, also known as the contiguous or near side of the adjacent finger (e.g., defect on ulnar side of index finger with donor site on radial side of middle finger), the pivot point can be at the bifurcation of the common digital artery, as a short pedicle would be sufficient. This pivot point can be approximately landmarked in the intermetacarpal space at the level of the distal palmar crease. The distance from this pivot point to the proximal edge of the defect can then be measured to determine the reach needed by the flap and hence the location of the proximal margin of the flap. If the flap is not coming from the contiguous side of the adjacent finger, it is likely that a more proximal pivot point would be required to ensure sufficient reach of the flap. The most proximal point would be the superficial palmar arterial arch, which can be approximated to the level of the proximal palmar crease in the relevant intermetacarpal space. In such situations, as mentioned previously, it will be necessary to ligate and divide the neighboring digital artery of the common digital artery that supplies the adjacent finger to maximize the reach of the flap.

Experience has shown that the reach of the flap increases by 10% once the digital artery is adequately mobilized. However, in the interests of safety and ensuring minimum tension in the pedicle, a 1:1 ratio should still be maintained for the length of the arterial pedicle during preoperative planning of flap surgery.

The timing for reconstruction depends on the pathology. As far as possible, early reconstruction (within 1 week) is preferred as it minimizes overall hand stiffness from prolonged disuse. For traumatic conditions, the reconstruction is ideally performed within 1 week. For postreplantation surgery with residual skin defects, the resurfacing is performed within 10 to 15 days when re-endothelialization of the vascular anastomoses is completed. Infection cases are ideally resurfaced within 4 to 7 days when the surrounding cellulitis and edema have subsided. In order to achieve this time line in infective cases, infection resolution should be achieved within one to two formal definitive excisional debridement surgeries in conjunction with appropriate intravenous antibiotics.

The surgery can be performed under general or regional anesthesia with sedation. The patient's general condition and coagulation profile should be optimized as per any reconstructive surgery. The patient should be consented and counseled as to the surgery, the postoperative course, and the duration of stay following surgery.

SURGERY

Anatomy

The common digital arteries in the hand (average diameter of 1.6 mm, range of 1.0 to 2.0 mm) arise from the superficial palmar arch. At the level of the metacarpophalangeal joint in the corresponding web spaces, the common digital arteries divide into radial and ulnar digital arteries of contiguous fingers. In general, the ulnar digital arteries of the index and middle finger are almost always larger than their radial counterparts. For the ring and little finger, the radial digital arteries are usually larger.

Patient Positioning

The patient should be in the supine position, and care should be taken to protect bony prominences with suitable pressure-relieving bolsters. The upper limb with the hand requiring reconstruction should be abducted to not more than 80 degrees at the shoulder to prevent excessive stretch to the nerves in the axilla. The elbow should be flexed slightly, so that the forearm can be placed transversely on a stable hand table. A pneumatic tourniquet should be applied to the most proximal part of the upper arm. If the surgery is expected to require two or more tourniquet inflations, a sterile tourniquet is recommended. It should be placed in the operative field outside of the drapes so that the Velcro of the tourniquet can be loosened by the surgical team during tourniquet breaks to avoid any tourniquet complications. Urinary catheterization should also be performed for long surgeries.

Technique

Tourniquet inflation should be done with the upper limb elevated but not exsanguinated. This is to facilitate identification and mobilization of the digital artery and the digital dorsal vein. The defect should be thoroughly debrided and irrigated. A template of the defect is made. This can be done by marking the edges of the defect with surgical marker and transferring that marking to a surgical wrapping paper moistened with an alcohol swab.

Using the template created, the appropriate dimension of the flap is then transferred onto the donor site. The flap should be centered on the lateral or dorsolateral side of the finger, depending on the width of flap required, to ensure the inclusion of the digital artery and a dominant digital dorsal vein. The maximum width of the flap should not exceed the midpalmar line and the middorsal line (a width of approximately 3 cm). The maximum length of the flap is from the base of the finger to the distal interphalangeal joint crease (usually 4 to 5 cm depending on the size of the finger). If necessary, the flap length may be extended 0.5 cm distal to the distal interphalangeal joint crease. Next, a palmar Z incision is drawn biased to the respective side of the finger to access the proximal part of the digital artery. This incision is carried into the palm to the level of the common digital artery. The location of the dominant dorsal digital vein is then verified and marked to ensure that it will drain the flap. Once this is completed, the flap is ready to be harvested.

HTA flap harvesting is performed with the aid of loupe magnification. The flap is first raised from its palmar margin (Fig. 24-1). If the palmar margin of the flap crosses any digital palmar flexion creases, a mini-Z cut can be made at these creases, to break up the resultant scar line. Superficial palmar veins can be carefully cauterized with bipolar electrocautery and divided. The dissection follows the digital artery from proximal to distal starting from the bifurcation of the common digital artery. The angle of dissection toward the neurovascular bundle is an oblique plane skiving dorsal to the digital nerve, which is more central and superficial compared to the digital artery. As far as possible, the nerve should be left undisturbed in its bed with a collar of fat kept around it. Besides ensuring that the nerve is not traumatized, the collar of fat also provides additional cushioning and enhances the take of the full-thickness skin graft at the donor site. Ideally, a collar of fat or soft tissue should also be kept around the digital artery to preserve the venae comitantes. Fortunately, in the HTA flap, this is not as critical, as the dorsal vein would provide the main conduit for venous drainage.

At this point, an intraoperative occlusion test can be performed using nontraumatic microsurgical vascular clamps to determine the integrity of the contralateral digital artery in the donor finger. If mobilization of the arterial pedicle to the level of the superficial palmar arch is necessary, a similar occlusion test should be performed on the bifurcated digital artery supplying the adjacent nondonor finger to ensure that it also has a healthy contralateral digital artery.

As mobilization of the digital artery progresses, the transverse palmar arches of the digital artery will be encountered. These are rather large and short. Sufficient room is developed and the arches can be carefully cauterized with bipolar electrocautery before division. Care should be taken to ensure that the bipolar electrocautery is applied at least 2 mm from the parent artery to prevent compromising flow in the main digital artery.

Dorsal dissection is performed next with proximal to distal dissection and mobilization of the dominant dorsal digital vein to ensure inclusion of the vein in the flap. The flap is dissected free from the extensor tendons in the plane superficial to the paratenon. Care should be taken not to damage the dorsal skin branches of the digital artery supplying the flap. At the distal margin of the flap,

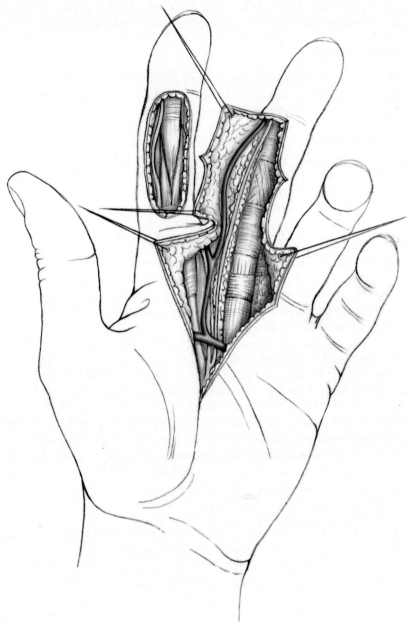

FIGURE 24-1

Completed palmar dissection of the HTA flap with the digital nerve left undisturbed in its bed with a collar of fat around it. Proximal dissection of the arterial pedicle is facilitated by a palmar Z incision into the palm.

the distal end of the dominant dorsal vein is ligated and divided, and the same is performed for the digital artery on the palmar side.

At this stage, the flap should be detached from distal to proximal. The adherent fibrous septa and Cleland's ligaments are divided. At the base of the digit, some dissection may be necessary to complete the division of subcutaneous tissues attached to the flap. The natatory ligament at the web space may also be divided to prevent kinking of the dorsal vein and lengthen the reach of the flap.

A generous subcutaneous tunnel is created between the donor and the recipient site. Tunneling is performed from the proximal edge of the recipient site into the palm to reach the pivot point of the flap. A hemostat forceps is used to gently enlarge the tunnel for easy flap delivery. The distal end of the flap is carefully grasped and gently maneuvered into the tunnel. A recommended method of flap delivery is to completely wrap the flap with tulle gras dressing and deliver the flap by grasping only on the tulle gras. This serves to prevent direct grasping of the flap and also protects the flap and pedicles from being avulsed if the delivery in the tunnel is inadvertently rough

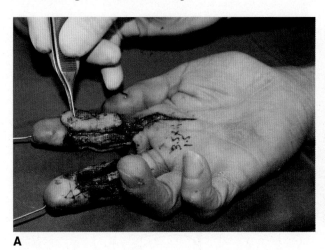
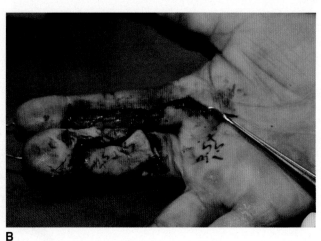

A   **B**

FIGURE 24-2

A: The raised HTA flap is shown with the arterial and dorsal venous pedicle. **B:** The HTA flap shown after transfer and inset.

or jerky. As the flap traverses the tunnel, care is taken to ensure that the digital artery and the dorsal vein do not become twisted or kinked. The flap should not be rotated more than a half turn. If there is any uncertainty, the flap should be redelivered to ensure its correct orientation (Fig. 24-2).

When a longer reach of the flap is required, and the bipedicled nature of the flap is restricting the transfer, the dominant dorsal vein may be divided before the transfer (Fig. 24-3) and anastomosed to the original vein or another vein over the dorsum of the hand in an area free of adversity, after the flap has been transferred (Fig. 24-4). When this procedure is performed, it is called the "partially free HTA flap" (Fig. 24-5).

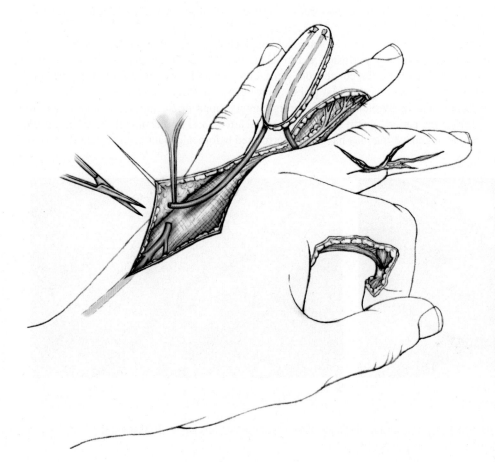

FIGURE 24-3

Completed dorsal and palmar dissection of the HTA flap with the flap completely islanded from the donor ring finger. The flap is now to be transferred. In this case, the defect requiring resurfacing is on the volar side of the index finger. The middle finger has a significant injury and is not suitable as a donor. The bipedicled nature of the flap will obstruct the transfer through the palmar subcutaneous tunnel. Thus, the venous pedicle of the flap has been divided over the dorsum of the hand to partially free the flap and convert it into a monopedicled flap.

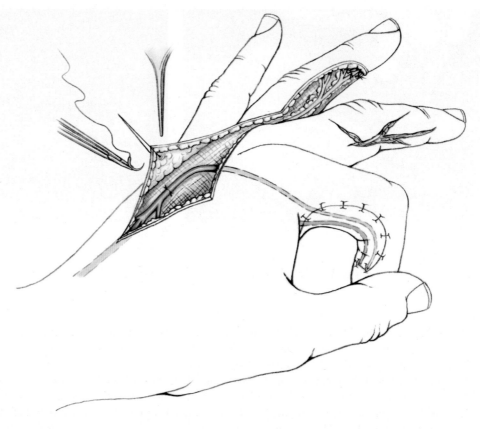

FIGURE 24-4

The partially free HTA flap after successful transfer to the defect site on the index finger. The venous pedicle of the flap has been tunneled back for microsurgical repair to the original draining vein over the dorsum of the hand.

After flap transfer, the flap is provisionally held in place with a few fine sutures. The tourniquet is then deflated to check for flap perfusion and to secure hemostasis. If flap perfusion does not return after 5 minutes or if there is flap congestion, some sutures may have to be removed. If this fails to improve flap color, kinks in the vascular pedicle may have to be located and relieved. If the vascular pedicle suffered mild inadvertent trauma during surgery, appropriate flap resuscitation measures such as warming the patient, warm saline soaks to the artery, and immersion of the arterial pedicle in 2% lidocaine or papaverine may have to be performed before adequate flap perfusion is restored.

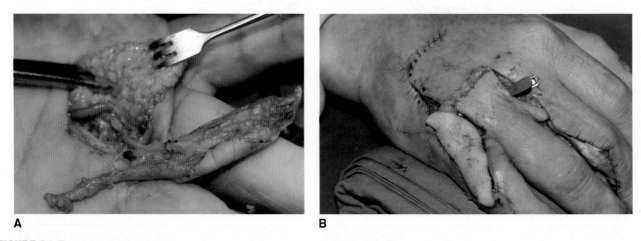

FIGURE 24-5

A: The "partially free HTA flap" with a divided dorsal vein to facilitate flap transfer to a noncontiguous finger. **B:** After transfer from the middle to the little finger, the dorsal vein of the HTA flap is reanastomosed.

Once adequate flap perfusion is restored, the flap is then fully inset with fine sutures, usually nonabsorbable monofilament 5-0 sutures, spaced not less than 3 to 5 mm apart. Care should be taken during the insetting to ensure that both the dorsal vein and the digital artery are not compressed or traumatized. The donor defect is resurfaced with a full-thickness skin graft. This can be taken from the medial proximal forearm, the anterior elbow, or groin if necessary. As early postoperative active rehabilitation is required, it is highly recommended to secure the skin graft with a cotton wool bolster and a meticulous tie-over dressing to prevent skin graft loss during therapy. The rest of the surgical wounds are closed with fine sutures with or without nonsuction drains. A bulky, nonconstrictive dressing is applied with a window left open for flap monitoring. Healthy flap perfusion should be confirmed before leaving the operating room.

Variants of the Heterodigital Arterialized Flap

Once the surgeon is familiar with the standard HTA flap, there are several variants of this flap that can extend its usefulness. The cross-finger HTA flap (Fig. 24-6) is particularly suited for coverage of dorsal defects distal to the proximal interphalangeal joint that cannot be reached by the reverse dorsal intermetacarpal flap or the Quaba flap. The cross-finger HTA flap can also be used in situations where proximal dissection of the digital artery in the hand is not advisable due to previous trauma or infection. The cross-finger HTA flap only requires dissection of the venous and arterial pedicle up to the level of the base of the finger and will allow transfer to any surface on the adjacent finger. The flap is accessed via midlateral incisions raising small dorsal and volar soft tissue flaps proximal to the donor site. Care should be taken not to extend these incisions into the web space or the lateral walls of the web commissure. A similar midlateral incision is performed proximal to the defect on the injured finger. The flap is directly transferred across the interdigital space and onto the defect (Fig. 24-7). This avoids the need to tunnel the pedicles and flap through the distal part of the hand and also allows the flap to reach a defect on any surface of the finger distal to the proximal interphalangeal joint. The dorsal and volar soft tissue flaps of the midlateral incisions are then sutured

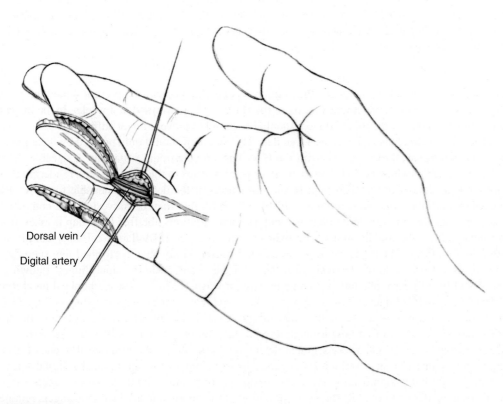

Dorsal vein

Digital artery

FIGURE 24-6

Cross-finger HTA flap from the ulnar side of the ring finger for transfer to a defect on the ulnar side of the distal little finger. Note that minimal pedicle length is required for this direct cross-finger transfer and there is no need to perform any pedicle dissection in the palm.

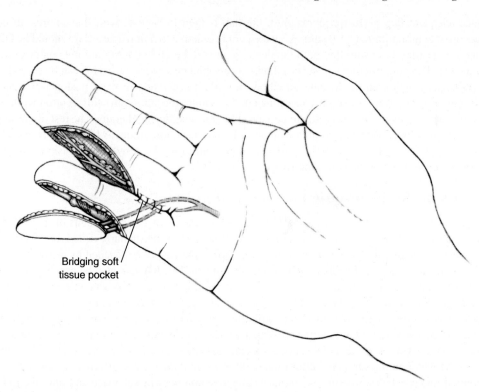

Bridging soft
tissue pocket

FIGURE 24-7

Cross-finger HTA flap after transfer to the defect site. The flap has been tunneled through volar tissue of the little finger. The vascular pedicles of the flap are now protected by a soft tissue skin bridge that has been created between the base of the ring and little finger. A full-thickness skin graft with a cotton wool bolus with tie over will be applied to the donor site. The soft tissue skin bridge, together with the HTA flap vascular pedicles, will be divided at 3 weeks postoperatively when the cross-finger HTA flap has established its own vascular supply in the reconstructed little finger.

together to create a soft tissue pouch that will protect the flap pedicle and prevent separation of the digits. Division of the cross-finger version of the HTA flap is performed at 3 weeks. In the interim, active rehabilitation of the joined fingers should be started to prevent finger stiffness.

The HTA flap may also be used as a free flap. This free flap should only be used by hand microsurgeons already well experienced with the HTA flap. In occasional situations, a sizeable defect exists in a hand in which there is concomitant or prior injuries to the other fingers, rendering them unsuitable as donors of the HTA flap. In such situations, if the defect is amenable for a free flap procedure and other free flaps are not available, the HTA flap may be harvested as a completely free flap from the uninjured contralateral hand. In such situations, the free HTA flap is taken from the ulnar side of the middle finger. The indication for the free HTA flap is certainly unique and rare. First performed in 1991, we have since found cause to only have performed five such flaps. In one case, it was used to electively resurface a sizeable defect on the small finger following a successful four-finger replantation. In another case, it was used to resurface a nonhealing chronic defect on the middle finger following an injury that also involved the other three fingers (Fig. 24-8). In two cases, there were acute concomitant injuries to the other fingers. In the last case, the free HTA flap was used as a free flow-through arterial flap, not only to reconstruct the skin defect but also to reconstruct a digital artery segment defect in a finger that had arterial insufficiency following an injury that also involved all the fingers. The excellent size matching of the digital arteries certainly contributed significantly to the success of the procedure. In all five cases, except for the mild cosmetic defect of the full-thickness skin graft at the donor site, all the donor fingers retained full and complete range of active motion and preservation of normal pulp sensation (Fig. 24-9). An important reason why the free HTA flap might have such an excellent result in the donor fingers might be due to the fact that there were no other injuries in the donor hand, which greatly facilitated active rehabilitation.

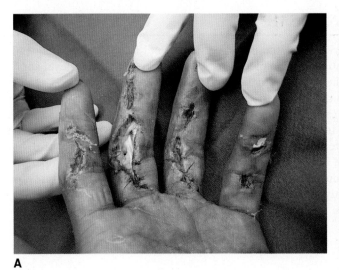

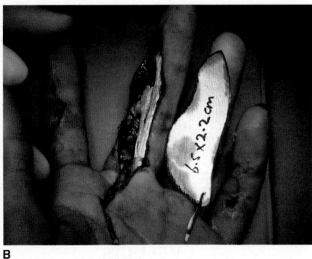

FIGURE 24-8

A: A patient referred from another hospital with a sizeable chronic nonhealing defect on his left middle finger with concomitant injuries to all the other fingers. **B:** After debridement, the true defect size is apparent (6.5 × 2.2 cm) with exposed bare flexor tendons. The patient will be undergoing free HTA flap procedure with the flap being harvested from the ulnar side of the right middle finger.

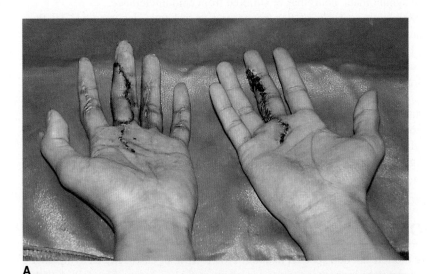

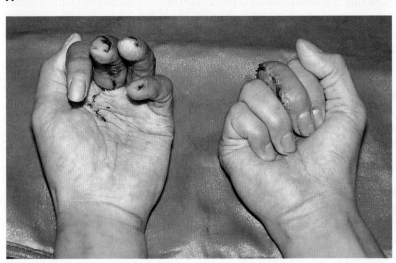

FIGURE 24-9

A: Two weeks after surgery with 100% survival of the free HTA flap with excellent primary healing in the reconstructed left middle finger. The full-thickness skin graft is also healing well on the donor site (ulnar side of the right middle finger). **B:** Full flexion of the right middle donor finger demonstrated. The stiffness that is apparent in the left hand is due to prolonged immobilization and disuse as a result of the chronic nonhealing wound. With successful and robust coverage of the defect in the left hand with excellent primary healing, aggressive rehabilitation of the hand can be started to alleviate the stiffness.

POSTOPERATIVE MANAGEMENT

The first 24 hours are the most critical for the flap. The flap should be monitored frequently with the hand placed in mild elevation. The ambient temperature can be raised to a level appropriate for the season at least for the first night depending on the surgeon's preference. Drains, if used, should be removed within the first 24 to 48 hours. Rehabilitation should commence on the second postoperative day but can be delayed if circumstances dictate. An early and active rehabilitation program is crucial in minimizing heterodigital donor finger morbidity. Active and passive range of motion exercises are instituted for both the recipient and donor digits. Regional anesthesia in the form of infusion blocks can be maintained during the postoperative period to assist with pain control during rehabilitation. The use of a cotton bolster ensures that the full-thickness skin graft is firmly secured so as to allow progressive hand therapy within the first week. Interval splinting of the donor digit between exercises may be necessary to prevent flexion contractures.

RESULTS

A total of 40 HTA flaps were performed between 1991 and 2001. Thirteen of these flaps involved division and repair of the dominant dorsal digital vein to extend the reach of the flap. Total active range of motion of the donor finger was excellent in 82.5%, good in 15%, and fair in 2.5% (one patient) according to Strickland and Glogovac's criteria for flexor tendon surgery. The fair result was due to the development of reflex sympathetic dystrophy and associated flexion contracture. Donor finger two-point discrimination was 3 to 5 mm, except in one case (6 mm). None of the donor fingers had hypersensitivity and symptomatic neuromas or suffered from cold intolerance.

Flap survival was 100% with no cases of flap congestion or ischemia documented. All flaps healed primarily and provided supple coverage of the defects. Full-thickness skin graft take was similarly successful at 100% in the donor fingers. Although a contour concavity is present at the time of removal of the cotton wool bolus on the fifth postoperative day, the concavity usually fills out within 3 months after surgery. None of the cases required any further surgery to the flap such as insetting or defatting.

We evaluated the total active motion in 22 fingers that had undergone reconstruction with the HTA flap. According to Strickland and Glogovac's criteria, 45.4% achieved excellent and good results, with the remainder achieving fair to poor results. It should be noted that the poorer outcomes in the reconstructed fingers are due to severe insults resulting in multiple tissue involvement with concomitant damage to joints, tendons, and/or ligaments and not due to contractures of the HTA flap.

COMPLICATIONS

Mild loss of total active motion can be expected in about 10% to 15% of cases. Reflex sympathetic dystrophy with flexion contracture is another serious complication that can occur. Flap failure, either partial or complete, is always a potential complication, but it has not occurred in our series. In the five cases of free HTA flap, we did not experience any vascular complications and all the free flaps survived completely. In dark-skinned races, the darker dorsal skin may be a poor cosmetic match for defects on the volar side of the hand.

PEARLS AND PITFALLS

- When elevating the flap, dissect the digital nerve off the digital artery. In this way, the soft tissue attachment between the pedicle and the flap can be preserved as much as possible as well as the venae comitantes of the digital artery.
- Some defatting at the edges of the flap can be performed to assist in the inset of the flap. If the flap is too thick, insetting can be tight and when combined with postoperative flap, swelling may lead to compromised flap viability.
- If the dorsal vein is restricting transfer of the flap, do not hesitate to divide the dorsal vein and transfer the flap as a partially free HTA. The dorsal vein can then be anastomosed to a dorsal vein over the back of the hand at the site of flap insetting.

RECOMMENDED READING

Adani R, Squarzina PB, Castagnetti C, et al. A comparative study of the heterodigital neurovascular island flap in thumb reconstruction with and without nerve reconnection. *J Hand Surg Br.* 1994;19B:552–559.

Brunelli F, Mathoulin C. Digital island flaps. In: Gilbert A, Masquelet AC, Hentz VR, eds. *Pedicle Flaps of the Upper Limb: Vascular Anatomy, Surgical Technique, and Current Indications.* London, UK: Martin Dunitz; 1992:169–176.

Buchler U. The dorsal middle phalangeal finger flap. *Handchir Mikrochir Plast Chir.* 1988;20:239–243.

Caffee HH, Ward D. Bipolar coagulation in microvascular surgery. *Plast Reconstr Surg.* 1986;78:374–377.

Chow SP, Zhu JK, So YC. Effect of bipolar coagulation and occlusion clamping on the patency rate in microvascular anastomosis. *J Reconstr Microsurg.* 1986;2(2):111–115.

Endo T, Kojima T, Hirase Y. Vascular anatomy of the finger dorsum and a new idea for coverage of the finger pulp defect that restores sensation. *J Hand Surg Am.* 1992;17A:927–932.

Henderson HP, Reid DA. Long term follow up of neurovascular island flaps. *Hand.* 1980;12(3):113–122.

Hirase Y, Kojima T, Matsuura S. A versatile one-stage neurovascular flap for fingertip reconstruction: the dorsal middle phalangeal finger flap. *Plast Reconstr Surg.* 1992;90(6):1009–1015.

Hood JM, Lubahn JD. Bipolar coagulation at different energy levels: effect on patency. *Microsurgery.* 1994;15:594–597.

Hueston J. The extended neurovascular island flap. *Br J Plast Surg.* 1965;18:304–305.

Isogai N, Kamiishi H, Chichibu S. Re-endothelialization stages at the microvascular anastomosis. *Microsurgery.* 1988;9(2):87–94.

Kumta SM, Yip KMH, Pannozzo A, et al. Resurfacing of thumb-pulp loss with a heterodigital neurovascular island flap using a nerve disconnection/reconnection technique. *J Reconstr Microsurg.* 1997;13(2):117–122.

Kurokawa M, Ishikawa K, Nishimura Y. A neurovascular island flap including a vein for the treatment of an acquired ring constriction. *Br J Plast Surg.* 1995;48(6):401–404.

Lee YL, Teoh LC, Seah WT. Extending the reach of the heterodigital arterialised flap by cross finger transfer. *Plast Reconstr Surg.* 2006;117(7):2320–2328.

Leupin P, Weil J, Buchler U. The dorsal middle phalangeal finger flap: mid-term results of 43 cases. *J Hand Surg Br.* 1997;22(3):362–371.

Littler JW. Neurovascular pedicle method of digital transposition for reconstruction of the thumb. *Plast Reconstr Surg.* 1953;12:303–319.

Lucas GL. The pattern of venous drainage of the digits. *J Hand Surg Am.* 1984;9A:448–450.

Moss SH, Schwartz KS, von Drasek-Ascher G, et al. Digital venous anatomy. *J Hand Surg Am.* 1985;10A:473–482.

Paterson P, Titley OG, Nancarrow JD. Donor finger morbidity in cross-finger flaps. *Injury.* 2000;31:215–218.

Quaba AA, Davison PM. The distally based dorsal hand flap. *Br J Plast Surg.* 1990;43(1):28–39.

Riordan DC, Kaplan EB. Surface anatomy of the hand and wrist. In: Spinner M, ed. *Kaplan's Functional and Surgical Anatomy of the Hand.* 3rd ed. Philadelphia, PA: Lippincott Williams & Wilkins; 1984:353.

Rose EH. Local arterialized island flap coverage of difficult defects preserving donor digit sensibility. *Plast Reconstr Surg.* 1983;72:848–858.

Roth JH, Urbaniak JR, Boswick JM. Comparison of suture ligation, bipolar cauterization, and hemoclip ligation in the management of small branching vessels in a rat model. *J Reconstr Microsurg.* 1984;1:7–9.

Strauch B, de Moura W. Arterial system of the fingers. *J Hand Surg Am.* 1990;15A:148–154.

Strickland JW, Glogovac SV. Digital function following flexor tendon repair in zone II: a comparison of immobilization and controlled passive motion techniques. *J Hand Surg Am.* 1980;5A:537–543.

Tay SC, Teoh LC, Tan SH, et al. Extending the reach of the heterodigital arterialized flap by vein division and repair. *Plast Reconstr Surg.* 2004;114(6):1450–1456.

Teoh LC, Tay SC, Yong FC, et al. Heterodigital arterialized flaps for large finger wounds: results and indications. *Plast Reconstr Surg.* 2003;111(6):1905–1913.

Weeks PM. Local arterialized island flap coverage of difficult hand defects preserving donor digit sensibility. *Plast Reconstr Surg.* 1983;72:858.

25 Homodigital Island Flaps

Mark Henry

Homodigital island flaps (HIFs) refer to flaps taken from the injured digit to reconstruct the injured digit. Heterodigital flaps refer to flaps taken from an adjacent or distant finger to reconstruct the traumatic defect. The major advantages of the HIF over other reconstructive options include the flap's proximity to the wound, avoidance of injuring other fingers, and the ability to reconstruct the defect with similar tissue. This chapter discusses the indications and use of homodigital flaps for soft tissue defects of the finger.

INDICATIONS/CONTRAINDICATIONS

HIFs are indicated for any digital wound defect that lacks a sufficient base of perfusion to support a full-thickness skin graft or has a critical exposure of raw tendon fibers, nerve, bone, joint, or hardware. Alternatives to the use of the HIF include heterodigital island flaps, dorsal metacarpal artery–based flaps, free flaps, random flaps, or dermal regeneration templates. Relative contraindications to HIFs include patients with peripheral vascular disease, uncontrolled diabetes, long-term heavy smoking, and a secondary zone of crush injury involving the pedicle. Absolute contraindications to HIFs include an actively infected wound, the expectation that flap harvest will induce terminal ischemia of the digit, patients in such poor medical health as to be unable to tolerate the surgery or heal the wounds, and patients unwilling to follow instructions and care for the flap postoperatively.

Anatomy

The arterial architecture of the digit is based on two proper digital arteries (PDAs) and two smaller dorsal digital arteries (DDA). The two PDAs communicate with each other in the coronal plane through a series of transverse branches that pass through the floor of the flexor sheath at the proximal metaphysis of each phalanx and at the neck of the proximal phalanx (P1) and middle phalanx (P2) (Fig. 25-1). Overlying P1, the DDAs are supplied by the longitudinal extensions of the dorsal metacarpal arteries, joined by the first dorsal branch of the PDA. Unlike the thumb, the finger DDAs inconsistently continue past the proximal interphalangeal (PIP) joint. The DDAs overlying P2 arise primarily from subsequent dorsal branches of the PDAs. The same is true passing the distal interphalangeal (DIP) joint.

Most HIFs involve at least one of the PDAs as part of the pedicle. It is possible to leave both PDAs undisturbed and transfer a flap based exclusively on one of the dorsal branches arising from the PDA. Such cases are rare, as the flap has a very limited arc of rotation. In such cases the flap must pivot based on the point of takeoff by the dorsal branch from the PDA, requiring the recipient site (primary defect) to be immediately adjacent to the donor site (secondary defect). The remainder of this chapter addresses flaps that involve mobilization of PDAs.

While arterial flow is in HIFs is free to course in any direction through communicating channels, the pedicle design will affect venous outflow. Unique circumstances exist where a superficial vein may be independently retained to drain the flap or anastomosed to supercharge drainage; however the majority of HIFs drain solely through the small comitant veins that adhere to the adventitia of the artery. For this reason, a perivascular cuff of tissue should be retained with the artery during pedicle dissection and transfer; this avoids skeletonizing the artery and damaging

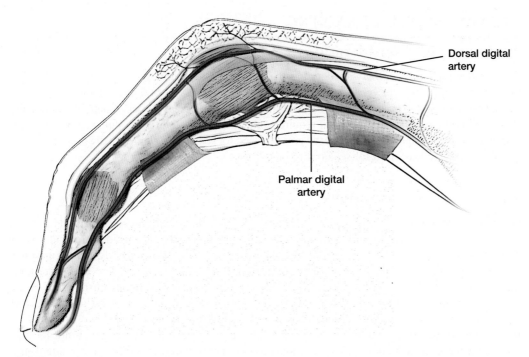

FIGURE 25-1

Schematic of the arterial supply to the digit. There are vascular connections between the dorsal and palmar blood supply surrounding the MCP and PIP joints. In addition, there are connections between the ulnar and radial arteries at the level of the neck of the proximal and middle phalanx. This arterial network allows for retrograde flow in cases of reverse homodigital flaps.

the venous comitants (Fig. 25-2). Flaps termed *antegrade* require venous return to flow only in the normal physiologic direction. Flaps termed *retrograde* require venous return to flow in the opposite direction. Retrograde venous flow forms the basis of many successful flap designs, but with some higher risk of venous congestion, rarely leading to complete flap loss. The remainder of this chapter addresses flaps draining exclusively through the comitant veins (with the terms antegrade and retrograde referring to the direction of flow, not whether the recipient site is proximal or distal relative to the donor site). The term *reverse* is most commonly applied to the situation where the pivot point of the pedicle is located between a distal recipient site and a proximal donor site.

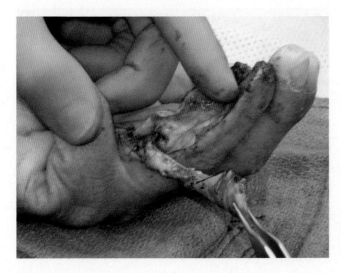

FIGURE 25-2

An antegrade flap based on the PDA (with all branches ligated) has been harvested with a wide cuff of perivascular tissue to protect the small comitant veins.

PREOPERATIVE PLANNING

Recipient Site Considerations

Preoperative planning begins with defining the recipient site requirements in terms of location, dimension, shape, skin type (glabrous/nonglabrous), and contour. The digit is fundamentally a cylinder. Depending on flap orientation during insetting, greater or lesser degrees of bending around this curve will prove necessary. Functional requirements differ by location. The pulp requires padding and resistance to compression and has the greatest need for sensibility, while the dorsal skin must be pliable but has the least need for sensibility (Fig. 25-3).

Donor Site Considerations

One advantage of selecting an HIF over alternative flaps is that the donor site morbidity remains confined to the already traumatized digit. Perhaps the most salient consideration, unique to homodigital flaps, is the sufficiency of residual perfusion to the distal digit following flap harvest. For instance, a flap based on a PDA will have robust flow compared to one based on a dorsal digital branch. But, harvesting the PDA to supply the flap robs the distal digit of the PDA's remaining distal blood supply. Depending on the exact level at which the PDA is harvested, transverse communicating branches from the contralateral PDA will need to supply the blood flow to the finger. Additional vascular damage in the traumatized ray may not be fully known until the time of surgery, and one must always be prepared to modify donor site design accordingly. The acoustic Doppler is a fairly reliable preoperative planning tool to determine PDA patency. One should map the remaining components of the arterial network to ensure adequate Doppler signals in the vessels that will support distal perfusion once the flap has been transferred. If both sets of vessels provide quality Doppler signals, one may proceed with the planned flap.

Other donor site considerations include the effect of planned incisions relative to postoperative contracture and painful scarring of nerves. We prefer to raise flaps using Bruner or midaxial incisions (Fig. 25-4). Donor sites should avoid exposure of flexor tendons, extensor tendons, or proper digital nerves (PDNs) in the secondary defect.

Need for Sensate Flap

HIFs that include a neurovascular pedicle will be sensate; alternatively, flaps can be reinnervated if a small expendable dorsal nerve is included in the flap design (Fig. 25-5). A small-caliber dorsal nerve branch associated with the skin paddle is connected to the free traumatized ending of the PDN

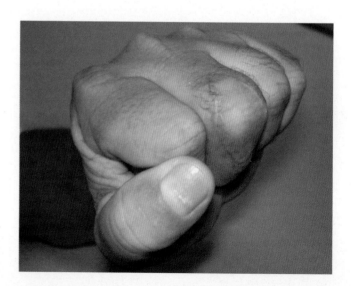

FIGURE 25-3

The primary recipient site requirement of a dorsal wound overlying the PIP joint is a thin supple flap capable of unrestricted flexion.

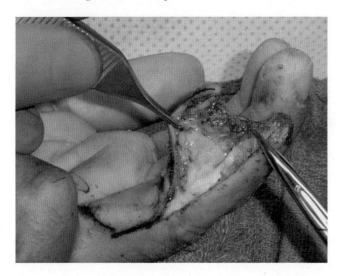

FIGURE 25-4

Antegrade HIF harvested with dorsal margin in midaxial line. Note the four titanium ligature clips dividing the transverse branches at the neck and base of P2.

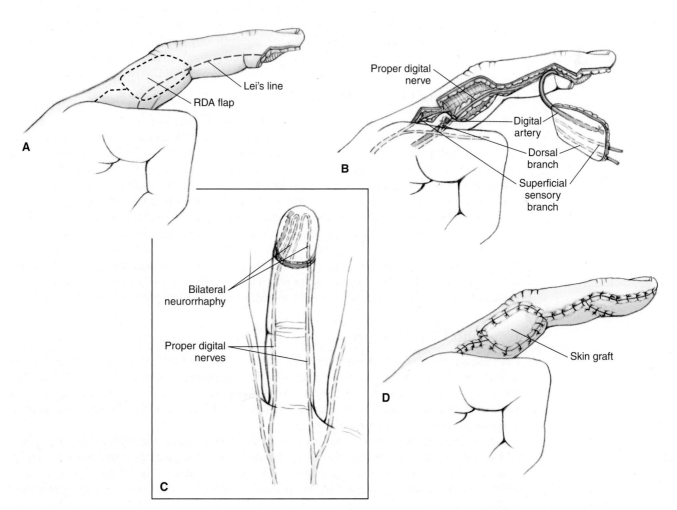

FIGURE 25-5

The required size of RDHDA flap is marked on the dorsolateral aspect of the involved proximal phalanx. **A:** The flap is based on the digital artery, which topographically courses under the dorsoventral skin junction line. **B:** The vascular pedicle is ligated at its proximal end. Both the dorsal branch from the proper digital nerve and the superficial sensory branch from the corresponding radial or ulnar nerve are sectioned proximally, leaving 1 cm nerve tails attached to the flap. **C:** The flap is transposed to the recipient wound. The attached sensory nerves of the flap are microanastomosed with both ulnar and radial digital nerves at the recipient wound. **D:** The flap donor site is resurfaced with a full-thickness skin graft. The pivot area of the vascular pedicle is also covered with a piece of skin to eliminate the pressure completely.

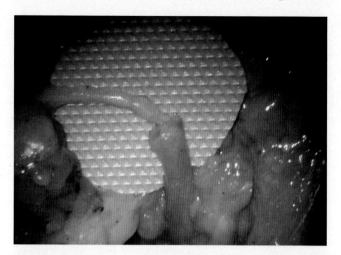

FIGURE 25-6

A reverse flap used for digital tip amputation may be reinnervated by coapting the small dorsal digital nerve branch to the traumatized end of the proper digital nerve, albeit with a substantial size discrepancy.

at the recipient site (Fig. 25-6). The quality of final sensibility is limited by the size of the dorsal digital nerve branch and the degree to which it actually serves the skin paddle. When this procedure is used for digital pulp defects, it may limit terminal neuroma formation in the PDN. Overall, it has been our experience that noninnervated flaps become indirectly reinnervated from the surrounding wound bed to a sufficient degree as to be functionally comparable to directly innervated flaps.

Guaranteeing Flap Perfusion

It is important to design the HIF over an area of known skin perforators. If the surgeon plans a large flap, the likelihood of capturing cutaneous branches is high and the flap will almost assuredly be perfused by default. When the surgeon plans a smaller flap, the skin island must be designed to capture at least one cutaneous branch or the skin will not be perfused. One way to assure that a cutaneous branch has been included is to look for the small perforators with high-powered loupes. At least one side of the flap has to be elevated before the surgeon has the opportunity to look for a branch. Ideally, the exact donor site is planned and marked prior to initiating any dissection; however, the handheld Doppler is not ideal for identifying these small perforators. Fortunately, the vascular anatomy follows a fairly reliable pattern and cutaneous branches lie directly opposite the transverse communicating branches previously described. As long as a part of the skin paddle overlies the neck level or proximal metaphyseal level of the proximal or middle phalanx in the axis of the source vessel, a cutaneous branch will be present within the flap.

Common Flap Designs

One common flap design is the antegrade HIF based on a single PDA. All branches of the PDA are ligated from the base of the digit to the distally located flap donor site (Fig. 25-7; see Fig. 25-2). This flap design is used to reconstruct distal tip amputations. One harvests a combined neurovascular pedicle for direct innervation of the flap by the PDN. The flap is transferred distally to the recipient site, requiring the pedicle to stretch.

A less commonly performed version of the antegrade HIF leaves the PDN in situ to innervate an intact digital tip, and the flap (harvested overlying distal to mid P2) is transferred to reconstruct a more proximal defect exposing the PIP joint or tendons (Fig. 25-8). In this instance, shortening the distance traversed by the pedicle requires a gentle curve, avoiding any focal kinking.

The other fundamental pattern of HIF is a retrograde flow flap, where the pivot point of the flap is the transverse communicating branch at the neck of P2. The flap donor site overlies mid to proximal P1, and flow between these two points is retrograde (Fig. 25-9). This flap is chosen over the antegrade flap for distal amputation defects when the slope is volar oblique. Such a transfer pattern is termed reverse, as the pivot point lies between a distal recipient defect and a proximal flap donor site. The retrograde HIF may also be transferred without reversing the pedicle orientation to a recipient site overlying the PIP joint or P2 (Fig. 25-10).

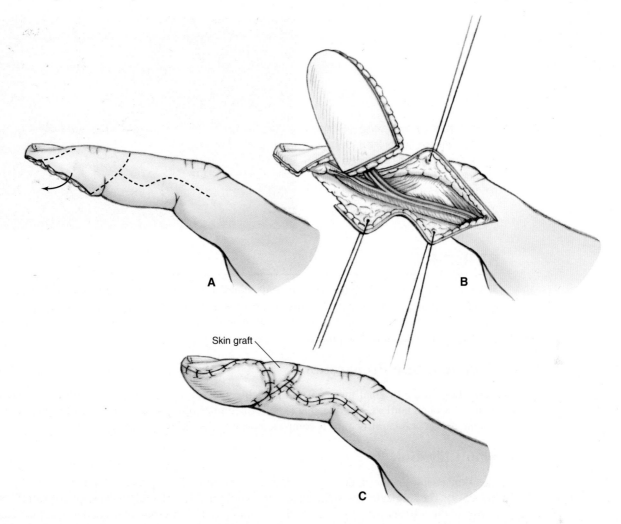

A

B

Skin graft

C

FIGURE 25-7

A: The design of the incision and distal dorsal homodigital (DDHD) neurovascular island flap. The axis of the flap curves obliquely and dorsally toward the contralateral side. **B:** The flap is elevated with its neurovascular pedicle and transposed obliquely into the defect. The typical wound suitable for a DDHDA flap has an intact tip and hypochium. **C:** The flap inset and grafted donor defect.

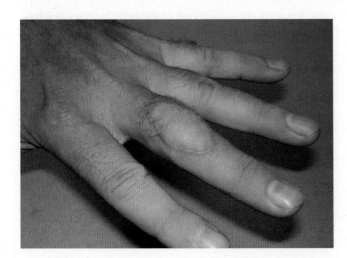

FIGURE 25-8

An antegrade HIF may be used for a recipient defect (PIP) located proximal to the flap donor site (P2 level).

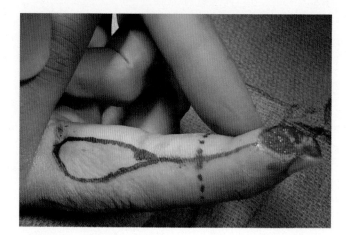

FIGURE 25-9

The pivot point for the reverse HIF flap lies at the intersection of the midaxial transfer wound and the transverse line drawn at the level of the neck of P2. The proximal aspect of the skin paddle should not transgress the web commissure.

SURGERY

The patient is positioned supine with the arm extended on a hand table and supinated. Local anesthesia is discouraged because it alters the tissue volume of the region. Limb block or laryngeal mask airway is preferred. The patient should be well hydrated in a warm ambient temperature. An upper arm tourniquet is used for the procedure.

Recipient Site Preparation

Depending on the original mechanism, a variable zone of secondary injury will exist in the surrounding wound borders. Debridement is performed to healthy tissue, and repair of any underlying tendon, nerve, or bone structures is completed prior to flap design.

Flap Elevation

The skin paddle at the donor site is drawn to the dimension planned for reconstruction (see Fig. 25-9). The surgical plan often includes the intentional use of a full thickness skin graft (FTSG) as part of the primary defect reconstruction to allow for the elevation of a smaller flap. Flap elevation may begin at the root of the pedicle to examine the quality of the vessel. In the rare event that the vessel proves unsuitable, only a small incision has been made and an alternative flap can be pursued. Otherwise, in most instances, the elevation begins longitudinally along one border of the flap. If the PDN is to be left in situ, first separate the nerve from the vascular pedicle before pursuing side branch ligation (Fig. 25-11). The surgeon confirms the orientation of the flap's skin paddle relative to the pedicle and, if necessary, locates branches from the pedicle to the skin to avoid the scenario of an unperfused flap. At this point, it is simply a matter of isolating the flap by cutting the remaining borders of the skin paddle and ligating all branches, including the PDA proximally for retrograde flaps (Fig. 25-12). Since the skin paddle is the portion of the flap handled during elevation and transfer (to avoid touching the pedicle), it is possible to cause traction injury to the small branches from the pedicle to the flap. Suturing the ligated end of the pedicle artery (farthest from the source of flow) to the flap with a 6-0 absorbable suture prevents traction injury. Ligation

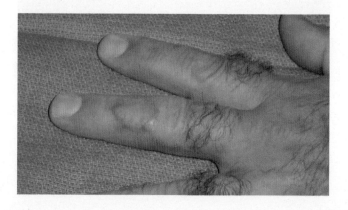

FIGURE 25-10

A retrograde flap may be used for recipient sites other than digital tip amputation such as tendon exposure at the P2 level.

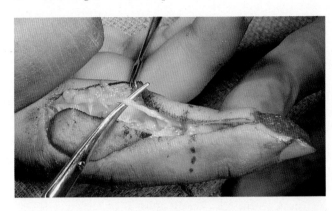

FIGURE 25-11

When left in situ, the PDN should be dissected free of the pedicle in a volar direction prior to pursuing side branch ligation.

of larger caliber branches off the pedicle should be done with titanium microclips or sutures (Fig. 25-4). Small-caliber branches can be cauterized with bipolar. The goal is to avoid any direct contact with the pedicle, traction stress, or kinking. *One of the worst dissection mistakes is to avulse a side branch off the artery, inducing often profound vasospasm and a leaking vessel.* Once all connections have been separated, but for the root of the pedicle, the flap is ready for transfer. From this point, the surgeon should never let go of the flap until at least two sutures have been inset. If a flap is dropped and dangled on its pedicle, when the surgeon picks it up again, the flap could easily be torsed 360 degrees and go unnoticed.

The pedicle can be transferred from donor to recipient through an open incision or a tunnel connecting the two wounds. The advantage of the tunnel is mostly cosmetic with less total length of incision. When dissecting the tunnel with scissors or hemostat, the passage may well seem wide open, and the pedicle can be confirmed to slide easily back and forth while the passage is held by retractors. But once the retractors are removed and the tunnel is allowed to collapse around the pedicle, there can be fascial bands (which had been previously retracted) that shift into a position to impinge or kink the pedicle and compromise flow. Although more laborious for the surgeon, an open incision from the donor site to the wound allows the pedicle to be gently placed in a trough carefully prepared free of any obstructions.

Flap Insetting

If the primary defect has a wide transverse dimension around the external circumference of the cylindrical digit, suturing every edge of the flap to the border narrows its deep concave surface, bunching together the subcutaneous fat and compressing the pedicle. At the same time, the convex outer surface of the flap can become stretched too tight over the volume of its own subcutaneous tissues to meet the borders of the defect. The excessive tension washes out the dermal plexus, rendering the skin paddle ischemic even if flow is maintained in the underlying pedicle. This effect is easily demonstrated while insetting with the tourniquet down. When adding a border suture that is slightly too tight, the surrounding skin will blanch for a distance around the suture but the rest of the flap will remain pink. If the suture is removed, the whole flap returns to pink. When adding a border suture that is excessively tight, the entire flap blanches and remains so until the tension is relieved by removing that suture or another suture at a key location. If one leaves the flap inset under such excessive tension, degrees of flap ischemia may result: superficial

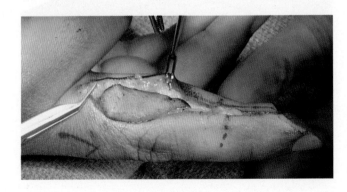

FIGURE 25-12

Ligation of larger side branches (including proximal PDA ligation) is easily accomplished with microsized titanium ligature clips.

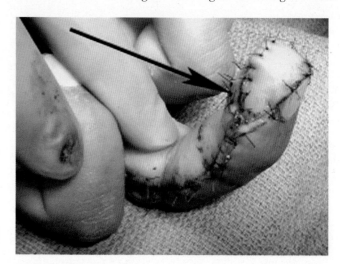

FIGURE 25-13

When the recipient defect is very large or requires a high degree of curvature, incorporating a planned FTSG (*arrow*) at the primary defect optimizes the result.

epidermolysis only, full-thickness necrosis of the flap's dermis with survival of the subcutaneous tissue surrounding the pedicle, or complete flap loss. Including an FTSG in the recipient wound permits reduction of tension while orienting the flap to cover the most important portion of the wound (Fig. 25-13).

Use of Skin Grafts at Recipient and Donor Sites

The decision to use a skin graft at the recipient site is usually made during the flap planning stages when evaluating the dimensions of the primary and secondary defects. Sometimes, the decision is made intraoperatively in response to an assessment of excess tension during insetting. Only FTSGs are used in digits; split-thickness skin grafts do not create the durable, shear-resistant result needed for an active hand. We take our FTSG from the ulnar border of the hand near the glabrous/nonglabrous border (Fig. 25-14). A purely glabrous graft is typically used, but a very elegant result can be achieved if the recipient site spans a glabrous/nonglabrous junction. The FTSG can be harvested part glabrous and part nonglabrous to perfectly match the recipient site. The skin graft needs firm approximation to the wound bed to revascularize, but cannot be sutured in a manner that compromises flap perfusion. Horizontal mattress sutures serve this purpose well.

Most secondary defects created by flap elevation at the donor site will require some amount of skin graft, even when the donor site is opposite the primary pathway of perfusion. Circumferential tension in the digit as a whole can still compromise flow in the PDA on the opposite side of the digit. Partial closure and reduction of the secondary defect are performed up to the point where the surgeon judges that any further direct closure may affect perfusion (once postoperative swelling sets in). The typical reduction in size of the secondary defect is around 50%. FTSG is applied to the remaining defect, using 5-0 horizontal mattress sutures.

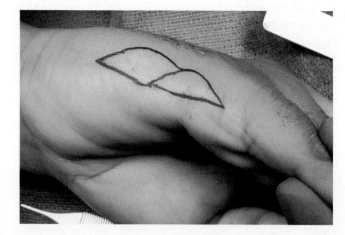

FIGURE 25-14

Two FTSGs (for primary and secondary defects) can be harvested together from the ulnar border of the hand, then separated, and inset.

POSTOPERATIVE MANAGEMENT

Dressing

The dressing can be confined to the hand only and should not include splints, even when underlying fracture fixation has been performed. The hard material of a splint has the potential to create focal compression. Every effort must be made to avoid compression to the flap and underlying pedicle. Surgeons less experienced with pedicle flaps may wish to leave a monitoring window to look at the flap or Doppler the pedicle.

Management of Physiologic Variables

We prefer to admit the patient for an overnight, 23-hour stay of intravenous hydration, a warm temperature room, rest, and good pain control. All of these efforts can limit vasospasm and encourage normal physiologic flow within the flap. One of the more powerful agents countering vasospasm is chlorpromazine, administered as 50 mg IM intraoperatively with two additional postoperative doses of 25 mg PO. The patient can be discharged the following day with instructions to rest, drink fluids, take pain meds, stay warm, and not smoke.

Rehabilitation

Rehabilitation begins within a week of surgery, focused on restoring range of motion, particularly at the PIP joint. Motion should be active or assisted, but passive motion is avoided in the early postoperative course. Passive motion can be added after initial wound and skin graft healing. Therapists need to be explicitly warned about placing any constricting dressings over the path of the pedicle. Both patient and therapist are also taught to avoid shear stress to any skin grafts until the grafts have been fully revascularized. External wrapping with cohesive bandages to limit edema should not be used until the third week and only distally (including over the flap itself) but not over the path of the pedicle leading to the flap. Contact desensitization training is initiated at 2 weeks. More aggressive therapy measures such as sustained passive stretch and static progressive splints are usually reserved for time points of 4 to 6 weeks postoperatively and beyond.

RESULTS

Most patients achieve full ROM (Fig. 25-15); however, PIP joint contractures can occur. If the wound lies in the midaxial line, but the surgeon differentially sutures the volar and dorsal wound

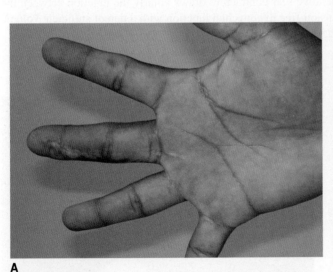
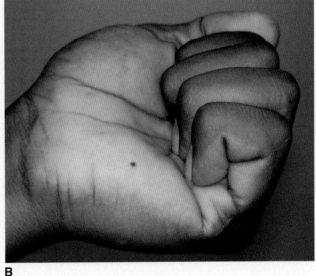

A   **B**

FIGURE 25-15

A: When properly harvested, transferred, and inset, an HIF need not restrict full digital extension or web spread. **B:** Use of neutral tension line incisions and proper insetting technique leads to full digital flexion in most cases.

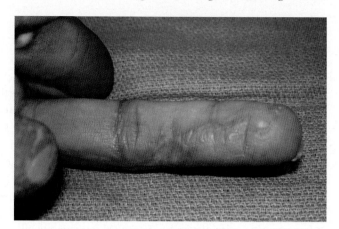

FIGURE 25-16

The unique morphology of the pulp and hyponychium are difficult to reproduce with a flap, where initial insetting and subsequent scar contracture must both be carefully calculated.

edges during the insetting and closure phase of the case with the digit resting in a flexed posture, a flexion contracture may be induced by the surgeon. Even with perfect surgical technique and a hardworking patient in therapy, incomplete motion may still occur in the setting of concomitant injury to tendon, fracture, or a patient's genetic predisposition to heavy scar formation or stiffness.

The sensibility achieved with HIFs ranges from 5 to 12 mm static two-point discrimination with an average of 9 mm. Flaps that are directly innervated by the PDN (antegrade flow flaps) typically achieve 5 to 8 mm of static two-point discrimination. Less sensibility occurs when flaps must be reinnervated, either directly or indirectly (retrograde flow flaps). Flaps directly reinnervated by the connection of a dorsal digital nerve branch to the traumatized end of the PDN can achieve anywhere from 6 to 10 mm static two-point discrimination. Return of sensibility to the skin surface of a flap that has no direct nerve connection is still possible through ingrowth from the surrounding wound. The higher range of static two-point discrimination (8 to 12 mm) is seen in these cases, with the result dependent on the size of the flap (better for smaller flaps, worse for larger flaps).

For flaps that simply cover a measured wound defect more proximally in the digit, the result is typically a well-balanced volume of flap tissue proportionate to the region. The challenge lies in recipient sites at the tip of the digit, where the unique conformation of the pulp and hyponychium is difficult to reproduce (Fig. 25-16). Inadequate tissue at the tip of the finger can generate a hook-nail deformity, as the process of postoperative scar contracture draws volarly the junction between the flap and the sterile nail matrix. A tension-free hyponychial junction with a flap of sufficient volume prevents hook-nail deformity (Fig. 25-17).

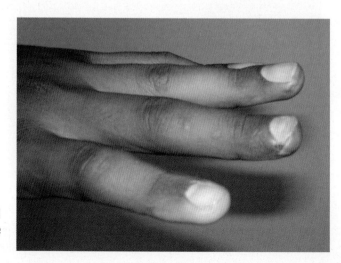

FIGURE 25-17

Hook-nail deformity can be avoided when the flap is inset tension free, at full volume, and with proper curvature at the hyponychium.

COMPLICATIONS

Venous Congestion: Superficial Epidermolysis

The venous drainage for HIFs is almost always the comitant veins accompanying a small-caliber artery. Venous congestion occurs more commonly in retrograde flaps. To minimize the chances of venous congestion, care must be taken to minimize tension in the transfer wound surrounding the pedicle (Fig. 25-18). If the drainage is only slightly impaired, the flap will look dusky and cool during the first week but can recover with no long-term harm. If venous congestion is more significant, the skin of the flap becomes compromised and undergoes superficial epidermolysis. The flap will develop a hard dark crust at the epidermal level that will later slough, leaving a discolored but viable dermis that eventually provides the necessary coverage. In the most extreme of cases, venous compromise may kill the dermis, but in our experience, the underlying subcutaneous fat that surrounds the pedicle survives. In this circumstance, the skin of the flap can be cut off and an FTSG applied to the residual viable tissue surrounding the pedicle.

Marginal Arterial Hypoperfusion

Arterial hypoperfusion, if present, usually manifests at the margins of the flap. Most flaps should be able to survive to all borders based on a single skin branch coming from the axial vessel. Two scenarios lead to marginal hypoperfusion; both are under the surgeon's control. The first is inadequate wound debridement, leading to marginal necrosis following flap inset. The second problem is tight flap insetting. In either case, the result is inadequate arterial perfusion of the margin. Unlike venous congestion, arterial hypoperfusion is usually full thickness, requiring surgical revision.

PIP Joint Contracture

Any flap whose pedicle dissection crosses the level of the PIP joint has the potential to cause loss of PIP motion. Midaxial incisions that follow the neutral tension lines in the digit minimize this risk. Ideally, the flap itself encompasses tissue entirely distal to the PIP or entirely proximal to the PIP, not including a width of tissue at the PIP level. Narrowing the circumference of wound closure at the PIP level or skin grafts that span the PIP level have greater potential for PIP stiffness compared to a linear midaxial incision that simply passes by the PIP. During surgery, as the flap is being inset, the PIP should be able to reach full extension and full flexion without inducing tension in either the pedicle or any of the wound borders. Early motion rehabilitation should place particular emphasis on the PIP joint.

Digital Nerve Hypersensitivity

Nerves may be deprived of segmental vascular supply when arteries are transferred away from the paired nerve. Small branches (terminal or lateral) may be separated from their receptors and form small neuromas. When planning the flap, one should design the wounds to minimize nerve

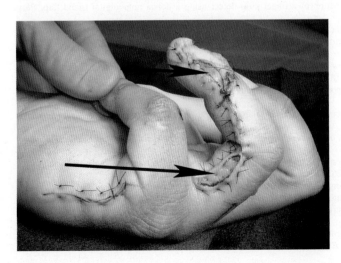

FIGURE 25-18

FTSG harvested from a combined donor site on the ulnar border of the hand serves to alleviate circumferential tension at both the secondary defect (*long arrow*) and in the transfer wound (*short arrow*).

exposure to postoperative scarring, particularly where scarring will subject the nerve to traction stress with motion. Progressive contact desensitization techniques are an important part of postoperative rehabilitation.

SUMMARY

HIFs are one of many strategies available to treat digital wound defects. The primary advantage of an HIF is that the whole reconstruction is confined to the same digit. Any piece of skin on the digit can be transferred to fulfill the reconstructive requirements, provided that the fundamental principles outlined in this chapter are satisfied.

PEARLS AND PITFALLS

- Perform an adequate debridement prior to designing the flap.
- If the pedicle is dissected through an area of previous trauma, the small comitant veins may be thrombosed despite sufficient flow in their accompanying artery. Avoid designing flaps whose pedicles run through areas of tissue trauma.
- HIF are most reliable when designed to include the skin overlying the digital arteries at the level of the proximal metaphysis of the proximal and middle phalanx and/or the neck of the proximal and middle phalanx.
- A perivascular cuff of tissue should be retained with the artery during pedicle dissection to preserve the venous comitants draining the flap.
- Suturing the ligated end of the pedicle artery (farthest from the source of flow) to the flap with a 6-0 absorbable suture prevents traction injury to the vessels during insetting.
- When suturing the skin graft to the flap, observe each suture placement carefully to avoid catching the pedicle.
- Never hesitate to take out sutures if the flap's blood supply looks compromised. Have a very low threshold for adding skin graft if the closure appears too tight. Have a low threshold to open the skin bridge between the wound and the flap as tunneling often places compression on the pedicle. Apply a nonconstrictive dressing at the completion of the case.
- Inset the flap with the finger in full extension; pause frequently to take the digit through a full range of motion, checking for any excess tension in sutures.

RECOMMENDED READING

Adani R, Busa R, Castagnetti C, et al. Homodigital neurovascular island flaps with "direct flow" visualization. *Ann Plast Surg.* 1997;38(1):36–40.

Adani R, Busa R, Pancaldi G, et al. Reverse neurovascular homodigital island flap. *Ann Plast Surg.* 1995;35(1):77–82.

Bektas G, Ozkan O, Cinpolat A, et al. Comparing the effects of pedicle torsion on axial or perforator flaps; Improving the perforator flap resistance to pedicle torsion with delay phenomenon. *J Reconstr Microsurg.* 2014;30:531–538.

Borman H, Maral T, Tancer M. Fingertip reconstruction using two variations of direct-flow homodigital neurovascular island flaps. *Ann Plast Surg.* 2000;45(1):24–30.

Chen C, Tang P, Zhang X. Sensory reconstruction of a finger pulp defect using a dorsal homodigital island flap. *Plast Reconstr Surg.* 2012;130(5):1077–1086.

Chen CT, Wei FC. Lateral-dorsal neurovascular island flaps for pulp reconstruction. *Ann Plast Surg.* 2000;45(6):616–622.

Henry M. Specific complications associated with different types of intrinsic pedicle flaps of the hand. *J Reconstr Microsurg.* 2008;24(3):221–225.

Henry M, Stutz C. Homodigital antegrade-flow neurovascular pedicle flaps for sensate reconstruction of fingertip amputation injuries. *J Hand Surg [Am].* 2006;31(7):1220–1225.

Huang YC, Liu Y, Chen TH. Use of homodigital reverse island flaps for distal digital reconstruction. *J Trauma.* 2010;68(2):429–433.

Karacalar A, Sen C, Ozcan M. A modified reversed digital island flap incorporating the proper digital nerve. *Ann Plast Surg.* 2000;45(1):67–70.

Kayalar M, Bal E, Toros T, et al. The results of reverse-flow island flaps in pulp reconstruction. *Acta Orthop Traumatol Turc.* 2011;45(5):304–311.

Kim KS, Yoo SI, Kim DY, et al. Fingertip reconstruction using a volar flap based on the transverse palmar branch of the digital artery. *Ann Plast Surg.* 2001;47(3):263–268.

Matsuzaki H, Kouda H, Yamashita H. Preventing postoperative congestion in reverse pedicle digital island flaps when reconstructing composite tissue defects in the fingertip: a patient series. *Hand Surg.* 2012;17(1):77–82.

Momeni A, Zajonc H, Kalash Z, et al. Reconstruction of distal phalangeal injuries with the reverse homodigital island flap. *Injury.* 2008;39(12):1460–1463.

Ozaksar K, Toros T, Sugun TS, et al. Reconstruction of finger pulp defects using homodigital dorsal middle phalange neurovascular advancement flap. *J Hand Surg Eur Vol.* 2010;35E(2):125–129.

Takeishi M, Shinoda A, Sugiyama A, et al. Innervated reverse dorsal digital island flap for fingertip reconstruction. *J Hand Surg [Am]*. 2006;31A(7):1094–1099.

Varitimidis SE, Dailiana ZH, Zibis AH, et al. Restoration of function and sensitivity utilizing a homodigital neurovascular island flap after amputation injuries of the fingertip. *J Hand Surg (Br)*. 2005;30(4):338–342.

Yang D, Morris SF. Vascular basis of dorsal digital and metacarpal skin flaps. *J Hand Surg [Am]*. 2001;26A(1):142–146.

Yazar M, Aydin A, Kurt Yazar S, et al. Sensory recovery of the reverse homodigital island flap in fingertip reconstruction: a review of 66 cases. *Acta Orthop Traumatol Turc*. 2010;44(5):345–351.

Yildirim S, Avci G, Akan M, et al. Complications of the reverse homodigital island flap in fingertip reconstruction. *Ann Plast Surg*. 2002;48(6):586–592.

26 First Dorsal Metacarpal Artery Island Flap

Michael Sauerbier and Günter Germann

Soft tissue defects in the hand, and particularly in the thumb, frequently present difficult reconstructive problems because of the restricted availability of local tissue. Although local skin flaps have been employed and time proven over decades, the philosophy of immediate wound closure of complex defects with exposure of tendon, bone, or joints has stimulated interest in anatomic research and the development of refined reconstructive techniques.

Traditional flaps have many disadvantages such as two-stage operations (i.e., cross-finger flap), tedious dissections with considerable donor site morbidity and loss of discriminative power (i.e., Littler flap), or limited arc of rotation and mobility (i.e., transposition flaps and the Moberg flap). On the other hand, more recent microsurgical reconstructions such as the free pulp flap require a significant amount of time and a familiarity with microsurgical technique. The first dorsal metacarpal artery (FDMA) island flap overcomes the disadvantages of traditional hand flaps and can provide a moderate-sized skin paddle on a long consistent vascular leash, allowing one-stage reconstruction for thumb and dorsal hand wounds without the need for microsurgical anastomosis.

The FDMA island flap was originally described by Hilgenfeldt in 1950 and subsequently refined by Paneva-Holevic in 1968 and finally described as a pure island flap ("kite flap") by Foucher and Braun in 1979. Many variations of the flap have since been described and established in daily clinical use based on the consistent anatomy of the dorsal metacarpal arterial arcade. Most of the flaps in recently published reports are raised from the dorsal aspect of the hand with only a few being found on the palmar surface.

The dorsum of the hand is supplied by the network of dorsal metacarpal arteries that are fed from the main forearm vessels: the radial, ulnar, and interosseus arteries. The FDMA consistently arises from the radial artery or the princeps pollicis artery and runs distally to the fascia of the interosseus muscle, frequently embedded in a fascial pocket. In most cases, the FDMA divides in the middle of the second metacarpal into three terminal branches. The radial branch of the FDMA goes to the thumb, while the intermediate branch runs to the first web space. Distally, the ulnar branch usually terminates at the level of the metacarpophalangeal joint and then arborizes into the dorsal skin of the index finger after giving off a perforating branch at the level of the metacarpal neck.

The exact location of the artery with respect to the first dorsal interosseous muscle may vary. Kuhlmann and de Frenne found the artery to run superficial to the muscle in 75% of specimens, while the FDMA was found within the muscle in 15% of specimens; in 10% of specimens, the artery ran within and on top of the muscle during its course. Dautel and Merle identified a superficial course of the FDMA in 36% of specimens, a suprafascial course in 23% of specimens, and a deep, intramuscular course in 56%. Despite its exact location, all authors agree on the consistency of an FDMA (Fig. 26-1).

Overall, the flap provides excellent sensibility, pliability, and stability for a variety of hand defects. We feel the first dorsal metacarpal island flap is one of the workhorses for reconstructive hand surgery.

INDICATIONS/CONTRAINDICATIONS

Indications

Indications for the FDMA flap ("kite flap") are based on the following criteria:

- Etiology, location, size, and condition of the defect
- Availability of the flap (i.e., previous injuries that may compromise the vascular pedicle)

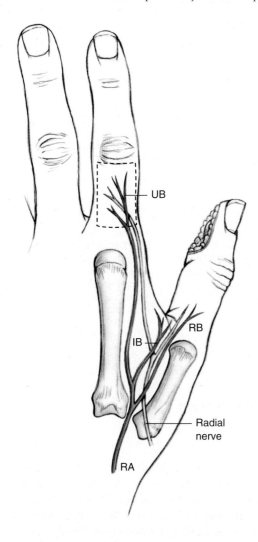

FIGURE 26-1

The three branches of the radial artery (*RA*). The radial branch of the FDMA (*RB*) goes to the thumb, the intermediate branch (*IB*) to the first web space, and the ulnar branch (*UB*) of the FDMA runs to the index finger.

- Suitability of the flap for the defect (e.g., size, arc of rotation)
- Inclusion of other tissue components (i.e., tendon, bony segment)
- Patient's wishes (donor site morbidity, aesthetic appearance)
- Surgeon's familiarity with the technique

Based on these decision-making criteria, the flap is indicated for primary or secondary reconstructions of:

- The dorsal aspect of the thumb
- Restoration of sensibility with pulp reconstruction in the thumb
- Skin defects at the dorsal aspect of the hand within the arc of rotation of the antegrade kite flap
- Palmar defects of the index finger
- Defects of the web space
- Defects around the wrist
- Defects at the base of the thumb or the middle finger ("retrograde kite flap")
- Complex flaps including various tissue components
- Microvascular flap transfer based on the vascular pedicle in the snuff box

The list of indications demonstrates the versatility of the flap: however, reconstruction of the thumb takes precedence as the main indication in most centers.

Following the pioneer work of Tränkle et al., the flap has replaced other sensate neurovascular island flaps for restoration of sensibility in the thumb due to the dissection technique, the discriminative power that can be achieved, and the acceptable donor site morbidity. Based on this study, the flap is now widely used for this indication (Fig. 26-2).

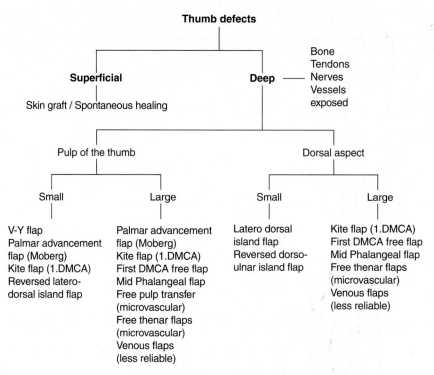

FIGURE 26-2

Decision-making algorithm for flap selection in treatment of thumb defects.

Contraindications

Contraindications for flap use include acute trauma or a history of significant trauma to the donor site. In addition, injury mechanisms such as crush avulsions, wringer injuries, and high-energy trauma (e.g., blast injuries or gunshot wounds) may limit the reliability of this flap if they have disrupted the course of the FDMA. If the tissue viability of the donor site cannot be estimated properly in the first hours of the trauma, wound closure should be delayed or a different flap should be used for wound coverage.

Burn injuries of the dorsum of the hand do not present a contraindication for the use of a FDMA flap in all cases. The dorsal metacarpal artery system is not damaged by deep partial-thickness burns that are excised and grafted. In 80% of patients with full-thickness burns, the dorsal metacarpal artery system is still intact. The potential for elevating a FDMA flap is therefore preserved after burn excision and grafting. Nevertheless, preoperative Doppler ultrasound examination is recommended before flap elevation.

PREOPERATIVE PLANNING

As in any surgical procedure, careful preoperative assessment and planning are key factors to success and the avoidance of complications or failure. Decision making follows an algorithmic approach in which the defect must be assessed for size, etiology, and characteristics.

The decision for flap selection is based on the criteria outlined previously (see indications). The patient should be thoroughly informed about the therapeutic options, and his or her expectations and wishes should also be discussed. Special attention should be paid to donor site morbidity including numbness over the radial aspect of the dorsum of the hand and the implications of a full-thickness skin graft to the donor site. The postoperative management and potential complications such as flap failure or impaired mobility of the fingers, impaired sensibility, and other possible undesirable results should be discussed with the patient. Donor site morbidity is an important issue that should also be discussed with the patient before surgery. The functional and aesthetic morbidity of the donor site is an issue often neglected in the choice of a flap, and it must be borne in mind that the donor area of a FDMA island flap is in a very exposed position.

Clinical examination should exclude prior injuries in the area of the vascular pedicle. In most cases, the artery is palpable, but Doppler ultrasound examination before flap elevation is mandatory since the course of the artery is variable (see previous discussion). The course of the artery should be marked on the skin preoperatively after Doppler examination.

SURGERY

The defect size is templated to the dorsum of the index finger. The course of the artery is marked on the dorsum of the hand with the aid of a handheld Doppler ultrasound device. Surgery is performed using either an axillary bloc, or general or regional anesthesia. The use of a pneumatic tourniquet and loupe magnification is necessary for the dissection. The flap is harvested from the dorsum of the index finger and includes the FDMA, a branch of the superficial radial nerve, and at least one subcutaneous vein (Fig. 26-3).

Dissection is performed starting with the vascular pedicle including a large subcutaneous vein, which has first to be identified and mobilized. Elevation of the flap starts radially by incising the interosseus fascia at the most radial edge of the muscle. The fascia is then peeled off the muscle toward the second metacarpal. Thereby, a wide pedicle including the subcutaneous vein, a branch of the superficial radial nerve, and the vascular pedicle is created. A vessel loop is used to mark this pedicle. The pedicle is traced back to its origin in the snuffbox. There is no need to isolate the vascular pedicle from the interosseus fascia, since this may injure the delicate vessels. Transillumination will verify the inclusion of the artery and the small accompanying veins in the pedicle.

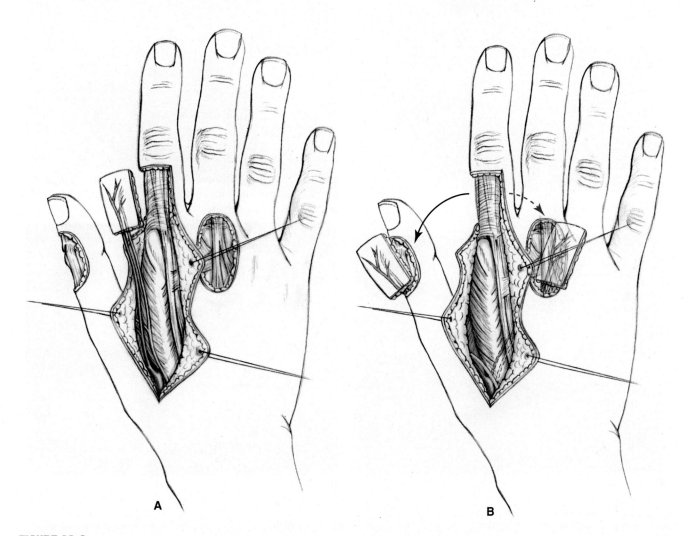

A   B

FIGURE 26-3

Schematic drawing of the dissected **(A)** FDMA flap and the FDMA flap with its pedicle passed distally under the skin tunnel **(B)**. (Redrawn from Germann G, et al. *Decision-making in Reconstructive Surgery—Upper Extremity*. Berlin, Germany: Springer-Verlag; 2000.)

Dissection now proceeds from the distal border of the flap. The flap is incised and dissected off of the paratenon of the extensor apparatus toward the proximal border of the flap. Care must be taken to preserve the paratenon in order to secure graft take at the donor site. A critical point in the dissection is the radial aspect of the extensor hood of the metaphalangeal joint where the vessels enter the subcutaneous network of the flap. It is recommended to include a small strip of extensor hood to secure the vessel entrance. This area can be easily repaired without any functional deficit by a 4-0 resorbable suture.

Once the flap is raised, the tourniquet is deflated to assess the blood supply of the flap. Occasionally, the flap may first appear pale but usually begins to turn pink within a few minutes. The flap may be passed through a subcutaneous tunnel into the defect. If the skin is too tight, the tunnel is opened and the pedicle is skin grafted. As a sensory island flap, the FDMA island flap allows a wide arc of rotation due to its pedicle length of up to 7 cm.

The donor defect of the index finger is covered with a full-thickness skin graft. A split-thickness skin graft may also be used; however, a full-thickness skin graft will provide a better color match. Full-thickness grafting will provide an aesthetically acceptable appearance at the donor site within a shorter period of time, although the long-term results using a split-thickness graft are comparable (Figs. 26-4 and 26-5).

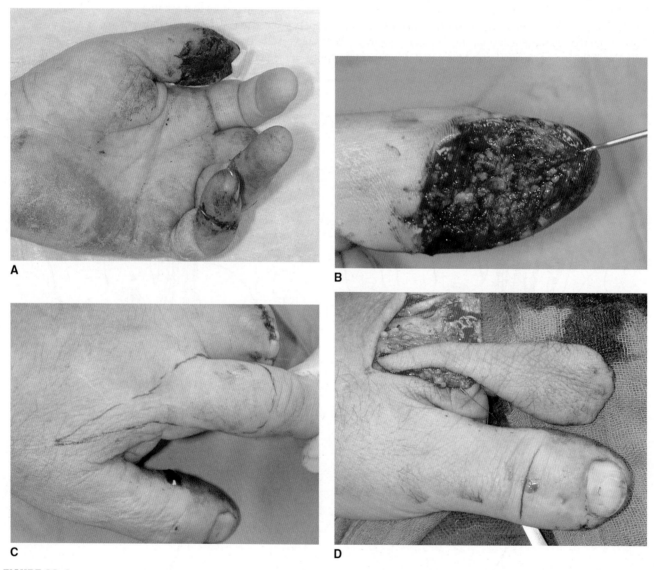

FIGURE 26-4

A: A 63-year-old man sustained a mutilating saw injury of the hand with avulsion of the palmar aspect of the distal phalanx of the left thumb (additional injuries in the middle and small fingers). Six days after the injury: complete necrosis of the pulp of the thumb. **B:** Intraoperative view after radical debridement. **C:** Flap design: the FDMA island flap is outlined over the dorsal aspect of the proximal phalanx of the index finger. **D:** The FDMA island flap is elevated. Note the "cutaneous tail" of the flap that allows primary skin-skin closure.

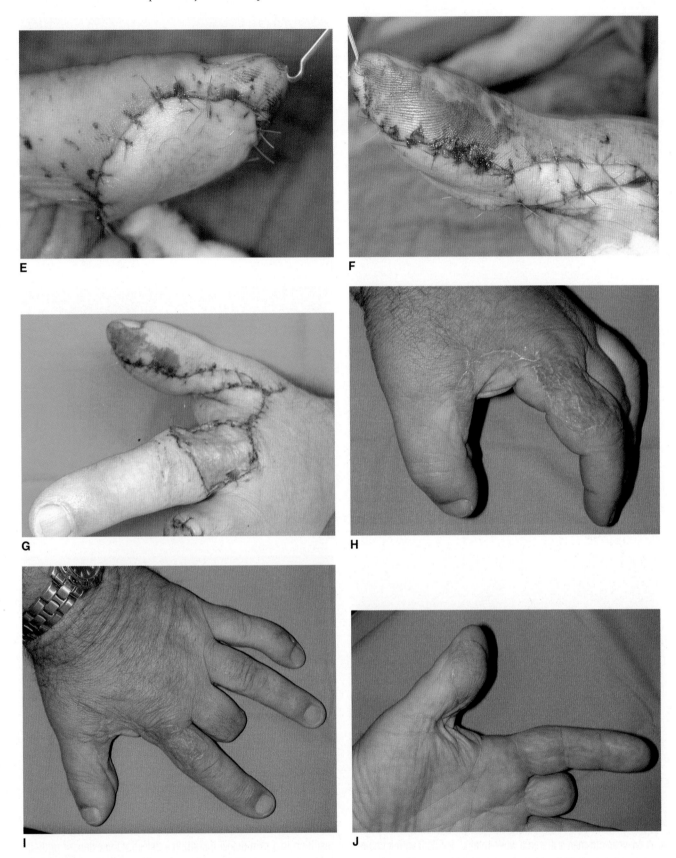

FIGURE 26-4 (*Continued*)

E, F: After tunneling the flap into the defect, primary skin-skin closure is achieved. **G:** Reconstruction of the donor site with skin graft.
H–J: Aesthetic and functional outcome 2 years postoperatively. Full extension of thumb and index finger. The patient describes cold intolerance of the donor site. Two PD of the flap: 6.5 mm; 2 PD of the donor site: 6 mm.

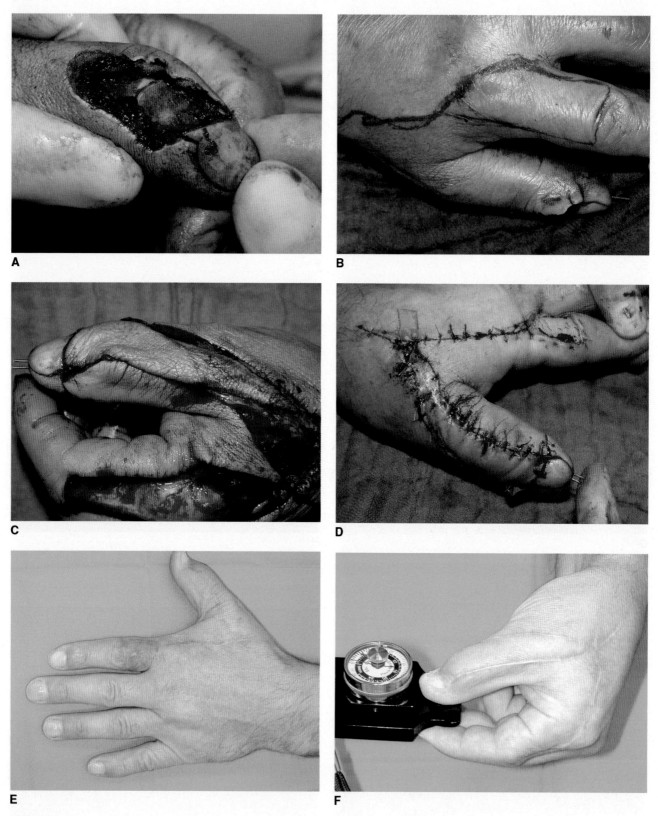

FIGURE 26-5

A: A 44-year-old man suffered a work-related accident with a chain saw, resulting in a skin defect including a defect of the extensor pollicis longus tendon at its insertion and exposure of the interphalangeal joint. **B:** Design of the FDMA island flap on the dorsal of the index finger. **C:** The FDMA island flap prior to insertion into the defect. **D:** Result after insetting of the first dorsal metacarpal island flap. The flap shows perfect capillary refill. The donor site has been diminished in size by mobilization of the surrounding skin. Aesthetic **(E)** and functional **(F)** outcome 2 years postoperatively. Excellent hand function and aesthetic appearance have been achieved. The patient returned to his previous employment without limitations.

Extensive experience with this flap has lead to some refinements. To avoid any tension on the pedicle, the subcutaneous tunnel has to be opened frequently. We now raise the flap constantly with a "cutaneous tail" extending from the proximal border of the flap to the radial aspect of the second metacarpal. This extension allows opening of the tunnel and direct skin-skin closure after flap transfer. This technique does not only provide a more stable skin closure but also a better aesthetic appearance (see Fig. 26-4C,F). In addition, segments of the second metacarpal or the extensor indicis proprius tendon can be included in the flap for more complex reconstruction.

The FDMA flap can also be raised as a microvascular free flap (Fig. 26-6). The flap is harvested using the same technique as the pedicled FDMA flap described previously. Dissection of the FDMA back to its origin from the radial artery provides an artery of adequate diameter for microvascular anastomosis. A long pedicle length facilitates microvascular reconstruction outside the area of trauma; inclusion of the cutaneous nerve permits reconstruction of sensibility. We believe that dissection of this flap is easier and faster than a toe and first web space flap.

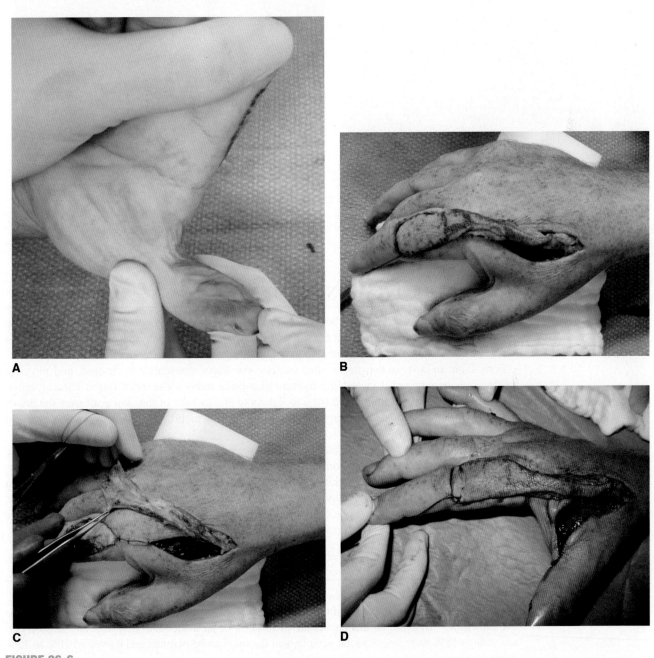

FIGURE 26-6

A: A 48-year-old policeman presented with an unstable and painful scar over the thumb pulp with associated hyperesthesia. **B:** The scar is excised and a FDMA flap is chosen for skin coverage. **C:** The flap is turned so the vessels may be visualized running within the fascia. **D:** The flap is well perfused after tourniquet release.

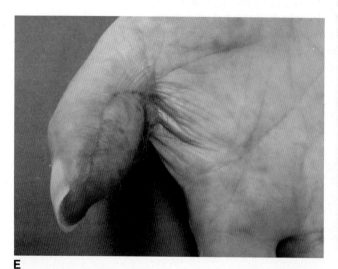

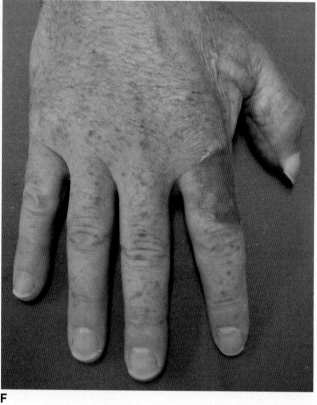

FIGURE 26-6 (Continued)

E: The thumb 1 year after surgery is pain free, and the patient was able to return to work. **F:** The contour of the hand looks good. The donor site of the index finger was covered with a full-thickness skin graft.

POSTOPERATIVE MANAGEMENT

The hand may be immobilized in a bulky dressing following surgery. A palmar plaster splint may be used to immobilize any concomitant fractures. A window is left in the dressing for evaluation of the flap. Care is taken not to apply the dressing too tight for fear of causing arterial or venous compromise.

Forty-eight to seventy-two hours after surgery, the flap's vascularity is ensured, and physical therapy may be initiated if underlying fracture fixation is stabile. The index finger metacarpophalangeal joint is usually immobilized for 5 to 7 days to ensure take of the skin graft over the donor site, but the proximal and distal interphalangeal joints may be mobilized as soon as possible to avoid postoperative stiffness.

Occupational therapy is also initiated for sensory reeducation of the flap. Initially, sensation in the flap will be perceived as coming from the dorsum of the index finger, or a dual sensation phenomenon may result. Cortical reorientation of sensation is possible with a structured sensory reeducation program. The FDMA island flap allows immediate restoration of sensibility even in older patients, among whom neuronal coadaptation of a pedicled or a free flap yields poorer results than in younger people.

COMPLICATIONS

Although the FDMA island flap has proven to be very reliable, various complications can occur. These complications include planning errors, complications during the operation, and postoperative difficulties. To avoid an inadequate arc of rotation or an inadequate flap size, the surgeon can add 10% to 15% more length to the pedicle, and the flap can be planned and harvested 10% to 15% larger in size.

Care should be taken to exert only gentle traction when passing the flap through the subcutaneous tunnel to close the thumb pulp defect. Excessive tension can cause a partial compression of the vessels, and marginal necrosis could result. Whereas vascular insufficiency on the arterial side is frequently the result of tunneling, a short pedicle or tight wound closure can compromise the venous outflow. In case of postoperative vascular insufficiency, sutures can be released, and leech therapy may be employed.

Donor site morbidity of dorsal metacarpal artery island flaps is low compared with axial homodigital island flaps. Neuromas are rare, and the patients report less hypersensitivity than in homodigital island flaps. However, one of the most important donor site problems of the FDMA island flap is a diminished protective sensation over the transplanted skin graft, and patients may complain of cold intolerance. Hypertrophic scars present a minor donor site problem. Functional limitation because of the donor site is negligible, and the range of motion of the donor finger reaches approximately 95% of the opposite index finger.

PEARLS AND PITFALLS

- The course of the FDMA should be marked on the skin preoperatively using a handheld Doppler.
- Template the flap 10% to 20% larger than the defect to minimize tension during insetting.
- Care must be taken to preserve the paratenon over the extensor tendon in order to secure graft take at the donor site.
- A critical point in the dissection is the radial aspect of the extensor hood of the metaphalangeal joint where the vessels enter the subcutaneous network of the flap. It is recommended to include a small strip of extensor hood to secure the vessel entrance. This area can be easily repaired without any functional deficit by a 4-0 PDS suture.
- Consider elevating a skin tail over the pedicle—this facilitates insetting and minimizes pressure on pedicle.
- Cover the donor site with a full-thickness graft and use a bolster to maximize graft take.
- The flap can be divided and used as a free flap if necessary.

RECOMMENDED READING

Adani R, Busa R, Castagnetti C, et al. Homodigital neurovascular island flaps with "direct flow" vascularization. *Ann Plast Surg.* 1997;38(1):36–40.
Adani R, Squarzina PB, Castagnetti C, et al. A comparative study of the heterodigital neurovascular island flap in thumb reconstruction, with and without nerve reconnection. *J Hand Surg Am.* 1994;19(5):552–559.
Baumeister S, Menke H, Wittemann M, et al. Functional outcome after the moberg advancement flap in the thumb. *J Hand Surg Am.* 2002;27A:105–114.
Bertelli JA, Catarina S. Neurocutaneous island flaps in upper limb coverage: experience with 44 clinical cases. *J Hand Surg Am.* 1997;22(3):515–526.
Chang SC, Chen SL, Chen TM, et al. Sensate first dorsal metacarpal artery flap for resurfacing extensive pulp defects of the thumb. *Ann Plast Surg.* 2004;53(5):449–454.
Chen C, Wie F. Lateral-dorsal neurovascular island flaps for pulp reconstruction. *Ann Plast Surg.* 2000;45:616–622.
Dautel G, Merle M. Dorsal metacarpal reverse flaps. *Br J Hand Surg.* 1991;16B:400–405.
Dellon AL. Sensory recovery in replanted digits and transplanted toes. *J Reconstr Microsurg.* 1986;2:123.
Early MJ, Milner RH. Dorsal metacarpal flaps. *Br J Plast Surg.* 1987;40:333–341.
Ege A, Tuncay I, Ercetin O. Foucher's first dorsal metacarpal artery flap for thumb reconstruction: evaluation of 21 cases. *Isr Med Assoc J.* 2002;4(6):421–433.
El-Khatib HA. Clinical experiences with the extended first dorsal metacarpal artery island flap for thumb reconstruction. *J Hand Surg Am* 1998;23A:647–652.
Elliot H. Small flap coverage of hand and digit defects. *Clin Plast Surg.* 1989;16:427–442.
Foucher G, Braun JB. A new island flap transfer from the dorsum of the index to the thumb. *Plast Reconstr Surg.* 1979;63:344–349.
Gebhard B, Meissl G. An extended first dorsal metacarpal artery neurovascular island flap. *J Hand Surg Am.* 1995;20(4):529–531.
Germann G. Principles of flap design for surgery of the Hand. *Atlas Hand Clin.* 1998;3:33–57.
Germann G, Funk H, Bickert B. The fate of the dorsal metacarpal arterial system following thermal injury to the dorsal hand: a Doppler sonographic study. *J Hand Surg Am.* 2000;25(5):962–967.
Germann G, Hornung R, Raff T. Two new applications for the first dorsal metacarpal artery pedicle in the treatment of severe hand injuries. *J Hand Surg Br.* 1995;20(4):525–528.
Germann G, Levin LS. Intrinsic flaps in the hand: new concepts in skin coverage. *Tech Hand Up Extrem Surg.* 1997;1(1):48–61.
Germann G, Raff T, Schepler H, et al. Salvage of an avascular thumb by arteriovenous flow reversal and a microvascular "kite" flap: case report. *J Reconstr Microsurg.* 1997;13:167–291.
Giessler G, Erdmann D, Germann G. Soft tissue coverage in devastating hand injuries. *Hand Clin.* 2003;19:63–71.
Grossman JAI, Robotti EB. The use of split-thickness hypothenar grafts for coverage of fingertips and other defects of the hand. *Ann Chir Main Memb Super.* 1995;14:239–243.
Holevich J. A new method of restoring sensibility to the thumb. *J Bone Joint Surg.* 1963;45B:496–502.

Inoue G, Maeda N, Suzudi K. Resurfacing of skin defects of the hand using the arterial venous flap. *Br J Plast Surg.* 1990;43(2):135–139.

Krag C, Rasmussen KB. The neurovascular island flap for defective sensibility of the thumb. *J Bone Joint Surg Br.* 1975;57(4):495–499.

Lassner F, Becker M, Berger A, et al. Sensory reconstruction of the fingertip using the bilaterally innervated sensory cross-finger flap. *Plast Reconstr Surg.* 2002;109(3):988–993.

Lister G. Local flaps to the hand. *Hand Clin.* 1995;1(4):621–640.

Marx, A, Preisser P, Peek A, et al. Anatomy of the dorsal mid-hand arteries-anatomic study and review of the literature. *Handchir Mikrochir Plast Chir.* 2001;33(2):77–82.

Masquelet AC, Gilbert A. *An Atlas of Flaps in Limb Reconstruction.* London, UK: Martin Duniz; 1995.

Oka Y. Sensory function of the neurovascular island flap in thumb reconstruction: comparison of original and modified procedures. *J Hand Surg Am.* 2000;25(4):637–643.

Pelzer M, Sauerbier M, Germann G, et al. Free "kite" flap: a new flap for reconstruction of small hand defects. *J Reconstr Microsurg.* 2004;20(5):367–372.

Prakash V, Chawla S. First dorsal metacarpal artery adipofascial flap for a dorsal defect of the thumb. *Plast Reconstr Surg.* 2004;114(5):1353–1355.

Preisser P, Marx A, Klinzig S, et al. Covering defects of the basal finger area by pedicled flaps anastomosed to the dorsal metacarpal arteries. *Handchir Mikrochir Plast Chir.* 2001;33(2):83–88.

Quaba AA, Davison PM. The distally based dorsal metacarpal artery flap. *Br J Plast Surg.* 1990;43:28–32.

Ratcliff RJ, Regan PJ, Scerri GV. First dorsal metacarpal artery flap cover for extensive pulp defects in the normal length thumb. *Br J Plast Surg.* 1992;45:544–546.

Rose EH. Local arterialized island flap coverage of difficult hand defects preserving donor digit sensibility. *Plast Reconstr Surg.* 1983;72(6):848–858.

Rose EH. Small flap coverage of hand and digit defects. *Clin Plast Surg.* 1989;16(3):427–442.

Sherif MM. First dorsal metacarpal artery flap in hand reconstruction. I Anatomical study. *J Hand Surg Am.* 1994;19A:26–31.

Sherif MM. First dorsal metacarpal artery flap in hand reconstruction. II Clinical application. *J Hand Surg Am.* 1994;19(1):32–38.

Shun-Cheng CH, Shao-Liang CH, Tim Mo Chen, et al. Sensate first dorsal metacarpal artery flap for resurfacing extensive pulp defects in the thumb. *Ann Plast Surg.* 2004;53:449–454.

Small JO, Brennen MD. The first dorsal metacarpal artery neurovascular island flap. *J Hand Surg Am.* 1988;15:145–148.

Tränkle M, Germann G, Heitmann C, et al. Defect coverage and reconstruction of thumb sensibility with the first dorsal metacarpal artery island flap. *Chirurg.* 2004;75:996–1002.

Tränkle M, Sauerbier M, Heitmann C, et al. Restoration of the thumb sensibility with the innervated first dorsal metacarpal artery island flap. *J Hand Surg Am.* 2003;28A(5):758–766.

Vlastou C, Earle AS, Blanchard JM. A palmar cross-finger flap for coverage of thumb defects. *J Hand Surg Am.* 1985;10(4):566–569.

Voche P, Merle M. Vascular supply of the palmar subcutaneous tissue of fingers. *Br J Plast Surg.* 1996;49(5):315–318.

Williams RL, Nanchahal J, Sykes PJ, et al. The provision of innervated skin cover for the injured thumb using the first dorsal metacarpal artery island flap. *J Hand Surg Am.* 1995;20B:231–236.

Yang D, Morris SF. Vascular basis of dorsal digital and metacarpal skin flaps. *J Hand Surg Am.* 2001;26(1):142–146.

27 Flap Reconstruction of the Thumb

David Elliot and Adam Sierakowski

The primary goals of thumb reconstruction are to restore length and sensation. A thumb should be of adequate length to allow for pinch to the index and middle fingertips and to achieve span grasp with all five digital tips. Adequate length is also essential for developing power grip. The surgeon aims to provide adequate cover of the deeper, vital structures with soft tissue and skin of good quality. Sensibility of the tip is of particular importance, being crucial to fine pinch. A tapered thumb tip, as in the normal thumb, can often be achieved surgically and is preferred to reconstruction of a tip that is broad, flat, and spatulate. A thumb post with no, or little, movement distal to the basal joint or with poor tip shape and sensation can still work to aid in hand use but will not allow for finesse of function.

In attempting to obtain optimal reconstruction, one should avoid shortening the thumb unless absolutely necessary. We encourage distal replantation or composite draft replacement and also look to homodigital flap reconstruction whenever possible. Care should be spent in nail bed preservation and repair. Any nail bed longer than one-third of its normal length should be retained, at least at primary surgery. Reconstruction of thumb defects with the use of skin grafts from elsewhere on the body can create patches of dissimilar color, texture, and thickness and a noticeably poor cosmetic result. Finally, with respect to mobility and rehabilitation, the time-honored plastic surgical techniques of cross-finger, thenar, groin, and cross-arm flaps should be avoided if possible, as they tether the injured thumb to another part of the body and prevent early mobilization, increasing the risk of long-term immobilization by fibrin-loaded edema.

Most of the techniques described here use homodigital reconstruction. Homodigital reconstruction involves rearrangement of the soft tissues of the injured digit to achieve healing without seeking tissue for reconstruction from outside that digit. This concept of reconstruction has definite advantages for thumb reconstruction. In particular, it reconstructs "like with like" and avoids the creation of further scarring and morbidity elsewhere on the hand or body. While homodigital reconstruction is advantageous in these respects, the availability of donor tissues within the thumb is obviously limited.

Perhaps the single most important surgical pearl to remember when employing homodigital reconstruction is that the digits have an astonishing ability to close skin defects of considerable size by a combination of wound contraction and re-epithelialization to give a cosmetic and functional result that cannot be bettered by any surgical procedure (Fig. 27-1).

Thus, if a portion of the wound can heal under moist antiseptic dressings through secondary intention, the surgeon can use the homodigital flaps to cover only those portions of the wound that contain exposed vital structures or to improve soft tissue coverage over bone. The flap does not have to cover the entire defect, only the essential components of the defect, considerably enlarging the possibilities of skin cover by homodigital techniques.

PREOPERATIVE PLANNING

Preoperative planning should include AP and lateral radiographs in addition to a thorough hand examination. Concomitant arterial and nerve injuries can often be identified prior to exploration within the operating room. Many thumb injuries will often occur in conjunction with other hand injuries and revascularization of injured digits takes precedence over coverage issues. Wounds should be debrided of all necrotic tissue and free of infection before embarking on soft tissue coverage.

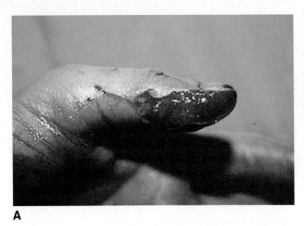
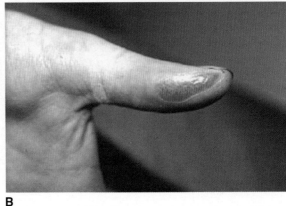

FIGURE 27-1

A: Industrial scalpel wound of the thumb tip. **B:** Same digital surface after healing by re-epithelialization under moist antiseptic dressings for 3 weeks.

PATIENT POSITIONING

Patients are positioned supine on the operating room table. General or regional anesthesia is used for most surgical procedures. Thumb or wrist blocks may be used when performing smaller flaps or debridement procedures. Surgery is always performed under tourniquet control, mostly at upper arm level, to aid visualization of vital structures.

RECONSTRUCTION OF PALMAR AND TIP DEFECTS

Neurovascular Tranquilli-Leali or Atasoy-Kleinert Flap

Indications/Contraindications

Historically, the original Tranquilli-Leali or Atasoy-Kleinert flap was described to cover partial amputation defects of the distal phalanges of the fingers. However, this flap does not work well on the thumb because of the inflexibility of the subcutaneous soft tissues. Laterally based, single pedicle flaps, vascularized in the same way by the small vessels beyond the trifurcations of the digital arteries, also move poorly. The *neurovascular* Tranquilli-Leali or Atasoy-Kleinert flap is designed to be much larger. It is islanded on both neurovascular pedicles (Fig. 27-2) and is designed to extend to, and across, the IP joint crease proximally.

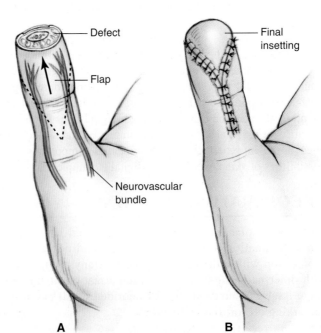

FIGURE 27-2

The neurovascular Tranquilli-Leali flap. **A:** The flap extends proximally beyond the IP crease and includes both the neurovascular bundles. **B:** Final insetting is performed in a V to Y fashion.

Although used primarily for minor transverse or oblique injuries of the distal phalanx, this flap can be used for stump reconstruction of any length of amputated thumb with exposure of bone and is more useful than the original Tranquilli-Leali flap. However, it moves less freely than on a finger, partly because of the fibrous nature of the subcutaneous tissues of the thumb and partly because of what has been described by Gaul as the "vertical dimension" of the thumb, that is, its palmar-dorsal width at the tip. On fingers, it can be used to reconstruct defects with a palmar slope of up to 30 degrees; on the thumb, it can only reconstruct defects with bone exposure that are dorsally facing, transverse, or palmar facing with less than 10 degrees of slope.

Surgical Technique

The incisions of the V cross the interphalangeal joint crease at an angle and thus do not cause contractures (Fig. 27-3). When designing the flap, one takes the V incisions out almost to the lateral nail folds distally. Having made the flap wide, the leading edge of the flap after advancement

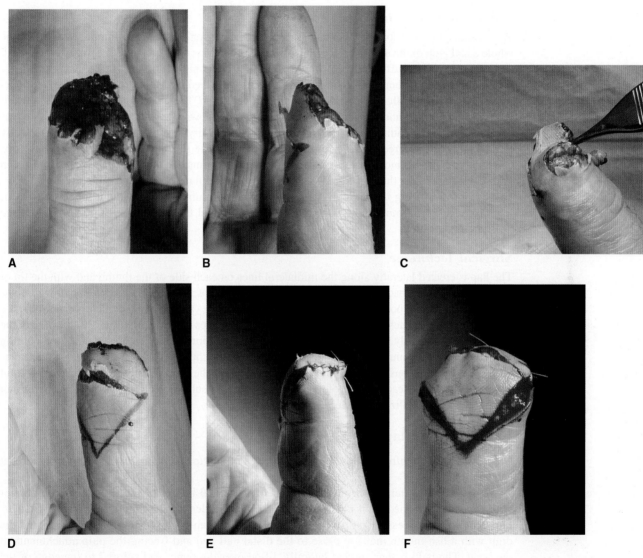

FIGURE 27-3

A, B: Dorsal sloping crush amputation of the right thumb tip of a 70-year-old man. **C:** Simple folding back of the palmar tissues after excision of the nail germinal matrix to suture the skin to the proximal nail fold is not possible because of the bulk of the pulp tissue. **D:** A neurovascular Tranquilli-Leali flap designed to allow easier folding back of the palmar tissues and shaping of the thumb tip. The transverse skin split just beyond the "V" was part of the injury but only skin deep so not affecting the vascularity of the tissues distal to it. **E, F:** The reconstructed shape after trimming the lateral points of the advanced flap to round the thumb tip. (Reproduced from Elliot D. Specific flaps for the thumb. *Tech Hand Up Extrem Surg.* 2004;8:198–211, with permission.)

is wider than the original thumb tip. Unless the lateral corners of the flap are excised, this results in a spatulate end to the digit. Cutting off the lateral corners and allowing the resulting raw edges and tip to epithelialize not only narrows the digital tip but also rounds it to achieve a good appearance. The flap is designed as a V at its proximal extremity and was conceived to close proximally as a Y after the flap has moved distally. Mostly, however, the proximal donor defect is left open to close under dressings as primary closure of the vertical limb of the Y tightens the thumb too much proximally over the vascular pedicles of the flaps and may compromise the vascularity of the flap.

A useful small addition to this flap was described more recently: if the flap does not quite advance easily enough to allow suture to the distal nail remnant without tension, a smaller V may be cut through the skin of the flap to create a flap within the flap, which is likened to Russian Matryoshka, or Gigogne, dolls, fitting inside each other. Effectively, this creates a true Tranquilli-Leali or Atasoy-Kleinert flap within the larger neurovascular flap.

Moberg Flaps

Indications/Contraindications

With greater losses of palmar thumb tissue, more sloping palmar oblique injuries, and when the whole distal pulp of the thumb has been avulsed, the neurovascular Tranquilli-Leali flap is too small and cannot advance sufficiently. For these larger defects confined to the distal phalanx, we favor use of a modified Moberg flap. The Moberg flap, as described by Moberg in 1964, is an advancement flap based on both neurovascular bundles of the thumb. The advantages of this flap are that it returns glabrous skin and sensation to the thumb tip. The downside of the original flap design was the IP joint flexion, leading to long-term contracture, necessary to achieve suture of the flap distally to the nail. Our preferred modification of the flap avoids the IP joint flexion of the original. It is, essentially, O'Brien's modification of the Moberg flap but using a V tail proximally instead of a skin graft at the base of the thumb (Fig. 27-4). This V-Y Moberg flap achieves the same excellent results as the original Moberg flap in terms of sensibility of the thumb tip but without the restrictions of interphalangeal joint movement associated with the original flap or the need for skin graft of the O'Brien modification.

Surgical Technique

The flap is created laterally along the midlateral lines on each side of the thumb and with the tip of the proximal V well back on the thenar eminence, at least as far proximally as a line drawn proximally from the radial border of the middle finger. This creates a large flap that incorporates the more lax subcutaneous tissues of the thenar eminence. Smaller flaps with the proximal V at the base of the thumb move less easily and less far distally. The wider and longer flap avoids any need for addition of techniques to accommodate tightness at the base of the thumb. The use of this flap is considerably extended in reconstructing palmar oblique defects if the pulp distally that is denuded of skin cover remains as the leading edge of the flap, with suture of subcutaneous tissue, not skin, to the nail distally then epithelialization under dressings.

Lateral Pulp Flaps

Other flaps have an infrequent use in reconstruction of the tip and palmar surface of the thumb but can be useful.

We devised the lateral pulp flap for losses of the radial border of the tip of the index finger with exposure of bone, but it is also useful on either borders of the thumb tip (Fig. 27-5). This flap exploits the excess of pulp in the digital tip. The flap is raised by opening the tip of the digit with a fish-mouth incision close to the distal nail bed and freeing the pulp attachments to the bone. The pulp is then moved laterally, lifted over the bone, and sutured to the edge of the nail. The deep edge of the pulp—not the superficial edge—is brought up to the nail bed to cover the bone. The pulp is then epithelialized under moist antiseptic dressings. This reconstruction creates a digital tip that is sensate but has no lateral nail fold. This seems to cause no functional problems and is less obvious than most lateral nail fold reconstructions, as these are usually too bulky.

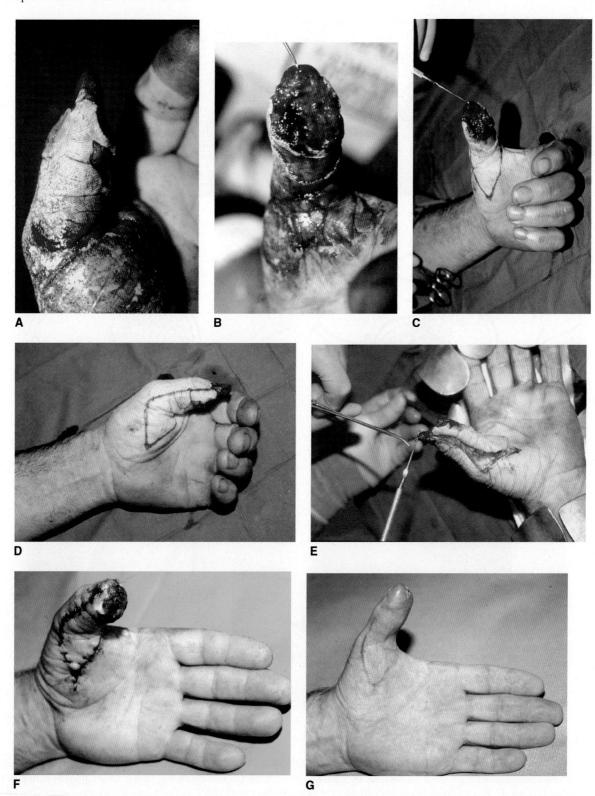

FIGURE 27-4

A, B: Preoperative views of the thumb of a 47-year-old man with a typical crush avulsion of the distal pulp. **C, D:** Markings of a V-Y modification of the Moberg flap shown preoperatively. **E:** Intraoperative view of the fully mobilized flap. **F:** Immediate postoperative view with the flap advanced to provide pulp cover of the distal bone. **G:** Final result after epithelialization of the tip under moist antiseptic dressings. (Reproduced from Elliot D, Yii NW. Homodigital reconstruction of the digits: the perspective of one unit. *Handchir Mikrochir Plast Chir.* 2001;33(1):7–19, with permission.)

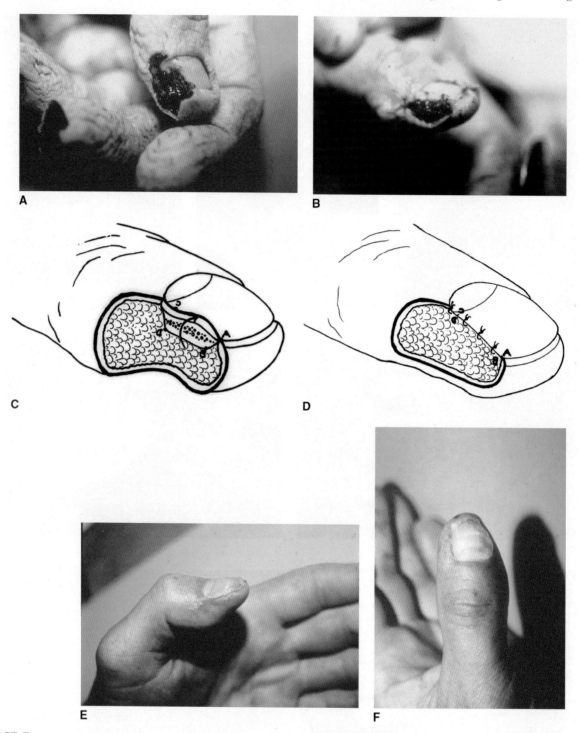

FIGURE 27-5

A: A slicing defect with loss of the radial lateral pulp, lateral nail fold, and lateral one-third of the nail of the thumb in a 50-year-old man.
B: Lateral pulp transposed to cover the distal phalanx. **C, D:** Diagrams to show the original injury and transposition of the pulp to cover the bone of the distal phalanx. **E, F:** Late views of the reconstruction, 1 year after the injury. (Reproduced from Elliot D, Jigjinni VS. The lateral pulp flap. *J Hand Surg Br.* 1993;18(4):423–426, with permission.)

Side-to-Side Switch Flaps

Side-to-side homodigital switch flaps, which reconstruct or reinnervate one side of a digital tip at the expense of the other side, can be useful to resurface areas of pulp sensibility in the hand that are critical for pinch activity after localized loss of tissue or irrevocable digital nerve injury

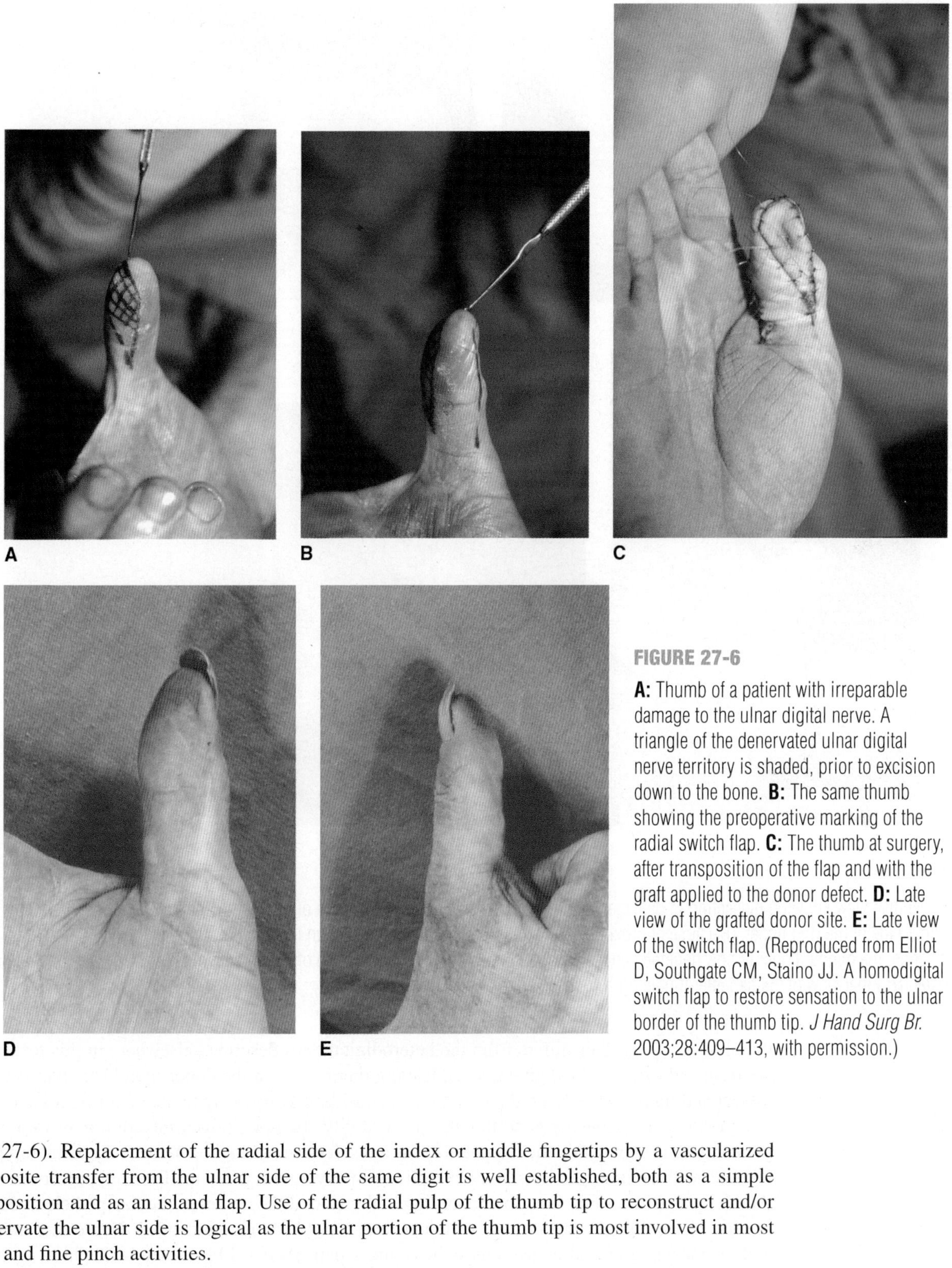

FIGURE 27-6

A: Thumb of a patient with irreparable damage to the ulnar digital nerve. A triangle of the denervated ulnar digital nerve territory is shaded, prior to excision down to the bone. **B:** The same thumb showing the preoperative marking of the radial switch flap. **C:** The thumb at surgery, after transposition of the flap and with the graft applied to the donor defect. **D:** Late view of the grafted donor site. **E:** Late view of the switch flap. (Reproduced from Elliot D, Southgate CM, Staino JJ. A homodigital switch flap to restore sensation to the ulnar border of the thumb tip. *J Hand Surg Br.* 2003;28:409–413, with permission.)

(Fig. 27-6). Replacement of the radial side of the index or middle fingertips by a vascularized composite transfer from the ulnar side of the same digit is well established, both as a simple transposition and as an island flap. Use of the radial pulp of the thumb tip to reconstruct and/or reinnervate the ulnar side is logical as the ulnar portion of the thumb tip is most involved in most gross and fine pinch activities.

Littler Flaps

The classic Littler flap was designed for thumb palmar and tip resurfacing. Unlike the flaps described above, this is a heterodigital flap, meaning that the donor site is tissue from the ulnar border of the middle or ring finger. Because of proximity to the thumb and the presence of an incomplete superficial palmar arch in up to 34% of hands, the middle finger is now generally chosen as the donor finger. The flap is transferred on its neurovascular bundle, allowing for sensate reconstruction of the

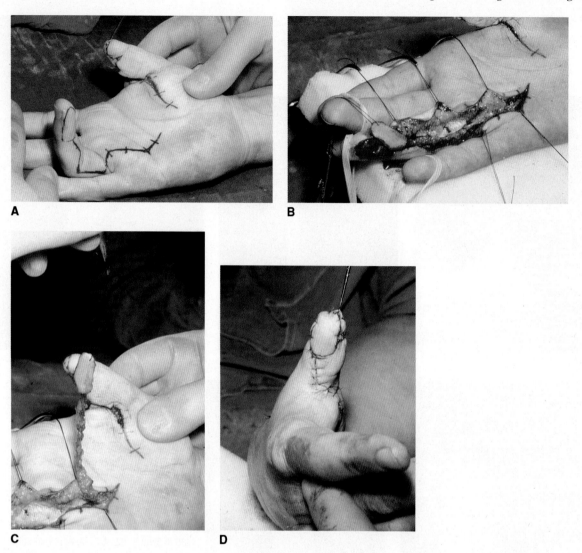

FIGURE 27-7

A: Intraoperative view showing dissection of damaged and denervated skin on the ulnar side of the thumb and the markings of a Littler flap on the ulnar side of the ring finger. (Because of proximity to the thumb and the presence of an incomplete superficial palmar arch in up to 34% of hands, the middle finger is now generally chosen as the donor finger.) **B:** Dissection of the pedicle of the flap. **C:** Demonstration of the transfer. **D:** Final view of the flap after tunneling across the palm and insetting.

thumb (Fig. 27-7). This differs from the heterodigital flaps described elsewhere in this text, which are designed to spare the digital nerves, leaving them intact in the donor digit. This flap is easy to dissect and transfer. However, the transfer can considerably downgrade the donor finger and it suffers problems of achieving good thumb tip sensibility. Two-point discrimination may well remain greater than 12 mm within the flap, perhaps as a result of stretching the nerve: very distal injuries of a thumb with an intact skeleton may be difficult to cover with this flap. To avoid perception of the thumb tip as still coming from the donor finger, division of the nerves in the flap pedicle and reconnection to the digital nerves of the recipient thumb has been recommended. Nerve disconnection and reconnection extend its usefulness in younger patients but, like all neurorrhaphies, gives less satisfactory tip innervation in middle-aged and elderly patients. Contraindications to use of this flap include injury to the neurovascular pedicle of the donor finger, its common vascular bundle or the superficial arterial arch in the palm.

Superficial Branch of the Radial Artery Flaps

A flap based on the superficial branch of the radial artery (SUBRA) and harvesting the thin skin of the thenar eminence was first described as a free flap in 1993. The size of this flap was subsequently increased by harvest of a long, narrow ellipse of skin along the interface between the thenar eminence and the palm. While use as a free flap has continued, both for reconstruction of the tips of the digits and for more extensive palmar resurfacing of the digits, use as a retrograde pedicled flap for thumb reconstruction was introduced in 1997. This pedicled flap may also be used with harvest of the thin skin of the flexor aspect of the wrist, lengthening the pedicle for thumb reconstruction. Although providing excellent skin and subcutaneous tissue replacement and good donor scars in the palm or at the wrist, this flap is viewed generally with some suspicion: the dissection is difficult and risks damage to the palmar cutaneous and recurrent motor branches of the median nerve. The presence of an incomplete superficial palmar arch can complicate raising a viable retrograde pedicled flap. Preoperative Doppler ultrasonography is advised and a need to convert to a free flap is a possibility. Surprisingly, closure of a palmar donor defect of up to 2 cm does not cause contracture of the palm in the way that scarring of wounds over the carpal tunnel does.

RECONSTRUCTION OF SMALL DORSAL DEFECTS

Hatchet Flaps

Indications/Contraindications

For the more common smaller, defects of the dorsum of the thumb of the size of a thumb nail, or slightly smaller, homodigital techniques are very useful. For many of these defects, usually round, or approximating to this shape, the Hatchet flap provides an easy reconstructive option. They are generally simple and quick to execute, avoid involvement of adjacent fingers, and can be used as far distally as the proximal nail fold.

Of 1,077 dorsal wounds of all digits we treated over a 6-year period, 154 digits required flap reconstruction. The dorsal V-Y flap accounted for 42% of the flaps used and was the commonest skin flap used on this surface of the digits, reflecting the relative incidence of defects of this size and shape.

These dorsal V-Y Hatchet flaps are also very useful in replantation, as they allow one to advance the dorsal veins of the proximal part of the thumb to the replant and achieve direct vein anastomoses under good skin cover without recourse to skeletal shortening, vein grafts, or a separate skin cover procedure.

Surgical Technique

The flap is designed as a random dorsal cutaneous flap (Fig. 27-8). A curvilinear incision is made over either the radial or ulnar aspect of the thumb, preserving a broad base on the opposite side of the thumb. As on the palmar surface when using a Moberg flap, a V-Y tail can be added to these flaps

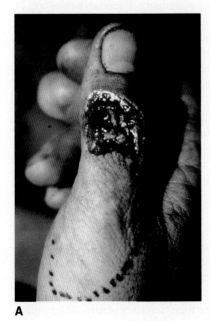

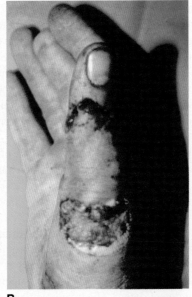

A   B

FIGURE 27-8

A: Preoperative view of a typical "small" skin defect on the dorsum of the thumb. A simple dorsal hatchet flap is marked. **B:** Closure of the defect with this flap, with split skin graft reconstruction of the donor defect. (Reproduced from Elliot D. Specific flaps for the thumb. *Tech Hand Up Extrem Surg.* 2004;8(4): 198–211, with permission.)

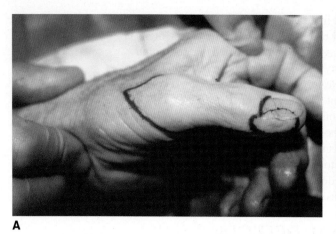

A

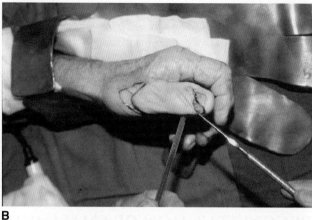

B

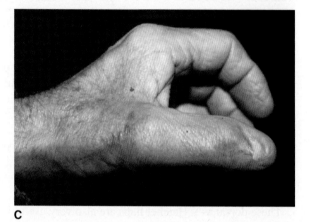

C

FIGURE 27-9

A: Preoperative view of the thumb of a 73-year-old man with a squamous cell carcinoma of the radial lateral fold of the nail. The thumb is marked with a dorsal V-Y hatchet flap for reconstruction. **B:** Intraoperative view of the flap being advanced. **C:** Late postoperative view.

to avoid the need to skin graft the donor site proximally (Fig. 27-9). On this surface of the digit, it is necessary to close the proximal V as a Y to protect the extensor paratenon from desiccation.

Longitudinal Bipedicle Flaps

Indications/Contraindications

About one-fifth of the dorsal digital defects we have reconstructed involved using a new variant of the old technique of longitudinal bipedicle flaps. These were used specifically for long narrow full-thickness dorsal defects following injuries by glass and rotating machinery. Because the dorsum of the digit is a convex surface and the injuring object presents a flat surface to this convexity, the deep structures are only exposed along and immediately adjacent to the midline, with the wound becoming progressively shallower laterally. Next to the central zone of complete loss of the integument is a zone, of variable width, in which the subcutaneous fat is preserved, alive but without skin cover. The extreme dorsolateral integument is commonly uninjured. While the parts of the dorsolateral tissues over which the skin is preserved are, by themselves, often too narrow to create bipedicle flaps that can be brought together successfully in the midline, inclusion, not debridement, of the more medial dorsolateral soft tissues, over which only the skin has been removed, gives a narrower central defect and wider bipedicle flap that allows dorsal closure defect.

Dorsal bipedicled strap flaps may be raised on any part of the digit and these flaps can be used to reconstitute the nail bed in more distal injuries in which a narrow length of the central part of the nail has been removed.

Surgical Technique

Midlateral incisions are made down to the skeleton, with division of Cleland ligaments, taking care to preserve the dorsal branches of the digital nerve that provide innervation of the flap. It is unnecessary to preserve the dorsal branches of the digital artery if they impede medial movement of the flap. The integument is mobilized by blunt dissection superficial to the extensor paratenon from the lateral incisions to the dorsal defect. The bipedicle flaps are then moved centrally with midline

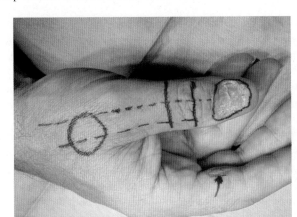

A

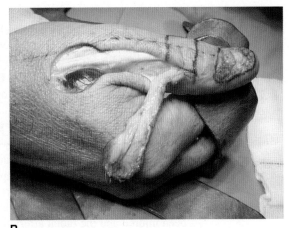

B

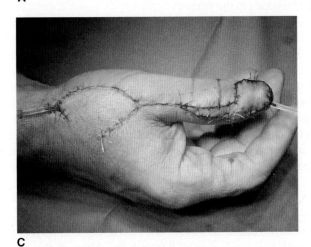

C

FIGURE 27-10

A: A thumb with a badly damaged nail before excision for biopsy. The Brunelli flap and its pedicle have been marked. **B:** The flap has been raised and shows the artery on which it is based on its undersurface. **C:** The flap inset after total excision of the nail complex. The flap has been taken with a "tail" to ease pressure on the pedicle beyond its turning point. The donor site has been closed with a dorsal V-Y hatchet flap. (Reproduced from Elliot D. Homodigital reconstruction of the digits: the perspective of one unit. *Indian J Plast Surg.* 2003;36:106–119, with permission.)

suture of skin or subcutaneous tissue to cover the extensor tendon. The lateral defects and any parts of the central closure that have no skin cover are re-epithelialized under moist antiseptic dressings while mobilizing the finger.

Brunelli (Reverse Dorsoulnar Artery) Flaps

Indications/Contraindications

In 1993, Brunelli and his colleagues in Paris described a very easily and quickly raised homodigital flap based on the dorsoulnar artery of the thumb that is useful for reconstruction of dorsal defects of the tip of the thumb involving all or parts of the nail complex (Fig. 27-10).

Surgical Technique

The presence of the artery may be verified preoperatively with a handheld Doppler probe but is very consistent in its path on the ulnar side of the extensor tendons. Alternatively, measurements illustrated in the original article allow precise location of the artery preoperatively. We raise the flap with a skin tail to reduce the risk of compression of the pedicle just proximal and lateral to the nail fold, which is the tightest part of its course.

Closure of the donor defect with a local V-Y hatchet flap avoids a graft on the obvious dorsal surface of the thumb.

It has more recently been redescribed carrying a segment of vascularized bone from the first metacarpal with it and may prove a useful means of placing vascularized bone at the tip of the thumb without microsurgical transfer from the foot.

Reverse Dorsoradial Flaps

A similar flap has been described that is based on the reversed dorsoradial artery of the thumb. Brunelli reported the dorsoulnar artery to be present in 100% of 25 dorsal thumb dissections and the dorsoradial artery to be present in only 52%, with the former always being the dominant artery and the latter being 'often extremely fine'. Most recent clinical series of these flaps have reported constancy of survival of this flap. While it has the theoretical advantage of avoiding any risk of first web space contracture from closure of the donor defect of the dorsoulnar artery flap, this has not been a problem in our experience. Both flaps can be innervated for reconstruction of the thumb tip but, like the other flaps of origin from the dorsum of the hand, carries skin with poor innervation.

RECONSTRUCTION OF LARGE DORSAL DEFECTS

A very few techniques of reconstruction suffice to cover almost all full-thickness soft tissue losses on the dorsum of the thumb. Complete loss of the dorsal surface cover can be replaced using the reverse radial artery flap or with a reverse posterior interosseous artery flap; both flaps are described in detail elsewhere in the text. The latter is particularly useful if the adjacent tissues of the wrist have been injured and the radial artery flap compromised. The reverse posterior interosseous artery flap can also carry vascularized bone (and tendon) to the thumb.

The posterior interosseous vessel is small and the dissection relatively difficult, requiring microsurgical instrumentation and expertise. However, this flap is mostly safe and does not involve sacrifice of a major blood vessel of the forearm. For which reason, it is preferred to use of the radial forearm flap for larger defects of the dorsum of the thumb, although the latter is useful for complete wraparound of the first ray. When used to reconstruct the dorsum of the thumb, the reverse posterior interosseous artery flap donor site can almost always be closed primarily and then heals with a fine, narrow scar that may be almost invisible in the hair of a male forearm. A modification that we use on all reverse posterior interosseous artery flaps is to construct them with a "tail." This ensures that more perforator branches of the artery reach the flap and reduces the risk of compression of the pedicle where it crosses the dorsum of the wrist, which is the tightest part of its course to the thumb or elsewhere in the hand.

POSTOPERATIVE MANAGEMENT

We remove all dressings and splints from reconstructed hand injuries on the day after surgery to allow washing and dressing of the raw wounds and verification of flap viability. Although this sometimes has to be done with care to avoid tension on flap pedicles, it allows the hand to be bathed in warm water. This both helps general cleaning and debridement of the wounds and is a comfortable environment in which to encourage early mobilization. The wounds are dressed as lightly as possible while maintaining a moist antiseptic presence around any areas without skin. Suture lines that are not oozing are not covered. Sometimes, homodigital and more distant reconstructions require that one or more joints be prevented from moving in a certain direction to take tension off the pedicle. For example, with all of the advancement flaps on the palmar surface, full extension will pull on the flap pedicles, so the thumb is splinted in slight flexion. Conversely, a slightly extended wrist position will ease tension on the pedicle of reverse posterior interosseous artery flaps. Protection of pedicles is continued during bathing and dressing changes by appropriate positioning and guarding with the other hand and between dressing changes by use of thermoplastic splints. Bathing and dressing changes are carried out twice a day with the patients learning to do this themselves as soon as possible.

REHABILITATION

The use of homodigital flaps allows for early mobilization. Motion will be restricted by concomitant tendon, nerve, and bony injuries. However, with stable skeletal fixation, most thumbs can be mobilized using limited active or passive motion protocols under the supervision of a hand therapist within the first 72 hours after surgery. Whenever possible, we avoid techniques of bandaging, splinting, and skeletal fixation that completely immobilize the reconstructed thumb. Over and above the early mobilization under water during dressing changes, mobilization of as much of the thumb and the rest of the hand as possible is continued from this early stage by exercises three or four times daily with the splint in place, albeit sometimes with loosening of some straps, if this is possible without loss of the protection of flap pedicles. The splint provides a solid resting position for the thumb at night and gives the patient confidence that the thumb will not suffer jarring by unexpected contact with external forces. Splints are generally used for 1 to 2 weeks. However, this period can be extended to 4 or 5 weeks, if required to protect structures repaired under the flap. Between activities, the hand is elevated. This regime of elevation and enthusiastic exercising is intended to eliminate edema from the hand as quickly as possible to minimize fibrin restriction of joint and extensor tendon movement. In respect of eliminating edema, open wound management is helpful as the edema leaks out of the open wounds instead of being retained in the digit.

COMPLICATIONS

Major complications include flap loss, partial flap post, infection, and iatrogenic injury to the digital arteries or nerves. Partial flap loss is often best managed by allowing the wound to heal by secondary intention. Total flap loss necessitates the use of a heterodigital island flap, such as the reverse first dorsal metacarpal artery flap, or a larger pedicled forearm flap, such as the posterior interosseous or radial forearm flap. Obviously, use of such flaps adds additional morbidity within the limb but are reliable means of providing soft tissue coverage. An additional downside to the use of heterodigital flaps is that they are often insensate or require a neurorrhaphy to re-establish sensation. Return of sensation in these situations may be dependent on the age of the patient.

RESULTS

The techniques described above have proved adequate to reconstruct the thumb defects we have seen in our practice over the last 20 years. The principle used in the smaller cases, particularly in reconstructing the tip of the thumb, has been to capitalize on the enormous healing capacity of digital skin and assist this, when necessary, by simple local flap reconstructions. These provide the best sensation possible and the best cosmetic profile to the thumb tip. For larger defects, we prefer to use homodigital techniques whenever possible, although there are upper limits to the size of defects that can be reconstructed by these. For any defect, our choice of flaps is, in part, determined by the site, size, and shape of the defect and, in part, by flap reliability and ease of use. The homodigital flaps described above have proved particularly versatile and reliable in the hands of surgeons of varying levels of experience within our unit, although requiring some familiarity with microsurgical technique and instrumentation. They are quick to perform, which can be an advantage following lengthy bony or soft tissue reconstructions. They allow early and independent mobilization of the thumb and the use of local tissue respects the cosmetic principle of reconstruction of "like with like." Donor site morbidity is also limited to the already injured part. When used for digital tip reconstruction, advancement homodigital flaps cannot achieve the sensibility of the original but are durable and intrinsically more likely to restore good sensory function in the tips than most of the reconstructive alternatives. For larger defects, the Littler transfer, the dorsum of the index ray, and the reverse posterior interosseous artery flap are our local work horses. These are discussed in subsequent chapters.

PEARLS AND PITFALLS

- Digits have an astonishing ability to close skin defects of considerable size by a combination of wound contraction and re-epithelialization to give a cosmetic and functional result that cannot be bettered by any surgical procedure.

Neurovascular Tranquilli-Leali or Atasoy-Kleinert Flaps

- Simple, entirely safe, and can be executed quickly for amputations at any length of the thumb to achieve distal bone cover.
- Leave good donor scars on the palmar aspect of the thumb.
- Achieve good sensibility of the thumb tip.
- Less useful in the thumb than in the fingers. In the former, it can only reconstruct defects that are dorsally facing, transverse, or palmar facing with less than 10 degrees of slope.
- Leading edge of the flap being sutured to the nail, or dorsal skin, is often subcutaneous tissue, not skin: provided the bone is covered, the former will epithelialize under moist dressings.
- The interphalangeal joint crease is crossed at an oblique angle to avoid scar contracture.
- The oblique incisions are made by pushing the subcutaneous tissue with the scalpel blade to cut the small subcutaneous fibers and then by gentle spreading of tenotomy scissors to avoid damage to the underlying digital arteries.

Moberg Flaps

- Achieve the best reconstruction of the thumb tip in respect of distal sensibility of the classical flaps.
- Leave good donor scars on the palmar aspect of the thumb.
- Can only provide distal cover for palmar-sloping defects limited to the distal phalangeal segment of the thumb.
- Must include the thenar skin as the proximal "V" of the flap as described above to achieve its full advancement potential and avoid a tight skin closure on proximal suture of the V-Y advancement.
- The flap should be advanced with the IP joint in full extension to reduce the risk of a flexion contracture of this joint.
- The digital nerves to the thumb are very superficial at the level of the MCP joint and care must be taken to identify them and avoid injury during the dissection.

Lateral Pulp Flaps

- Simple, entirely safe, and can be executed quickly.
- Leave no donor scars.
- Useful only for reconstruction of a specific distal thumb injury with soft tissue and skin loss, which is not common.

Side-to-Side Switch Flaps

- Simple, entirely safe, and can be executed quickly.
- Useful only for reconstruction of a specific distal injury with soft tissue and skin loss, which is not common and where reinnervation of the ulnar side of the thumb tip after proximal nerve injury of the ulnar digital nerve is not possible, also a rare injury.

Littler Flaps

- May provide thumb tip sensation when the distal thumb defect is too large for a Moberg-type flap and toe-to-hand transfer is not possible.
- Can give rise to scar contracture where the neurovascular pedicle crosses the palm.
- Leave a less than perfect donor finger, cosmetically and functionally.
- Two-thirds of these flaps do not achieve thumb tip sensation, which is perceived to be always at the tip of the thumb rather than at the tip of the donor finger.
- Nerve disconnection-reconnection reduces the sensibility of the thumb tip.
- A generous cuff of fatty tissue is included around the neurovascular bundle in the flap pedicle. This fat contains the venae comitantes, which are vital to venous drainage of the flap.
- Placing the donor site more laterally on the digit makes the grafted donor site less obvious and reduces the risk of linear scar contracture.

SUBRA Flaps

- Provide good skin and subcutaneous tissue replacement for the palmar aspect and tip of the thumb.
- Leave good donor scars in the palm or at the wrist.
- Can be used as a flow-through flap in cases of segmental digital artery loss.
- The palmar cutaneous branch of the median nerve or a branch of the superficial radial nerve can be connected to a proximal digital nerve of the thumb to provide sensation. However, this risks donor nerve end-neuroma formation and satisfactory sensation can also be obtained without neurorrhaphy, probably as a result of neurotization.
- Difficult and deep dissection, risking local nerve damage in the thenar eminence donor site: advised that a copy of the original paper be reread before raising this flap.
- Take a relatively narrow, small flap in order to achieve donor site closure.

Hatchet Flaps

- Simple, entirely safe, and can be executed quickly.
- Useful in a large number of cases of dorsal digital skin loss.

- Can be used along the length of the dorsum of the thumb.
- Very useful adjunct to replantation/revascularization surgery.
- Blood supply of these flaps is the dorsal branches of the digital arteries; these must be preserved during advancement of the flap, particularly if Cleland ligaments are divided to increase flap advancement.
- The V-to-Y advancement must be sutured to preserve the underlying extensor paratenon from desiccation.

Longitudinal Bipedicle Flaps

- Simple, entirely safe, and can be executed quickly.
- Deal easily with a defect of longitudinal shape, which is not easily reconstructed by other flaps.
- Leaving the lateral skin defects open allows early egress of edema fluid, speeding mobilization of the finger.
- Achieve an excellent cosmetic and functional end point.
- Useful only for reconstruction of a specific shape of dorsal injury, which is not common.

Brunelli (Reverse Dorsoulnar Artery) Flaps

- Good reconstruction of dorsal injuries or resections of the thumb nail bed.
- Closure of the donor defect with a hatchet V-Y flap from the adjacent tissues of the first web space and base of the thumb improves the cosmesis of the donor defect.
- Dissection needs to follow Brunelli's instructions carefully to ensure that the very small dorsal ulnar artery and its distal connection to the ulnar digital artery of the thumb are included in the pedicle (we advise that a copy of the original article be reviewed before raising this flap).
- Poor innervation, so does not achieve a good thumb tip reconstruction in respect of sensibility.

Reverse Dorsoradial Flaps

- Good reconstruction of dorsal injuries or resections of the thumb nail bed.
- Closure of the donor defect with a hatchet V-Y flap from the adjacent tissues of the first web space and base of the thumb improves the cosmesis of the donor defect.
- Has no particular advantage over use of the reverse dorsoulnar artery flap, with a questionable constancy of its feeding artery.

RECOMMENDED READING

Allen MJ. Conservative management of finger tip injuries. *Hand.* 1980;12:257–265.

Atasoy E, Ioakimidis E, Kasdan ML, et al. Reconstruction of the amputated finger tip with a triangular volar flap. *J Bone Joint Surg Am.* 1970;52:921–926.

Bakhach J, Guimberteau JC, Panconi B. The Gigogne flap: an original technique for an optimal pulp reconstruction. *J Hand Surg Eur.* 2009;34:227–234.

Bao QY, Xiao CW, Peng F, et al. Restoration of thumb sensibility with innervated reverse homodigital dorsoradial flap. *J Reconstr Microsurg.* 2014;30:15–20.

Brunelli F, Gilbert A. Vascularisation of the thumb. *Hand Clin.* 2001;17:123–138.

Brunelli F, Vigasio A, Valenti P, et al. Arterial anatomy and clinical application of the dorsoulnar flap of the thumb. *J Hand Surg Am.* 1999;24:803–811.

Cavadas PC. Reverse osteocutaneous dorsoulnar thumb flap. *Plast Reconstr Surg.* 2003;111:326–329.

Costa H, Smith R, McGrouther DA. Thumb reconstruction by the posterior interosseous flap. *Br J Plast Surg.* 1988;41:228–233.

Elliot D, Moiemen NS, Jigjinni VS. The neurovascular Tranquilli-Leali flap. *J Hand Surg Br.* 1995;20:815–823.

Elliot D, Jigjinni VS. The lateral pulp flap. *J Hand Surg Br.* 1993;18:423–426.

Elliot D, Southgate CM, Staino JJ. A homodigital switch flap to restore sensation to the ulnar border of the thumb tip. *J Hand Surg Br.* 2003;28:409–413.

Elliot D, Wilson Y. V–Y advancement of the entire volar soft tissue of the thumb in distal reconstruction. *J Hand Surg Br.* 1993;18:399–402.

Elliot D. Specific flaps for the thumb. *Tech Hand Up Extrem Surg.* 2004;8:198–211.

Gaul JS. A palmar-hinged flap for reconstruction of traumatic thumb defects. *J Hand Surg Am.* 1987;12:415–421.

Iwuagwu FC, Orkar SK, Siddiqui A. Reconstruction of volar skin and soft tissue defects of the digits including the pulp: experience with the free SUPBRA flap. *J Plast Reconstr Aesthet Surg.* 2015;68:26–34.

Kamei K, Ide Y, Kimura T. A new free thenar flap. *Plast Reconstr Surg.* 1993;92:1380–1384.

Littler JW. Neurovascular pedicle transfer of tissue in reconstructive surgery of the hand. *J Bone Joint Surg Am.* 1956;38:917.

Moberg E. Aspects of sensation in reconstructive surgery of the upper extremity. *J Bone Joint Surg Am.* 1964;46:817–825.

Moschella F, Cordova A. Reverse homodigital dorsal radial flap of the thumb. *Plast Reconstr Surg.* 2006;117:920–926.

O'Brien B. Neurovascular island pedicle flaps for terminal amputations and digital scars. *Br J Plast Surg.* 1968;21: 258–261.

Pelissier P, Pistre V, Casoli V, et al. Dorso-ulnar osteocutaneous reverse flow flap of the thumb: anatomy and clinical application. *J Hand Surg Br.* 2003;26:207–211.

Pilz SM, Valenti PP, Harguindeguy ED. Free sensory or retrograde pedicled fasciocutaneous thenar flap: anatomic study and clinical application. *Handchir Mikrochir Plast Chir.* 1997;29:243–246.

Sun YC, Chen QZ, Chen J, et al. Reverse dorsoradial flaps for thumb coverages show increased sensory recovery with smaller flap sizes. *J Reconstr Microsurg.* 2015;31:426–433.

Yii NW, Elliot D. Bipedicle strap flaps in reconstruction of longitudinal dorsal skin defects of the digits. *Plast Reconstr Surg.* 1999;103:1205–1211.

Yii NW, Elliot D. Dorsal V–Y advancement flaps in digital reconstruction. *J Hand Surg Br.* 1994;19:91–97.

Zheng D-W, Li Z-C, Shi R-J, et al. Thumb reconstruction via a pedicled flap based on the superficial radial artery from the wrist crease area. *J Plast Reconstr Aesthet Surg.* 2015;68:1581–1587.

PART V

MANAGEMENT OF SOFT TISSUES OF THE LOWER EXTREMITY

28 Soft Tissue Management Following Traumatic Injury to the Femur

Thomas F. Higgins and Lance Jacobson

Open injuries of the femur and thigh are common. However, the need for major soft tissue coverage in this area in the setting of trauma is uncommon, due to the generous surrounding muscular envelope. Soft tissue coverage of the femur can be a concern in certain situations such as power takeoff injuries or pedestrians struck by motor vehicles; however, the majority of these defects may be covered with skin grafts, and the need for vascularized free tissue transfer is unusual. Despite this, there are several components to soft tissue management in this area that may be used during exposure to the proximal and distal portions of the femur. Simple alterations in established techniques can lead to improved postoperative contour, improved soft tissue coverage of hardware, and decreased rates of postoperative infection and stiffness following both elective and emergent surgical procedures.

This chapter covers four major areas of concern with regard to soft tissue management in the thigh:

- The approach to the proximal femoral shaft and intertrochanteric zone
- The approach for the repair of supracondylar and intra-articular distal femur fractures
- Exposure for the treatment of open femur fractures
- The management of posttraumatic arthrofibrosis of the knee with the use of a Judet quadricepsplasty

APPROACH TO THE LATERAL PROXIMAL FEMUR

Indications/Contraindications

Fractures of the proximal femur, whether femoral neck or intertrochanteric, constitute the majority of all femur fractures. The soft tissue management issues in this portion of the proximal femur are the relative dearth of coverage over the greater trochanter and the area of the femur just distal to the vastus lateralis. Frequently, plate and screw implants (such as dynamic hip screw) and laterally based orthopedic constructs will be prominent and symptomatic, particularly in thin patients. An approach that maximizes soft tissue coverage over the lateral aspect of the proximal femur and restores the most normal anatomy will be described. Rather than a direct lateral approach cutting through the vastus lateralis, which has been frequently advocated for this operation, a simple modi-fication provides a more anatomic dissection and a friendlier soft tissue reconstruction.

Patient Positioning

The patient is positioned as desired for ultimate reduction and fixation goals.

Surgery

A direct lateral approach begins 1 cm proximal to the vastus ridge and extends as far distally as necessary for osteosynthesis. On the sagittal plane, the incision should be 1 cm posterior to the midcoronal point of the femur (Fig. 28-1). Dissection is taken down to the iliotibial band, and this is divided sharply in line with its fibers with a knife, slightly longer than the skin incision (Fig. 28-2).

A gentle sweeping motion with a sponge will clear trochanteric bursa or areolar soft tissue that lies in this layer. Particularly fibrotic bursal tissue may need to be excised with scissors (Fig. 28-3). This will reveal quite clearly the proximal extent of the vastus lateralis and its insertion at the vastus ridge and the confluence with the distal extent of the vastus medialis tendon. Rather than directly incising the vastus lateralis in the midsagittal point of the femur, a J-shaped incision is performed. Leaving several millimeters of the vastus lateralis tendon still attached to the vastus ridge, the ten-don is incised from its anterior extent posteriorly until connecting with the lateral intermuscular septum (Fig. 28-4). The dissection is then taken through the most posterior fibers of the vastus lateralis extending from proximal to distal, just anterior to the lateral intermuscular septum. The vastus tendon is tagged with a heavy braided nonabsorbable suture before being detached from the vastus ridge (see Fig. 28-4A). As the dissection extends greater than 5 cm distal to the vastus ridge, the first perforating branch off the profunda femoris will be encountered penetrating the lateral

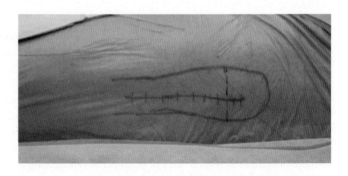

FIGURE 28-1

Incision drawn over the greater trochanter. *Dotted transverse line* represents the vastus ridge.

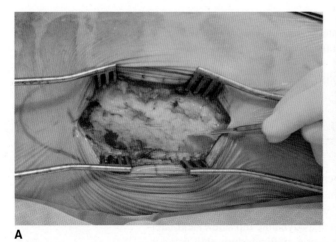

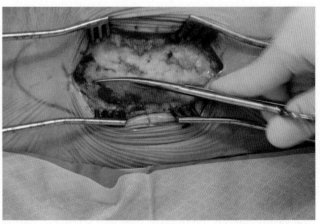

A   B

FIGURE 28-2

A: The iliotibial band is incised in line with its fibers. **B:** Alternatively, the iliotibial band is divided from proximal to distal with curved Mayo scissors.

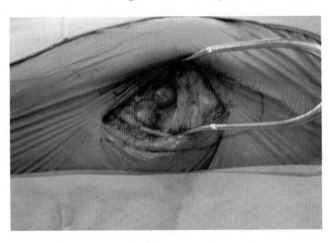

FIGURE 28-3
Fibrotic trochanteric bursa may need to
be excised.

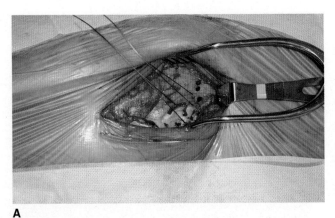

A

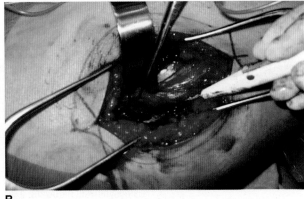

B

FIGURE 28-4

A: Proximal tendon of vastus lateralis is to be incised in a posteriorly based "J" shaped incision. **B:** Vastus lateralis origin is elevated in along the "J" shaped incision.

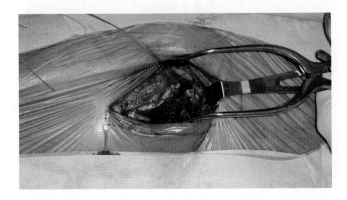

FIGURE 28-5
Lateralis is retracted anteriorly with
tagging sutures.

intermuscular septum. Care should be taken to isolate and ligate or cauterize these perforators prior to their transection. The dissection through the vastus muscle should be slightly anterior to the lateral intramuscular septum at this level, so that any perforators of the profunda femoris that are divided do not retract to the posterior aspect of the septum, which is difficult to access from here. A gentle sweeping motion under the muscle with an elevator from posterior to anterior along the proximal femur will allow reflection of the vastus lateralis in an anterior direction (Fig. 28-5). The periosteum and deepest soft tissues should not be stripped off the femur. For ideal visualization at this point, a Bennett retractor is placed anterior to the femur, and an assistant holds this forward (Fig. 28-6). Osteosynthesis proceeds as planned.

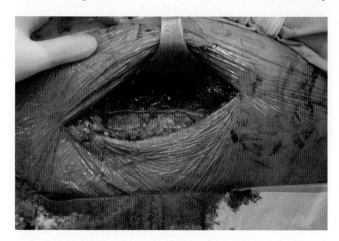

FIGURE 28-6

Bennett retractor is used to reflect the vastus anteriorly.

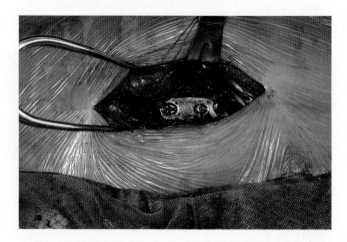

FIGURE 28-7

Osteosynthesis hardware, after placement, is covered by vastus.

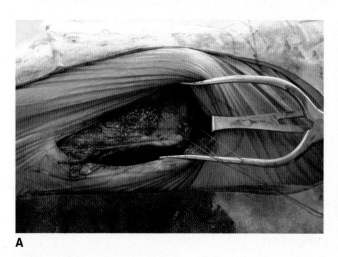

A

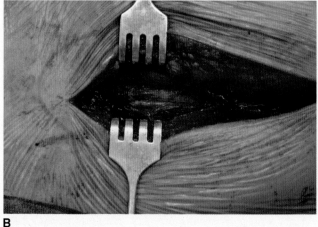

B

FIGURE 28-8

A: Vastus lateralis pulled back to its origin at the vastus ridge. **B:** Through the closing iliotibial band, repair of the vastus origin can be visualized.

The Bennett retractors make for easy retraction and permit reduction and fixation. At the conclusion of the procedure, Bennett retractors are simply removed, and gravity allows the vastus to fall back into place, padding and directly covering the implant (Fig. 28-7). The most proximal origin of the vastus lateralis is then repaired back to its tendinous origin with a heavy braided nonabsorbable suture (Fig. 28-8). The posterior aspect of the vastus lateralis does not need to be repaired. The iliotibial band is repaired with interrupted nonabsorbable suture, and the skin may be closed according to surgeon preference (Fig. 28-9).

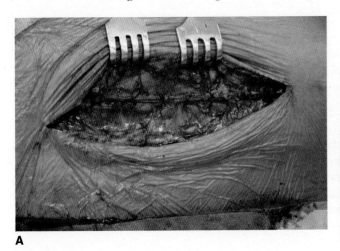

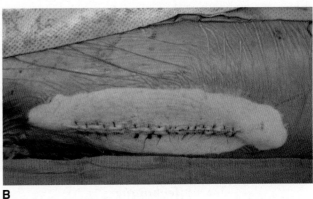

A   B

FIGURE 28-9

A: Iliotibial band is repaired with interrupted nonabsorbable suture. **B:** Skin closure at completion of intertrochanteric fracture osteosynthesis.

This approach is most helpful for the placement of a dynamic hip screw, blade plate, or laterally based femoral plating construct. It offers less scarring, as the muscle belly has not been interrupted. This should also be a more functional repair, as less damage presumably has been done to the vastus origin by dividing it and repairing it, rather than by directly insulting it with a midgastric approach.

Postoperative Management

In the elderly population with intertrochanteric hip fractures, patients are generally allowed to bear weight as tolerated to facilitate mobilization. The first 2 weeks postoperatively focus on range of motion of the hip and knee and gait training with assistive devices as necessary. At 2 weeks postoperatively, strengthening of the abductors, hip flexors, and quadriceps is added to the regimen.

In younger patients, or fractures with a subtrochanteric component, weight bearing may be protected initially and advanced as desirable by the treating surgeon.

Complications

Complications of operations through this approach are generally related to the osteosynthesis, and these may be avoided somewhat with careful attention to achieving reduction and adherence to correct placement of implants.

APPROACH TO THE DISTAL FEMUR AND KNEE

Indications/Contraindications

Multiple variations on parapatellar and lateral parapatellar approaches have been described. Similar to the muscle-sparing approach described for the proximal femur, the "swashbuckler" approach described by Starr et al. at Parkland Hospital offers excellent visualization of the joint for anatomic fixation of intra-articular fractures while preserving the vastus and quadriceps with no intramuscular dissection. Criticism of this approach has centered on soft tissue stripping of the distal femoral metaphysis, but this is by no means mandatory. Simply put, this is a "vastus-sparing" approach to the lateral distal femur.

This approach offers the advantage of not interfering with or dividing the extensor mechanism while gaining adequate visualization of the joint space. With proximal and distal retraction, the intervening metaphyseal soft tissues should be left largely undisturbed to enhance healing of comminuted metaphyseal bone.

Recently, Beltran described a "mini-swashbuckler" approach. As described by the author, this approach utilizes a similar deep dissection as the traditional swashbuckler but uses a smaller lateral skin incision. This allows access to the articular surface of the distal femur, including the medial compartment and posterior condyles, without further extensile measures. Using this limited approach in a cadaveric model, they were able to visualize 87% of the articular surface compared to the traditional swashbuckler approach.

Below, the more traditional lateral vastus-sparing approach is described in detail.

Surgery

Patient Positioning

The patient is positioned supine. A bump may be placed under the hip to facilitate internal rotation of the lower extremity, if this is desired. The author prefers to not bump up the ipsilateral hip, so that the rotational profile of the lower extremity may be accurately assessed at the conclusion of fixation. The lower extremity is prepared and draped free. A sterile bump may be used under the knee to facilitate exposure and/or reduction.

Technique

The skin incision starts at the insertion of the patellar ligament and extends directly cephalad to the apex of the patella. It then extends lateral and proximal toward the lateral intermuscular septum (Fig. 28-10). A full-thickness flap of skin and subcutaneous tissue is elevated off the extensor fascia. The lateral margins of the patella and patellar ligament are identified distally. Proximally, the lateral margin of the vastus lateralis is identified.

The knee capsule is incised immediately along the lateral aspect of the patellar ligament (Fig. 28-11). Care must be taken not to cut the anterior horn of the lateral meniscus. Dissection

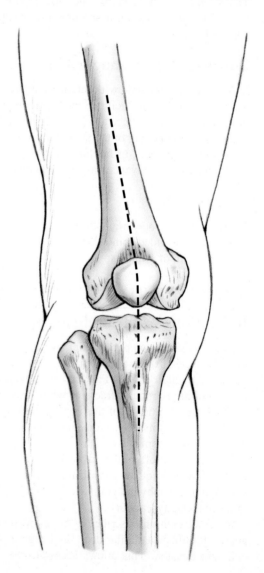

FIGURE 28-10

The skin incision for the "swashbuckler" approach to the distal femur. (Redrawn from Starr AJ, Jones AL, Reinert CM. The "swashbuckler": a modified anterior approach for fractures of the distal femur. *J Orthop Trauma.* 1999;13(2):138–140.)

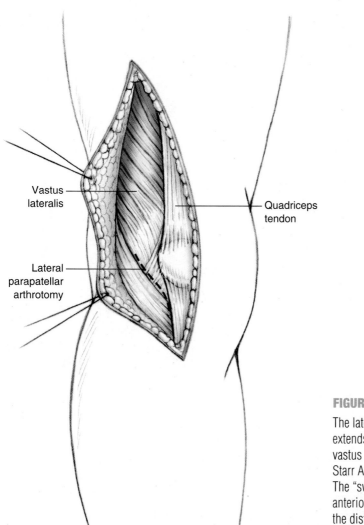

Vastus
lateralis

Quadriceps
tendon

Lateral
parapatellar
arthrotomy

FIGURE 28-11

The lateral parapatellar arthrotomy
extends to the lateral margin of the
vastus lateralis. (Redrawn from
Starr AJ, Jones AL, Reinert CM.
The "swashbuckler": a modified
anterior approach for fractures of
the distal femur. *J Orthop Trauma*.
1999;13(2):138–140.)

is taken directly along the lateral margin of the patella, leaving a small cuff of tissue for eventual repair. At the superolateral shoulder of the patella, the deep dissection extends laterally toward the lateral intermuscular septum. The vastus lateralis is thus spared and is elevated anteriorly off the lateral intermuscular septum. As dissection nears the femur, perforating branches of the profunda femoris artery must be identified and ligated. These will be located every 3 to 4 cm approximately 1 cm lateral to the femoral cortex.

Right angle retractors may be placed at the level of the quadriceps tendon for medial excursion of the quadriceps and patella (Fig. 28-12). These retractors in combination will allow adequate visualization of the femur for reconstruction. If possible, no retractors at all should be placed medially at the level of the metaphysis, as most techniques demand preservation of the medial soft tissues to promote healing of metaphyseal comminution. Adequate visualization may easily be achieved with retractors placed proximal and distal to this area.

For full visualization of the femoral condylar articular surface, the patella may be everted. This may be facilitated by elevating a small proximal portion of the most lateral insertion of the patellar ligament off the tibia. This must be done with care not to elevate so much of the ligament that it will jeopardize the continuity of the extensor mechanism or slow rehabilitation. Osteosynthesis is then performed.

Closure is achieved with an interrupted nonabsorbable braided suture repair of the lateral parapatellar retinaculum and capsule lateral to the patellar ligament. If desired, a drain may be placed in the knee and run along the lateral intermuscular septum, exiting the skin proximally. Subcutaneous tissue and skin are repaired according to surgeon preference.

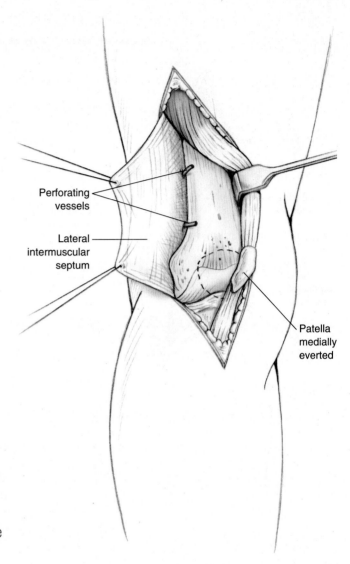

Perforating vessels

Lateral intermuscular septum

Patella medially everted

FIGURE 28-12

With quad retracted and patella everted, visualization of the distal femur is excellent. (Redrawn from Starr AJ, Jones AL, Reinert CM. The "swashbuckler": a modified anterior approach for fractures of the distal femur. *J Orthop Trauma.* 1999;13(2):138–140.)

Postoperative Management

Assuming stable osteosynthesis has been achieved, immediate range of motion is initiated. A physical therapist may perform passive supervised range of motion, 0 to 90 degrees, with no strengthening and no active quadriceps. Alternatively, a continuous passive motion machine may be used. Quadriceps strengthening begins at 6 weeks postoperatively, and weight bearing is advanced according to surgeon judgment.

Complications

Potential complications of complex distal femur fractures include infection, nonunion, and arthrofibrosis. Judet quadricepsplasty for loss of knee motion will be addressed later in this chapter.

SURGICAL EXPOSURE OF OPEN FEMORAL FRACTURES

Indications/Contraindications

Given the wide girth of soft tissues around the femur, an open fracture by definition implies a high-energy injury. There are compelling data to support early irrigation and debridement of higher-grade open fractures for the prevention of infection. Small lacerations or puncture wounds are often the telltale signs of an open fracture and should not be overlooked; these relatively small surface injuries often disguise a significant deeper soft tissue insult. Open fractures of the distal femur in particular will present with a very small opening of the skin where the femoral shaft has pistoned distally to penetrate the vastus medialis obliquus or the vastus lateralis and the skin (Fig. 28-13).

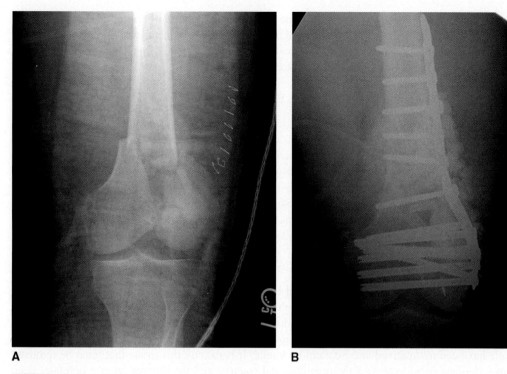

A   B

FIGURE 28-13

A: The skin staples demonstrate the length of the *inadequate* incision used to debride this open intracondylar distal femur fracture. **B:** This inadequate index debridement leads to a long and complicated course of treatment, including a deep infection and the placement of antibiotic beads.

Frequently, the treatment of open intra-articular distal femur fractures will necessitate an aggressive irrigation and debridement at the time of presentation and transarticular spanning external fixation for temporizing stabilization. Even in the hemodynamically unstable trauma patient, early stabilization of the femur is often advantageous. Prolonged maintenance of a patient in Hare traction is not advisable given the attendant complications of skin breakdown and sciatic nerve palsy, and so spanning external fixation is recommended over prolonged traction.

The initial management of these fractures should not include the placement of a pulsatile irrigation catheter through the small traumatic wound. This may succeed only in further embedding debris in an open fracture site and will certainly not provide an adequate debridement of the injured soft tissues that would ultimately be responsible for the development of a deep infection. Adequate debridement of an open femoral fracture *demands* significant surgical extension of the trauma wounds.

Based on the most recent results of the FLOW trial, following extension of the wound, the choice of device used to deliver irrigation does not show statistical significance. Reoperation rates following open fracture are similar whether using high, low, or very low pressure devices. With regard to irrigation solution, the same study shows that normal saline is a low-cost, effective alternative that may have lower rates of complications when compared to castile soap.

Surgical debridement is paramount in open fracture management. The goal is a clean wound with removal of any nonviable tissues. A sterile tourniquet may be applied but should only be used when necessary. Not inflating the tourniquet allows identification of viable tissues and minimizes ischemia to the already traumatized tissues. Skin and subcutaneous tissues should debrided back to bleeding edges. Using a muscle's bleeding, color, consistency, and contractility can help identify viability. Cortical bone fragments that have lost vascularity may be used to assist with reduction. However, completely stripped nonarticular skeletal elements should be discarded prior to final osteosynthesis. Effort should be made to preserve articular fragments, however, provided they are large enough to assist in reconstruction of the involved joint.

How aggressive to be with debridement of open femur fractures remains unclear. Recently, a less aggressive protocol has been supported by Ricci et al. This protocol involved debridement of grossly contaminated bone with retention of other bone fragments and no use of antibiotic cement spacers. This resulted in increased healing after the index procedure, less reoperations, and no difference in infection rates when compared to a more aggressive protocol. Although this lends support for a less aggressive debridement, rigidly defining the "extent of debridement" is difficult, and further studies are needed to clarify the matter.

The author's preferred technique is detailed below.

Preoperative Planning

Initial debridement entails some insight by the initially treating surgeon into the definitive fixation plan. Frequently, the entire approach for the eventual repair of an open femur fracture may be performed at the time of debridement, particularly if this will include plating of a distal femur fracture. Open fractures of the femoral diaphysis may still be treated quite successfully with intramedullary nailing after wound extension and debridement. Regardless of eventual fixation plan, proximal and distal extension of soft tissue wounds is always necessary.

Surgery

Extension of the skin laceration is performed both proximally and distally down to the investing fascia of the thigh, which is always torn due to the preexisting trauma. Fracture exposure will often require intramuscular dissection. Specific landmarks or structures to avoid will vary depending on location of the open wounds. Extensive dissection through muscle may be required, but most of this muscle has been traumatized and may not be viable. It is exactly this tissue that must be removed for the adequate debridement of the open femoral fracture and the prevention of a potential deep infection.

If, following aggressive irrigation and debridement, it is determined that a transarticular spanning external fixation is going to be used for definitive or temporary stabilization, consideration must be given to the underlying soft tissues. In applying joint spanning external fixation, one should be careful to place the femoral pins proximal enough that the eventual internal fixation is not communicating with the pin sites if at all possible. Femoral pins may be introduced directly anterior through the quadriceps, anterolateral, or directly lateral. Tibial pins are generally introduced anteromedially. Spanning external fixation may be maintained for several weeks while waiting for physiologic or soft tissue stabilization. Nowotarski et al. demonstrated in nonspanning external fixation that patients could safely undergo one-stage conversion to internal fixation without significant infectious problems. However, waiting much longer than 3 weeks may create problems in having to take down interval callus formation and makes the articular reconstruction more difficult.

Postoperative Management

In an effort to stabilize the soft tissue envelope, initiation of range of motion may be delayed after open fracture of the distal femur. If an open distal femur fracture has been spanned with an external fixator, subsequent debridements may be necessary, and the exact timing of definitive internal fixation is at the surgeon's discretion.

If a thorough debridement and immediate intramedullary nailing of an open diaphyseal fracture has been completed, range of motion and weight bearing may be initiated right away.

Complications

The prompt and aggressive debridement of open fractures is an attempt to avoid the most obvious complication, osteomyelitis. Further complications from open fractures include knee stiffness and nonunion. In cases with a segmental bone loss, or a high degree of metaphyseal comminution, patients may be informed at the time of definitive fixation that an elective bone grafting procedure will be performed 4 to 6 weeks later. The author prefers to use proximal tibial cancellous autograft, as it is biologically active, is a low-morbidity harvest site when compared to iliac crest, and limits the affected area of the patient to a zone already involved in the injury. For large segmental defects, a cement spacer may be placed at the time of index fixation, with the plan to exploit the "biologic membrane" formed around this spacer to promote healing at the time of subsequent bone grafting.

JUDET QUADRICEPSPLASTY

Indications/Contraindications

Frequently, patients who have suffered comminuted intra-articular injuries of the distal femur or supracondylar femur will suffer from poor range of motion secondary to posttraumatic scarring and contracture. Various methods have been proposed for the treatment of this loss of flexion at the knee. Arthroscopic lysis, closed manipulation, and quadriceps tendon lengthening have all been advocated. For particularly stubborn cases of posttraumatic arthrofibrosis and quadriceps contracture leading to loss of knee flexion, the author finds the Judet quadricepsplasty to be the most effective way to regain functional motion of the knee.

This approach recognizes that, in addition to the skeletal injury apparent on the radiographs, there was great soft tissue damage sustained at the time of distal femoral fracture. It is this damage to the rectus and vastus musculature that is at least in part responsible for the subsequent loss of range of motion. Arthrofibrosis and capsular contracture also contribute to posttraumatic stiffness and are addressed by this operation.

Judet attributed the stiffness of the knee to four principal anatomic reasons. First was adhesion of the suprapatellar pouch deep to the quadriceps with tethering of the patella. Second was retraction of the parapatellar fibrous elements and intra-articular adhesions. Third was adherence of the vastus intermedius muscle of the femur. Fourth was degenerative fibrosis of the quadriceps. The surgical procedure is based on a sequential release of these various parts of the contracture. Range of motion is to be assessed after each stage, and the operation proceeds until the desired results are achieved or maximum range of motion is achieved after completion of all steps.

Preoperative Planning

An epidural catheter is placed preoperatively. General and epidural anesthetic are used intraoperatively, but the regional anesthesia will help with patient compliance and tolerance with postoperative continuous passive motion. The operation entails extensive excision of scar tissue, and blood loss may be significant. Type and crossmatch should be obtained prior to initiation of surgery. The patients should be counseled that they will make gains in range of motion but will likely end up maintaining somewhat less flexion than that which was achieved intraoperatively.

Surgery

Range of motion is assessed on administration of the general anesthetic (Fig. 28-14). Two incisions are generally used (Fig. 28-15). The sterile prep should include the entire hindquarter, as the final steps of the surgery require access to the anterior hip. A sterile tourniquet may be applied in the field, for use intermittently to diminish blood loss, but this restricts excursion of the quad and as such cannot be used throughout the operation.

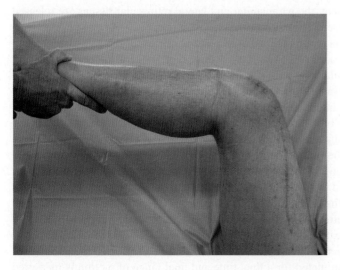

FIGURE 28-14

Range of motion is assessed preoperatively.

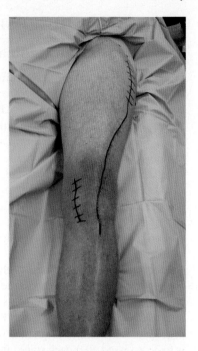

FIGURE 28-15
Two incisions planned preoperatively for Judet quadricepsplasty.

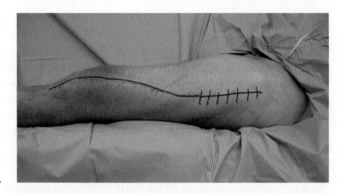

FIGURE 28-16
Lateral incision planned as extension
(*dotted line*) off existing scar (*solid line*).

The first is a medial parapatellar approach. This allows access to the medial aspect of the patellar tendon, the suprapatellar pouch medially, and the medial gutter. The medial retinaculum is released, and adhesions of the medial joint and suprapatellar pouch are excised directly with a knife.

The second incision often follows the lateral incision made for the operative repair of the fracture (Fig. 28-16). This will usually follow the lateral aspect of the patella ligament through the lateral patellar retinaculum and proximal up along the lateral intramuscular septum to the level of the greater trochanter. In the distal segment, the parapatellar and lateral retinacular tissues are released and intra-articular adhesions are excised. The patella is freed until it may be easily lifted off the femoral condyles (Fig. 28-17). Scar tissue along the medial and lateral aspects of the patellar ligament, particularly distally, would likewise need to be excised. At this point, range of motion is checked, and the quadriceps should be manipulated at each subsequent step to assess progress in knee range of motion. The vastus lateralis is elevated from the linea aspera, and perforating vessels are ligated as they are encountered. The vastus intermedius is then lifted extraperiosteally from the front and side of the femur (Fig. 28-18). Much of the intermedius may be replaced by scar and fibrotic tissue, and this may be excised without significant functional impact (Fig. 28-19). Frequently, one will find heterotopic bone formation within the muscle bellies, and this may be excised along with fibrotic muscle tissue in an effort to regain length. Once again, the knee is manipulated and range assessed.

Next, the vastus lateralis is released from its femoral origin superolaterally, and the rectus femoris may be released from its origin on the anterior capsule and anterior inferior iliac spine. Adequate exposure here is difficult and may often be best obtained with large right angle retractors held by an assistant positioned on the opposite side of the table (Fig. 28-20). The proximal quad origin release allows distal excursion of much of the quadriceps mechanism in an effort to regain range of motion at the knee. The knee is manipulated for a final time and final range of motion is measured

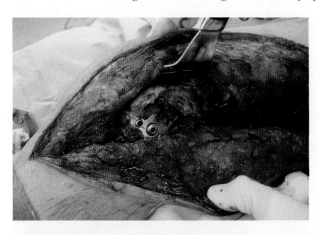

FIGURE 28-17
Supracondylar zone shows dense fibrotic scar tissue.

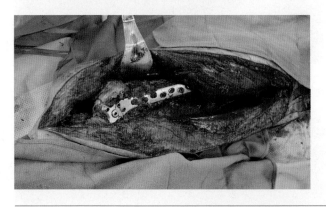

FIGURE 28-18
Scar tissue release mobilizes the extensor mechanism off the anterior femur.

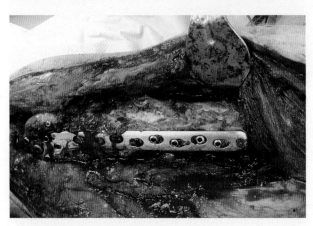

FIGURE 28-19
Heterotopic bone may scar the quadriceps to the femur and must be excised.

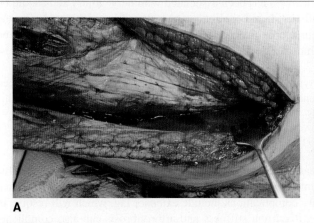

A   B

FIGURE 28-20
A: Dissection may be extended up to the level of the vastus lateralis origin and the rectus origin anteriorly. **B:** With release of the rectus proximally, ultimate excursion of the extensor mechanism may be achieved.

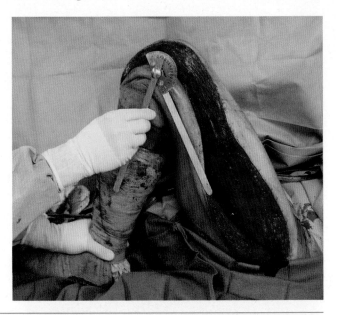

FIGURE 28-21

Ultimate range of motion should be assessed before and after closure.

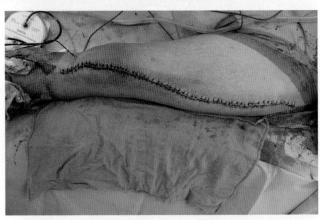

FIGURE 28-22

Final skin closure of the lateral incision.

(Fig. 28-21). Only the skin is closed, and a drain is used (Fig. 28-22). Given the somewhat sanguineous nature of the dissection along the well-perfused margins of scar tissue, postoperative hematoma must be guarded against, and drain use is encouraged.

Postoperative Management

The knee may be immobilized in a position of flexion so that, on awakening from anesthetic, the patient may have some idea of what the range of motion may be achieved. However, immobilization in hyperflexion (greater than 100 degrees) has been associated with nerve injury and should be avoided. Epidural anesthetic is generally used, and continuous passive motion is initiated after the recovery room. The drain is removed in approximately 48 hours. Due to the bleeding that may be encountered in dissection of scar and muscle, we have found that blood transfusion is often necessary before discharge.

No postoperative immobilization is typically used at the time of discharge, and patients may need crutches for ambulation, as they frequently will have a functional extensor lag postoperatively. This extensor lag usually resolves over time.

Complications/Results

The most common immediate complication following this procedure is hematoma formation. This complication can be minimized with intraoperative hemostasis and with the routine use of closed suction drains in all patients. Secondary complications include extensor lag, which will resolve in most cases with postoperative therapy. Recurrent stiffness and arthrofibrosis can also complicate postoperative results; however, the results of this operation in the literature have been encouraging, with total gains in range of motion between 55 and 69 degrees in the largest studies.

SUMMARY

The soft tissue around the femur and thigh segment is adequate enough to sustain extensive trauma without requiring free tissue transfer. Some of the techniques listed in this chapter may facilitate the correct handling of the soft tissues, help to prevent infection in the setting of open fracture, or help patients to regain motion after a comminuted knee injury.

PEARLS AND PITFALLS

- During the approach to the proximal femur, use of a posteriorly based J-shaped incision rather than direct lateral incision of the vastus lateralis provides less disruption of the muscle improving soft tissue coverage of the implant.
- When positioning the patient for lateral approach to the distal femur, the lower extremity should be draped free and bumps should be avoided to allow an accurate assessment of the rotational profile of the femur.
- In the lateral vastus-sparing approach to the distal femur, medially placed retractors at the level of the metaphysis should be avoided to prevent injury to the blood supply (and healing) of metaphyseal comminution.
- In open fractures, proximal and distal extension of soft tissue wounds is always necessary. With advanced planning, the approach for eventual fixation of the fracture may be accomplished at the time of initial debridement.
- Given the sanguineous nature of the dissection during Judet quadricepsplasty, preoperative type and crossmatch is mandatory and postoperative drain use is encouraged.
- Following Judet quadricepsplasty, epidural anesthesia and continuous passive motion devices can be used to maintain the hard-won knee range of motion.
- During the approach to the proximal femur, posterior dissection of the vastus lateralis right off the lateral intramuscular septum could result in transection of perforator vessels behind the septum, making hemostasis difficult.
- In distal femur intra-articular fractures, the articular surface should be reduced before reducing the condyles to the shaft or the exposure of the joint becomes much more difficult.
- Following Judet quadricepsplasty, immobilization in hyperflexion (greater than 100 degrees) has been used to maintain the newly gained flexion. This should definitely be avoided, and this has been associated with nerve injury.

RECOMMENDED READING

Ali AM, Villafuerte J, Hashmi M, et al. Judet's quadricepsplasty, surgical technique, and results in limb reconstruction. *Clin Orthop Relat Res.* 2003;(415):214–220.
Bellemans J, Steenwerckx A, Brabants K, et al. The Judet quadricepsplasty: a retrospective analysis of 16 cases. *Acta Orthop Belg.* 1996;62(2):79–82.
Beltran MJ, Blair JA, Huh J, et al. Articular exposure with the swashbuckler versus a "mini-swashbuckler" approach. *Injury Int J Care Injured.* 2013;44:189–193.
Daoud H, O'Farrell T, Cruess RL. Quadricepsplasty: the Judet technique and results of six cases. *J Bone Joint Surg Br.* 1982;64(2):194–197.
Giannoudis PV, Papakostidis C, Roberts C. A review of the management of open fractures of the tibia and femur. *J Bone Joint Surg Br.* 2006;88(3):281–289.
Gustilo RB, Anderson JT. Prevention of infection in the treatment of one thousand and twenty-five open fractures of long bones: retrospective and prospective analyses. *J Bone Joint Surg Am.* 1976;58(4):453–458.
Gustilo RB, Merkow RL, Templeman D. The management of open fractures. *J Bone Joint Surg Am.* 1990;72(2):299–304.
Judet R. Mobilisation of the stiff knee. *J Bone Joint Surg Br.* 1959;41B:856–857.
Koval KJ, Sala DA, Kummer FJ, et al. Postoperative weight-bearing after a fracture of the femoral neck or an intertrochanteric fracture. *J Bone Joint Surg Am.* 1998;80(3):352–356.
Martinet O, Cordey J, Harder Y, et al. The epidemiology of fractures of the distal femur. *Injury.* 2000;31(suppl 3):C62–C63.
Merchan EC, Myong C. Quadricepsplasty: the Judet technique and results of 21 posttraumatic cases. *Orthopedics.* 1992;15(9):1081–1085.
Nowotarski PJ, Turen CH, Brumback RJ, et al. Conversion of external fixation to intramedullary nailing for fractures of the shaft of the femur in multiply injured patients. *J Bone Joint Surg Am.* 2000;82(6):781–788.
Oliveira VG, D'Elia LF, Tirico LE, et al. Judet quadricepsplasty in the treatment of posttraumatic knee rigidity: long-term outcomes of 45 cases. *J Trauma Acute Care Surg.* 2012;72(2):E77–E80.
Pelissier P, Masquelet AC, Bareille R, et al. Induced membranes secrete growth factors including vascular and osteoinductive factors and could stimulate bone regeneration. *J Orthop Res.* 2004;22(1):73–79.

Ricci WM, Collinge C, Streubel PN, et al. A comparison of more and less aggressive bone debridement protocols for the treatment of open supracondylar femur fractures. *J Orthop Trauma.* 2013;27(12):722–725.

Starr A, Bucholz R. *Fractures of the Shaft of the Femur.* Philadelphia, PA: Lippincott Williams & Williams; 2001.

Starr AJ, Jones AL, Reinert CM. The "swashbuckler": a modified anterior approach for fractures of the distal femur. *J Orthop Trauma.* 1999;13(2):138–140.

The FLOW Investigators. A trial of wound irrigation in the initial management of open fracture wounds. *N Engl J Med.* 2015;373(27):2629–2641.

Wang JH, Zhao JZ, He YH. A new treatment strategy for severe arthrofibrosis of the knee. A review of twenty-two cases. *J Bone Joint Surg Am.* 2006;88(6):1245–1250.

Warner JJ. The Judet quadricepsplasty for management of severe posttraumatic extension contracture of the knee: a report of a bilateral case and review of the literature. *Clin Orthop Relat Res.* 1990;(256):169–173.

29 Management of Soft Tissue Defects Surrounding the Knee and Tibia: The Gastrocnemius Muscle Flap

Karim Bakri and Steven L. Moran

Soft tissue defects involving the proximal tibia, knee joint, or patella are usually encountered as a consequence of trauma or as a complication of knee arthroplasty. The options for soft tissue coverage are dependent on the size of the wound, its location, and the extent of the surrounding injury. The gastrocnemius muscle flap is a workhorse flap that can be used to cover a majority of defects around the knee, proximal leg, lower thigh, and patellar region. Its vascular and musculoskeletal anatomy is very consistent, and this allows for a straightforward surgical technique as well as predictable and reliable outcomes.

ANATOMY

The muscles of the leg are arranged in four compartments—anterior, lateral, and two posterior compartments (superficial and deep). The superficial posterior compartment of the leg contains three muscles (soleus, plantaris, and gastrocnemius), of which the gastrocnemius is the most superficial. The gastrocnemius muscle has two heads, and these arise from the posterior aspect of the medial and lateral condyles of the femur (Fig. 29-1). The two muscle bellies join at the level of the fibular head to form a bipennate muscle with a clearly visible longitudinal median raphe that delineates the neurovascular territory of each head. Distally, the gastrocnemius muscle unites with the tendon of the soleus in the middle third of the leg to form the Achilles tendon, which inserts on the posterior aspect of the calcaneus.

The medial and lateral gastrocnemius muscle flaps exhibit a type 1 vascular anatomy (each having one dominant pedicle). The medial gastrocnemius is supplied by the medial sural artery, and the lateral gastrocnemius is supplied by the lateral sural artery. These arteries originate from the popliteal artery approximately 4 cm above the level of the fibula head.

Each muscle head is innervated by a direct branch that arises from the tibial nerve in the popliteal fossa. Before diving deep to the gastrocnemius, the tibial nerve also gives off a superficial sensory branch, the medial sural cutaneous nerve. This nerve exits between the two heads of the gastrocnemius, courses obliquely over the lateral head of the muscle, and runs superficially in the posterior aspect of the leg, with the short saphenous vein, behind the lateral malleolus. The medial sural cutaneous nerve can be easily injured during exposure and division of the muscle, resulting in

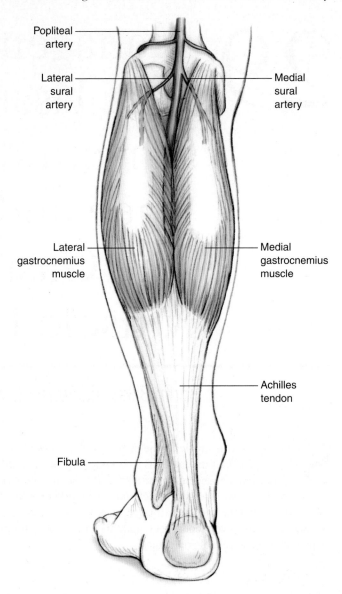

FIGURE 29-1

The medial and lateral gastrocnemius muscles as seen from the posterior approach.

paresthesia of the lateral aspect of the foot. The common peroneal nerve also arises from the sciatic nerve in the popliteal fossa and winds superficially around the proximal end of the lateral gastrocnemius and the fibular head. It gives off a lateral sural cutaneous nerve that runs superficially in the posterior leg and joins the medial sural nerve in the midportion of the leg to form the sural nerve proper. The common peroneal and lateral sural cutaneous nerves can be easily damaged during dissection and rotation of the lateral gastrocnemius flap.

INDICATIONS/CONTRAINDICATIONS

The medial and lateral gastrocnemius muscle flaps are most commonly used as proximally based, pedicled, rotation flaps. They are usually used independently but may be used in conjunction with each other for more extensive defects. The medial gastrocnemius is the larger and longer of the muscle heads and is used more commonly than its lateral counterpart. It will cover the inferior thigh, medial knee joint, patella, and proximal tibia. The lateral head may be used for coverage of lateral tibial defects or distal thigh wounds; however, the muscle belly is much shorter and narrower than the medial head. For defects at the level of the midportion of the tibia, the gastrocnemius muscle may not provide adequate coverage, and the soleus muscle is preferred for coverage of middle third defects. For defects involving the distal third of the tibia and ankle, free tissue transfer or pedicled perforator flaps are usually required.

Contraindications to the use of the gastrocnemius muscle flap include clinically evident infection, injury, or vascular disease of the popliteal artery and vascular pedicles and massive defects requiring a larger amount of tissue transfer. Direct trauma to the posterior calf may result in muscle destruction and should be ruled out prior to proceeding with flap elevation. Radiation to the knee following tumor extirpation may compromise the vascular pedicle, increasing the chance of total or partial muscle necrosis following transfer. The muscle should not be used if the soleus and contralateral gastrocnemius muscle are no longer functional, as this will create postoperative difficulty with plantar flexion. A history of a recent deep venous thrombosis within the involved extremity is a relative contraindication for the use of the flap, although we have used the flap successfully in such situations.

Distally based gastrocnemius muscle flaps have been described for coverage of lower leg defects. Vascular supply to the muscle in these cases is through crossing anastomotic arterial connections between the medial and lateral gastrocnemius muscle bellies extending across the midline raphe. Use of the flap in this manner is not common, and more reliable methods of middle third and lower leg coverage are recommended including the soleus muscle flap, the sural flap, pedicled fasciocutaneous perforator flaps, and free flap coverage.

PREOPERATIVE PLANNING

The preoperative management of severe open fractures involves stabilization of the patient, tetanus prophylaxis, and broad-spectrum antibiotics. Nonviable or heavily contaminated tissue requires aggressive debridement. Serial debridements may be needed if tissue viability is uncertain. Flap coverage may proceed when the wound is clean, preferably at the earliest opportunity. Preoperative physical examination should focus on determining the function of the remaining muscles of the lower leg to determine if sacrifice of the gastrocnemius could result in a significant loss of plantar flexion following muscle transfer. A vascular examination should also be performed to assess for the patency of the popliteal artery. In those patients with a history of peripheral vascular disease or a history of popliteal arterial trauma, an angiogram or CT angiogram can confirm patency of the sural arteries prior to surgery.

SURGERY

Patient Positioning

The patient should receive either general or spinal anesthesia and may be positioned supine, lateral, or prone, depending on the location and extent of the defect and the anticipated approach. After sterile preparation, the entire extremity is draped and fully exposed. A thigh tourniquet may facilitate dissection, especially in lateral gastrocnemius harvest where the peroneal nerve should be identified and protected during flap elevation.

If the patient is prone, a stocking seam or midposterior S-shaped incision is made and significantly facilitates proximal extension for exposure of the muscle's origin posteriorly over the femoral condyle. The posterior approach is made with an incision starting 3 cm below the popliteal crease and extending down to the distal end of the muscle belly. More commonly, however, for anterior traumatic defects around the patellar and tibial region, the patient is positioned in the supine position with the leg internally or externally rotated to facilitate exposure of the medial or lateral heads, respectively. An oblique incision can be made extending from the edge of the end toward the medial or lateral aspect of the posterior calf depending on which head is to be used. Lateral decubitus positioning is also an option for lateral gastrocnemius muscle elevation.

The ipsilateral or contralateral thigh should be prepared for a skin graft donor site. Appropriate preoperative antibiotics should be given prior to incision.

Technique

Medial Gastrocnemius Muscle Flap

A longitudinal skin incision is made where the separation of the bellies of the gastrocnemius and soleus muscle can be palpated. This should parallel the medial border of the tibia and can be curved proximally in a posterior direction to facilitate exposure and dissection of the proximal portion of

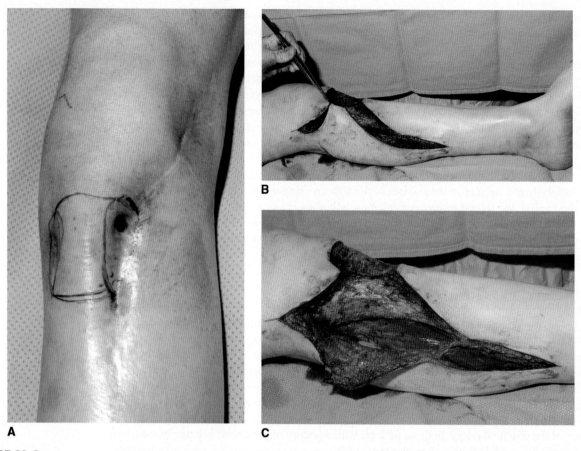

FIGURE 29-2

A: A 53-year-old patient with long-standing osteomyelitis of the tibia requiring debridement and soft tissue coverage. **B:** The skin surrounding the defect is excised. The bone is debrided and filled with antibiotic beads. The skin defect is incorporated into the skin incision for exposure of the gastrocnemius muscle. The skin incision is curved posterior approximately 4 cm beyond the medial border of the tibia. **C:** This incision gives excellent exposure of the posterior compartment, especially the medial gastrocnemius. Note that the saphenous vein has been preserved at the inferior extent of the skin incision.

the muscle. The incision should extend from the level of the tibial plateau to 10 cm above the medial malleolus. If the flap is to be tunneled into position on the anteromedial aspect of the leg, a skin bridge of at least 7 cm must be maintained to prevent skin necrosis. For more anterior defects, or preexisting peripatellar defects, a curved incision can be extended both proximally and distally from the defect site to a line 4 cm medial to the edge of the tibia (Fig. 29-2A, B). During initial subcutaneous dissection, the long saphenous vein is identified and preserved (Fig. 29-2C).

The underlying deep investing fascia of the leg is then opened to expose the plane between the gastrocnemius and soleus muscles (Fig. 29-3). In most patients, the plantaris tendon is located in this interval and should be left intact. This plane is easily opened with blunt finger dissection. The plane between the external fascia of the muscle and the overlying skin should also be opened using blunt dissection. Large perforating vessels can be identified running from the muscle to the overlying skin. These vessels serve as the main blood supply to the skin paddle of a gastrocnemius musculocutaneous flap, which is rarely used. These vessels should be ligated in the gastrocnemius muscle flap dissection. The medial sural nerve and lesser saphenous vein can be exiting between the medial and lateral heads of the gastrocnemius muscle and should be preserved.

Dissection is then continued medially between the plane of the gastrocnemius and the soleus until the midline raphe of the gastrocnemius muscle is identified. Often this raphe will be identified by decussation of the muscle fibers distally. If the raphe is not clearly visualized distally, the two heads may be easily identified and separated proximally before they unite. The sural nerve will be identified within the gastrocnemius raphe and should be preserved. Using cautery, the raphe can be divided and the gastrocnemius can be separated from the Achilles tendon. The inferior margin of the muscle is divided from the Achilles tendon with a 2-cm cuff of gastrocnemius tendon, which

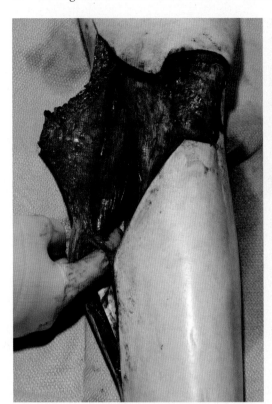
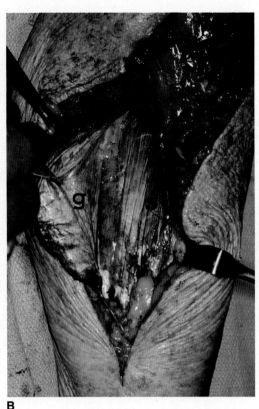

A   **B**

FIGURE 29-3

The deep investing fascia of the leg is divided, and the plane between the gastrocnemius (*g*) and the soleus (*s*) muscles may be identified using finger dissection. Figure **(A)** shows plane between gastrocnemius muscle (*left of the thumb*) and soleus muscle (*right of the thumb*). The preserved saphenous vein lies above the thumb. Figure **(B)** shows close up of gastrocnemius muscle retracted medially as muscle is mobilized from soleus muscle.

facilitates insetting of the muscle. This cuff of tendon is also valuable for reconstruction of the terminal extensor mechanism of the quadriceps muscle.

At this point, the muscle may be pedicled and mobilized for coverage of the upper one-third of the lower leg. If the knee or distal thigh requires coverage, the origin of the muscle will require release. For release from the femoral condyle, posterior extension of the skin incision significantly facilitates visualization of the muscle's vascular pedicle, which runs on the underside of the muscle belly. Skeletonization of the sural vessels from the deep surface of the muscle will also allow further mobilization of the muscle. The muscle can be inset with either its deep or superficial surfaces exposed. Cross-hatching or removal of the fascia will allow for further mobility and advancement of the muscle without impairing blood supply (Fig. 29-4).

The fascia is then inset into the defect using horizontal mattress sutures, pulling the muscle beneath the overlying skin on the far side of the defect. Prior to inset, a 10-mm flat or round drain can be placed under the flap; a second drain should be placed at the donor site prior to closure.

A meshed skin graft should then be placed on the exposed muscle flap, followed by a nonadherent dressing and bolster or negative pressure dressing (Fig. 29-5). The remainder of the wound should be covered with sterile dressings and the leg placed in a knee immobilizer or Robert Jones dressing. The skin graft donor site may be dressed with a single-layer transparent dressing.

Lateral Gastrocnemius Muscle

The lateral gastrocnemius muscle will cover the inferior thigh, knee, and proximal tibia. For harvesting of the lateral gastrocnemius, the skin incision is made at the posterior midline of the lower calf extending to the lateral popliteal fossa. The proximal mark is placed 2 or 3 cm posterior to the fibula. Once again, an adequate skin bridge must be maintained between the traumatic defect and the incision to avoid skin bridge necrosis. Alternatively, the existing skin defect may be extended proximally and distally over the posterior margin of the fibula to allow for exposure of the muscle (Fig. 29-6).

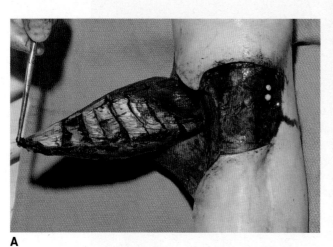
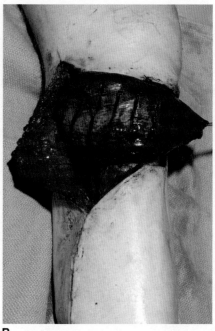

A   **B**

FIGURE 29-4

Once the medial head of the gastrocnemius is mobilized, the anterior and posterior fascia may be transversely scored or cross-hatched **(A)** to allow for easier insetting **(B)**.

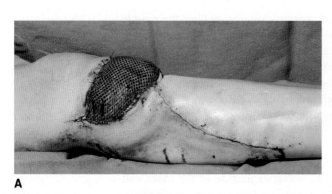
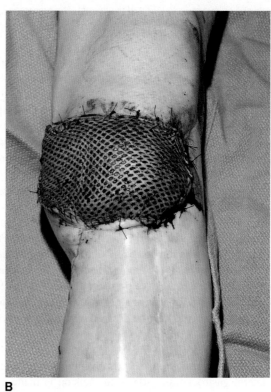

A   **B**

FIGURE 29-5

After the muscle is inset, it is covered with a split-thickness skin graft. The leg incision is closed over a suction drain. Figures **(A)** and **(B)** show appearance after final insetting.

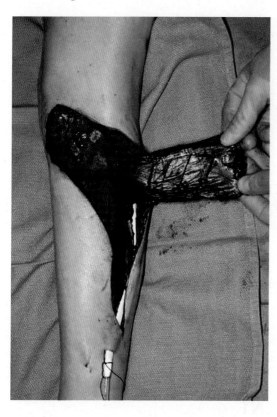

FIGURE 29-6

The incision for exposure of the lateral gastrocnemius muscle flap is made 2 to 3 cm posterior to the fibula.

Dissection begins five to six fingerbreadths below the fibular head so as not to encounter the peroneal nerve. Once the plane between the soleus and gastrocnemius is clearly identified, super-ficial dissection can begin between the gastrocnemius and the investing fascia of the lower leg. The common peroneal nerve must be identified at the level of the neck of the fibula and protected throughout the rest of the dissection. Since the common peroneal nerve passes between the lateral head of the gastrocnemius and the tendon of the biceps femoris, particular attention should be paid to identify the nerve during this portion of the dissection. The muscle is then separated as described for the medial gastrocnemius muscle flap and may then be pedicled into the overlying defect site (Fig. 29-7). To extend the reach of the lateral gastrocnemius, and for more proximal defects, the

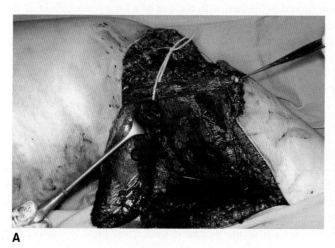

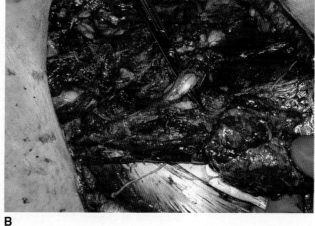

A   **B**

FIGURE 29-7

A: A traumatic lateral tibial and patellar defect in a 28-year-old woman. The lateral gastrocnemius muscle has been harvested with a posterior and inferior incision extended from the original defect site. Note that the common peroneal nerve has been identified and marked with blue vessel loop. The soleus muscle belly (*s*) can be seen below the gastrocnemius muscle (*g*). **B:** The common peroneal nerve (seen here running above the scissors) must be identified prior to pedicling the flap into the defect site to ensure it is not inadvertently compressed or injured during flap insetting.

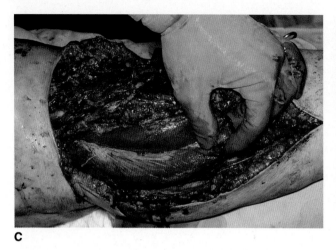

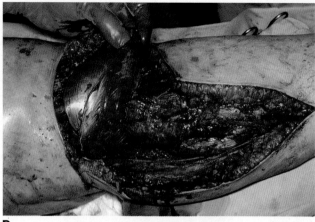

C   D

FIGURE 29.7 (*Continued*)
C, D: Once the lateral gastrocnemius muscle is isolated from midline raphe, it can easily reach the lateral aspect of the peripatellar region.

common peroneal nerve may be dissected with extreme caution, and the flap can be passed under the nerve to allow more proximal reach. This approach is not routinely required and should be reserved for special circumstances, as significant neuropraxia or even avulsion injury can result from the dissection, resulting in a footdrop.

POSTOPERATIVE MANAGEMENT

The patient should be maintained on bed rest for 5 days. The bolster dressing may be removed on postoperative day 5 to ensure adequate skin graft "take." Following this, nonadherent dressing changes are performed daily until the skin graft has matured, at which point the patient is encouraged to keep the skin graft lubricated with a petroleum-based lotion to prevent desiccation of the newly grafted skin. If immediate postoperative motion is essential, the origin of the gastrocnemius muscle should be divided to minimize forces across the flap in the early postoperative period. A vacuum assisted compressive sponge may also aid in securing skin grafts if immediate motion is essential.

The drains are removed once drainage is less than 30 mL/day. Gentle range of motion should then begin at 10 to 14 days, increasing the motion by 5 or 10 degrees per day. Ambulation can begin on postoperative day 10, but knee flexion should be limited with the use of a knee immobilizer. If the flap is inset under tension or if the healing environment is less than ideal, the knee immobilizer can be maintained for an additional week to prevent excessive tension on the margins of the muscle flap.

Postoperative swelling is minimized with the use of elastic wraps or supportive stockings. Compression stockings worn long-term can facilitate flap contouring. Muscle flaps undergo a process of atrophy over 6 to 12 months; patient concerns regarding scarring or flap contour should not be addressed surgically until 12 to 24 months following the initial reconstructive surgery (Fig. 29-8).

COMPLICATIONS

Complications following the use of the gastrocnemius muscle flap include bleeding, infection, nerve injury to the common peroneal or sural nerves, injury to the Achilles tendon, and flap loss. Bleeding (hematoma) and infection are most common problems, though rare if meticulous hemostasis is achieved at closure and aggressive debridement of the wound is performed prior to muscle flap transfer.

Partial flap necrosis or complete flap loss is usually associated with technical error, including injury to the vascular pedicle and/or excessive tension causing marginal flap ischemia. If flap ischemia is suspected intraoperatively, the vascular pedicle should be examined for signs of kinking or injury to the sural artery. Small areas of skin graft loss may be seen postoperatively, but can be conservatively managed with topical ointments and wound care without the need for further surgical intervention.

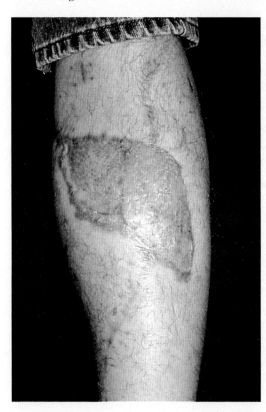

FIGURE 29-8

A 2-year follow-up of a 35-year-old man who underwent medial gastrocnemius muscle coverage for exposed tibia following a motor vehicle accident. Significant improvement in contour is obtained with long-term use of a compression wrap or compression stocking.

In order to avoid iatrogenic injuries, the surgeon should appreciate the relationship of the common peroneal nerve, medial sural nerve, and saphenous veins to the surgical field. Nerve injury is uncommon with meticulous dissection; however, injury to the sural nerve can occur during separation of the medial and lateral heads of the gastrocnemius muscle. Injury to the common peroneal nerve may occur during elevation of the lateral gastrocnemius flap. The saphenous nerve may be ligated inadvertently with the saphenous vein during exposure of the posterior compartment; attempts should be made at nerve identification and preservation during flap dissection.

The gastrocnemius muscle provides plantar flexion of the foot and flexion of the knee joint. Removal of the muscle does not usually result in significant morbidity, although some loss of plantar flexion may lessen jumping and leaping ability. Either or both heads may be used with little functional deficit as long as the soleus muscle is preserved and uninjured.

PEARLS AND PITFALLS

- The medial gastrocnemius has a larger and longer muscle belly than its lateral counterpart and is more useful for the majority of knee defects.
- The anatomy of the common peroneal and sural nerves should be specifically appreciated to avoid injury during flap dissection.
- The median raphe can be found by identifying the divergent muscle fibers each head, by identifying the muscles proximally prior to their decussation, or by identifying the medial sural nerve that lies on the raphe.
- A longer reach or wider arc of rotation can be achieved by dividing the origin of the muscle at the femoral condyle.
- The tendinous fascia on the underside of the muscle belly can be removed or aggressively cross-hatched to allow the muscle to stretch and cover a broader surface area.
- Preserving a portion of the distal gastrocnemius tendon and a rim of fascia on the muscle facilitates suturing the muscle flap to the surrounding tissues.
- If the lateral gastrocnemius is passed under the common peroneal nerve to extend its proximal reach, meticulous and tedious mobilization of the nerve is necessary to avoid excessive traction, avulsion, or compression injury to the nerve.

- The major contribution of the soleus muscle to the Achilles tendon should be identified and preserved to avoid unnecessary morbidity from division of the true Achilles tendon when mobilizing the distal aspect of the gastrocnemius.
- Overaggressive or blind blunt dissection of the underside of the flap should be avoided proximally, so as not to injure the vascular pedicle.

RECOMMENDED READING

Arnold PG, Mixter RC. Making the most of the gastrocnemius muscles. *Plast Reconstr Surg*. 1983;72:38.

Bengston S, Carlsson A, Relanber M, et al. Treatment of the exposed knee prosthesis. *Acta Orthop Scand*. 1987;58:662.

Bos GD, Buehler MJ. Lower-extremity local flaps. *J Am Acad Orthop Surg*. 1994;2:342–351.

Dibbell DG, Edstrom LE. The gastrocnemius myocutaneous flap. *Clin Plast Surg*. 1983;7:43.

Ger R. The management of pretibial skin loss. *Surgery*. 1968;63:757–763.

Hersh CK, Schenck RC, Williams RP. The versatility of the gastrocnemius muscle flap. *Am J Orthop*. 1995;24:218–222.

Mathes SJ, Nahai F. *Reconstructive Surgery Principles, Anatomy, and Technique*. New York: Churchill Livingstone; 1997.

McCraw JB, Arnold PG. *McCraw and Arnold's Atlas of Muscle and Musculocutaneous Flaps*. Norfolk, VA: Hampton Press Publishing; 1986:491–543.

Pico R, Luscher NJ, Rometsch M, et al. Why the denervated gastrocnemius muscle flap should be encouraged. *Ann Plast Surg*. 1991;26:312–324.

30 Revision and Infected Total Knee Arthroplasty

David J. Jacofsky and Oren Goltzer

Success and knee salvage in cases of revision and infected total knee arthroplasty (TKA) is dependent on adequate healing of the soft tissues and preservation of an intact extensor mechanism. Without uneventful soft tissue healing, complication rates increase and the ultimate benefit of the operation is diminished. In this chapter, we review important factors that should be considered in the preoperative, intraoperative, and postoperative setting to improve soft tissue healing in cases of revision and infected TKA.

INDICATIONS/CONTRAINDICATIONS

While any patient who undergoes revision TKA should be considered at risk for soft tissue complications, some patients will have greater risks due to certain host factors. A healthy patient with just one prior knee surgery and aseptic loosening is at less risk than a patient with diabetes and peripheral vascular disease who has a chronically infected total knee replacement. If the soft tissues are severely compromised preoperatively due to multiple incisions or open draining wounds and the surgeon is not experienced in flap techniques, a preoperative plastic surgery consultation should be considered for help with incisional planning and consideration of prophylactic flap coverage at the time of surgery. Once the risks have been evaluated, a decision to proceed with revision TKA surgery should be based on the individual circumstances, since absolute indications and contradictions are difficult to define. In each case, the current symptoms, including pain and disability, presence or absence of prosthetic infection, as well as the age and activity demands of the patient must be evaluated in the context of the potential risks of revision arthroplasty.

Absolute contraindications for revision TKA include irreversible medical comorbidities that raise the risk of perioperative mortality to unacceptable levels, an avascular extremity where revascularization options have been exhausted, uncontrolled sepsis, and neurologic injuries with no motor function of the extremity. Relative contraindications include failed prior soft tissue flaps, massive bone loss, recurrent prosthetic infection, extensor mechanism disruption, and unstable medical comorbidities that require optimization. When the potential risks are too great, alternative procedures including permanent resection arthroplasty, knee arthrodesis, or amputation may be required.

PREOPERATIVE PLANNING

Preoperative planning is critical for minimizing soft tissue problems about the knee. Both systemic factors and the characteristics of the knee and leg should be considered before revision knee surgery.

Patient-specific medical comorbidities should be assessed and treated before surgery (Table 30-1). While medical optimization of these conditions appears to reduce the risk of developing wound complications after revision TKA, the increased risk is multifactorial and may not return to baseline. For example, the increased risks of delayed wound healing and infection noted in patients with diabetes appear to be caused by both deficiencies in polymorphonuclear neutrophil cell function as well as hyperglycemia, which has been shown to inhibit collagen synthesis, disrupt fibroblast proliferation, and slow capillary ingrowth. Similarly, the increased risk of soft tissue complications in patients with rheumatoid arthritis is likely due to numerous factors including the long-term sequelae of corticosteroid use, which regulates macrophage function, reduces collagen synthesis, and delays vascular ingrowth, as well as direct causes of the disease itself such as skin atrophy, decreased albumin, and vasculitis.

TABLE 30-1 Complicating Comorbidities

Condition	Evaluation	Management
Diabetes	Blood glucose	Optimize diet and medications
Inflammatory arthritis	Review disease-modifying medications	Hold medications, if possible, until wound healing has occurred
Tobacco use	Serum cotinine level if poor abstinence/compliance	Avoid tobacco use 4–8 wk before surgery and postoperatively until wound healing has occurred
Malnutrition	Total lymphocyte count <1,500 mm³ Serum albumin <3.4 g/dL	Nutritional supplements before surgery
Anemia	Hgb/Hct	Correct before surgery with erythropoietin injections
Hypoxia	SaO₂	Optimize pulmonary function
Peripheral vascular disease	Peripheral pulses, Doppler ultrasound, arteriogram	Revascularization prior to revision TKA
Obesity	BMI	Avoid significant weight loss in the immediate pre- or postoperative periods
Cancer	History	Avoid elective surgery, if possible, while on chemotherapeutic agents
Chronic corticosteroid use	History	>2 y duration appears to increase risks of wound complications

BMI, body mass index; TKA, total knee arthroplasty.

Another important risk factor in the preoperative and postoperative periods is the use of tobacco products. Nicotine and its metabolites cause vasoconstriction, which interferes with microcirculation; however, the effects on wound healing are more profound than from vasoconstriction alone. Other constituents of tobacco smoke, such as carbon monoxide, decrease the oxygen-carrying capacity of hemoglobin, which reduces tissue oxygenation. Nicotine also appears to have a direct effect on fibroblast and immune function. The optimal time for smoking cessation is 4 to 8 weeks preoperatively, but even a week of abstinence appears to reduce the risk of complications. Abstinence in the entire postoperative period is also critical. For elective procedures, all patients who use tobacco products should be counseled to stop. In some circumstances, professional services are utilized to achieve this goal. The use of nicotine delivery substitutes such as lozenges and patches is controversial, as these do not eliminate the patient's use of nicotine but do eliminate the toxic substances that are inhaled in tobacco smoke, such as carbon monoxide and hydrogen cyanide. Therefore, while not an optimal solution, in certain circumstances, these substitutes may be preferable to smoking to reduce the overall risk.

SURGERY

Anatomy

In revision TKA, a thorough understanding of the anatomy will help minimize wound complications. The local vascular anatomy of the knee can be unforgiving in comparison to the hip, where wound necrosis is rarely a problem. In part, this is because the cutaneous blood supply is distinct from the blood supply to the patella and there is little interconnection between the two. Most of the perfusion to the skin is derived from perforator vessels that originate below the level of the deep fascia. Therefore, when raising skin flaps about the knee, the dissection should be below the level of the deep fascia rather than in the subdermal plane to avoid damaging this superficial plexus. *The importance of raising flaps that are fasciocutaneous in preference to subcutaneous flaps cannot be overstated.* While the peripatellar vascular plexus has been well described and is formed by the medial and lateral, superior and inferior genicular arteries, the majority of the inflow to the skin appears to be derived from the medial side of the knee in the distribution of the saphenous and descending genicular arteries. With this in mind, general guidelines for selection and placement of skin incisions follow.

Surgical Exposure

The orthopedic surgeon must be proficient in techniques that allow adequate exposure in revision TKA that minimizes risks to the skin and extensor mechanism. General principles to optimize wound healing and avoid complications include meticulous soft tissue handling in every case. Prolonged local tension from self-retaining retractors or from vigorous stretching due to attempts to perform mini-incision surgery should be avoided; in addition, undermining along the margins of the incision should be minimized. Intraoperatively, the importance of optimizing component positioning to avoid the need for a lateral patellar release that is associated with increased wound problems is also important. The use of a tourniquet is controversial, as evidence suggests that postoperative tissue oxygenation is reduced in patients in whom a tourniquet is used. Certainly, in patients with significant peripheral vascular disease, especially those in whom either a bypass has already been performed, or the lateral radiograph shows extensive calcification of the popliteal vessels, consideration should be made to perform the knee replacement without a tourniquet. In addition to the previously noted principles, numerous techniques exist for facilitating surgical exposure and relieving tension on the extensor mechanism to reduce the risk of iatrogenic tendon rupture or patellar fracture. These techniques, along with the results and complications that are specific to each, are reviewed in later sections this chapter. All of these procedures, except where noted, are performed during revision TKA with the patient positioned supine.

SUPERFICIAL APPROACH THROUGH SKIN

A single, longitudinal anterior midline incision provides the most extensile exposure and is preferred for all revision and infected total knee replacement cases. In consideration of the increased incidence of wound healing complications in revision TKA, incisional length should be generous enough to prevent excessive tension placed on the tissue edges. Prior incisions about the knee should be carefully evaluated in terms of their age, length, and orientation. Horizontal or oblique incisions should be crossed perpendicularly in order to avoid acute angles, which increase the risk of skin necrosis. When a single, prior longitudinal anterior incision exists, it should be used. If placement of this prior incision is not directly midline, the proximal and distal ends of the incision may be extended back toward the midline to reduce tension on the wound. In these cases, subcutaneous dissection should be minimized, and full thickness, fasciocutaneous flaps should be created to allow adequate exposure of the extensor mechanism. If the prior incision is located far from midline and would necessitate creation of a large laterally based subcutaneous flap, one may consider using a new incision. In these circumstances, skin bridges greater than 5 cm should be maintained between the new and old incisions. When multiple, fully healed, longitudinal incisions are present, the most lateral incision should generally be used since the blood supply to the skin travels from the medial to the lateral side of the knee.

CAPSULAR APPROACH

Prior to arthrotomy, the entire extensor mechanism including the quadriceps tendon, patellar borders, patellar tendon, and tibial tubercle should all be adequately exposed. Extension of the incision into native tissue beyond the edge of the scar will help to locate and allow development of the tissue planes. While there are multiple descriptions of arthrotomies including the von Langenbeck and subvastus approaches, in the revision setting the medial parapatellar approach should be utilized. During the approach, the medial and lateral gutters should be recreated, and any fibrotic tissue in the suprapatellar pouch should be freed to allow mobilization of the extensor mechanism. Similarly, in cases of arthrofibrosis, a quadricepsplasty may be employed to free the extensor mechanism from the anterior aspect of the femur. The specific techniques described below generally progress from less extensile to more extensile.

Medial Parapatellar Arthrotomy and Proximal Tibial Peel

The medial parapatellar arthrotomy is versatile, allows the optimal exposure in revision TKA, and is compatible with each of the more extensile exposures detailed in subsequent sections. This exposure should be incorporated into every revision and provides the foundation for obtaining adequate visualization and access in order to safely remove the existing components and reconstruct the knee. The arthrotomy is begun at the proximal end of the quadriceps tendon approximately 6 to 8 cm proximal to the superior pole of the patella and continues distally leaving at least a 3- to

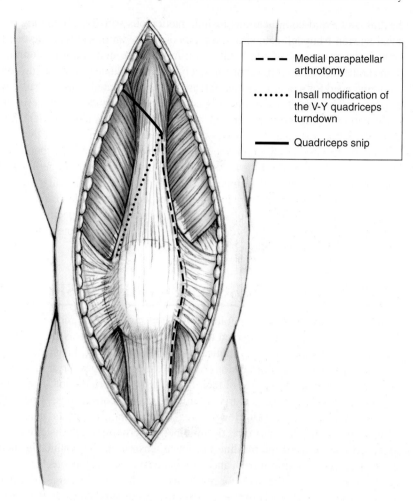

┌─────────────────────────────────────┐
│ ─ ─ ─ Medial parapatellar   │
│   arthrotomy   │
│   │
│ ······· Insall modification of   │
│   the V-Y quadriceps   │
│   turndown   │
│   │
│ ───── Quadriceps snip   │
└─────────────────────────────────────┘

FIGURE 30-1

The medial arthrotomy (*dashed line*) is the standard exposure for revision TKA. This can be extended with a quadriceps snip (*solid line*) if the extensor mechanism is tight. The Insall modification of the V-Y quadriceps turndown (*dotted line*) allows extensile exposure in the stiff knee but is associated with postoperative extensor lag.

5-mm cuff of medial quadriceps tendon to repair at the time of closure (Fig. 30-1). An arthrotomy should be generally based in the center of the tendon to allow for extensile procedures proximally if needed. The arthrotomy is extended distally and curved around the medial border of the patella and carried distally along the medial edge of the patellar tendon. Insall described this incision to continue distally over the patella in a relatively straight fashion with the quadriceps expansion over the anterior patella peeled subperiosteally before continuing distally adjacent to the medial border of the patellar tendon. The standard medial parapatellar approach is similar to Insall's description; however, at the level of the medial border of the patella, a small cuff of retinaculum is left on the patella to allow for subsequent repair during the closure. Either of these approaches is acceptable during revision TKA.

Once the arthrotomy is made, the periosteum of the medial tibia is elevated sharply beginning at the medial border of the arthrotomy at the level of the joint, initiating the medial release. Working carefully, the entire medial periosteum is elevated approximately 5 to 7 cm distally and to the level of the semimembranosus tendon in the midcoronal plane. A periosteal elevator can be used once the flap of periosteum has been raised. Patellar subluxation is generally preferred over eversion as it allows adequate exposure of the knee while minimizing risk to the patellar tendon insertion. The extensor mechanism must be protected through the case since fibrosis, osteolysis at the tibial tubercle, and noncompliant soft tissues increase the risk of iatrogenic avulsion. At this stage, the knee is flexed, and the tibia is gradually externally rotated while the subperiosteal elevation is continued to the posteromedial corner. In many cases where this tissue plane was not violated in the primary replacement, the semimembranosus insertion on the posteromedial corner will be well defined, and this expansile insertion should be released in the subperiosteal plane. As the dissection continues, externally rotating the tibia will cause it to subluxate from underneath the femur. Often, this will allow access to the modular tibial polyethylene, which can be removed at this time. This relaxes the flexion and extension gaps, improves the exposure and mobility of the soft tissues, and in many cases allows sufficient exposure for revision surgery. At this point, if patellar subluxation and knee flexion to 110 degrees causes excessive tension on the patellar tendon, a more extensile approach should be employed.

Quadriceps Snip

Technique

The quadriceps snip is an excellent first choice for additional exposure. Originally described by Insall and now with several modifications, the quadriceps snip facilitates the exposure of stiff knees in the primary and revision setting. This technique is a proximal (and lateral) extension of a medial parapatellar arthrotomy (see Fig. 30-1). Beginning distal to the musculotendinous junction of the rectus femoris at the proximal apex of the standard arthrotomy, the incision is extended at a 45- to 60-degree angle proximally and laterally into the fibers of the vastus lateralis. This extension not only relieves the tension on the extensor mechanism in a stiff knee that can aid in exposure of the joint but also allows the patella to be everted more easily during patellar preparation if this is required. The arthrotomy and this proximal extension are closed in routine fashion once the arthroplasty has been completed. In distinction to many of the alternative techniques for optimizing exposure in difficult cases, there is no need to modify or restrict postoperative rehabilitation. It is important during the initial exposure of knee and during the initial arthrotomy to stop short of the musculotendinous junction proximally, as extension into the rectus muscle makes it impossible to perform the quadriceps snip without transecting rectus muscle fibers and makes the repair far more difficult.

Results

Insall's clinical experience in 16 patients who had bilateral TKA with a quadriceps snip on only on one side has been reported. In these patients, no differences in quadriceps strength were observed postoperatively between the two sides. In a similar study, no difference was identified between patients who had undergone a quadriceps snip versus those in whom a standard medial parapatellar arthrotomy had been performed. Sun et al. reported that outcomes with a quadriceps snip were similar to those with tibial tubercle osteotomy in revision knee arthroplasty.

Tibial Tubercle Osteotomy

Technique

First described by Dolin in 1983 and subsequently popularized by Whiteside in 1995, the tibial tubercle osteotomy facilitates exposure in particularly stiff or difficult cases and can still be used even after a quadriceps snip has already been performed. The tibial tubercle osteotomy allows access to the tibial canal, which may be helpful in revision or infected TKA when well-fixed stemmed, tibial components must be removed. Additionally, the benefits of the osteotomy include bone-to-bone healing, improved exposure distally, and potential preservation of the patellar blood supply. Lastly, during fixation, the tubercle can be moved to improve its position in cases of patella baja or maltracking. Therefore, if the surgeon is confident that access is needed to the tibial canal, a quadriceps snip should be deferred, as it likely will not be required in conjunction with the osteotomy. The technique involves first incising the periosteum 1 cm medial to the tubercle for a length of approximately 6 to 10 cm starting 1 cm distal to the joint line. The osteotomy is then performed with an oscillating saw from medial to lateral, creating a wedge of bone that is approximately 2 cm wide and 6 to 10 cm long. The osteotomized wedge should taper from a thickness of about 1 cm proximally, to the level of the anterior cortex distally (Fig. 30-2). This minimizes the stress riser specifically at the distal end of the anterior tibia. In addition, at the proximal end, a step "dovetail" cut should be created, which acts as a buttress to resist proximal migration of the osteotomized wedge after it has been reattached at the end of the case. Proximal migration is also resisted by the periosteum and musculature that should remain attached to the lateral edge of the osteotomized piece. During the revision knee arthroplasty, the lateral soft tissues act as a hinge that allows the osteotomized segment to be everted and displaced laterally. In the multiply revised knee, the proximal shelf of bone may be absent at the time of repair, and the lip of the tibial component may be used to prevent proximal migration. At the time of closure, the osteotomy can be repaired with either screws or three to four 18-gauge cerclage wires.

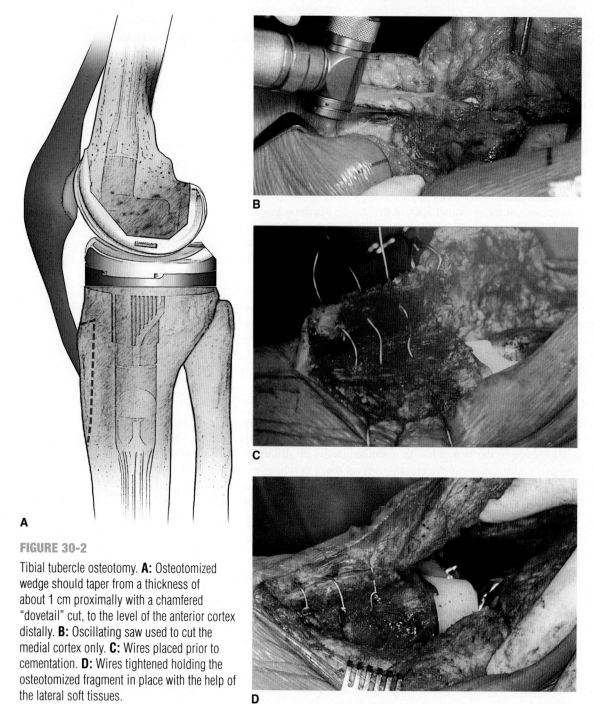

FIGURE 30-2

Tibial tubercle osteotomy. **A:** Osteotomized wedge should taper from a thickness of about 1 cm proximally with a chamfered "dovetail" cut, to the level of the anterior cortex distally. **B:** Oscillating saw used to cut the medial cortex only. **C:** Wires placed prior to cementation. **D:** Wires tightened holding the osteotomized fragment in place with the help of the lateral soft tissues.

If wires are used, they are passed through drill holes in the medial tibia and then brought up through the lateral aspect of the tubercle shingle. They are then brought distally and medially over the tibial crest and tightened on the medial side of the tibia. Tightening the wires tethers the osteotomy distally and counters the proximal pull of the patellar tendon. In most cases, we favor long-stemmed revision tibial components that bypass the distal extent of the osteotomy by at least two cortical diameters. If a cemented stem is used, it is helpful to remember to pass the wires before insertion of cement, and care must be made to prevent cement extravasation into the osteotomy site, which could potentially interfere with bone healing. This can be achieved with the use of a shield on the inner edge of the osteotomy to prevent the cement from being extruded into the space where the tibial shingle will subsequently be replaced. A dampened metal suture wrapper removed after the cement is very doughy can function as such a dam. The wires are then tightened, and bone graft may be applied to the osteotomy if significant defects exist. The arthrotomy is then closed in a standard fashion.

Results

Whiteside reported his experience with the tibial tubercle osteotomy in 136 patients; he found an overall complication rate of 7% with only two patients experiencing a residual extensor lag. A complication rate of 5% to 10% is reported in the current literature and includes postoperative fixation failure with proximal migration of the osteotomized tubercle, patellar tendon disruption, painful hardware, tibial shaft fracture, and extensor lag. Despite these unique problems, we favor the use of tubercle osteotomy when adequate exposure cannot be obtained with a standard arthrotomy and/or quadriceps snip. When rigid fixation is obtained and the patient has reasonable bone stock, full weight bearing and unrestricted range of motion are allowed postoperatively.

Femoral Peel

Technique

If arthrofibrosis continues to obstruct exposure of the knee components, a medial femoral peel can be performed as described by Windsor and Insall. It may be especially helpful for visualizing the femoral component and posterior aspect of the femoral condyles after significant medial-sided contraction has occurred, such as during reimplantation following static spacer use for infection. Initially, the proximal medial tibia is exposed subperiosteally, preserving the origin of the medial collateral ligament on the tibia and on the femur. Then, the distal medial femur is skeletonized by subperiosteal dissection, and care is taken to preserve the soft tissue sleeve medially in its entirety (Fig. 30-3). This allows access to the medial side, the posterior knee, and allows safe subperiosteal dissection of the posterior capsule off the femur if required. During closure, the medial soft tissue sleeve is allowed to fall back to its normal position, and no alteration in postoperative rehabilitation is required. If the sleeve is intact, no fixation of the sleeve is required on the medial side. This technique can be used on the lateral side when needed, although this is far less commonly required.

Results

Although the soft tissue sleeve, including the medial and lateral stabilizing structures, is preserved, joint stability may be compromised by the extensive dissection; in these cases, a constrained knee prosthesis implant may be required. Additionally, the extensive dissection may result in devascularization of the distal femur, although this is quite rare. In a series of 116 revision cases in which the femoral peel was utilized, Lavernia reported significant improvement in Knee Society scores in all patients, however, with an overall complication rate of 17%. An alternative to the femoral peel is the medial epicondylar osteotomy, whereby a 1-cm-thick wafer of bone is hinged off the medial epicondyle and preserved as a bony fragment within the soft tissue flap. During the planning stage, care must taken to ensure osteolysis of the medial femoral condyle is minimal, as an osteotomy may result in a large uncontained femoral bone defect and/or fibrous union after fixation. Most experienced surgeons find the peel to be adequate and generally avoid medial epicondylar osteotomy due to the possibility of creating an uncontained defect coupled with the increased incidence of

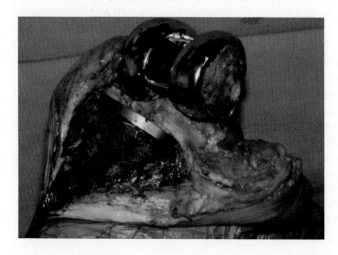

FIGURE 30-3

Femoral peel of the knee in a patient with severe arthrofibrosis demonstrating medial soft tissue sleeve maintained in continuity.

both heterotopic bone formation and the possibility of symptomatic nonunion of the epicondyle. However, this is a useful technique if the soft tissue sleeve is so poor that a peel will result in disruption of the medial sleeve continuity and subsequently will lead to medial instability.

V-Y Quadriceps Turndown

Technique

Although this technique allows excellent exposure and releases excessive tension on the extensor mechanism during surgery, patients may develop an extension lag or other complications postoperatively. Therefore, the indications for the V-Y turndown are now very limited in the context of other available extensile approaches. The V-Y quadriceps turndown was originally described by Coonse and Adams and subsequently modified by Insall. In both techniques, an inverted V-shaped flap incorporating the quadriceps tendon is created. Insall's modification described creating a second incision beginning at the apex of a standard medial parapatellar arthrotomy that is extended distally and laterally at a 45-degree angle along the tendinous portion of the vastus lateralis (see Fig. 30-1). In addition to allowing excellent exposure, the inverted V of tissue may be lengthened at the time of closure, forming an inverted Y shape, which is useful in the cases of severe quadriceps tendon contracture.

Results

Trousdale et al. reported the Mayo Clinic experience with this technique. Patients who had undergone bilateral TKA with a V-Y quadriceps turndown in one knee, and a standard medial parapatellar arthrotomy in the contralateral knee, underwent postoperative strength testing. In these patients, the results did not show any statistical differences between the strength of the two legs. However, 5 of 14 patients with the V-Y quadriceps turndown had a persistent extensor lag. Furthermore, use of the V-Y quadriceps turndown requires alterations in the postoperative rehabilitation protocol that includes restricted range of motion, use of a brace, and partial weight bearing for about 6 weeks. Due to the high rate of lag and the increased recovery time associated with the use of the V-Y turndown, we favor the graded progression of quadriceps snip followed by tibial tubercle osteotomy and medial femoral peel to obtain adequate exposure. The turndown is especially contraindicated in the multiply revised knee where fibrosis of the quadriceps can lead to inability to safely repair the tendon, as well as quadriceps necrosis. This exposure is very rarely used and is generally indicated only when lengthening of the extensor mechanism is a major need and goal of the revision procedure.

SOFT TISSUE PROCEDURES

In circumstances in which the skin and subcutaneous tissues are atrophic due to systemic conditions or have been severely damaged by prior surgery, trauma, radiation exposure, or infection, preoperative soft tissue management techniques may be required and are described in following sections.

Sham Incision

Technique

The sham incision or delay procedure is reviewed primarily for its historical significance as an early attempt to manage patients considered at risk for wound healing problems after TKA. Approximately 10 to 14 days before the planned knee procedure, the intended skin incision is made and extended to the level of the extensor mechanism. Next, the extensor mechanism is exposed as required for the upcoming knee replacement, and the incision is then closed and observed. If the wound heals without complications, the intended knee procedure is subsequently performed. If skin necrosis occurs, a soft tissue flap is performed before knee replacement. The main advantage in these cases is that the knee joint has not been violated, and there is no prosthesis at risk for infection. Furthermore, increased collateral flow caused by the incision due to the delay phenomenon was theorized to reduce the risk of subsequent wound healing problems. More contemporary soft tissue expansion techniques have, for the most part, eliminated the use of the sham incision and, although mentioned for the sake of historic interest, is likely no longer indicated.

Results

There is little except anecdotal evidence to support the use of this technique. Rothaus has detailed the outcomes in a small group of 12 patients, with multiple prior incisions, in whom this technique was used. In all 12 patients, the incisions healed, and TKA was successfully performed without wound healing problems.

Soft Tissue Expanders

Technique

The concept of tissue expansion is not new and has been successfully used in a variety of soft tissue reconstructive procedures throughout the body. Despite the challenges posed by the unforgiving nature of the vascular supply around the knee, the use of tissue expanders is a relatively new concept with only a limited number of large patient series.

Tissue expansion has three important benefits that aid wound healing in the overlying soft tissues. First, and probably most important, it stimulates neovascularization of the overlying soft tissue; this improves the capillary inflow that directly promotes healing. Second, it physically expands the overlying skin and subcutaneous tissue allowing larger areas, due to correction of malalignment or limb lengthening, to be covered. This also reduces the tension on the wound. This expansion is not simply a stretching and thinning of the overlying soft tissue, which would leave the flap less resilient, but actually a hypertrophy of the dermis and epidermis due to fibroblast stimulation, leading to an increase in the quantity of tissue available. Third, a fibrous capsule develops around the expander, and this thick, robust, vascular tissue is very useful as a "pseudofascial" layer to close over the joint and is particularly helpful in the area of the proximal medial tibia where the periosteum and soft tissue layer can be thin.

The technique for soft tissue expansion over the knee is begun approximately 6 to 8 weeks prior to the intended TKA (Fig. 30-4). Typically, two to four 200 to 300 mL expanders are placed in pockets deep to the subcutaneous layer, just above the fascia (see Fig. 30-4C). These pockets are strategically placed based on the location of prior incisions and characteristics of the overlying subcutaneous tissue and skin. The first step involves infiltrating the deep subcutaneous layer with a dilute solution composed of 1,000 mL Ringer lactate, 50 mL 1% lidocaine, and 1 mL 1:1,000 epinephrine to create a pocket.

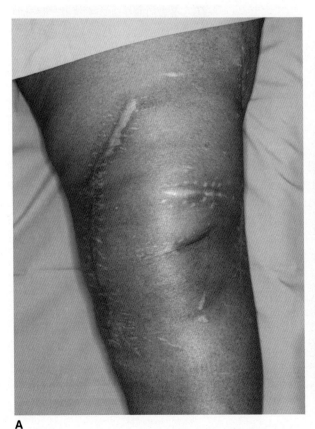
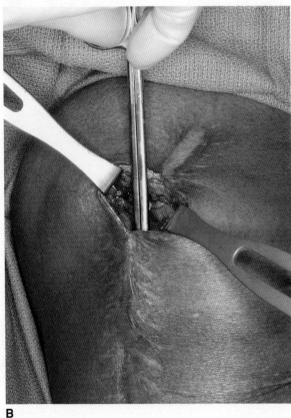

A   **B**

FIGURE 30-4

A: Knee with multiple prior vertical and horizontal incisions at risk for poor postoperative wound healing after TKA. **B:** Creation of subcutaneous pocket for soft tissue expander.

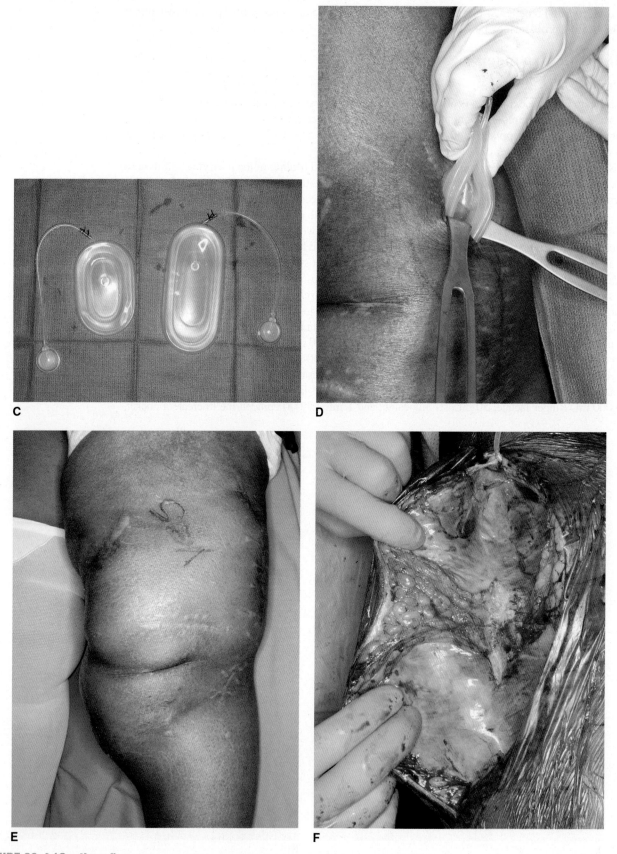

FIGURE 30-4 (*Continued*)

C: Saline expanders demonstrating access portals for infusing saline. **D:** Insertion of the deflated saline soft tissue expander. **E:** Knee after tissue expansion process is complete. **F:** Fibrous, vascular membrane that surrounds the expander cavity after removal of the expander at the time of TKA.

Typically, injection of 250 to 300 mL of this solution is sufficient to produce the hydrodissection that separates the skin and subcutaneous tissue from the underlying fascia to create a pocket. Also, use of the local anesthetic helps with postoperative pain relief. Next, through a short incision placed in one of the prior incisions, scissors are used to bluntly define and enlarge this plane within the deep subcutaneous tissue to create a pocket (see Fig. 30-4B). The uninflated expander is then inserted through the same incision (see Fig. 30-4D). The access port to the expander is then tunneled through the subcutaneous tissue to an easily accessible site. The port should be accessed prior to skin closure and saline injected to ensure that the port is functional and that the expander was not damaged during the insertion. After this initial expansion, the incision is closed and a sterile dressing applied. Most patients are admitted for an overnight stay and treated with 24 hours of intravenous antibiotics. Patients are typically placed in a knee immobilizer for a week and allowed to bear weight as tolerated. Subsequently, each week, about 10% to 15% of the volume of the expander is infused with the patient as an outpatient, via the access port. If at any time the overlying skin blanches and doesn't recover after a few minutes of observation, or if the patient experiences significant pain, saline must be removed until the problem is alleviated.

At the time of the intended TKA, the expanders are extracted through the incision used for the procedure (see Fig. 30-4F). The subcutaneous tissue and skin flaps should be protected during the TKA. At the end of the procedure, a superficial drain is placed in each individual expander pocket. These drains are removed individually once output is less than 10 mL per 8 hours or 30 mL per 24 hours. This protocol appears to reduce the risk of subcutaneous hematoma formation. Early in the experience of tissue expansion about the knee when subcutaneous drains were not routinely employed, hematomas occurred more frequently and occasionally had to be drained to reduce tension on the overlying tissue. During wound closure, the expansion process may have created excessive amounts of soft tissue that need to be excised. In these cases, the edge of the flap, especially focusing on old widened scars, can be trimmed or removed. However, the tension on the wound should not be increased by resecting too much surplus tissue.

Results

Few large series of tissue expansion in association with TKA have been published, with most reports presenting only a handful of cases. The morbidity associated with the use of tissue expanders has been previously reported and includes infection, hematoma, expander rupture or deflation, and skin necrosis. In an initial study, no significant complications occurred during the expansion process in a small group of 10 patients.

In a second larger group of 29 knees, 6 (21%) minor wound complications occurred during expansion, including mild erythema or skin blistering. These complications were successfully managed by reducing the volume in the expander and delaying further expansion until the problem resolved. In this same group, one major complication occurred after the insertion of the soft tissue expanders; this involved full-thickness skin necrosis in a patient with a history of radiation to the anterior knee. The knee replacement was subsequently not performed, as the patient declined to accept a prophylactic muscle flap, choosing to endure her arthritic symptoms. In this series, following the knee replacement, 5 (18%) of 29 patients experienced minor complications; three knees developed persistent drainage, and two knees developed subcutaneous hematomas. The persistent drainage resolved after wound compression, and immobilization was initiated. The two subcutaneous hematomas required surgical evacuation, and it was these problems that prompted the use of subcutaneous drains in the expander pockets.

In a more recent study that included patients from the previously described study, a consecutive series of 64 soft tissue expansion surgeries were performed on patients who on average 3.5 previous surgeries. The expansion took an average 70 days during which there were 14 (22%) minor complications that required local care, antibiotics, or removal of fluid. There were 7 (11%) major complications that required reoperation with all but 1 of the patients going on to TKA. The authors concluded that "soft tissue expansion is an effective prophylactic prearthroplasty option to reduce the risk of wound healing complication after TKA."

SOFT TISSUE FLAP COVERAGE PROCEDURES

Soft tissue flap procedures about the knee have been used both prophylactically and for salvage of wound complications about the knee. Although a large number of different techniques have been described, including simple skin grafts, random or axial pattern skin flaps, fasciocutaneous flaps, and rotational or free muscle flaps, the most reliable and most frequently used tissues about the knee include medial gastrocnemius muscle flaps and free latissimus dorsi or rectus abdominis flaps. In addition to these techniques, the development of musculocutaneous perforator flaps during the past decade has provided another alternative for coverage about the knee. The principles involved in these three types of techniques are described following in ascending order of the extent of the area that can be adequately managed.

Musculocutaneous Perforator Flaps

The development of musculocutaneous perforator flaps in plastic surgery occurred during the 1990s as an extension of the generally very favorable experience with musculocutaneous flaps during the 1980s. Perforator flaps were based on the principle that neither the underlying fascial plexus nor muscle was required if the vessel that perforated through the muscle was carefully dissected. The major advantage of musculocutaneous perforator flaps versus musculocutaneous flaps is that the functional and cosmetic morbidity due to transfer of the underlying muscle could be avoided by transferring only the overlying skin. Therefore, the thin musculocutaneous perforator flap is used for resurfacing shallow wounds when bulk is considered a disadvantage.

Although perforator flaps can provide additional vascularized tissue in an area that may be deficient or fibrotic, their use in the setting of infection is controversial, and in these cases, traditional muscle flaps are preferred. Their use is best reserved for aseptic cases with a deficient or scarred soft tissue envelope.

Technique

The wound is first debrided to remove all necrotic tissue (Fig. 30-5A, B). Next, elevation of the perforator flap requires careful microsurgical dissection of the musculocutaneous perforator vessels

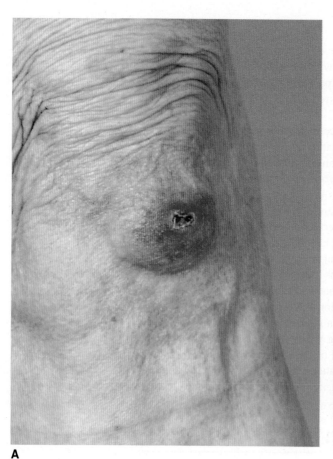
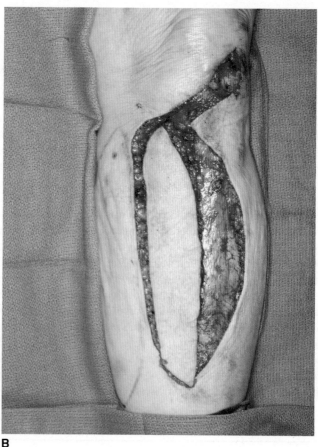

A   B

FIGURE 30-5

A: Prepatellar bursa with central necrosis and recurrent infection that failed numerous attempts of local wound care. **B:** A perforator flap has been harvested after identifying the vessel, and the prepatellar area has been debrided.

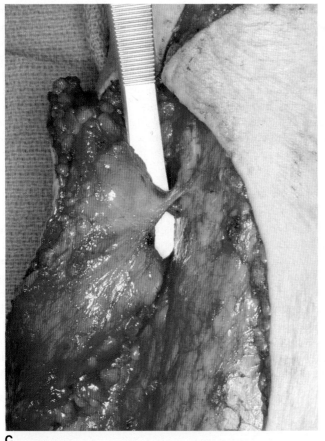

C

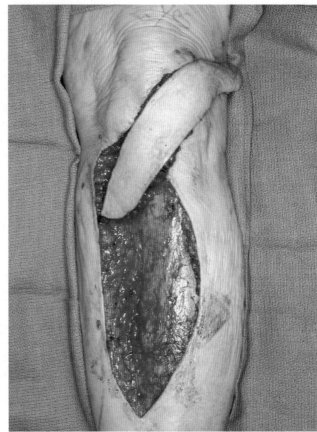

D

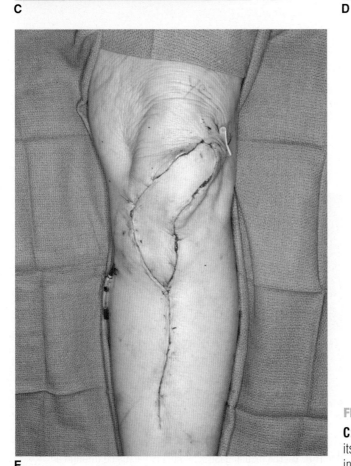

E

FIGURE 30-5 (*Continued*)

C: Perforator vessel to flap. **D:** The flap is rotated 180 degrees on its pedicle and transferred to the area of the defect. **E:** Harvest site incisions have been closed primarily and the flap sutured in place.

(Fig. 30-5C). Due to anatomical variability of these perforating vessels, Doppler ultrasound is used to locate the perforator before elevation of the flap. Once isolated, the perforator flap can be rotated about the vascular pedicle or transferred as a free flap (Fig. 30-5D). The donor site can be managed with either primary closure or split-thickness skin grafts depending on the specific perforator flap used (Fig. 30-5E). A number of perforator flaps have proven quite reliable for managing soft tissue problems in the lower extremity; these include flaps based on the muscle perforators of the vastus lateralis, tensor fascia lata, sartorius, gracilis, and medial gastrocnemius. Unfortunately, due to the volume of tissue required in many cases associated with failed TKA, these muscle perforator flaps often would not provide enough soft tissue to cover the defect; in these circumstances, one of the alternative techniques must be considered.

Medial Gastrocnemius Flap

Technique

Although both the lateral and medial heads of the gastrocnemius muscle can be used to provide soft tissue coverage about the knee, both the quantity of tissue provided by the lateral gastrocnemius and its shorter vascular pedicle restrict its use. The lateral head is generally 3 to 4 cm shorter than the medial head, and its transfer can place the common peroneal nerve at risk for injury as the muscle is passed across the proximal fibula. Therefore, the medial gastrocnemius rotational flap has been the preferred option for treating wound problems in association with total knee replacement (Figs. 30-6 and 30-7). In cases of more severe soft tissue loss, the lateral gastrocnemius can be used in conjunction with the medial-sided flap. First, the wound is debrided to healthy margins. Next, the medial gastrocnemius muscle flap is developed through a posteromedial incision, separating the muscle belly away from the deep tissue superficially

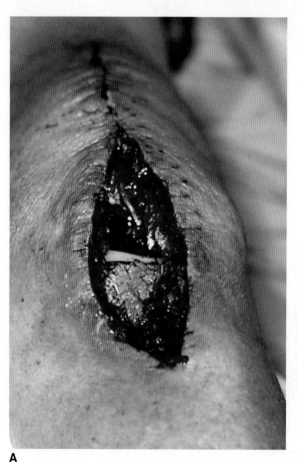
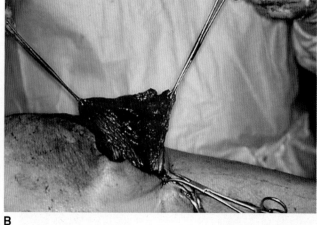

A　　　　　　　　　　　　　　　　　　　**B**

FIGURE 30-6

A: Debrided wound after full-thickness necrosis over proximal tibia after TKA. **B:** The medial gastrocnemius is harvested through a posteromedial incision of the calf and then tunneled under a skin bridge to the debrided area.

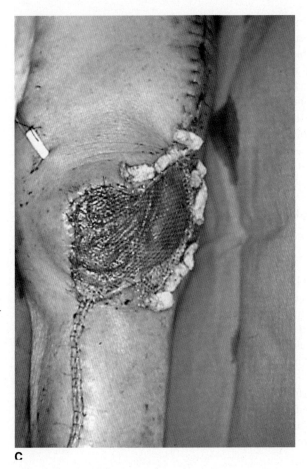

C

FIGURE 30-6 (*Continued*)
C: The muscle flap is covered with a split-thickness skin graft.

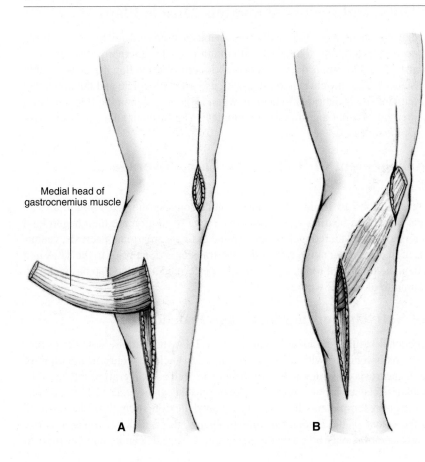

Medial head of
gastrocnemius muscle

A

B

FIGURE 30-7

A: The medial head of the gastrocnemius muscle is harvested through a medial calf incision.
B: The muscle is then rotated and delivered a skin bridge into the defect.

and the underlying soleus muscle along its deep surface. The plantaris tendon, which courses between the medial head of the gastrocnemius muscle and the soleus muscle in the midportion of the leg, provides an excellent landmark. The medial head is separated from the lateral head along its decussation, which does place the sural nerve at risk for injury. The vascular pedicle is based proximally on the sural artery, which is the first branch of the popliteal artery. The muscle is then divided distally at the musculotendinous junction and folded proximally. Next, the flap is tunneled under a medial skin bridge to cover the defect, where it is sutured in place (see Fig. 30-7). If added length is needed, radial scoring of the fascia along the undersurface of the muscle can be performed at 1-cm intervals to increase its arc of rotation. Once transferred, the muscle flap is covered with a split-thickness skin graft that can be performed either primarily, or at a later date; in most circumstances, the donor site can be closed primarily. Alternatively, the flap may be harvested as a musculocutaneous flap, where the entire soft tissue flap including the skin, subcutaneous tissue, fascia, and muscle is rotated about the vascular pedicle. In these cases, the donor site must be skin grafted.

Results

In association with infected or exposed total knee prostheses where wound breakdown has occurred, use of medial gastrocnemius flaps has been quite successful, considering the complexity of the problems. In one series, Gerwin et al. reported their experience from the Hospital for Special Surgery; successful salvage of an infected or exposed total knee prosthesis with a medial gastrocnemius flap was achieved in 10 of 12 patients. Similar results have been reported by McPherson et al., with successful reimplantation in 20 of 21 patients who had chronically infected total knee replacements and compromised soft tissues about the knee.

Utilization of the gastrocnemius muscle for knee coverage results in little functional morbidity, with no significant deficits at walking speed and only mild deficits as demand increases. The use of flaps when concern about soft tissue viability exists should be liberal, especially if an implant is underlying the envelope. Surgeons will rarely regret having done a flap when concern exists, but many a surgeon will wish they had.

Free Latissimus Dorsi and Rectus Abdominis Muscle Flaps

In cases where the medial gastrocnemius flap has been previously used and failed, or when the extent of the soft tissue necrosis is too large to manage with rotational flaps, alternative flaps must be considered. The free transfer of a latissimus dorsi or rectus abdominis muscle flap has been reliable in these difficult circumstances. The muscle is harvested with its vascular pedicle and the donor site primarily closed. The recipient site is debrided to healthy wound edges, and then the free muscle is sutured into the defect after the vascular anastomosis is complete. The vascular anastomosis is typically performed to the popliteal vessels.

Postoperative Management of Soft Tissue Flap Coverage Procedures

Immobilization with elevation for 7 to 10 days to reduce venous congestion is common to all flap coverage procedures. Partial weight bearing and progressive range of motion are then begun on a case-by-case basis. Factors to be considered include any wound drainage, marginal necrosis, venous congestion, and success of the overlying skin graft. If the flap transfer is done prior to the TKA as a prophylactic measure, then the total joint replacement may be performed after the flap has matured, which is generally a minimum of 8 to 12 weeks.

Complications of Soft Tissue Flap Coverage Procedures

In addition to poor functional results associated with revision TKA that require soft tissue procedures, other complications associated with all types of flaps can include recurrent infection or wound problems, marginal necrosis or complete loss of the flap, as well as skin graft problems at the donor or graft sites. Weakness caused by transfer of the donor muscle can also occur. For example, after medial gastrocnemius transfer, patients have reduced plantar flexion strength of the involved ankle; however, given the extent of the associated knee problems, the functional limitations due to loss of the medial gastrocnemius may be clinically irrelevant. Cosmesis can be another issue as the flaps may be quite bulky; however, this concern must be considered relative to the presenting problem and only occasionally debulking or thinning of a mature flap may be undertaken where atrophy of the muscle was less than anticipated.

EXTENSOR MECHANISM DYSFUNCTION

Quadriceps Tendon Rupture

Technique

Fortunately, the incidence of quadriceps tendon rupture after TKA is very low with approximately 1 case per 1,000 reported, as this problem has proven to be difficult to manage. In distinction to the native knee, where primary repair of the tendon to its attachment on the superior pole of the patella with nonabsorbable sutures passed through vertical tunnels in the patella has proven quite successful, the same results have not been achieved in the setting of TKA due to patellar components and poor soft tissue quality. Therefore, the preferred technique includes a repair of the tendon with augmentation of the repair using autologous hamstring tissue or a synthetic mesh. Cadaveric dermal tissue can be utilized as well, as a patch to reinforce the repair. First, the distal end of the tendon is resected back to healthy tissue. Then, two no. 5 nonabsorbable sutures are woven through the avulsed tendon in a Krackow-type technique and passed through vertical tunnels in the patella using a suture passer or straight needle. These sutures are then tied with the knee completely extended. An autologous semitendinosus or gracilis graft, or a synthetic surgical mesh, is then used to augment the repair. Postoperatively, the patient is immobilized in full extension for 6 to 8 weeks; motion is then increased by 30-degree increments at 2-week intervals, with the goal of 90 degrees by 3 months postoperatively. During this time, the leg is protected in a hinged brace. Patients with postoperative partial quadriceps tendon rupture after TKA can be adequately managed by the same nonoperative protocol as described for those patients with complete tears who have undergone surgical reconstruction.

Results

Patients with partial quadriceps tears after TKA treated nonoperatively, as described previously, have generally done well, with all seven patients in one recent series achieving good results. In distinction, nonoperative treatment for patients with complete quadriceps tears has been poor, with patients generally requiring drop lock knee braces to ambulate. Furthermore, patients with complete tears treated with simple repair alone also had poor results. Six of ten patients in this group had unsatisfactory outcomes, including four reruptures. Other complications included knee recurvatum and instability, and deep infection. These generally dismal results prompted the changes in surgical techniques noted previously.

Patellar Tendon Disruption

Technique

In association with TKA, postoperative patellar tendon rupture is an uncommon but potentially catastrophic complication that presents a difficult reconstructive problem. Nonoperative management is associated with loss of extensor power in the involved extremity, usually requiring the use of a drop lock brace or walker. Surgical intervention has also been associated with poor results when simple primary repair has been attempted. More recently, successful salvage of a functional extremity has been made possible with allograft reconstruction using an entire extensor mechanism as described by Burnett et al. The technique is performed through a midline incision when possible. A midline arthrotomy passing over the medial patella allows the native patella to be shelled out from the retinaculum. If the prior patella has fragmented and there are numerous thin fragments of bone embedded in the soft tissue sleeve, these may be left in situ to prevent causing extensive damage to the retinaculum. Distally, over the proximal tibia, the native tendon remnants and retinacular tissue should be elevated subperiosteally, both medially and laterally, for a distance of 7 to 10 cm from the joint line to expose the entire tubercle area. This exposure creates two sleeves of tissue that will be closed over the allograft at the end of the procedure. If revision TKA needs to be simultaneously performed, the procedure is then performed at this stage. It is important to ensure that component positioning is optimal to minimize stress and shear forces on the graft.

Preparation of the host site begins with creating a trough about 6 cm long and just under 2 cm wide and deep with a burr, saw, or osteotome close to the location of the native tubercle. If possible, a bridge about 1.5 to 2 cm high should be left between the tibial surface proximally and the proximal end of the trough, although in some revision TKA cases, this may not be possible when the bone is deficient. The proximal end of the trough should have an oblique cut that creates a small overhang that will lock in the bone block of the graft and resist proximal migration due to the pull from the quadriceps.

While the host site is being prepared, a second team prepares the allograft. The fresh frozen extensor allograft must include a tibial bone block that is at least 6 to 8 cm long and 2 cm wide and deep, the entire patellar tendon, the patella, and at least 5 to 6 cm of the quadriceps tendon. Distally, a block about 6 cm long and 2 cm wide and deep is prepared. The prepared block should be slightly larger than the trough in the host tibia, and chamfered, to facilitate a solid press fit. The proximal end of the block should also have an oblique "dovetail" cut that is directed proximal and posteriorly that will help lock in the block, as previously noted (Fig. 30-8). In the proximal part of the allograft, two no. 5 nonabsorbable braided sutures are stitched through the medial and lateral portions of the quadriceps tendon using a Krackow technique. The free ends of the suture should exit from the proximal end of the quadriceps tendon.

Insertion of the graft begins by weaving two additional no. 5 nonabsorbable sutures into the distal end of the native medial and lateral quadriceps tendon remnants using a Krackow technique. Next, the bone block is gently press fit and then tamped into the trough. The proximal portion of the bone block should first be wedged under the oblique step in the native bone and then the distal end gently impacted to ensure the best fit. If the bone block needs to be trimmed at this stage, either a burr or bone rongeur can be used. Once the block is tapped in place, the block is fixed with two bicortical screws that should be countersunk. Certainly, use of screws creates stress risers in the graft and theoretically increases risk of graft resorption or weakening; however, loss of fixation anecdotally appears to be reduced. Alternatively, two or three 18-gauge wires can be used, as is customary with a standard tibial tubercle osteotomy. However, in these allograft cases, the surgeon must ensure that the proximal lock between the block and trough that is produced by the oblique cuts is solid, or proximal migration may occur. The risk of migration in these cases can be higher due to lack of the native lateral soft tissue attachments that help resist proximal migration of the block and longer time to union. After the block is secure, the sutures that were previously woven through the allograft quadriceps tendon are pulled proximally by an assistant. While under maximum tension, these sutures are passed under, and then up through the native quadriceps tendon remnants. The native tissues are simultaneously pulled distally using the other Krackow-type sutures that were previously

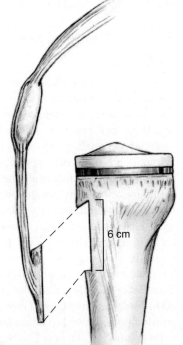

FIGURE 30-8

The trough in the host tibia should be made with a proximal overhang, underneath which the oblique cut of the extensor allograft bone block can be wedged.

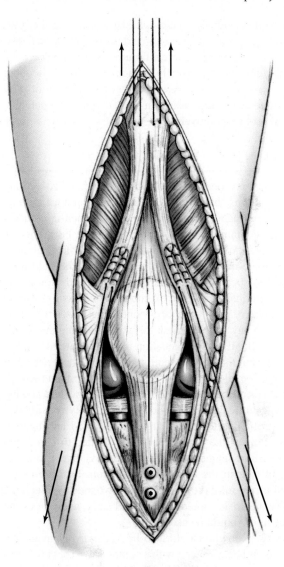

FIGURE 30-9

The extensor allograft should be tensioned and sutures tied with maximal proximal and distal directed forces applied to the allograft and native quadriceps, respectively.

woven through the medial and lateral sleeves (Fig. 30-9). While the knee is held in full extension and maximal proximal and distal forces are applied, the sutures that are attached to the allograft quadriceps tendon are tied. Additional no. 5 sutures are then placed into the native and allograft tendon to stitch the graft in place. The native medial and lateral tissue sleeves are then closed over the allograft in a "pants-over-vest" technique using a combination of no. 0 and no. 1 sutures. These grafts must be overtightened, as they stretch and creep over time due to hysteresis.

Postoperatively, these patients are immobilized in full extension in a well-fitting brace or cylinder cast for 6 to 8 weeks. Factors including the patient compliance, shape of the leg, and wound care issues must be considered in selecting the optimal method of immobilization. Patients may ambulate with partial weight bearing during this period. After 6 to 8 weeks, flexion is advanced by 30 degrees every 2 weeks, with the goal of 0 to 90 by 3 months postoperatively. Typically, a hinged knee brace with flexion stops is used to protect the patient during this period, and the brace is locked in full extension during ambulation.

Results

The results of simple repair of patellar tendon ruptures after TKA have been poor with high failure rates. Furthermore, early attempts at patellar tendon reconstruction after TKA, using extensor allografts with techniques that tensioned the graft in varying degrees of flexion, have also been associated with high rates of extensor lag. Other complications of all techniques include infection and wound healing problems. However, knee stiffness has not been a significant concern, and changes in the intraoperative technique, described previously, that emphasize tensioning the graft in maximal extension, in conjunction with prolonged immobilization in extension postoperatively, have been associated with better results. Burnett et al. reported clinical failures, with an average lag of 59 degrees, in all seven patients in whom the graft was minimally tensioned. In the subsequent 13 patients in whom the graft was maximally tensioned, all were successes with a mean of only 4 degrees lag. Modern techniques have led to quite acceptable results in these challenging patients, but patient expectations must be reasonable and set preoperatively.

POSTOPERATIVE MANAGEMENT

A number of factors have been reported to influence postoperative wound healing after TKA. Many of these factors include the same systemic conditions that need to be optimized preoperatively. Similarly, postoperatively, it is imperative that significant pulmonary disease and anemia, in addition to tobacco use, are aggressively managed to maintain optimal tissue oxygenation. Furthermore, nutritional requirements must be met, and management of diabetes should maintain blood glucose levels within tight control. When possible, immune-modifying medications should be held until primary wound healing has occurred. Other factors specific to the postoperative period should also be considered, especially in patients with other significant risks. For example, tight dressings should be avoided as these may compromise local capillary flow. Use of a continuous passive motion machine for extended periods should be avoided in any patient at risk for wound healing problems, as flexion beyond 40 degrees is known to reduce the tissue oxygenation along the lateral wound, and greater than 60 degrees also compromises medial tissue oxygenation. Indeed, a short period of immobilization should be instituted in patients who develop problem wounds. Development of a significant postoperative hematoma may also reduce tissue oxygenation; in cases where wound healing problems occur in conjunction with a hematoma, surgical drainage should be carefully considered.

When wound healing problems occur, the problem should be carefully followed and aggressively managed to avoid secondary bacterial seeding of the joint. Small areas limited to 1 to 2 mm of marginal superficial skin necrosis that involve short segments of the wound (less than 1 to 2 cm) may be observed and treated with local wound care in the absence of infection. In these cases, immobilization should be used and activity minimized until the margins of the wound have declared themselves. Wound breakdown or full-thickness necrosis should be debrided early, and one of the previously described soft tissue coverage procedures should be used.

Prolonged wound drainage, without wound breakdown, should also be aggressively managed. Significant serous drainage beyond 3 or 4 days should be managed with a compressive (but not tight) dressing, immobilization, and bed rest. Failure to respond within 48 hours should prompt surgical drainage if a seroma is suspected. In cases where there is significant bloody drainage, initial treatment is the same as for serous drainage. However, in this second group of patients, persistent bloody drainage after TKA is suggestive of capsular dehiscence. Failure to respond to nonsurgical treatment should prompt a return to the operating room for an evacuation of the hematoma and closure of the arthrotomy. Certainly, substantial drainage beyond a week from surgery should cause concern and requires careful observation and early intervention if quick resolution doesn't occur.

Incisional Negative Pressure Wound Therapy

Although as of yet there are no large randomized controlled trials investigating incisional negative pressure wound therapy (NPWT) in revision TKA, some high-risk patients may benefit from its application in the immediate postoperative period. In a prospective randomized multicenter clinical trial, Stannard et al. demonstrated that application of incisional NPWT after high-risk lower extremity fractures resulted in a decreased incidence of wound dehiscence and total infections. The proposed benefits of incisional NPWT include an increase in tissue perfusion, reduction in edema, seroma and hematoma mass, and stretching of cells leading to cell growth and expansion. Combined, these mechanisms may facilitate improved speed, strength, and quality of wound healing, therefore reducing risk of infection and/or dehiscence. Additionally, the sterilely applied incisional NPWT can be left in place for several days, therefore decreasing the need to expose the wound for dressing changes in the postoperative period. It is important to use as narrow a sponge strip as possible and interpose a nonadhesive but permeable dressing between the skin and sponge in order to avoid tissue maceration and blistering.

SUMMARY

In order for successful revision TKA to be accomplished, early wound healing is required. Numerous factors in the preoperative, intraoperative, and postoperative periods can influence this process. While many of these factors are beyond the control of the orthopedic surgeon, several are not. Careful preoperative evaluation helps identify and manage potential problems to minimize the risks. Furthermore, the orthopedic surgeon needs to be aware of the plastic and orthopedic surgery techniques that not only help reduce complications but also help salvage these knees when these potentially devastating problems occur.

PEARLS AND PITFALLS

- In revision TKA, preoperative planning in consideration of the patient's systemic factors and characteristics of the knee and leg is critical for minimizing soft tissue problems about the knee.
- For the superficial dissection, the importance of raising thick fasciocutaneous flaps as opposed to subcutaneous flaps cannot be overstated.
- Extension of the incision into native tissue beyond the edge of the scar will help to locate and allow development of the tissue planes.
- For the deep dissection, the medial parapatellar arthrotomy is versatile, allows the optimal exposure in revision TKA, and is compatible with each of the more extensile exposures.
- Following medial parapatellar arthrotomy, a medial tibial peel is performed. Often, the combination of these two techniques is sufficient to allow removal of the tibial polyethylene; this relaxes the flexion and extension gaps, improves the exposure and mobility of the soft tissues, and in many cases allows sufficient exposure for revision surgery.
- If additional exposure is required, the quadriceps snip is an excellent first choice as strength is not affected, and there is no need to modify or restrict postoperative rehabilitation.
- Alternatively, the tibial tubercle osteotomy facilitates exposure in particularly stiff or difficult cases and can still be used even after a quadriceps snip has already been performed. The tibial tubercle osteotomy allows access to the tibial canal, which may be helpful in revision or infected TKA when well-fixed stemmed, tibial components must be removed.
- There are various methods described within this chapter to achieve soft tissue coverage when primary closure is impossible or fails.
- Incisional NPWT should be considered in some high-risk patients as it may facilitate improved speed, strength, and quality of wound healing, therefore reducing risk of infection and/or dehiscence.

RECOMMENDED READING

Barrack RL, Smith P, Munn B, et al. Comparison of surgical approaches in total knee arthroplasty. *Clin Orthop.* 1998;356:16–21.

Burnett SJ, Berger RA, Della Valle CJ, et al. Extensor mechanism allograft reconstruction after total knee arthroplasty: surgical technique. *J Bone Joint Surg.* 2005;87A(suppl 1, pt 2):175–194.

Clarke HD, Craig-Scott S, Scott WN. Tissue expanders in total knee arthroplasty. *Tech Knee Surg.* 2005;4:12–18.

Garvin KL, Scuderi G, Insall JN. Evolution of the quadriceps snip. *Clin Orthop.* 1995;321:131–137.

Geddes CR, Morri SF, Neligan PC. Perforator flaps: evolution, classification, and applications. *Ann Plast Surg.* 2003;50:90–99.

Gerwin M, Rothaus KO, Windsor RE, et al. Gastrocnemius muscle flap coverage of exposed or infected knee prosthesis. *Clin Orthop.* 1993;286:64–70.

Haertsch P. The blood supply to the skin of the leg: a post-mortem investigation. *Br J Plast Surg.* 1981;34:470–477.

Insall J. A midline approach to the knee. *J Bone Joint Surg Am.* 1971;53(8):1584–1586.

Johnson DP. Midline or parapatellar incision for knee arthroplasty: a comparative study of wound viability. *J Bone Joint Surg.* 1988;70B:656–658.

Johnson DP, Eastwood DM. Lateral patellar release in knee arthroplasty: effect on wound healing. *J Arthroplasty.* 1992;7(suppl):407–431.

Karlakki S, Brem M, Giannini S, et al. Negative pressure wound therapy for management of the surgical incision in orthopaedic surgery: a review of evidence and mechanisms for an emerging indication. *Bone Joint Res.* 2013;2:276–284.

Lavernia C, Contreras JS, Alcerro JC. The peel in total knee revision: exposure in the difficult knee. *Clin Orthop Relat Res.* 2011;469(1):146–153.

Long WJ, Wilson CH, Scott SMC, et al. 15-year experience with soft tissue expansion in total knee arthroplasty. *J Arthroplasty.* 2012;27(3):362–367.

McPherson EJ, Patzakis MJ, Gross JE, et al. Infected total knee arthroplasty: two-stage reimplantation with a gastrocnemius rotational flap. *Clin Orthop.* 1997;341:73–81.

Mendes MW, Caldwell P, Jiranek WA. The results of tibial tubercle osteotomy for revision total knee arthroplasty. *J Arthroplasty*. 2004;19(2):167–174.

Rothaus KO. Plastic and reconstructive surgery. In: Insall JN, ed. *Surgery of the Knee*. New York: Churchill-Livingstone; 1993:1200–1201.

Sanna M, Sanna C, Caputo F, et al. Surgical approaches in total knee arthroplasty. *Joints*. 2013;1(2):34–44.

Stannard JP, Volgas DA, McGwin G, et al. Incisional negative pressure wound therapy after high-risk lower extremity fractures. *J Orthop Trauma*. 2012;26(1):37–42.

Sun Z, Patil A, Song EK, et al. Comparison of quadriceps snip and tibial tubercle osteotomy in revision for infected total knee arthroplasty. *Int Orthop*. 2015;39(5):879–885.

Trousdale RT, Hanssen AD, Rand JA. V–Y quadricepsplasty in total knee arthroplasty. *Clin Orthop*. 1993;286:48–55.

van den Broek CM, van Hellemondt GG, Jacobs WCH, et al. Step-cut tibial tubercle osteotomy for access in revision total knee replacement. *Knee*. 2006;13(6):430–434.

Weiss AP, Krackow KA. Persistent wound drainage after primary total knee arthroplasty. *J Arthroplasty*. 1993;8:285–289.

Whiteside LA. Exposure in difficult total knee arthroplasty using tibial tubercle osteotomy. *Clin Orthop*. 1995;321:32–35.

Windsor RE, Insall JN. Exposure in revision total knee arthroplasty: the femoral peel. *Tech Orthop*. 1988;3:1–4.

Younger AS, Duncan CP, Masri BA. Surgical exposures in revision total knee arthroplasty. *J Am Acad Orthop Surg*. 1998;6(1):55–64.

31 Pedicled Soleus Muscle Flap for Coverage of the Middle and Distal Third of the Tibia

Salvatore C. Lettieri and Steven L. Moran

Soft tissue defects involving the middle and lower third of the leg may occur following trauma, tumor extirpation, and osteomyelitis. Anteriorly, the skin and subcutaneous tissue overriding the middle third and lower third of the tibia are thin, and exposed bone and tendon may result from soft tissue injury or open fractures. Historically, middle third defects have been covered with the pedicled soleus muscle flap, while attempts have been made more recently to extend to soleus flap to cover defects of the lower third of the leg.

The soleus muscle, according to the Mathes and Nahai schema, is a type II muscle, containing dominant pedicles from the popliteal, peroneal, and posterior tibial arteries and minor segmental pedicles from the posterior tibial artery. The muscle lies in the superficial posterior compartment extending the entire length of the lower leg. The soleus originates from the posterior surface of the tibia, the interosseous membrane, and the proximal third of the fibula. The muscle runs deep to the gastrocnemius muscle in the upper third of the leg (Fig. 31-1). In the middle third of the leg, the muscle joins with the gastrocnemius muscle and is adherent to the calcaneal tendon. The soleus is a bipennate muscle with the medial and lateral muscle bellies each receiving an independent neurovascular supply; this allows the lateral and medial portions to be mobilized independently while preserving some function within the remaining soleus muscle. The medial head originates from the tibia and receives the majority of its blood supply from the posterior tibial artery. The lateral head originates from the fibula and receives the majority of its blood supply from the perineal artery, although 16% of muscles may be nourished entirely by the posterior tibial artery. The lateral and medial heads are fused proximally, while a septum divides the muscle distally. This septum is an extension of the calcaneal tendon and soleus tendon. Dividing the muscle longitudinally at the level of the septum allows for the elevation of the medial and lateral hemisoleus flaps.

In the distal one-third of the muscle, the soleus receives segmental arterial perforators from the posterior tibial artery (Fig. 31-2). These distal perforators may be absent in up to 26% of patients; in these cases, distal perfusion to the muscle is provided by axial blood flow from more proximal perforators. The diameter and position of these distal perforators are variable, but, if present and of large enough caliber, these perforators can allow for a portion of the muscle to be harvested in a reverse fashion. The muscle may then be rotated 90 to 180 degrees, based on its distal perforators, allowing coverage of the lower third of the tibia and ankle region.

The soleus functions to stabilize the ankle and assist in plantarflexion. The muscle works synergistically with the gastrocnemius and tibialis posterior muscle to provide plantarflexion, while the flexor hallucis longus, flexor digitorum longus, and tibialis posterior all help to provide ankle stability and resist dorsiflexion.

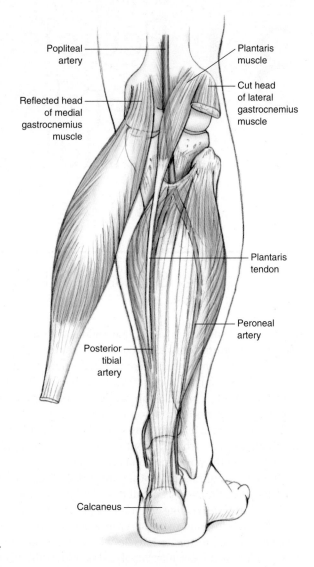

FIGURE 31-1

Schematic anatomy of the posterior leg showing the soleus located deep to the gastrocnemius muscle bellies. The plantaris tendon helps define the plane between the soleus and the gastrocnemius muscle bellies. The blood supply to the soleus is from the popliteal, posterior tibial, and perineal arteries.

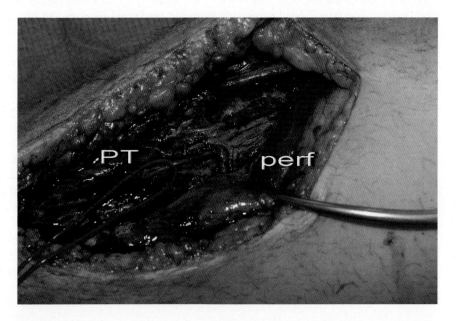

FIGURE 31-2

The posterior tibial artery (PT) as it approaches the ankle gives off several arterial perforators (perfs) to the distal soleus muscle. If these perforators are of adequate caliber, the muscle can be dissected free and rotated as a distally based flap.

INDICATIONS/CONTRAINDICATIONS

The primary indication for the use of the soleus muscle flap is coverage of soft tissue defects in the middle third of the leg. Distal third defects have historically been covered with free flaps; however, for small defects and in patients with significant comorbid disease, which would prohibit prolonged anesthesia times, a reverse soleus muscle flap may be considered as an alternative to free tissue transfer.

There are several factors that may prohibit the successful transfer of the soleus muscle and these are:

- Size of the defect
- Status of the soleus muscle belly
- Status of surrounding tissue and bone
- Size and location of existing perforators

Size of the Defect

The soleus muscle has a limited surface area and a limited arc of rotation (Fig. 31-3). Large defects occupying the majority of the middle third and lower third of the leg are best covered with free tissue

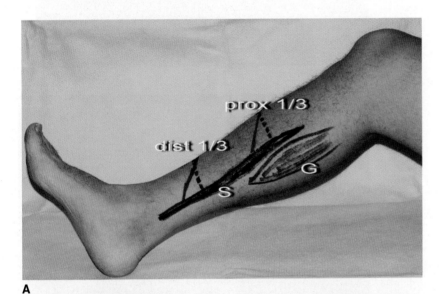

A

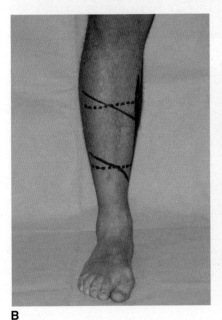

B

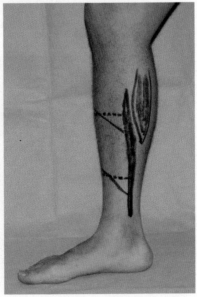

C

FIGURE 31-3

A: The soleus muscle (S) runs anterior to the gastrocnemius muscle (G) and to the area just proximal to the medial malleolus. The arc of rotation of the medially based soleus muscle is limited due to its deep origin and broad proximal attachments. This makes coverage of more laterally and inferiorly based middle third defects difficult. **B, C:** The *solid red line* shows the actual safe arc of rotation for the medially based soleus muscle flap, with the *dashed line* depicting the superior and inferior margins of the "middle third" of the leg.

transfer. In addition, the distal aspect of the muscle can be unreliable if it must be stretched or inset under significant tension. In such cases, alternative methods of closure should be considered or the soleus may be used in conjunction with another flap.

The soleus can be used in conjunction with the medial or lateral gastrocnemius muscles for larger defects spanning the upper aspect of the lower leg, but this will compromise remaining plantarflexion (Fig. 31-4). When the defect is so large as to require more than just the soleus and medial

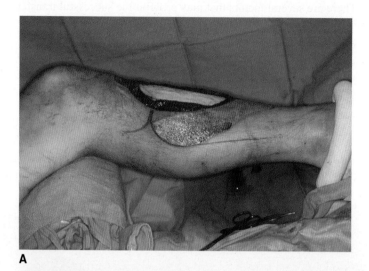

A

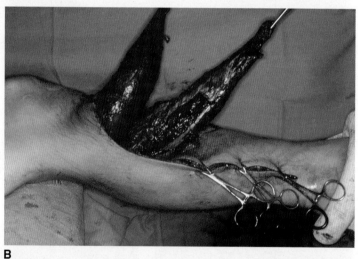

B

FIGURE 31-4

Figure **(A)** shows defect encompassing the upper and middle third of the leg. **B:** The gastrocnemius muscle and soleus muscle are elevated in preparation for defect coverage. **C:** This large defect is easily covered by elevating both the medial gastrocnemius muscle and the soleus muscle.

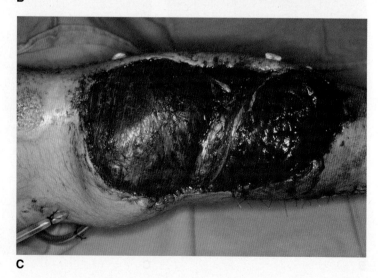

C

gastrocnemius flaps, a free flap should strongly be considered as a means of soft tissue coverage; this will also allow for preservation of remaining posterior compartment function. Defects that are to be covered with a reversed soleus muscle flap should be less than 50 cm^2 while the standard soleus flap can cover most defects under 75 cm^2.

Status of the Muscle

Because the soleus muscle is closely adherent to the deep posterior surface of the interosseous membrane, tibia, and fibula, it can often be significantly traumatized following comminuted fractures of the tibia and fibula. During initial wound evaluation and debridement, the muscle can often be inspected through the soft tissue defect. If the muscle is significantly lacerated by fracture fragments or contains a significant amount of intramuscular hematoma, it is most prudent to use another flap for soft tissue coverage. In addition, any associated injury to the popliteal, peroneal, or posterior tibial arteries can adversely affect the survival of the soleus muscle.

Status of Surrounding Tissue and Bone

Preexisting damage to the surrounding skin and deeper tissue of the middle third of the leg is also a relative contraindication to soleus muscle flap use. A history of previous radiation therapy, previous surgery, or penetrating trauma to the area surrounding the middle third of the leg should alert the surgeon to potential problems with the use of this flap. The soleus muscle has been shown to provide a source of collateral arterial flow between the posterior tibial and perineal arterial systems. In patients with vascular occlusions of the perineal or posterior tibial arteries, use of the soleus muscle may further compromise limb vascularity by sacrificing important arterial collaterals to the lower leg and foot.

Size and Location of Existing Perforators

Indications for use of the soleus for distal third defects are based on the work of Pu and include (a) defect size less than 50 cm, (b) defects located over the anterior or medial portion of the distal tibia, (c) the presence of large perforators in distal 4 to 5 cm of muscle, and (d) a soleus muscle that is nontraumatized on initial exploration. If these factors are met, a reversed hemisoleus flap may be attempted for lower third defects; otherwise, a free flap is chosen for distal third defects. In addition, patients who have a smoking history, peripheral vascular disease, and history of lower leg radiation therapy should be considered high risk for a reversed soleus muscle flap.

PREOPERATIVE PLANNING

Close inspection of the lower leg is necessary prior to surgery. Even though the soleus occupies the same compartment as the gastrocnemius, it can be more significantly damaged in open fractures due to its adherence to the tibia and interosseous membrane. If there is significant ecchymosis or swelling of the posterior compartment, in conjunction with significant displacement of the tibia and fibula on lateral radiographs, one must assume significant damage to the soleus muscle. In this case, free tissue transfer would provide a better alternative for coverage of the middle third of the tibia. If the patient has had previous surgeries, such as fasciotomies for trauma, this may also preclude reliable rotation of the flap, since the level of the fasciotomies and also the location of the injuries may have injured the underlying flap (Fig. 31-5).

A noninvasive vascular exam should be performed on the lower leg, verifying patency of the posterior, peroneal, and anterior tibial arteries. If the patient has a history of significant peripheral vascular disease or long-standing diabetes, a CT angiogram may verify patency of the posterior and perineal arteries prior to flap transfer.

SURGERY

Patient Positioning and Surgical Preparation

The patient is placed in the supine position for anterior defects, the lateral decubitus position for lateral defects, and prone for posterior defect coverage. As part of the surgical preparation, the entire lower extremity is prepped and draped in the usual fashion. For anterior midtibial defects, a sterile

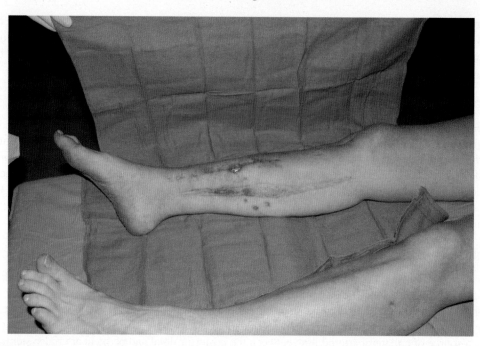

FIGURE 31-5

This patient had lower leg fasciotomies performed at the time of the original tibial injury. The patient now presents with osteomyelitis and exposed hardware over the middle third of the tibia. The defect is located within the arc of coverage of the medial soleus muscle flap; however, there is significant scarring and injury to the superficial posterior compartment secondary to the fasciotomies and previous split-thickness skin grafting. Because of concerns of the reliability of the soleus muscle in this situation, this patient underwent coverage of exposed hardware with a free tissue transfer.

"bump" is placed beneath the distal thigh region to allow for slight external rotation of the leg and bending of the knee; this can facilitate identification of the muscle. The muscle may be harvested with the use of spinal or general anesthetic. A tourniquet on the upper leg allows for a relatively bloodless field during muscle dissection.

Technique

Medially and Proximally Based Soleus Flap

The soleus is harvested through an incision that runs from the upper third of the leg to just above the medial malleolus. The incision is made 2 to 3 cm posterior to the medial palpable margin of the tibia. The defect site is incorporated into this incision (Fig. 31-6). Skin bridges are avoided. Dissection is carried down to the investing fascia of the superficial posterior compartment. The saphenous vein is identified and preserved during the dissection. The deep fascia is then opened longitudinally to expose the posterior compartment.

The muscle itself is most easily identified proximally, deep to the gastrocnemius muscle. The plane between the two muscles is relatively avascular with the exception of some small perforators, which may be ligated. The plantaris runs in the plane between the two muscles and can be used as a landmark in cases of severe trauma where hematoma may obscure the tissue planes.

The soleus fuses with the calcaneal tendon in the middle third of the leg. Here, sharp dissection is required to separate the soleus from the common calcaneal tendon as it extends toward the heel. This dissection is aided by placing medial traction on the edge of the Achilles tendon with the use of several clamps (Fig. 31-7). In the distal aspect, the muscle readily separates from the calcaneal tendon. Dissection from the calcaneal tendon is carried to the midline raphe for hemisoleus elevation. The midline septum does not extend the entire length of the muscle but should be used as guide for hemisoleus elevation. Once the soleus is elevated from the calcaneal tendon, the space between the gastrocnemius muscle and the soleus muscle is easily entered and there is a transverse junction point, which is easily cut with scissors or a knife. This will free the entire posterior aspect of the soleus muscle.

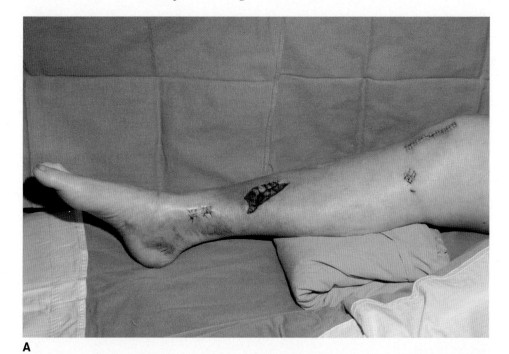

A

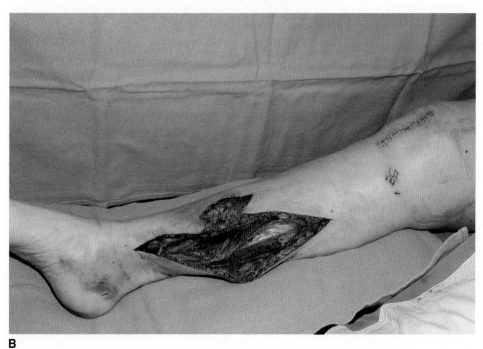

B

FIGURE 31-6

A: A middle third defect in the right leg of a 66-year-old diabetic woman following a Gustilo type IIIB fracture of the tibia. The fracture has been stabilized with an intramedullary rod and the wound has been covered with an antibiotic beads pouch following initial debridement at the time of fracture fixation. **B:** An incision is made slightly posterior to the medial tibial margin and then carried inferiorly. The open wound is incorporated into the incision to avoid creating a skin bridge.

The posterior tibial artery is identified in the plane between the soleus and flexor digitorum longus. Inferiorly, a finger can be passed beneath the soleus muscle but superficial to the posterior tibial vessels. A cautery is then used to separate these medial attachments of the soleus to the tibia. Once the medial aspect of the muscle is mobilized, the space between the soleus and the deep posterior compartments is readily opened with blunt dissection and the lateral aspect of the muscle is identified.

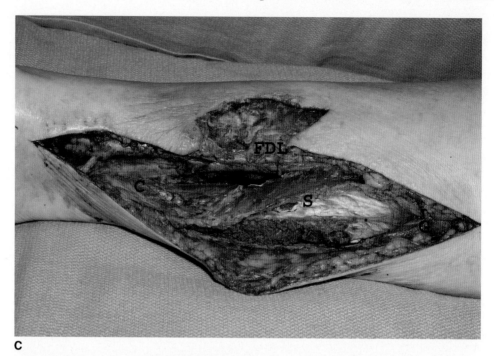

C

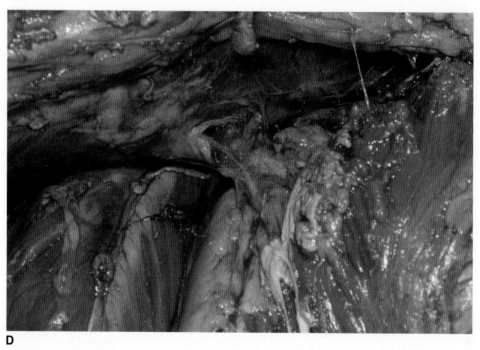

D

FIGURE 31-6 (*Continued*)

C: The soleus muscle (S) has been dissected free of the calcaneal tendon (C) and separated from the gastrocnemius muscle (G) and flexor digitorum longus muscle (FDL). **D:** Large perforators from the posterior tibial artery can be seen entering the muscle.

Once the posterior tibial artery and nerve are identified and the superficial and deep attachments of the muscle have been mobilized, the muscle may be divided distally. Distal perforators from the posterior tibial artery and perineal vessels are then sequentially ligated to allow for mobilization of the muscle. There can be multiple small diameter perforators off the posterior tibial artery; these vessels should be clipped or ligated and not cauterized, as thermal injury may be propagated to the posterior tibial vessels.

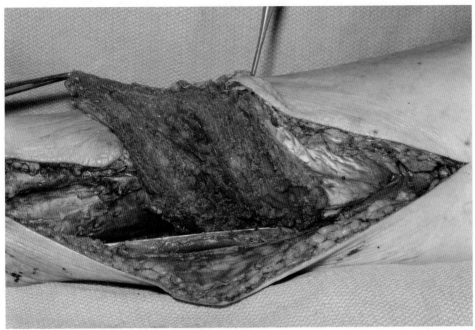

E

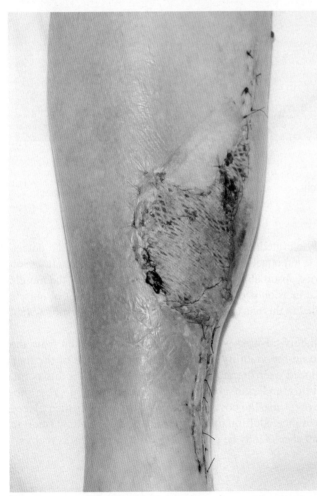

F

FIGURE 31-6 (*Continued*)

E: The muscle is now divided at its distal attachment and pedicled to cover the open defect. Because the soleus is elevated off the common calcaneal tendon, the superficial surface of the muscle is devoid of fascia. The muscle is "fanned out" and inset with half-buried absorbable sutures. **F:** The donor incision is closed up to the rotated muscle and the exposed muscle is covered with a split-thickness skin graft.

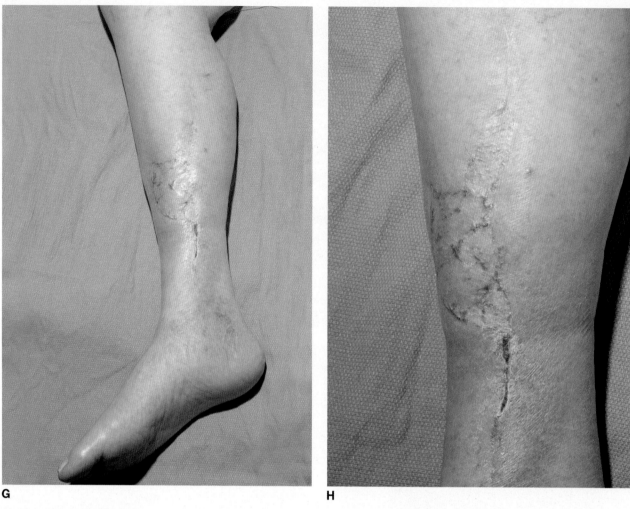

G

H

FIGURE 31-6 (*Continued*)
G, H: At 2 months, the patient has a well-healed wound with excellent contour.

Once the muscle has been completely elevated, it is rotated into position to cover the defect. Generally, the fascia on the deep surface is left attached to the muscle, but there will be no fascia on the superficial surface. Multiple half-buried absorbable sutures can be used to "fan out" the muscle and inset it into the defect site. The distal incision is closed over a drain up to the point of muscle rotation. The muscle should not be tunneled as this can contribute to distal venous congestion within the flap (Figs. 31-6 and 31-7).

The muscle flap can then be immediately covered with a meshed skin graft taken from the upper thigh. If there is any question about the viability of the soleus, or a portion of the flap, a negative pressure dressing may be placed over the muscle for 24 to 48 hours. At this point, the muscle can be reassessed for viability and skin grafted in a delayed fashion. Vaseline-impregnated gauze or a Xeroform dressing is used to cover the skin graft. The leg is then placed in a large Robert-Jones–type dressing with the addition of a posterior splint. A window is left in the dressing overlying the muscle so flap checks may be performed while the patient is recovering on the ward.

Laterally and Proximally Based Soleus Flap
Though the arc of rotation for this muscle is limited, the lateral approach can be advantageous for some lateral middle third defects. The incision is made just inferior to the lateral border of the fibula. The deep fascia is incised just below the fibula, and the plane between the gastrocnemius

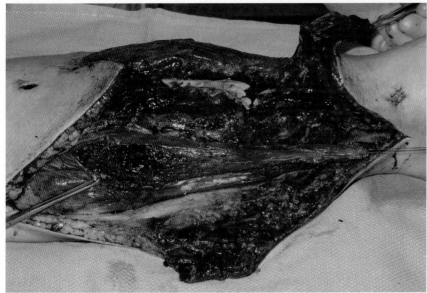

A

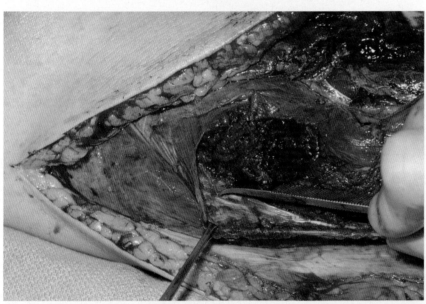

B

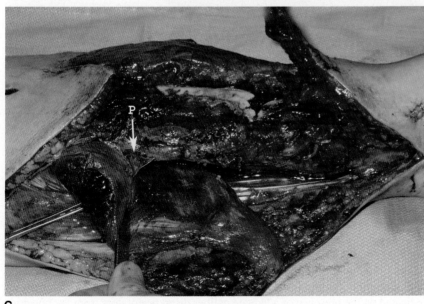

C

FIGURE 31-7

A: Middle to lower third Gustilo IIIB injury following a motor vehicle accident in a 58-year-old man. The soleus has been separated from the flexor digitorum longus as well as the gastrocnemius muscle. The muscle has just been divided distally and a stay suture has been placed in the distal aspect of the muscle. **B:** A Carroll elevator is used to facilitate dissection of the soleus muscle off the common calcaneal tendon as medial traction is applied to the edge of the tendon with Alice clamps. **C:** The muscle is dissected proximally until enough length is available for defect coverage. Large arterial perforators from the posterior tibial artery are preserved to perfuse the flap (P).

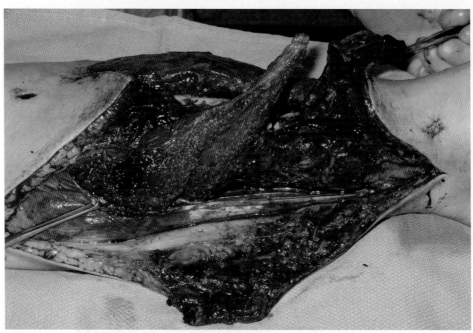

D

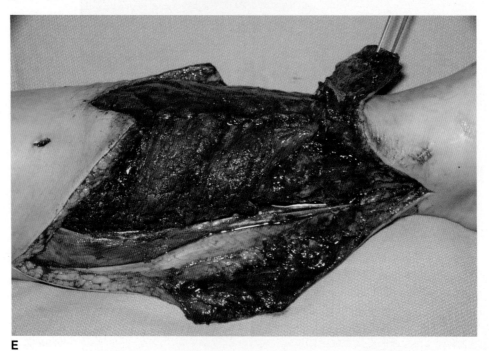

E

FIGURE 31-7 (*Continued*)

D, E: The flap is then pedicled into position and covered with a split-thickness skin graft.

muscle and soleus is created with blunt dissection. Distally, the soleus is again sharply dissected from the calcaneal tendon. Deep proximal dissection involves separating the soleus from its tough attachments to the fibula. During proximal dissection, one must be cognizant of the common perineal nerve running close to the fibular head. Once elevated, the muscle is inset as previously described.

Reverse Soleus Muscle Flap

The reverse soleus muscle flap modification (Fig. 31-8) is used to cover small distal defects over the medial anterior aspect of the tibia or medial superior aspect of the medial malleolus. The success of this operation is predicated on the presence of adequate caliber distal perforators from the posterior

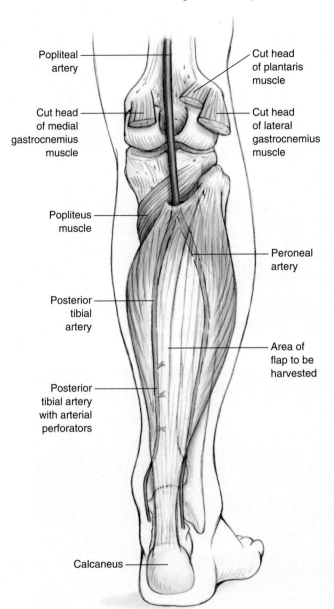

Popliteal
artery

Cut head
of plantaris
muscle

Cut head
of medial
gastrocnemius
muscle

Cut head
of lateral
gastrocnemius
muscle

Popliteus
muscle

Peroneal
artery

Posterior
tibial
artery

Area of
flap to be
harvested

Posterior
tibial artery
with arterial
perforators

Calcaneus

FIGURE 31-8

Schematic drawing of the distally based reverse soleus flap. The flap's arterial supply is from perforators found at the distal portion of the posterior tibial vessels. If present, these vessels may be used to supply a strip of soleus muscle, which is cut from the medial margin of the soleus muscle.

tibial artery. If during the surgical procedure these perforators are injured or are of insufficient quality, the procedure must be abandoned and the defect should be covered with a free tissue transfer. A preoperative angiogram has been recommended by some authors to verify the position of the distal perforator prior to surgery.

Dissection is performed under tourniquet control. The same incision is made as for the proximally based soleus flap (Fig. 31-9). The incision is 2 cm medial to the medial border of the tibia. The existing wound is incorporated into the incision. The medial portion of the soleus is identified as described above and is separated from the gastrocnemius muscle, calcaneal tendon, and the flexor digitorum longus muscle. The posterior tibial artery is identified and the distal perforators are examined to make sure they are adequate. As many distal perforators should be preserved as possible but the authors have had success with the preservation of one or two perforators alone if they are of adequate caliber (vein greater than 1.5 mm and artery of 1 mm or greater). Once the perforatus are determined to be of adequate size, the soleus is then split at the level of the central raphe and divided at the junction of the proximal and middle third. The muscle is then divided longitudinally using the cautery or scissors until the inferior perforator is reached. The muscle is then rotated 90 to 180 degrees. Additional arterial pedicle dissection may be required to prevent vessel kinking. The flap is then inset into the defect with half-buried mattress sutures and covered with a split-thickness skin graft (Fig. 31-10).

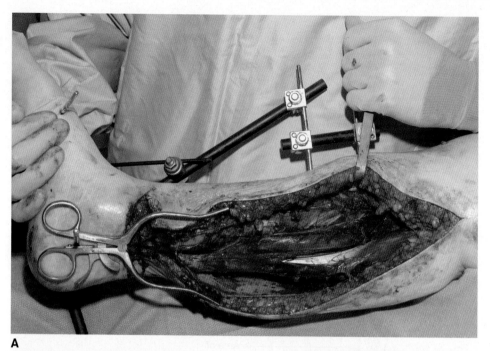

A

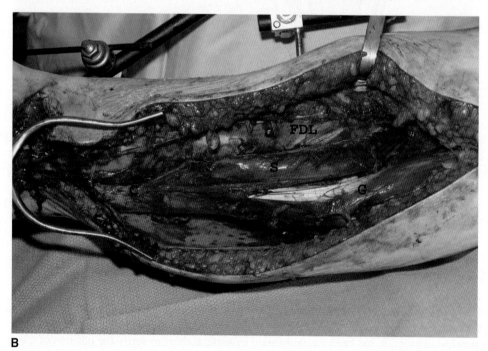

B

FIGURE 31-9

A: A 61-year-old woman with a distal defect overlying the superior medial margin of the malleolus. An incision was made at the medial posterior margin of the tibia. **B:** The gastrocnemius (G), soleus (S), flexor digitorum longus (FDL), and calcaneal tendon (C) are identified.

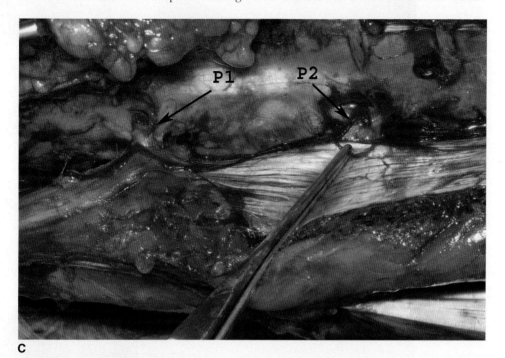

C

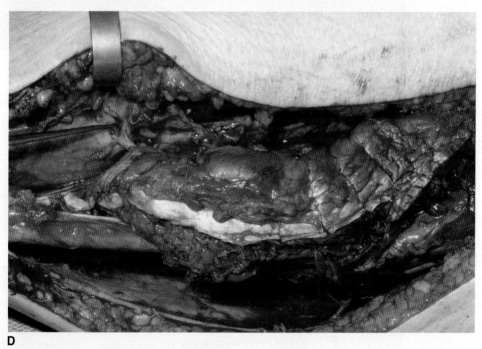

D

FIGURE 31-9 (*Continued*)

C: Exploration of the posterior tibial vessels, in preparation for free tissue transfer, revealed that the patient had two (P1 and P2) large distal perforators to the soleus muscle. Because of this, the patient was felt to be an excellent candidate for a distally based soleus muscle flap. **D:** A medial strip of soleus is then elevated from the common calcaneal tendon, gastrocnemius muscle, and flexor digitorum longus muscle. The nerve hook points to the preserved distal perforator.

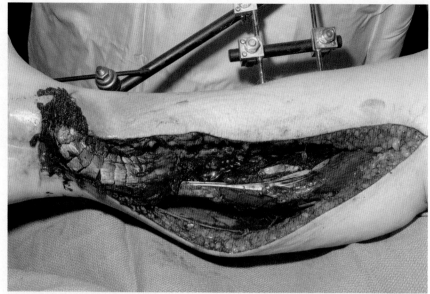

E

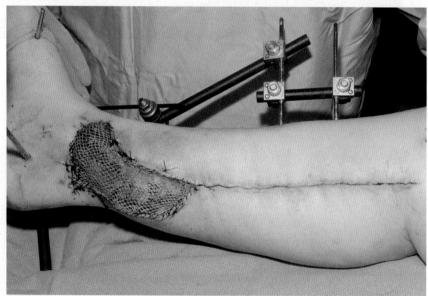

F

FIGURE 31-9 (*Continued*)

E: The muscle is then rotated 180 degrees to cover the distal defect. Care is taken to dissect the proximal perforator back to its origin on the tibial artery to prevent kinking of the artery or vein. **F, G:** The muscle is covered with a split-thickness skin graft and the remaining portion of the external fixator is attached to provide needed stabilization.

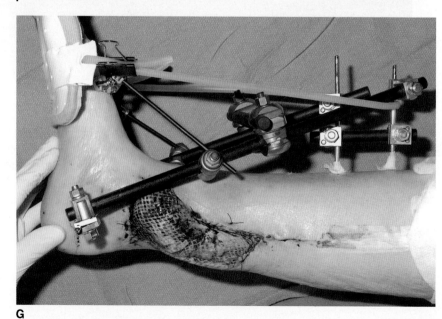

G

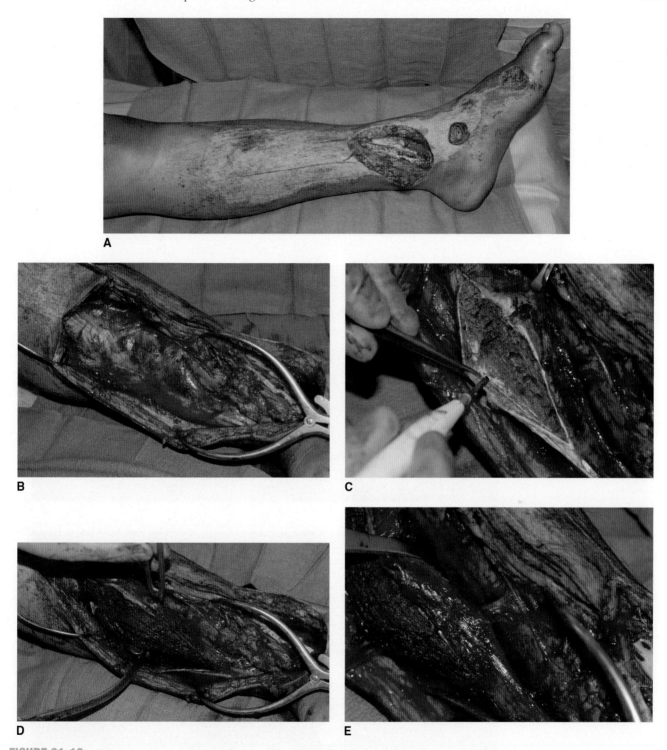

FIGURE 31-10

A: Distal third soft tissue injury in a 30-year-old man. **B:** Exposure of the posterior compartment revealed an uninjured soleus muscle with a very distal extension of the muscle belly. It was decided to perform a reverse soleus flap elevated on a distal third posterior tibial perforator. **C:** The muscle was carefully separated from the terminal tendon with the aid of a cautery device. **D.** The muscle was then separated from the raphe and remaining lateral muscle (retractor placed behind medial muscle). **E:** A large distal perforator was present to supply perfusion to reverse-based flap.

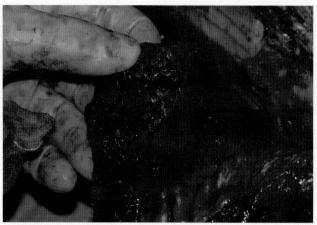

F

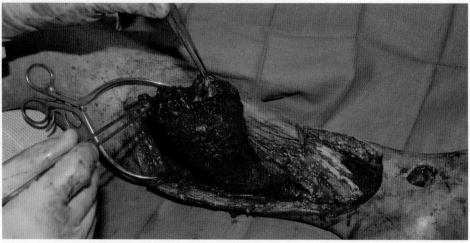

G

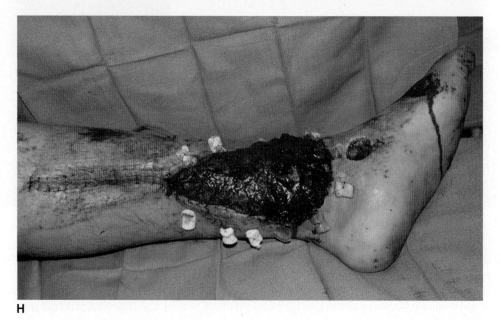

H

FIGURE 31-10 (*Continued*)

F: After division of the proximal portion of the muscle, the perfusion to the end of the flap was evaluated prior to rotation of the muscle into defect. **G:** The flap was rotated 180 degrees into defect. **H:** The flap was carefully inset with the use of soft tissue pledgets on the native skin to avoid skin breakdown.

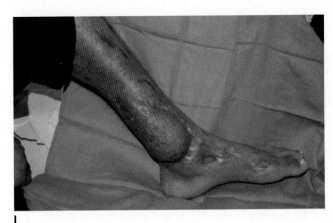

FIGURE 31-10 (*Continued*)

I: Final results at 3 months.

POSTOPERATIVE MANAGEMENT

The patient should be maintained on bed rest in a posterior splint or knee immobilizer for 4 to 5 days to allow time for skin graft inosculation and to minimize dependent edema in the leg. The bolster dressing may be removed on postoperative day 5 to ensure adequate skin graft "take." Until this time, the flap may be monitored through a window in the postoperative dressing. If the skin graft is adherent to the underlying muscle, the patient may begin to mobilize and bear weight as tolerated, barring any underlying fractures. Gentle range of motion should then begin, increasing the motion by 5 or 10 degrees per day. Ambulation can begin on the 10th postsurgical day. If the flap is inset under tension or if the healing environment is less than ideal, the knee immobilizer can be maintained for an additional week to prevent undue tension on the margins of the muscle flap. The drains are removed once drainage is less than 30 mL a day.

Once the original dressing is removed from the skin graft, dressings may be changed daily. This should include the application of topical antibiotic ointment and nonadherent gauze followed by a lightly compressive wrap to minimize edema. Dependent leg position is limited to 30 minutes an hour for the first 2 weeks to minimize edema. On the 3rd postoperative week, the patient is fitted for compressive stockings, which help the patient continue to manage lower extremity edema and help in the flap contouring.

Rehabilitation

Knee and ankle motion may begin once the skin graft is adherent to the underlying muscle bed. Weight-bearing status is determined by the stability of the underlying fractures.

Results

In a study by Hallock of 29 soleus flaps, 24 of 29 flaps were used for coverage of high-energy impact defects. All soleus muscle flaps in this study were based on a proximal pedicle. Complication rates were low. Similar results were reported by Pu, who found no cases of total flap loss when the flap was based on a proximal pedicle for coverage of middle third tibial defects.

COMPLICATIONS

Major complications include total and partial flap necrosis. Total flap loss can occur from injury to the vessels at the time of dissection, use of a flap that has been significantly injured with the surrounding bony trauma, or use of the flap in a situation where the posterior tibial vessels and peroneal vessels were compromised or injured. In such cases, a free tissue transfer is often needed for leg salvage.

Partial necrosis most often occurs at the distal most margin of the flap. If the partial flap necrosis results in exposure of vital structures, another flap will be required for coverage; most commonly, a free flap is used but local fasciocutaneous advancement flaps may be used to cover smaller defects. If the bone is completely covered and the defect is just along the periphery, the wound may be debrided and treated with dressing changes. The remaining wound can then heal through secondary intention.

Skin graft loss may occur due to infection or sheering. Such cases are treated with dressing changes until the underlying muscle bed appears capable of accepting another skin graft. Other minor complications include hematoma in the donor bed and injury to the tibial nerve or the posterior tibial vessels during flap dissection. Both complications may be avoided with meticulous hemostasis and clear identification of the anatomical landmarks prior to muscle division. Limitations in plantarflexion are minimized if the muscle is taken in isolation.

PEARLS AND PITFALLS

- If the preoperative evaluation reveals significant comminution to tibia or excessive hemorrhage or damage to the soleus muscle, another flap should be chosen for closure of the defect.
- Preoperative CT and MRI can often visualize the length of the soleus muscle helping the surgeon decide if is possible to use in defects at the junction of the middle and distal third of the leg.
- A reverse soleus muscle flap should be reserved for small defects (less than 50 cm²) surrounding the medial malleolar region.
- If one is preparing to use a reverse soleus flap, it is recommended that the distal perforator coming into the muscle for the posterior tibial artery be at least 1 mm in diameter and be associated with a healthy venous commitantes.
- If the flap looks compromised or portions do not appear to bleed after insetting the flap, delay skin grafting for 24 to 48 hours.

RECOMMENDED READING

Beck JB, Stile F, Lineaweaver W. Reconsidering the soleus muscle flap for coverage of wounds of the distal third of the leg. *Ann Plast Surg.* 2003;50;631–635.

Bos GD, Buehler MJ. Lower extremity local flaps. *J Am Acad Orthop Surg.* 1994;2:342–351.

Hallock GG. Getting the most from the soleus muscle. *Ann Plast Surg.* 1996;36:139–146.

Houdek MT, Wagner ER, Wyles CC, et al. Reverse medial hemisoleus flaps for coverage of distal third leg wounds: a technical trick. *J Orthop Trauma.* 2015;16.

Kauffman CA, Lahoda LU, Cederna PS, et al. Use of the soleus muscle flaps for coverage of distal third tibial defects. *J Reconstr Microsurg.* 2004;20:593–597.

Mathes S, Nahai F. *Reconstructive Surgery: Principles, Anatomy and Technique.* 1st ed. New York: Churchill Livingstone; 1997:1473–1487.

Pu LLQ. Medial hemi soleus muscle flap: a reliable flap for soft tissue reconstruction of the middle third tibial wound. *Int Surg.* 2006;91:194–200.

Pu LLQ. Soft tissue reconstruction of an open tibial wound in the distal third of the leg. *Ann Plast Surg.* 2007;58:78–83.

Pu LLQ. The reversed medial hemi soleus muscle flap and its role in reconstruction of an open tibial wound in the lower third of the leg. *Ann Plast Surg.* 2006;56:59–64.

Taylor GI, Gianoutsos MP, Morris SF. The neurovascular territories of the skin and muscles: anatomic study and clinical implications. *Plast Reconstr Surg.* 1994;94:1–36.

Tobin GR. Hemi soleus and reversed hemi soleus flaps. *Plast Reconstr Surg.* 1985;76:87–96.

32 Sural Artery Flap

Michael Sauerbier and Annika Arsalan-Werner

S oft tissue defects of the lower third of the leg and the calcaneal region remain difficult recon-structive problems. Because of the limited mobility of the skin and the superficial course of the anatomic structures in the lower third of the leg, exposure of vital structures such as nerves, ten-dons, bone, and hardware are common clinical problems following trauma. To prevent infection and provide stable coverage in these situations, flap reconstruction is necessary in many trauma patients.

Historically, free flaps have been the gold standard for the coverage of acute and chronic soft tissue defects in the lower third of the leg. Free flaps such as the gracilis flap, latissimus dorsi flap, or anterolateral thigh flap are frequently used to cover these defects; however, the downside of free tissue transfer includes the need for general anesthesia, microsurgical expertise, sophisticated equip-ment, extended operative times, and higher costs. For the coverage of large defects, a free flap may be the only option, but for coverage of smaller defects, pedicled flaps can be an effective alternative to free tissue transfer (Fig. 32-1; Table 32-1).

A pedicled flap that we have found effective for coverage of defects of the lower third of the leg is the distally based sural artery flap. The distally based sural artery flap is perfused by reverse flow through the anastomosis between the superficial sural artery (SSA) and the lowermost perforator of the peroneal artery. The advantages of this thin fasciocutaneous flap are that it can be performed quickly, and the flap provides durable soft tissue coverage, produces minimal postoperative discom-fort, and has an acceptable donor site. Finally, the flap can be performed without sacrificing any major vessels within the leg.

INDICATIONS/CONTRAINDICATIONS

The sural artery flap can be used for the successful coverage of moderate-sized defects (less than 9 cm × 12 cm) of the posterior and inferior surface of the heel, the Achilles tendon, the middle and distal third of the leg, the dorsum of the foot, and the lateral and medial malleolus (Tables 32-2 and 32-3). It can be harvested with a small piece of gastrocnemius muscle if needed for deeper defects but is ideal for coverage of more superficial structures such as the heel, Achilles tendon, and flexor tendons of the foot. The sural artery flap is an insensate flap so it should not be used if the recovery of sensation is mandatory in the area of reconstruction (such as the weight-bearing heel). Furthermore, the sacrifice of the sural nerve, which is included in the flap, will result in an area of hyposensitivity on the lateral border of the foot.

Absolute contraindications to flap use include absence or damage to the perineal artery (or its lowermost perforators), which supplies the flap (see Table 32-2). Additionally, as perfusion of large flaps (over 9 cm × 12 cm) is unreliable, it is not deemed suitable for coverage of extensive defects of the lower third of the leg. Higher complication rates should be anticipated in patients with comorbid-ities such as peripheral artery disease (PAD), diabetes mellitus, and venous insufficiency. Extreme care should also be exercised when using this flap in patients with lower extremity lymphedema, severe obesity, or venous insufficiency.

PREOPERATIVE PLANNING

A thorough clinical and radiologic examination of the donor and the recipient sites is mandatory. In patients suffering from chronic or infected wounds or diabetic gangrene, additional osteitis or osteomyelitis must be considered. Conventional radiographs and/or magnetic resonance imaging (MRI)

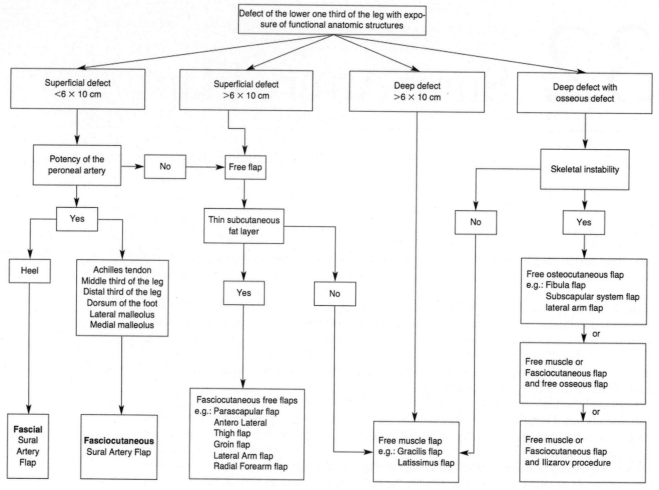

FIGURE 32-1

Treatment algorithm. Small superficial defects of the lower third of the leg can be treated by a sural artery flap if the defect size is smaller than 9 cm × 12 cm. Larger superficial defects can be reconstructed by fasciocutaneous free flaps, whereas deep defects, especially in combination with osseous defects, should be reconstructed by muscle flaps. Defects in the weight-bearing area of the heel should be reconstructed by fascial sural artery flaps to prevent pathologic movement of the subcutaneous layer. For alternative pedicled flaps to the lower limb, see Table 32-1.

scans can help to prove the existence or extent of altered osseous structures. The wound needs to be thoroughly debrided prior to flap closure. Radical debridement may result in an enlargement of the defect, and in some cases, debridement may create a wound too large for coverage with the sural flap. Although there are no studies addressing absolute maximum flap dimensions with regard to safety, small and moderate-sized defects up to 9 cm × 12 cm can be reconstructed successfully using sural artery flaps.

The patency of the sural artery flap pedicle should be verified preoperatively by examining the patency of the peroneal artery and the lesser saphenous vein. This is most easily accomplished

TABLE 32-1	Flaps and Their Indications According to Location
Flap	**Indications**
Soleus flap	Middle third of the leg
Flexor digitorum communis flap	Distal third of the leg
Flexor hallucis longus flap	Distal third of the leg
Peroneus flap	Achilles tendon
Lateral supramalleolar flap	Dorsum of the foot/heel (nonweightbearing)
Dorsalis pedis flap	Foot/distal third of the leg
Extensor digitorum brevis flap	Premalleolar area/dorsum of the foot and toes
Medial plantar flap	Heel (weightbearing)

TABLE 32-2 Advantages and Disadvantages of the Sural Artery Flap

Advantages	Disadvantages
Constant anatomy	Increased morbidity in patients with comorbidities
Thin flap with ideal contouring	Sacrifice of the sural nerve
Quick procedure	Susceptible to venous congestion
Durable soft tissue coverage	Insensate flap
Low donor site morbidity	Split-thickness skin grafts for donor site closure in
Acceptable donor site scar in small flaps (<4 cm)	large flaps (>4 cm)
No sacrifice of major vessels	

through the use of handheld Doppler probe examination. The lowermost perforators between the peroneal artery and the flap pedicle can be identified with a handheld Doppler 4 to 7 cm proximal to the tip of the lateral malleolus. In patients with comorbid conditions such as diabetes mellitus and peripheral vessel disease, a conventional digital subtraction angiography (DSA), magnetic resonance arteriography (MRA), or computed tomographic angiography (CTA) can be performed to verify peroneal artery patency. DSA is an invasive procedure and associated with a higher risk of complications compared to MRA or CTA; however, it allows angioplasty by dilatation or stenting in case of severe arterial stenosis. The peroneal artery should be patent for safe elevation of the flap; however, a recent case report suggests that retrograde flow in a proximally occluded peroneal artery provides enough perfusion for flap survival. If the perforators are patent in patients with PAD, the sural artery flap is a good treatment option as no major vessels are sacrificed to use this flap.

Finally, prior to surgery, the surgeon should provide the patient with detailed account of the surgical procedure and postoperative management. Information regarding the postoperative function and donor site morbidity should be explained. In particular, the surgeon should discuss the loss of sensation over the lateral border of the foot, the possibility of neuroma formation at the end of the cut sural nerve, and the potential for skin grafting the donor site in flaps wider than 4 cm (Table 32-4).

SURGERY

Anatomy

The reverse flow sural artery flap is based on the vascular network along the sural nerve. The nutrient artery is the SSA. It arises from the popliteal artery proximal to the medial and lateral sural arteries in about 65% of cases. In some cases, the artery can originate directly from the medial (20%) or lateral (8%) sural artery or sometimes from the common trunk of the sural arteries. The artery descends posteriorly for 2 to 3 cm before joining the medial sural nerve passing between the two heads of the gastrocnemius muscle. The medial sural nerve anastomoses with the communicating branch of the lateral sural nerve to become the sural nerve. Both the medial sural nerve and the SSA pierce the crural

TABLE 32-3 Indications for Sural Artery Flap Reconstruction

Healthy patients with no comorbidities (diabetes mellitus, peripheral artery disease, venous insufficiency)
Skin and soft tissue defects up to 9 cm × 12 cm:
    Chronic and diabetic ulcers
    Pressure sores
    Chronic infection
    Traumatic defects
    Unstable scars
    Exposure of viable structures (neurovascular bundles, tendons, bone, osteosynthesis material)
One of the following locations:
    Middle and lower third of the leg
    Posterior surface of the heel
    Inferior surface of the heel
    Achilles tendon
    Dorsum of the foot
    Lateral malleolus
    Medial malleolus

TABLE 32-4   **Preoperative Planning for Sural Artery Flap Reconstruction**
Clinical examination
Defect size (after debridement)
Peripheral function (to determine destruction of functional structures [nerves, tendons, blood vessels])
MRI or conventional radiographs of the recipient site (fractures, extension of osseous or soft tissue defects, osteitis)
Examination of patency of the lesser saphenous vein and peroneal artery
Doppler ultrasound probe in healthy patients
Conventional angiography or MRI angiography if available
Detailed information of the patient
Sacrifice of the sural nerve (hyposensitivity of the lateral border of the foot)
Neuroma formation
Split-thickness skin grafting of the donor site

fascia at the junction of the proximal and middle third of the leg to become subcutaneous. The SSA courses alongside the sural nerve to the lateral malleolus in 65% of all patients, while in 35% of cases, the artery fades into a vascular network at the distal third of the leg. Regardless of the termination, the SSA has a constant distal anastomosis from the lateral malleolar arteries, which in turn arises from the peroneal artery. The distally based sural artery flap is dependent on this anastomosis, and its perfusion is reverse flow through the SSA and its cutaneous branches at the distal two-thirds of the leg (Fig. 32-2).

The venous drainage of the sural artery flap is dependent on small comitant veins but primarily on the short saphenous vein, which accompanies the sural nerve at the distal two-thirds of the leg. Theoretically, reverse flow in this vein is impossible due to the presence of valves; however, clinical findings disprove this theory. Duplex scans of the small saphenous vein generally show a continuous or phasic reverse flow postoperatively. Several theories exist regarding these findings. Some authors stress the existence of bridging veins between the short saphenous vein and the comitant veins, thus bypassing the valves. Moreover, denervation of the short saphenous vein due to the surgical procedure and increased venous pressure due to the altered flow are thought to be responsible for

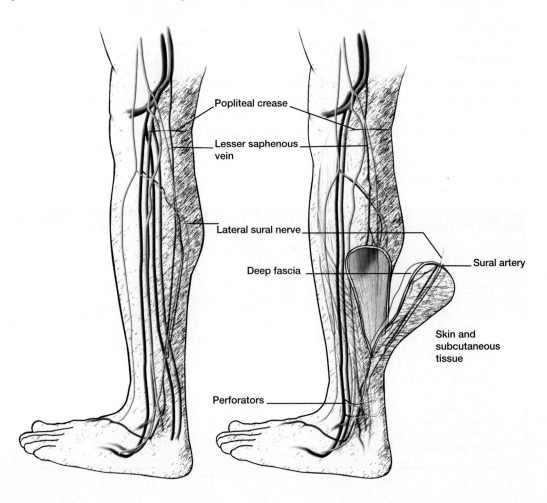

FIGURE 32-2

Anatomy of the sural artery flap.

venous dilatation, which renders the valves insufficient. Overall, the sural artery flap exhibits a constant anatomy with reliable arterial perfusion and venous drainage.

Patient Positioning

Surgery is usually performed under general anesthesia; however, in elderly patients or because of comorbidities, epidural or spinal anesthesia may also be utilized. Depending on the defect location, the patient is placed in prone position or lateral decubitus position.

Technique

The recipient site is prepared first. In patients with chronic wounds, infections, diabetic gangrene, or wound colonization, a radical debridement is mandatory. Analogous to the principles of oncologic resections, complete resection of the entire infected or altered tissue should be performed to increase the chance of successful reconstruction. After debridement, the recipient defect may be too large for a sural artery flap reconstruction. In such cases, a temporary wound closure (e.g., vacuum-assisted closure therapy) or other therapeutic options such as free flaps need to be considered.

The authors prefer to perform flap harvest under pneumatic tourniquet to aid in visualization of the vessels. In patients who have a history of deep vein thrombosis or severe peripheral arterial disease, raising the flap without the application of a tourniquet should be considered. Flap dissection is aided by the use of loupe magnification (2.5 to 4 times magnification). The defect size is measured and a skin island with adequate dimensions is centered along the line of the short saphenous vein. The proximal limit of the flap should not exceed a boundary of 20 cm proximal to the lateral malleolus. The skin island is planned in the middle or distal third of the leg, according to the required pedicle length (Fig. 32-3). Because of its thicker subcutaneous tissue, the skin

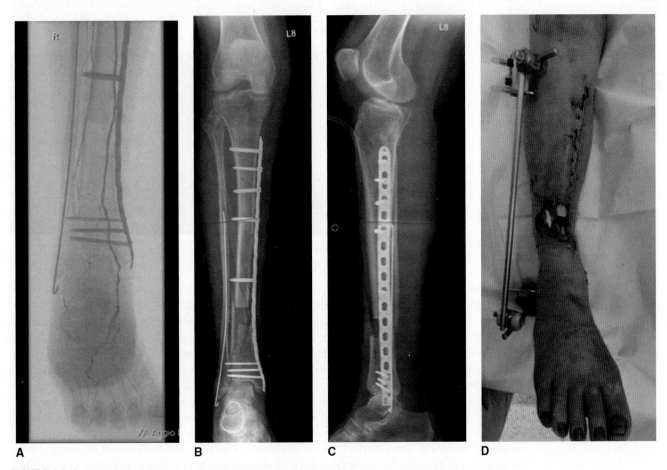

A   B   C   D

FIGURE 32-3

A–C: A 68-year-old woman with open lower leg fracture. The angiography shows a complete stenosis of the anterior tibial artery. **D–F:** After debridement, the soft tissue defect in the distal anterior third of the tibial region is reconstructed by a distally pedicled sural artery flap. Skin grafting was necessary to close the donor side.

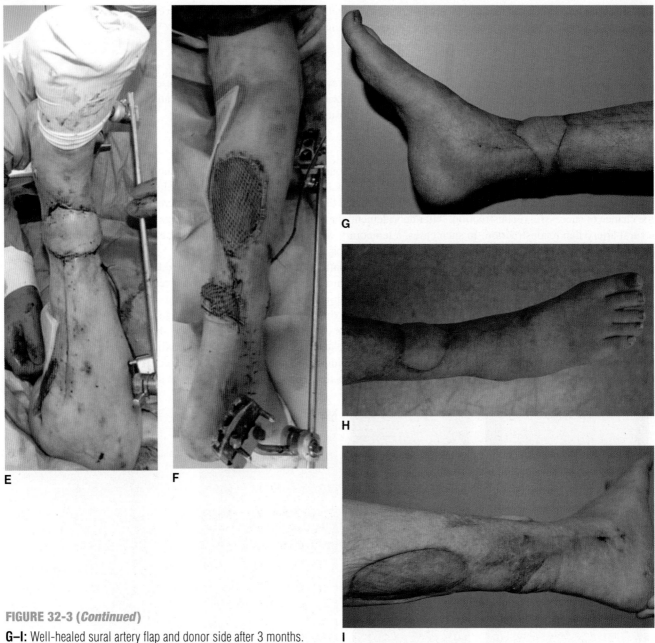

FIGURE 32-3 (*Continued*)

G–I: Well-healed sural artery flap and donor side after 3 months.

island should be designed slightly larger than the recipient defect to facilitate skin-to-skin closure of the defect with minimal tension. The maximum size of the skin island should not exceed 9 cm × 12 cm. The pivot point is marked approximately 4 to 5 cm above the tip of the lateral malleolus to include the branches that anastomose with the peroneal artery. The skin incision starts distally to localize the pedicle. Correction of the flap position is still possible if the skin island is not centered correctly. After locating the pedicle, the dissection proceeds in the proximal portion of the flap to identify the lesser saphenous vein and the sural nerve. At this point, the lesser saphenous vein, the sural nerve, and the SSA are ligated, divided, and included into the flap. The proximal stump of the nerve is coagulated or clipped to prevent symptomatic neuroma formation. Burying the nerve stump in the surrounding gastrocnemius musculature also helps to avoid symptomatic neuroma formation. Some authors report raising the flap and sparing the sural nerve to prevent neuroma formation and foot hyposensitivity. In our opinion, this strategy jeopardizes the vascular supply of the flap and is unnecessary because the morbidity of harvesting the flap with the sural nerve is minimal.

Dissection proceeds distally in the plane below the deep fascia, so that inclusion of the pedicle in the flap is easily accomplished and the nutrient anastomosis of the flap can be preserved. Two to three constant and direct perforators from the gastrocnemius muscle to the vascular axis of the sural nerve are identified and ligated with ligature clips. Electrocoagulation of these perforators might increase the risk of pedicle destruction. The fascial and subcutaneous pedicle, which includes the SSA, the sural nerve, and the short saphenous vein, should be at least 3 cm in width. The paratenon of the underlying Achilles tendon should carefully be preserved to facilitate skin graft take if grafting is required over the donor site. The flap procedure remains simple if care is taken to avoid dissection too close to the pedicle and is only extended to the demarcated limit of 4 to 5 cm above the tip of the lateral malleolus. During elevation of the flap, near this lower limit of dissection, efforts should be made to preserve the large perforating septocutaneous vessels.

After flap elevation, transposition of the skin island to the recipient defect can be performed. Under normal conditions (e.g., a sufficient amount of elastic skin), the flap can be transposed through a subcutaneous tunnel. However, in case of tight skin, a subcutaneous tunnel is not recommended and a direct skin incision to the defect site should be made to allow the pedicle to rest without external compression on the pedicle. The risk of pedicle compression increases with edema formation, surrounding scars, or skin induration. Two approaches should be considered in patients with these risks. First, a skin extension ("cutaneous tail") overlying the pedicle can be added to the flap design. This additional skin over the pedicle of the flap can be inset into the incision connecting the flap elevation site and the defect site, thus avoiding a skin tunnel. Second, the bridge over the subcutaneous tunnel can be opened and the pedicle of the flap can be covered with a split-thickness skin graft. Another approach discussed in the literature is a "distally based sural artery interpolation flap." This involves transposition of the flap to the defect without tunneling. The pedicle is exteriorized and skin grafted. In the interpolated flap procedure, the pedicle can be thinned or excised to improve cosmesis once the flap has developed collateral flow from the surrounding tissue (3 to 6 months). The authors have no experience using this approach, but there appears to be no distinct advantage of this approach over other options. Indeed, it has the disadvantage of being a two-step procedure.

If signs of insufficient perfusion or venous congestion occur after flap transposition, one should first verify there is no kinking in the vascular pedicle. If there are still concerns about venous congestion, the flap can be placed back into its donor site bed and a delay procedure can be performed. Delaying the flap transfer by 48 to 72 hours allows additional venous channels to open within the flap, which improves drainage. When performing the delay procedure, a powder-free glove or soft silicone low-adherence mesh (e.g., Mepitel® Soft Silicone Wound Contact Layer, Mölnlycke Health Care US, Norcross, GA) is placed between the elevated flap fascia and the gastrocnemius muscle. A temporary dressing may be placed over the defect site to keep it clean and the flap transfer may be performed in 2 to 4 days (Figs. 32-4 to 32-6).

Many modifications to the flap exist. For deep defects, portions of the gastrocnemius muscle can be included in the flap. Flap harvest is similar to the procedure described previously. The only difference is that a portion of the gastrocnemius muscle is taken from the lower part of the muscle without separating the fascia from the muscle. For very thin defects, the flap may be elevated without a skin island and include only vascularized fascia; this is the preferred approach of some authors in patients with heel defects. In these cases, the flap is covered by split-thickness skin grafting. Finally, the flap may be performed as a free microvascular flap for distant defects or in cases where the surgeon wishes to use the sural nerve as vascularized nerve grafts.

Primary donor site closure with acceptable functional and aesthetic outcome is possible when a skin island of less than 4 cm in width is harvested. Larger donor site defects have to be closed by split-thickness skin grafting. In these cases, the aesthetic outcome of the donor site scar is questionable, particularly among obese patients and females.

POSTOPERATIVE MANAGEMENT

Preventing compression of the vascular pedicle is the most important postoperative issue. This can be achieved either by an adequately elevated position of the leg or by the use of conventional splints with an opening over the flap. However, the authors prefer using an external fixation device. This allows treatment of concomitant fractures, prevention of an equinus, and an elevated positioning of the leg.

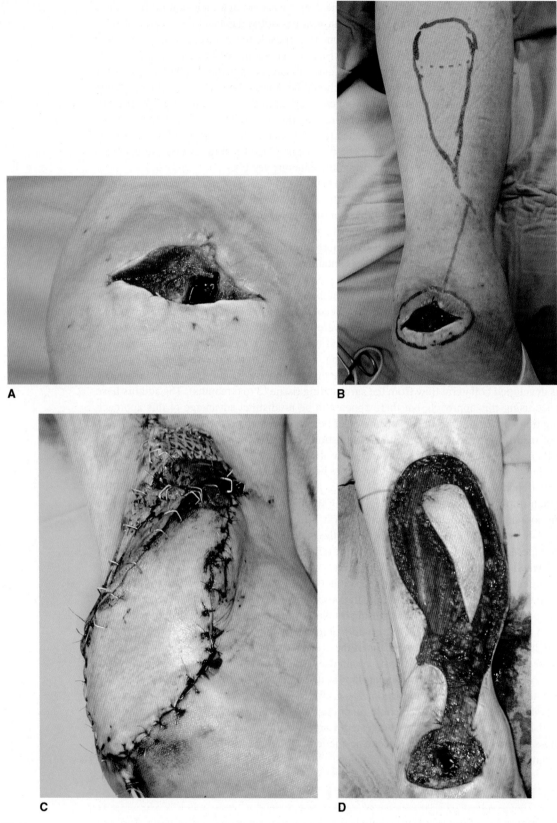

FIGURE 32-4

A: Male patient suffering from a combined soft tissue and osseous defect in the heel. **B:** After debridement, soft tissue reconstruction was planned by a sural artery flap. Flap transposition was performed to the defect **(C)** after flap harvest **(D)**. Split-thickness skin grafting of the donor site was necessary.

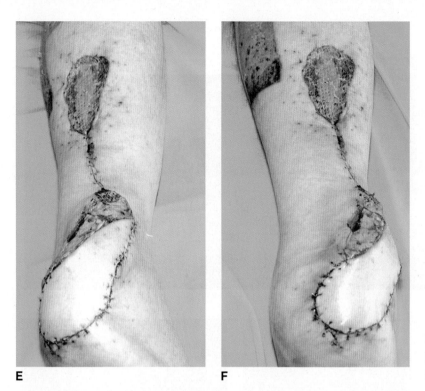

FIGURE 32-4 (*Continued*)

E, F: Postoperative course and wound healing were uneventful.

E

F

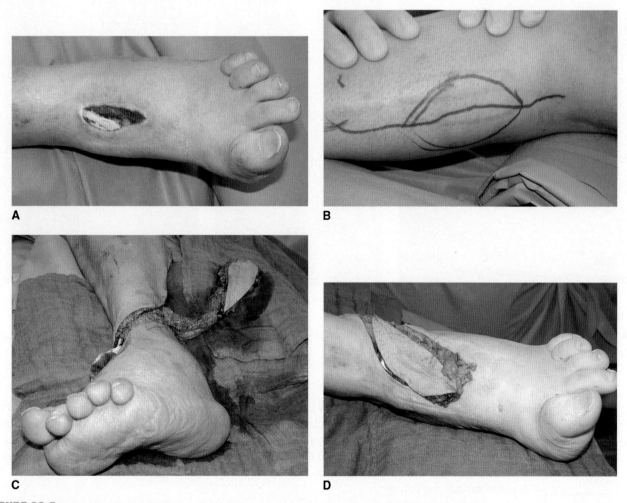

A

B

C

D

FIGURE 32-5

A 34-year-old man with a chronic ulcer of the dorsum of the foot. **A, B:** A sural artery flap was planned to reconstruct the defect with exposed tendons. **C, D:** After complete flap harvest, the skin island is transposed to the defect.

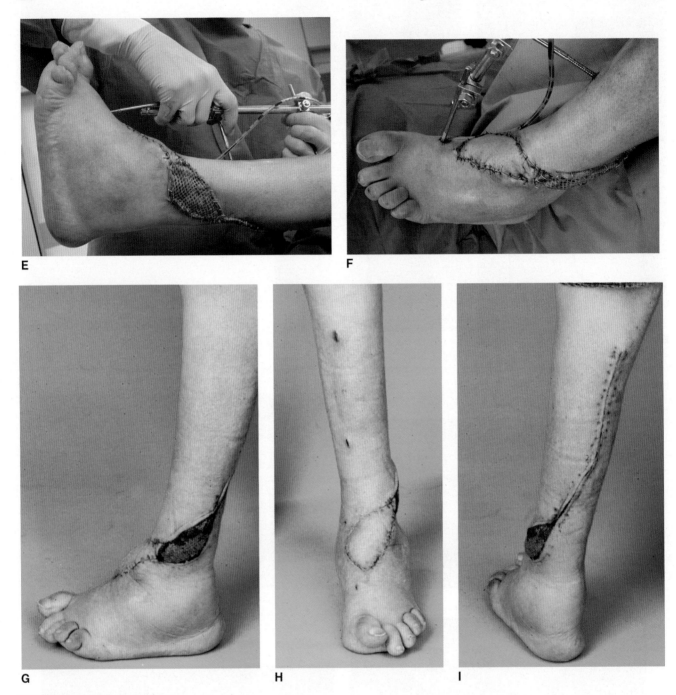

FIGURE 32-5 *(Continued)*

E, F: The skin over the pedicle is incised and split-thickness skin grafted to reduce pressure on the nutrient vessels. **G–I:** The functional and aesthetic results are excellent 2 weeks after surgery.

Administration of anticoagulants after pedicled flap reconstruction remains controversial. To the authors' knowledge, there is no scientific evidence of beneficial effects of anticoagulation therapy in terms of flap survival or thrombosis rates. On the contrary, anticoagulation might increase postoperative morbidity due to bleeding and hematoma. Thus, in our center, as in many other centers, anticoagulation usage is limited to low molecular weight heparin or unfractionated heparin for thrombosis prevention.

All patients are treated with antibiotics (cephalosporin or according to the specific bacteria) perioperatively. Antibiotic treatment is prolonged if the patient shows an increased risk of postoperative wound infection or persistent infection.

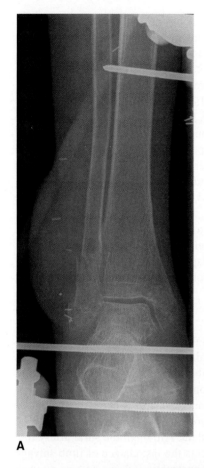

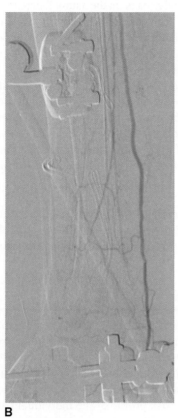

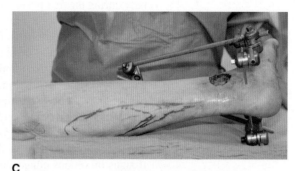

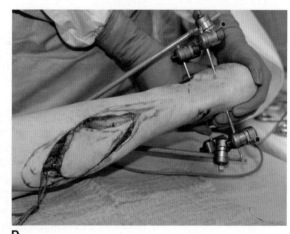

A   **B**   **C**

                                                             D

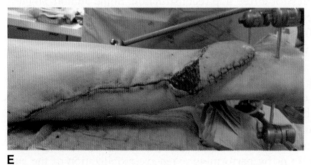

E

FIGURE 32-6

A: Radiograph of a 78-year-old woman with an open ankle
fracture. **B:** The angiography shows a complete stenosis of
the anterior tibial artery. **C:** Defect reconstruction after radical
debridement was planned by a distal pedicled sural artery flap.
The outline of the flap is sketched after a Doppler investigation
of the lower saphenous vein. **D:** The flap is raised with a visible
proximal pedicle on the left marked by the red vessel loop. **E:**
Transposition of the flap for defect reconstruction and primary
closure of the donor side. The small area around the pivot point
(3 cm superior to the lateral malleolus) was closed by split-
thickness skin graft. **F, G:** Result after 2 years with complete
healing of the flap and donor side.

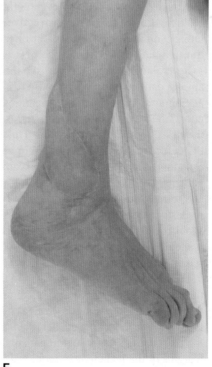

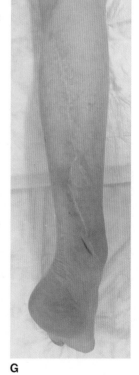

F   **G**

Surveillance of flap perfusion in terms of arterial as well as venous flow must be performed regularly during the first postoperative days. In the authors' department, the capillary refill is tested every 2 hours for the first 48 hours. Thereafter, the intervals between testing are increased.

A revision procedure should be performed if any signs of poor arterial perfusion or venous congestion are identified or bleeding and hematoma formation are detected. New positioning of the vascular pedicle or decompression of the nutrient vessels may facilitate flap salvage. Moreover, the flap may be laid back in the donor site bed if these options fail. Medicinal leeching and hyperbaric oxygen may increase flap survival in cases of venous congestion.

Patients should be out on bed rest for 3 to 5 days. After this period, mobilization begins with letting the leg hang down for 5 minutes and extending the time over the next days. The tolerance of the flap to this treatment (as well as accompanying injuries) determines the next stages of mobilization. If signs of venous congestion or poor perfusion are recognized, the mobilization protocol may be prolonged.

In most cases, patients are completely mobilized after 7 to 10 days. If the patient does not suffer from severe PAD, further use of a compression garment is obligatory for a period of at least 6 months after discharge to improve contouring of the flap and avoid hypertrophic scarring. Secondary corrections at the recipient or the donor site should not be performed until at least 6 months postsurgery.

COMPLICATIONS

Partial or complete necrosis of the sural artery flap is the main reason for failure of this procedure. Necrosis rates between 5% and 36% have been described in the literature. The different findings are most likely caused by different patient populations. Patient's age and systemic diseases such as diabetes mellitus, peripheral arterial disease, and venous insufficiency are considered to be risk factors for partial or total flap failure. Therefore, necrosis rates should always be interpreted in relation to the risk profile of the individual patient. Although the sural artery flap might have a lower success in these patients, it often represents the last chance of limb salvage in patients who are not suitable candidates for a free flap reconstruction. Some authors suggest that in cases of partial and even complete necrosis, the sural artery flap can serve as a valuable biologic dressing. The reconstructive surgeon sometimes experiences a well-vascularized granulating wound after debridement of the necrotic flap that allows successful split-thickness skin transplantation.

Several technical guidelines should be followed to prevent perioperative morbidity, particularly among patients with an increased risk of flap necrosis: (a) use of the Doppler ultrasound and angiography in preoperative planning, (b) inclusion of the sural nerve in the flap, and (c) paying attention to the subcutaneous layer. A bulky subcutaneous layer at the recipient site may increase the risk of pedicle compression. This can be prevented by designing the flap slightly larger than the defect to facilitate skin-to-skin closure or by performing extensive mobilization of the surrounding skin. This, however, can cause wound healing disturbances. Especially in less compliant patients, we recommend the use of an external fixation device to prevent pedicle compression and to facilitate postoperative care. Tunneling of the vascular pedicle should only be performed if elastic skin surrounds the defect; otherwise, the pedicle should be grafted or the skin paddle should be planned in a teardrop shape to facilitate pedicle coverage (see previously). Furthermore, it should be taken into consideration that a more proximal donor site is associated with a greater risk of flap necrosis.

Further complications described in the literature are not specific to sural artery flaps but relate to the underlying defect or the surgical procedure, respectively. Wound infection and persistent infection are common findings as well as hematoma, delayed healing, or persistent osteitis (which itself is usually due to incomplete debridement). As described previously, inelastic skin and induration are familiar findings especially in patients with comorbidities. Therefore, the skin surrounding the flap margins or the pedicle may require skin grafting for wound closure. Edema formation is common, especially in patients with venous insufficiency. In these cases, application of compression bandages may help improve local trophicity.

Donor site morbidity is generally low. The most common findings are neuroma of the sural nerve and scarring. In these patients, secondary corrections should be performed. Neuromas have to be resected, and the nerve stump has to be buried in the surrounding musculature.

PEARLS AND PITFALLS

- The sural artery flap is a thin and quick option for reconstruction of defects up to 9 cm × 12 cm.
- Proper preoperative planning with Doppler ultrasound and angiography will help you to design your flap and find the pivot point.
- The nerve and artery should be included in the flap when starting to dissect proximally.
- After planning the skin incisions, the flap might not be centered correctly over the pedicle but can still be adjusted after localization and careful dissection of the pedicle at the proximal edge of the flap.
- If you identify poor arterial perfusion or venous congestion during the operation, do not complete the flap transfer. A delayed procedure with transposition of the flap in 2 to 4 days can help improve perfusion to the flap and allow for successful transfer.
- Some patients are less compliant than others and might compress the flap's blood supply due to excessive postoperative movement. Consider using an external fixation device.

RECOMMENDED READING

Almeida MF, da Costa PR, Okawa RY. Reverse-flow island sural flap. *Plast Reconstr Surg.* 2002;109:583–591.

Arnez ZM, Kersnic M, Smith RW, et al. Free lateral arm osteocutaneous neurosensory flap for thumb reconstruction. *J Hand Surg Br.* 1991;16:395–399.

Baumeister SP, Spierer R, Erdmann D, et al. A realistic complication analysis of 70 sural artery flaps in a multimorbid patient group. *Plast Reconstr Surg.* 2003;112:129–140.

Bocchi A, Merelli S, Morellini A, et al. Reverse fasciosubcutaneous flap versus distally pedicled sural island flap: two elective methods for distal third leg reconstruction. *Ann Plast Surg.* 2000;45:284–291.

Cavadas PC, Bonanad E. Reverse-flow sural island flap in the varicose leg. *Plast Reconstr Surg.* 1996;98:901–902.

Cormack GC, Lamberty BG. A classification of fascio-cutaneous flaps according to their patterns of vascularisation. *Br J Plast Surg.* 1984;37:80–87.

Costa-Ferreira A, Reis J, Pinho C, et al. The distally based island superficial sural artery flap: clinical experience with 36 flaps. *Ann Plast Surg.* 2001;46:308–313.

De Blacam C, Colakoglu S, Ogunleye AA, et al. Risk factors associated with complications in lower-extremity reconstruction with the distally based sural flap: a systematic review and pooled analysis. *J Plast Reconstr Aesthet Surg.* 2014;67(5):607–616.

Dolph JL. The superficial sural artery flap in distal lower third extremity reconstruction. *Ann Plast Surg.* 1998;40:520–522.

Donski PK, Fogdestam I. Distally based fasciocutaneous flap from the sural region: a preliminary report. *Scand J Plast Reconstr Surg.* 1983;17:191–196.

Erdmann D, Gottlieb N, Humphrey JS, et al. Sural flap delay procedure: a preliminary report. *Ann Plast Surg.* 2005;54:562–565.

Fraccalvieri M, Verner G, Dolcet M, et al. The distally based superficial sural flap: our experience in reconstructing the lower leg and foot. *Ann Plast Surg.* 2000;45:132–141.

Germann G, Bickert B, Steinau HU, et al. Versatility and reliability of combined flaps of the subscapular system. *Plast Reconstr Surg.* 1999;103:1386–1399.

Germann GK. Invited discussion. The simple and effective choice for treatment of chronic calcaneal osteomyelitis: neurocutaneous flaps. *Plast Reconstr Surg.* 2003;111:761–762.

Goldberg JA, Adkins P, Tsai TM. Microvascular reconstruction of the foot: weightbearing pattern, gait analysis and long term follow-up. *Plast Reconstr Surg.* 1993;93:904–911.

Hasegawa M, Torii S, Katoh H, et al. The distally based superficial sural artery flap. *Plast Reconstr Surg.* 1994;93:1012–1020.

Huisinga RL, Houpt P, Dijkstra R, et al. The distally based sural artery flap. *Ann Plast Surg.* 1998;41:58–65.

Hyakusoku H, Tonegawa H, Fumiiri M. Heel coverage with a T-shaped distally based sural island fasciocutaneous flap. *Plast Reconstr Surg.* 1994;93:872–876.

Imanishi N, Nakajima H, Fukuzumi S, et al. Venous drainage of the distally based lesser saphenous-sural-veno-neuroadipofascial pedicled fasciocutaneous flap: a radiographic perfusion study. *Plast Reconstr Surg.* 1999;103:494–498.

Jeng SF, Wei FC. Distally based sural island flap for foot and ankle reconstruction. *Plast Reconstr Surg.* 1997;99:744–750.

Jeng SF, Hsieh CH, Kuo YR, et al. Distally based sural island flap. *Plast Reconstr Surg.* 2003;111:840–841.

Kneser U, Brockmann S, Leffler M, et al. Comparison between distally based peroneus brevis and sural flaps for reconstruction of foot, ankle and distal lower leg: an analysis of donor-site morbidity and clinical outcome. *J Plast Reconstr Aesthet Surg.* 2011;64(5):656–662.

Koshima I, Fukuda H, Utunomiya R, et al. The anterolateral thigh flap: variations in vascular pedicle. *Br J Plast Surg.* 1989;42:260.

Le Fourn B, Caye N, Pannier M. Distally based sural fasciomuscular flap: anatomic study and application for filling leg or foot defects. *Plast Reconstr Surg.* 2001;107:67–72.

Lin SD, Lai CS, Chiu CC. Venous drainage in the reverse forearm flap. *Plast Reconstr Surg.* 1984;74:508–512.

Lin TS, Jeng SF, Wei FC. Temporary placement of defatted plantar heel skin in the calf and subsequent transfer to the heel using distally based sural artery flap as a carrier. *Plast Reconstr Surg.* 2002;109:1358–1360.

Lozano DD, Stephenson LL, Zamboni WA. Effect of hyperbaric oxygen and medicinal leeching on survival of axial skin flaps subjected to total venous occlusion. *Plast Reconstr Surg.* 1999;104(4):1029–1032.

Maffi TR, Knoetgen J Jr, Turner NS, et al. Enhanced survival using the distally based sural artery interpolation flap. *Ann Plast Surg.* 2005;54:302–305.

Malokov, S, Casanova, D, Magalon, G, et al. Sural flap vascularization in arteritic patients: an anatomic study of 24 amputation specimens. *Surg Radiol Anat.* 2003;25:372–378.

Masquelet AC, Romana MC, Wolf G. Skin island flaps supplied by the vascular axis of sensitive superficial nerves: anatomic study and clinical experience in the leg. *Plast Reconstr Surg.* 1992;89:1115–1121.

Mueller JE, Ilchmann T, Lowatscheff T. The musculocutaneous sural artery flap for soft tissue coverage after calcaneal fracture. *Arch Orthop Trauma Surg.* 2001;121:350–352.

Nakajima H, Imanishi N, Fukuzumi S, et al. Accompanying arteries of the lesser saphenous vein and sural nerve: anatomic study and its clinical applications. *Plast Reconstr Surg.* 1999;103:104–120.

Ögun TC, Arazi M, Kutlu A. An easy and versatile method of coverage for distal tibial soft tissue defects. *J Trauma.* 2001;50:63–69.

Price MF, Capizzi PJ, Watterson PA, et al. Reverse sural artery flap: caveats for success. *Ann Plast Surg.* 2002;48:496–504.

Rajacic N, Darweesh M, Jayakrishnan K, et al. The distally based superficial sural flap for reconstruction of the lower leg and foot. *Br J Plast Surg.* 1996;49:383–389.

Satoh K, Fukuya F, Matsui A, et al. Lower leg reconstruction using a sural fasciocutaneous flap. *Ann Plast Surg.* 1989;23:97–103.

Sauerbier M, Erdmann D, Bruner S, et al. Covering soft tissue defects and unstable scars over the Achilles tendon by free microsurgical flap-plasty. *Chirurg.* 2000;71:1161–1166.

Schepler H, Sauerbier M, Germann GK. The distally pedicled suralis flap for the defect coverage of posttraumatic and chronic soft tissue lesions in the "critical" lower leg. *Chirurg.* 1997;68:1170–1177.

Singh S, Naasan A. Use of distally based superficial sural island artery flaps in acute open fractures of the lower leg. *Ann Plast Surg.* 2001;47:505–510.

Tajsic N, Winkel R, Husum H. Distally based perforator flaps for reconstruction of post-traumatic defects of the lower leg and foot: a review of the anatomy and clinical outcomes. *Injury.* 2014;45(3):469–477.

Torii S, Namiki Y, Mori R. Reverse-flow island flap: clinical report and venous drainage. *Plast Reconstr Surg.* 1987;79:600–609.

Touam C, Rostoucher P, Bhatia A, et al. Comparative study of two series of distally based fasciocutaneous flaps of the lower one-fourth of the leg, the ankle and the foot. *Plast Reconstr Surg.* 2001;107:383–392.

Yilmaz M, Karatas O, Barutcu A. The distally based superficial sural artery island flap: clinical experiences and modifications. *Plast Reconstr Surg.* 1998;102:2358–2367.

33 Propeller Flaps and Keystone Flaps in the Lower Extremity

Anita T. Mohan and Michel Saint-Cyr

The last several decades have seen a growing body of anatomic, radiologic, and clinical research that has extended our knowledge of vascular anatomy of the integument of the human body. This has propagated the development of perforator flaps, island pedicled flaps, and a spectrum of innovations in flap design in lower extremity reconstruction. Pedicled perforator flaps can obviate the need for microsurgical anastomosis, replace "like with like" tissue, limit donor site morbidity, and avoid the sacrifice of a major source vessel. Each perforator has a unique vascular territory that it supplies. Dominant (or large) perforators tend to be arranged in clusters throughout the body. We refer to these high-density areas as "hot spots." Flaps can be elevated on the perfusion territory of a dominant perforator outside the zone of injury and then rotated into the area of trauma. Alternatively, multiple perforators can be included in a flap that is advanced into a tissue defect, as is the case in a VY flap.

The published success of local perforator flaps has changed traditional thinking for flap choices for the lower leg soft tissue reconstruction. Propeller and keystone flaps based on perforators can be used reliably and an alternative for free tissue transfer or traditional pedicled muscle workhorse flaps; however, cases must be appropriately selected and the use of the muscle flaps must be kept in consideration during flap planning to act as a potential lifeboat.

PROPELLER FLAPS

The Tokyo Consensus defined the propeller flap as an island flap that reached the recipient site through axial rotation around its source perforator. Finding the location of perforator hot spots and understanding the vascular network within the skin and subcutaneous tissues are pertinent to the success of propeller flap utilization.

The lower extremity has many potential perforators that can be incorporated into flaps. The thigh contains the highest density of cutaneous vessels that afford a large caliber and long pedicle length, which can facilitate the arc of rotation and movement of the flap. Individual large perforators of the thigh, for example from the profunda artery perforator and superficial femoral artery or to the anterolateral thigh, can supply large vascular territories and support large dimensions of skin and subcutaneous tissue that can be used for local reconstruction in the thigh or proximal leg. Anatomic studies of perforasomes of the lower leg have demonstrated large clinically relevant perforator locations in the lower leg (Fig. 33-1) and that the perforators of the peroneal or posterior tibial artery can potentially perfuse approximately 40% of the whole lower leg surface with evidence of inter-perforator flow between perforators from same source and adjacent source arteries. However, exact flap dimensions based on individual perforasomes in the clinical setting have yet to be determined.

Indications/Contraindications

Assessment for a propeller flap begins with consideration of the quality of the local surrounding tissue: this includes previous radiation, previous trauma or degloving, previous surgeries, the timing of the surgery (immediate or delayed reconstruction), available tissue laxity, and history of vascular compromise at the time of injury. Patient factors such as other concomitant injuries, comorbidities, nicotine dependence, patient expectations, motivations, and compliance must all be incorporated in

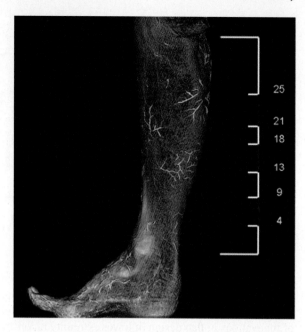

FIGURE 33-1

Anatomic study following a vascular injection with barium sulfate of the lower leg and computed tomographic angiography viewed with 3D volume rendering software and scale to illustrate intervals of clinical relevant perforators.

the preoperative planning stage in patient selection. Complication rates of propeller flaps have been found to be comparable to free flaps. Age, sex, etiology of the defect, arc of pedicle rotation, flap size, and comorbidities, including diabetes, smoking, and vascular disease, do not always correlate with complication rates. Traditionally, distal third leg defects are managed with free tissue transfer, but reconstructive practice has evolved such that a propeller flap may be a viable option in these cases.

Contraindications to locoregional reconstruction may include moderate to large defects since there is limited donor tissue available. However, for defects in the proximal lower leg, large flaps from the thigh may be harvested as propeller flaps for soft tissue coverage (Fig. 33-2). Other negative prognostic factors include defects associated with extensive local degloving, using a perforator within the zone of trauma, and using a flap when no local perforators can be identified. Propeller flaps are not appropriate options in cases in which there is segmental tissue or bone loss, crush injury, or vascular compromise.

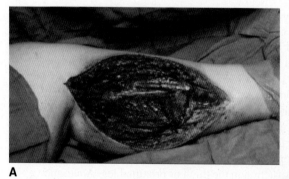

A

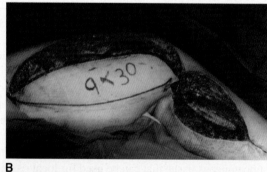

B

FIGURE 33-2

A: Large proximal calf defect following sarcoma resection creating a composite defect including partial resection of the medial head of the gastrocnemius muscle. **B:** Exploratory incision in the anteromedial thigh identified a large perforator from the superficial femoral artery and a large flap planned from the medial thigh donor site. **C:** Early postoperative clinical result and demonstrating healing of a split skin graft placed over the proximal portion of the flap to avoid direct closure over the pedicle and undue tension.

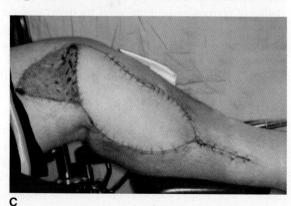

C

Preoperative Planning

Defect Size and Location

The wound or defect must be assessed to determine the size and extent of the injury, including degloving and damage to the underlying bone and neurovascular structures. Adequate debridement is essential to decrease the risk of infection, obtain a true size of the defect, and allow better visualization of the tissue planes. In lower extremity trauma, it may be better to convert multiple defects into a simpler single defect (Fig. 33-3).

Identify Suitable Perforators

Dominant perforators are generally clustered in predictable locations in the body in regional "hot spots" (Fig. 33-4). An understanding of the relevant blood supply to the region of the defect can

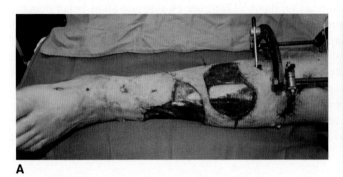
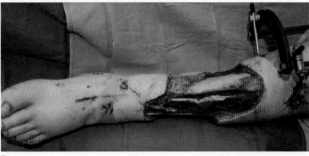

A   **B**

FIGURE 33-3

Left lower leg soft tissue defect with underlying fracture following trauma and external fixator in situ. **A:** Debridement of the wound and intervening skin bridge between two moderately sized soft tissue defects. **B:** Excision of the intervening skin bridge to create a single large defect that can be assessed for soft tissue reconstruction.

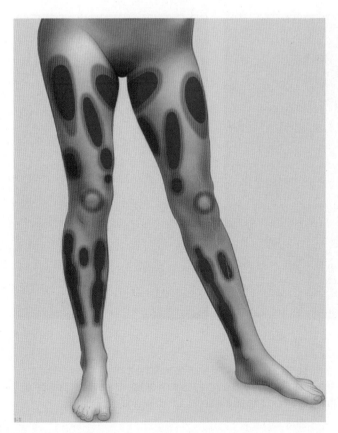

FIGURE 33-4

General hot spots of dominant perforators in the lower extremity.

provide more design options and greater freedom in flap harvest. Suitable perforators close to the defect can be assessed with a handheld Doppler. This is routine in our clinical practice especially in the setting of immediate soft tissue coverage following oncological resection. Computed tomographic angiography or magnetic resonance angiography (MRA) can also be used for preoperative imaging and give detailed information about regional perforators, location of dominant perforators, and their anatomical course. In trauma, the preoperative computed tomographic angiography runoff scans will determine distal vascular injury. If external devices are to be placed, it is important that these devices do not interfere with potential flap options being considered.

Assessment of Donor Tissue

The surrounding potential donor tissue must be assessed for signs of concomitant damage and laxity. It is vital to use a donor site that is outside the zone of injury; therefore, an assessment is required for scarring, undermining, trauma, and radiation damage. Flap selection and design should be based on resting skin tension lines and tissue laxity; this will facilitate closure and allow better concealment of incisions that would lie within a natural skin crease or an aesthetic unit. Following tumor extirpation with significant undermining of the skin edges, the skin flaps may have a small degree of vascular compromise and this area should not be considered a principal part of the flap design. The vascularity can be assessed clinically by the presence of fresh dermal bleeding, capillary return on the skin surface and color, or alternatively using intraoperative adjuncts for perfusion assessment, for example, laser-assisted indocyanine green fluorescence angiography (LA-ICGFA). Similarly, areas of irradiated tissue, scarring, and trauma should not be included in the flap design. The presence and orientation of scars should also be documented as previous surgeries may have damaged local perforators.

Consider Your Lifeboats

It is critical to always consider a lifeboat in planning and design of propeller flaps. The lifeboat options may be an underlying muscle flap, another regional fasciocutaneous flap, or a free flap (Fig. 33-5). The lifeboat flap choice will vary depending on the location, size, and anatomy of the defect. Incisions should be placed appropriately to maintain these secondary options if there is a complication with the initial surgery.

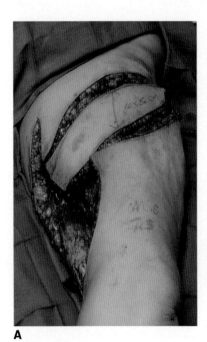 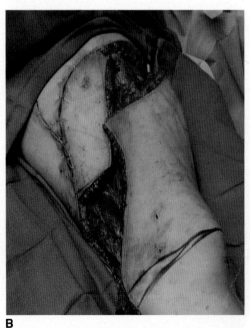 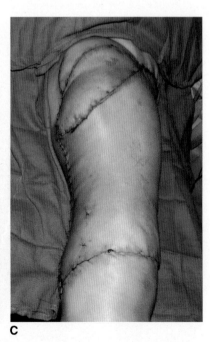

A   B   C

FIGURE 33-5

A: Medial thigh sarcoma resected and reconstructed with a proximal freestyle perforator flap based on a superficial femoral artery perforator. **B:** The lateral portion of the perforator flap was poorly perfused and excised intraoperatively leaving a residual defect in the distal portion of the medial thigh. **C:** A laterally based large keystone flap was harvested to assist in closure as a lifeboat, which healed uneventfully.

Surgery

Flap Design

Designing the skin paddle over the "hot spots" will ensure that either the dominant or as many perforators are incorporated within the flap; this will help maximize interperforator flow via direct and indirect linking vessels. Handheld Doppler can be used to identify perforators close to the defect. The perforator will become the pivot point for the flap.

To identify hot spots, a line can be drawn over the path of dominant axial vessels, for example, the posterior tibial artery, anterior tibial artery, or descending branch of lateral circumflex femoral artery. The handheld Doppler probe is then used to identify perforators along this vessel. The location of each perforator is marked on the skin, and the quality of the sound is noted. This information can be correlated with any preoperative imaging if available. The skin paddle should be orientated parallel to the axial vessel within the limb, but the design may also be influenced by local tissue laxity.

Patient Positioning

The patient should be positioned to ensure the flap design is accessible and that there will be adequate exposure for perforator assessment and dissection and to facilitate flap inset.

Technique

(See Video 1, Planning and harvest of a peroneal artery perforator flap for a lower leg traumatic defect with exposure of bone.) An initial wide exploratory incision that is incorporated in the flap design without interfering with a potential secondary reconstructive (or backup) option is made. The dissection can be performed either subfascially or suprafascially; however, subfascial dissection is more straightforward. Perforators are identified and reassessed, and the most dominant perforator with the best pivot point is selected (Figs. 33-6 and 33-7). This perforator can be situated eccentrically within the flap to optimize the pivot point and allow a wider angle of rotation to cover the defect. An eccentric flap design will permit a slightly smaller flap requirement compared to using a perforator that is central within the flap. Once the perforator is selected, the pedicle is dissected toward the source vessel to an appropriate length needed to allow a gentle arc of rotation. Small adhesions or fascial ligaments should be released as required to prevent kinking or twisting of the pedicle. Skeletonization of the pedicle is not routinely required but the pedicle can be freed by ligating small side branches to increase length and allow a greater degree of rotation and additional advancement of the propeller flap.

Once the pedicle is dissected, the final flap design can be confirmed and flap dimensions can be marked using reverse planning and determining the arc of rotation. The surface area of the flap should be designed 10% to 15% larger than the recipient site defect to avoid tension during inset and to accommodate postoperative swelling. The width at the base of the flap should be designed with a relatively broad angle to capture a greater number of linking vessels (direct, indirect, and communicating branches) that increases the overall perfusion along the axiality of the flap. Following flap dissection, the remainder of the flap can be circumferentially incised and raised. The flap is then rotated into the defect in the direction that offers the least amount of pedicle twisting (see Fig. 33-7). A handheld Doppler is used to confirm good arterial and venous signals prior to final

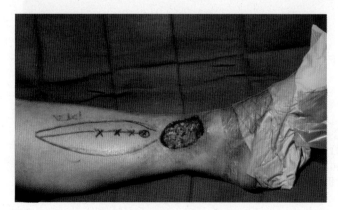

FIGURE 33-6

A small distal third medial defect and perforators identified along the axis of the posterior tibial artery and planned propeller flap design.

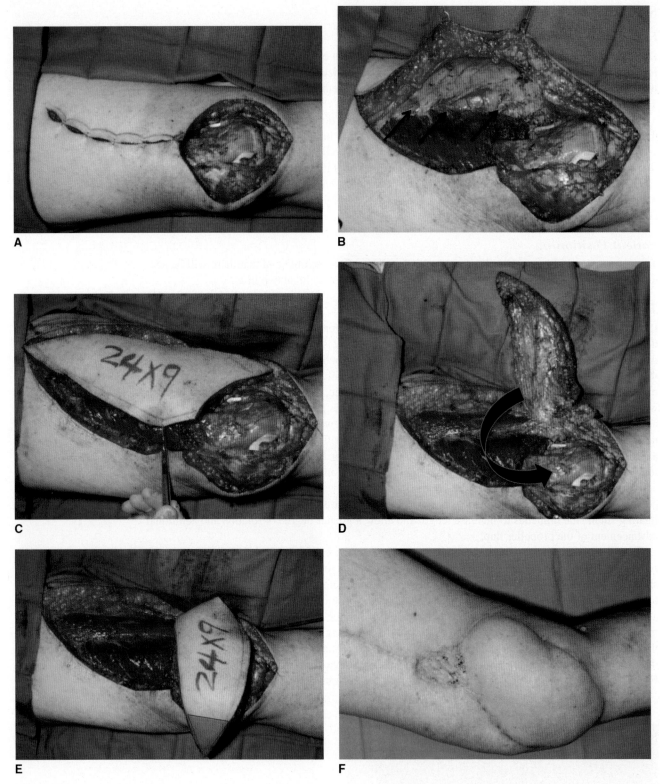

FIGURE 33-7

A: Perforators identified through an anterior exploratory incision from the superficial femoral artery in the medial thigh for a planned SFAP flap for a composite knee defect. **B:** Three perforators identified following a subfascial dissection (*black arrows*) with the perforator closest to the defect selected to provide the optimum pivot and arc or rotation. **C–E:** Once the perforator is selected and the pedicle is dissected, the remainder of the flap may be circumferentially incised **(C)**, raised **(D)**, and finally rotated into the defect **(E)**. The use of intraoperative laser-assisted fluorescence angiography allowed identification of reduced perfusion at distal edge of flap, which was excised intraoperatively (*purple shaded* area in **E**). **F:** Early postoperative result with well-healed flap and small healed skin graft over the pedicle to prevent tension on pedicle during closure.

flap inset. If intraoperative imaging is available such as LA-ICGFA, the perfusion of the flap can be confirmed at the most distal aspect of the propeller flap. The threshold for skin grafting near the pedicle should be low to prevent compression (see Figs. 33-2 and 33-7). It is crucial that there are no constrictive forces on the pedicle when insetting the flap. Tunneling of flaps should be avoided in the lower extremity as this can create unwanted constrictive forces, which may be made worse by postoperative swelling.

Once the flap is inset, it should be secured with minimal tension to take into account postoperative swelling. Flap inset is normally carried out with 3-0 Monocryl in the deep dermal layer and 4-0 Monocryl subcutaneous, but interrupted skin sutures can be used instead. A 5-0 nonabsorbable nonbraided suture is used to mark the Doppler signal. It is important to listen for a venous and arterial signal with the Doppler probe. The donor sites are closed with progressive tension sutures, and skin grafting of the donor site may be required if donor site closure compromised the flow within the perforator. A small Penrose or J-P drain is used for all propeller flaps and removed usually at 7 days.

Postoperative Management

It is important to standardize a postoperative plan and management protocol, which includes analgesia and follow-up plans. All patients receive long-acting local anesthetic at the flap and donor site margins at the end of the operation. Noncompressive soft bulky dressings should be applied avoiding any pressure over the flap and the pedicle. A window can be created to allow monitoring of the entire flap within the dressing. Depending on the nature of the injury, concomitant injuries, and location of the defect, the limb may need to be stabilized with splints if there is no external fixator. In the thigh reconstructions, gentle mobilization is commenced on postoperative day 1 as tolerated. However, in the lower leg, there is high variability in surgeon preferences in postoperative mobilization protocols. If there is no skin graft, we commence a modified "dangling" protocol, which generally involves progressive increase in time the leg is allowed to hang down from the edge of the bed at regular intervals. We start with 5 minutes three times a day and increase this to 10, then 15, and then 20 minutes. Both the time and frequency the leg is allowed to dangle are increased each day. Skin grafts, if used, are examined at 4 to 5 days, and then mobilization is commenced. At 1 week, the patient is followed up in the clinic for removal of the drain and splints. At 2 weeks, sutures are removed and a soft compression ACE bandage is applied to help with swelling.

Complications/Results

The most common immediate complication may be venous compromise, which may be related to hematoma formation, or kinking of the pedicle. This complication can be minimized by maintaining a bloodless field; this minimizes postoperative hematomas and minimizes pedicle compression. If signs of congestion or ischemia are observed intraoperatively, derotation of the flap can be attempted and release of any constricting fascial attachments to the pedicle. Postoperatively, if flap congestion is seen, the sutures can be removed or leech therapy can be initiated. Another potential complication is partial necrosis at the distal portion of the flap. This area may need to be excised and a secondary smaller procedure may be required such as skin graft or another local flap. Total flap loss is relatively uncommon but can be distressing to the patient and stressful for the surgeon. In such cases, a free flap or lifeboat option needs to be considered. Recent systematic reviews of the literature have demonstrated that complication rates in propeller flaps are comparable to free flap reconstruction. Complications such as delayed healing or wound complications can usually be managed conservatively with dressing changes.

KEYSTONE ISLAND PERFORATOR FLAPS

For defects not amenable to a single perforator flap, a keystone flap may be considered. The keystone perforator island flap was originally described in 2003 by Behan. The flap has a trapezoidal shape resembling the keystone in Roman arches and is designed to work ideally with an elliptical defect. They are classically divided into four types (Fig. 33-8). Keystone flaps, similar to propeller flaps, can obviate the need for microsurgical techniques. These flaps are executed as a single multiperforator fasciocutaneous advancement flap based on random fasciocutaneous or musculocutaneous perforators. The keystone flap design permits redistribution of tissue laxity and tension over the entire flap to cover the defect with a reduction in the longitudinal axis of the flap and an increase in its short axis, which is the point of greatest tension through a process of tissue creep and stress relaxation.

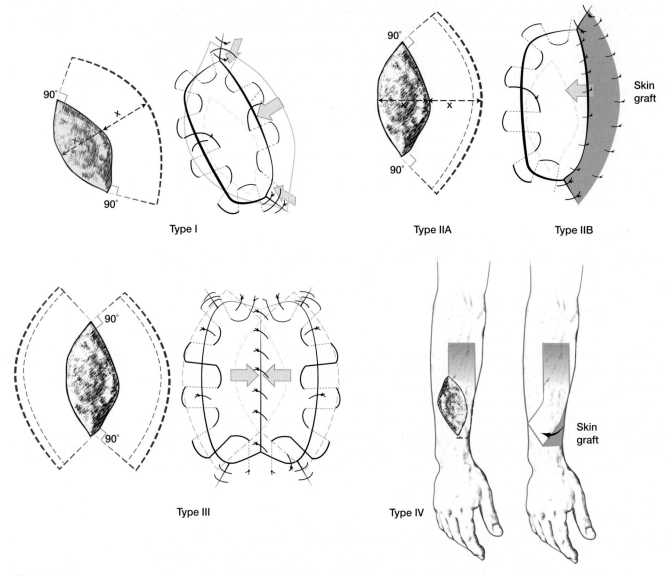

FIGURE 33-8

Traditional classification of keystone island perforator flaps as described by Behan in 2003. I: Skin incision only. IIA: Division of the deep fascia along the outer curvilinear line. IIB: Division of the deep fascia and a skin graft to the secondary defect. III: Opposing keystone flaps designed to create a double keystone flap. IV. Keystone flaps with undermining of up to 50% of the flap subfascially.

Indications/Contraindications

Indications for keystone flaps are similar to use of propeller flaps. They provide reliable reconstruction for simple and complex wounds and have greatest utility in patients who are high risk for longer microsurgical procedures or for patients that have multiple comorbidities. Flaps can be harvested in 20 to 30 minutes, and their use allows for early mobilization.

The flap can be used as the sole reconstructive technique, or it may be used in combination with other flaps. Although initially described for smaller defects, over the years the flap's indications have been extended for a growing number of clinical applications, including trauma defects and following oncological resections. More recent reports note its success in reconstructing defects in the trunk, limb, inguinal, perineal, and head and neck area. Reconstruction can be performed using a single keystone or bilateral opposing keystone flaps to cover defects. We have found these flaps useful in small lower leg defects (e.g., following resection of skin cancers) as they provide better contour and more durable reconstructions when compared to skin grafts.

Relative contraindications for flap use include an inflamed wound bed, flap design over irradiated tissue, or degloving injuries, or when defects have been extensively undermined at the edges.

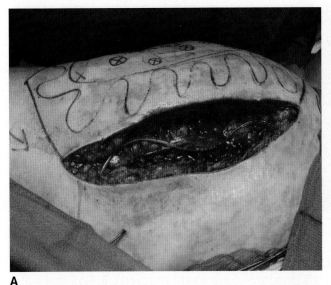

A

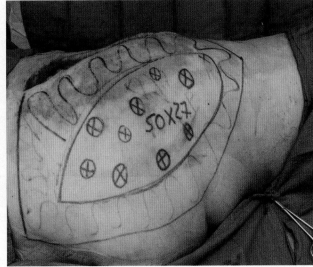

B

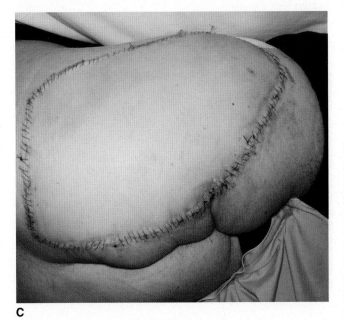

C

FIGURE 33-9

A: Anterior view following removal of an infected right hip prosthesis, inflamed surrounding tissue undermining of the adjacent skin, and resultant defect over the greater trochanter. **B:** A large posteriorly based keystone flap was designed centered over multiple perforators that were identified with handheld Doppler on the table and marked in an area of maximal laxity and noninflamed tissue, with the flap axis predominantly orientated in a longitudinal axis of the lower limb. **C:** Early postoperative result prior to suture removal demonstrating a health flap providing robust coverage and healing well.

However, in some circumstances, these complex wounds have been successfully reconstructed with keystone flaps following careful selection, planning, and execution (Fig. 33-9).

Preoperative Planning

Traditional Flap Design

The original keystone flap design represents two opposing VY flaps orientated parallel to the longitudinal axis of the defect. The lesion is excised in an elliptical fashion. Flap design should occur over the side of the lesion with maximal skin laxity. The limbs of the keystone flap are drawn at 90 degrees to the side of the defect, and the curvature of the flap is parallel to the defect. The width of the flap has a 1:1 ratio to the defect. The initial advancement of the VY is at the corners of the keystone flap design in the longitudinal axis of the flap (parallel to the defect). This creates residual laxity to allow horizontal translation or advancement of the flap into the defect (Fig. 33-8). The original flap design was based on random perforators.

Modifications in Flap Design

Smaller flaps for skin cancer reconstruction generally followed the 1 to 1.5:1 width ratio (Fig. 33-10). But for complex wounds and irradiated wound beds, the width of the flap often exceed this ratio to 3:1, or even to 4:1 and 5:1 ratios, depending on locoregional tissue laxity (Fig. 33-11;

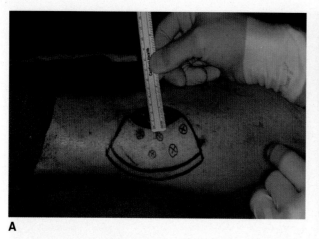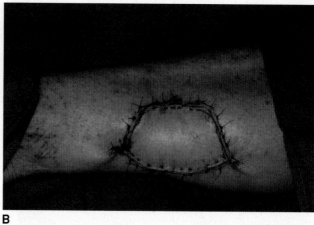

A   **B**

FIGURE 33-10

Keystone island perforator flap reconstructions in the lower leg. **A:** A pretibial defect following excision of a lesion and planning of keystone flap design, where a larger design will help recruit more tissue posteriorly and spread tension over a wider surface area. **B:** Final inset and closure of the keystone flap providing a stable and robust coverage and replacing "like with like."

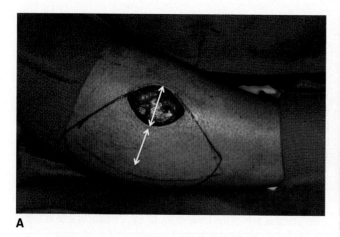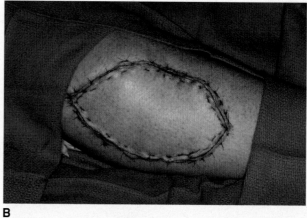

A   **B**

FIGURE 33-11

Pretibial defect after excision of a lesion in the lower leg. **A:** To optimize posterior tissue laxity and ensure a tension-free closure, a greater than 1:1 defect to flap ratio was designed (*white arrows*). **B:** Final inset of the flap.

see Fig. 33-9). Greater flap dimensions are recommended if tissue quality adjacent to the defect is compromised or the wound has been undermined, radiated, or inflamed; greater flap dimensions allow one to recruit well-vascularized tissue for robust coverage without significant tension. Areas of undermining are not considered part of the primary flap design. A second or opposing keystone flap may be designed if concern exists on closing tension and is of course dependent on local tissue laxity (Fig. 33-12). Larger flap designs can create conspicuous scarring, and when feasible, flap incisions should be designed along the aesthetic units on the side of maximal skin laxity, away from the traumatized field. The limbs of the flap in the traditional design are usually drawn at 90 degrees to the longitudinal axis of the defect; however, an asymmetric limb design may be required to avoid lymphatic basins or exposure of critical structures and to avoid crossing any joint creases (Fig. 33-13).

In smaller defects, one does not need to routinely map out nearby perforators; however, in larger defects, identification of dominant perforators with a handheld Doppler allows the surgeon to center the flap over the major perforators thus maximizing flap perfusion. The longitudinal axis of the flap should follow the maximal axiality of the flow from the dominant perforators, for example, along the longitudinal axis of the lower extremity. More aggressive undermining can be performed remotely from dominant perforators in "cold spots" (away from the major perforators), without compromising flap vascularity.

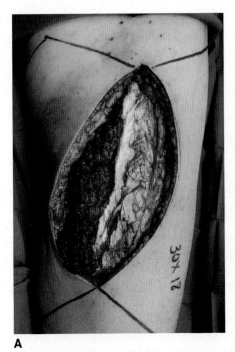
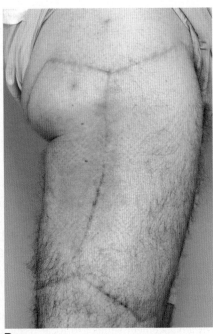

FIGURE 33-12

A: Lateral right thigh following sarcoma resection in a previously irradiated field and a second keystone flap was planned to minimize closing tension and overcome adjacent inelasticity of tissues. **B:** Early postoperative result at 1 month demonstrating well-healed scars.

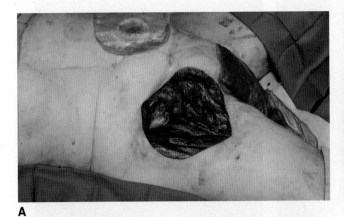
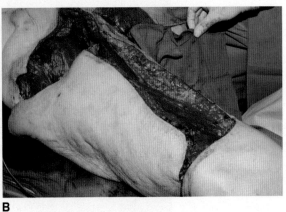
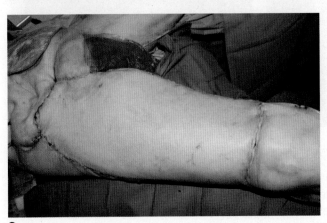

FIGURE 33-13

A: After resection of a right squamous cell sarcoma extending into the lower abdominal cavity, a large inguinal defect resulted. **B:** A large anterior keystone flap was harvested with asymmetric limbs to avoid crossing the knee joint and designed within the aesthetic unit of the thigh and near circumferential incision of the deep fascia, providing extensive movement over the muscle bellies in the thigh. **C:** Final inset with placement of closed suction drains and closure with progressive tension sutures. Part of the flap adjacent to the defect was de-epithelialized to obliterate dead space in the groin.

Modifications

Modifications include maintaining a skin bridge, partial undermining, folding of the flap into an omega (Ω), or rotation into a yin-yang bilateral configuration. Part of the keystone flap can also be de-epithelialized for obliteration of dead space together with progressive tension sutures for the final closure.

Surgery

Patient Positioning

This is dependent on the defect location, size, and proposed flap designs.

Technique

The traditional technique involves excising the lesion in an elliptical fashion and the flap is designed as described above. An initial incision is made through the skin and subcutaneous tissue down to the deep fascia. Advancement can be assessed prior to division of the deep fascia. If more advancement is needed, the deep fascia can be incised in a stepwise approach, starting with the longitudinal edge of the flap that is furthest from the defect. Although a progressive approach is used, a circumferential incision provides greatest freedom of movement and moderate flap stretch. This is commonly done for large defects and complex wounds for sarcoma or other soft tissue defects (with preservation of the proximal and distal fascia connections). However, when flaps are designed over mobile muscle bellies, for example, in the proximal thigh, release of the deep fascia even on one side can provide significant advancement subject to local tissue quality. Partial undermining of the flap below the deep fascia and away from "hot spots" of dominant perforator can further mobilize the flap.

The keystone flap may be designed as the primary reconstructive option, or it can be used as a lifeboat or adjunct flap in combination with regional perforator flaps (Fig. 33-14; see Fig. 33-5).

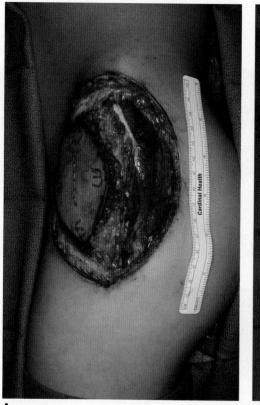
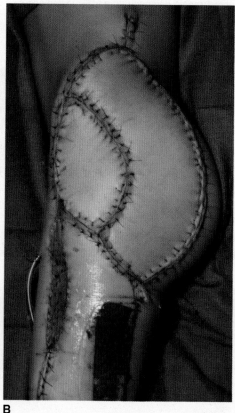

A   **B**

FIGURE 33-14

A: Planned resection of a chondrosarcoma in a child creating a resultant defect over the left hip with exposure of the anterior superior iliac spine. **B:** Immediately after flap inset of a pedicled anterolateral thigh flap and a posterior-based keystone flap to provide soft tissue coverage. (Case care of S. Moran.)

TABLE 33-1	Modifications in Keystone Flap Harvest and Potential Advantages
Key Points of Flap Harvest	**Potential Advantages**
Exceeding flap to defect ratios (1:1)	● Takes advantage of areas of greater donor laxity ● Incorporate well-vascularized tissue zone of injury/inflammation
Broad flap design	● Includes adjacent linking vessels and perforator territories, increasing the overall vascular integrity of the flap
Flap orientation	● Parallel to the dominant axiality of flow, in the extremities this is parallel to its longitudinal axis.
Aesthetic units	● May better redistribute tissue and contour irregularities ● More conspicuous scarring when aligned with aesthetic units of the body
Centered on known dominant perforators	● Allows for better vascular integrity, inclusion of dominant linking vessels ● Permits more aggressive undermining away from perforators and maintains vascular integrity
Routine fascial incision	● Routine incision of the fascia ● Near or complete circumferential incision combined with flap undermining greatly increases versatility
Multiple options	● Use bilateral keystone flaps. ● Combinations of transposition, rotation, and advancement ● Combined with other local flaps, pedicled or free flaps ● De-epithelialization of flap for dead space obliteration

For defects involving the inguinal region, excess tissue of the fasciocutaneous flap may be de-epithelialized and used for dead space obliteration in groin defects with or without local muscle transposition for protection of exposure vessels and progressive tension sutures during closure.

Intraoperative tools for assessment of perfusion, such as laser-assisted indocyanine green fluorescence angiography, may provide an initial assessment of skin perfusion adjacent to the defect following tumor ablative surgery or debrided wounds. This can influence the final design and reconstructive plan.

Progressive tension sutures have been increasingly adopted to redistribute tension during final closure and obliterate dead space. In some cases, the secondary donor site defect may require a small split skin graft if there is tension during primary closure or insufficient laxity. The use of surgical drains is based on the oncological or lymph node resection.

Table 33-1 illustrates modifications in flap harvest and execution in keystone island perforator flap design and harvest. Video 2 is an example of intraoperative planning and keystone flap harvest for an anterior thigh sarcoma resection defect.

Postoperative Management

A soft bulk dressing is applied but no flap monitoring is required. Patients are encouraged to mobilize early unless the oncological ablative surgery or comorbidities may influence a longer in-hospital stay.

Complications/Results

Partial and total flap loss can occur though they are uncommon. Delayed healing and wound dehiscence can in most cases be managed conservatively. Cases of total flap loss will require moving to a free flap or distant local flap. Cutaneous sensation has been previously described as well preserved, which can be attributed to the design within dermatome segments that can mirror the regions of dominant perforators and distribution of perforating cutaneous nerves within the flap design.

PEARLS AND PITFALLS

Propeller Flaps

● There is an associated learning curve in the planning and execution of local propeller flaps in lower extremity reconstruction.
● Know the regional anatomy and blood supply. Center the flaps over dominant perforators and orientate the longitudinal axis of the flap parallel to the dominant linking vessels, which typically follow the course of the source vessels and in the longitudinal axis of the lower limb. However, in the proximal thigh, transverse orientated skin paddles can be designed based on local skin laxity.

- Use an initial exploratory incision to allow identification and assessment of suitable perforators close to the defect in the region for the proposed flap design.
- Identify the septum early when appropriate, and start raising flaps in subfascial plane, which will facilitate dissection and allow early exposure of critical structures.
- Consider the lifeboat options and plan incisions that do not impede or violate the potential harvest of these second flap options.
- If the dominant blood supply is not available, such as no suitable perforators are available, consider exploring the adjacent vascular territory before considering lifeboat options.
- Avoid tunneling; any constrictive pressure or tension on the pedicle in the lower extremity had a low threshold for skin grafting to reduce closing tension when required; this can be later revised.
- The dissection of the perforator still requires careful microsurgical techniques for the flap harvest.
- The vascular territory of individual perforators is not fully defined, including the influence of interperforator flow and absolute flap size limitations that can be harvested safely in individual patients.
- Incorrect harvest of local flaps may interrupt superficial veins and cutaneous nerves that can lead to edema and neuromata.
- The key perforators or dominant perforators may be close to the zone of injury and therefore near the required pivot point. Careful assessment of the extent and nature of the zone of injury must be made to determine if local flap reconstruction is appropriate and feasible.
- Skeletonization of the pedicle should only proceed as required to gain the movement and rotation required, with removal of any fascial adhesions that may lead to torsion of the pedicle and compromise either inflow or outflow.
- The donor site following propeller flap harvest should ideally be closed primarily, but sometimes skin grafts are still required for wound closure that can significantly impact contour and cosmesis.

Keystone Flaps

- Modification to the traditional keystone flap description involves centering the flap over known perforator "hot spots."
- Larger flaps exceeding the 1:1 ratio incorporate the maximal density of perforators, creating a multiperforator advancement flap, and recruit well-vascularized tissue remote from the defect site.
- Smaller flaps should be avoided when extensive undermining has occurred adjacent to the defect.
- Areas of undermining should not be considered part of the primary flap design.
- Consider local skin laxity, and in irradiated fields, design bigger flaps.
- Avoid violation of lymph node regions.
- Use progressive tension sutures for closure.
- Consider bilateral keystone flaps for larger defects or when there is limited laxity.
- Design the flap along aesthetic units when possible and design on the side of maximal skin laxity that is distant to injury, inflammation, or irradiation.

RECOMMENDED READING

Angrigiani C, Grilli D, Thorne CH. The adductor flap: a new method for transferring posterior and medial thigh skin. *Plast Reconstr Surg.* 2001;107:1725–1731.

Behan F, Findlay M, Lo CH. *The Keystone Perforator Island Flap Concept.* Sydney, Australia: Churchill Livingstone; 2012.

Behan F, Sizeland A, Gilmour F, et al. Use of the keystone island flap for advanced head and neck cancer in the elderly: a principle of amelioration. *J Plast Reconstr Aesthet Surg.* 2010;63:739–745.

Behan F, Sizeland A, Porcedu S, et al. Keystone island flap: an alternative reconstructive option to free flaps in irradiated tissue. *ANZ J Surg.* 2006;76:407–413.

Behan FC. The keystone design perforator island flap in reconstructive surgery. *ANZ J Surg.* 2003;73:112–210.

Behan FC, Lo CH, Shayan R. Perforator territory of the keystone flap: use of the dermatomal roadmap. *J Plast Reconstr Aesthet Surg.* 2009;62:551–553.

Behan FC, Paddle A, Rozen WM, et al. Quadriceps keystone island flap for radical inguinal lymphadenectomy: a reliable locoregional island flap for large groin defects. *ANZ J Surg.* 2013;83:942–947.

Behan FC, Rozen WM, Azer S, et al. 'Perineal keystone design perforator island flap' for perineal and vulval reconstruction. *ANZ J Surg.* 2012;82:381–382.

Behan FC, Rozen WM, Lo CH, et al. The omega—Ω—variant designs (types A and B) of the keystone perforator island flap. *ANZ J Surg.* 2011;81:650–652.

Behan FC, Rozen WM, Tan S. Yin-yang flaps: the mathematics of two keystone island flaps for reconstructing increasingly large defects. *ANZ J Surg.* 2011;81:574–575.

Cormack GC, Lamberty BGH. Fasciocutaneous vessels. *Anat Clin.* 1984;6:121–131.

Georgescu AV. Propeller perforator flaps in distal lower leg: evolution and clinical applications. *Arch Plast Surg.* 2012;39:94–105.

Gir P, Cheng A, Oni G, et al. Pedicled-perforator (propeller) flaps in lower extremity defects: a systematic review. *J Reconstr Microsurg.* 2012;28:595–601.

Grover R, Nelson JA, Fischer JP, et al. The impact of perforator number on deep inferior epigastric perforator flap breast reconstruction. *Arch Plast Surg.* 2014;41:63–70.

Hallock GG. A paradigm shift in flap selection protocols for zones of the lower extremity using perforator flaps. *J Reconstr Microsurg.* 2013;29:233–240.

Hallock GG. The propeller flap version of the adductor muscle perforator flap for coverage of ischial or trochanteric pressure sores. *Ann Plast Surg.* 2006;56:540–542.

Hu M, Bordeaux JS. The keystone flap for lower extremity defects. *Dermatol Surg.* 2012;38:490–493.

Hyakusoku H, Yamamoto T, Fumiiri M. The propeller flap method. *Br J Plast Surg.* 1991;44:53–54.

Khouri JS, Egeland BM, Daily SD, et al. The keystone island flap: use in large defects of the trunk and extremities in soft-tissue reconstruction. *Plast Reconstr Surg.* 2011;127:1212–1221.

Martinez J-C, Cook JL, Otley C. The keystone fasciocutaneous flap in the reconstruction of lower extremity wounds. *Dermatol Surg.* 2012;38:484–489.

Maruyama Y, Iwahira Y. Popliteo-posterior thigh fasciocutaneous island flap for closure around the knee. *Br J Plast Surg.* 1989;42:140–143.

Miyamoto S, Kayano S, Kamizono K, et al. Pedicled superficial femoral artery perforator flaps for reconstruction of large groin defects. *Microsurgery.* 2014;34:470–474.

Mohan AT, Rammos CK, Akhavan AA, et al. Evolving concepts of keystone perforator flap (KPIF): principles of perforator anatomy, design modifications and extended clinical applications. *Plast Reconstr Surg.* 2016;137(6):1909–1920.

Mojallal A, Boucher F, Shipkov H, et al. Superficial femoral artery perforator flap: anatomical study of a new flap and clinical cases. *Plast Reconstr Surg.* 2014;133:934–944.

Moncrieff MD, Bowen F, Thompson JF, et al. Keystone flap reconstruction of primary melanoma excision defects of the leg-the end of the skin graft? *Ann Surg Oncol.* 2008;15:2867–2873.

Morris SF, Tang M, Almutari K, et al. The anatomic basis of perforator flaps. *Clin Plast Surg.* 2010;37:553–570.

Nelson JA, Fischer JP, Brazio PS, et al. A review of propeller flaps for distal lower extremity soft tissue reconstruction: is flap loss too high? *Microsurgery.* 2013;33:578–586.

Pignatti M, Ogawa R, Hallock GG, et al. The 'Tokyo' consensus on propeller flaps. *Plast Reconstr Surg.* 2011;127:716–722.

Pignatti M, Pasqualini M, Governa M, et al. Propeller flaps for leg reconstruction. *J Plast Reconstr Aesthet Surg.* 2008;61:777–783.

Rao AL, Janna RK. Keystone flap: versatile flap for reconstruction of limb defects. *J Clin Diagn Res.* 2015;9:PC05–PC057.

Saint-Cyr M, Schaverien M, Arbique G, et al. Three- and four-dimensional computed tomographic angiography and venography for the investigation of the vascular anatomy and perfusion of perforator flaps. *Plast Reconstr Surg.* 2008;121:772–780.

Saint-Cyr M, Schaverien M, Wong C, et al. The extended anterolateral thigh flap: anatomical basis and clinical experience. *Plast Reconstr Surg.* 2009;123:1245–1255.

Saint-Cyr M, Wong C, Schaverien M, et al. The Perforasome theory: vascular anatomy and clinical implications. *Plast Reconstr Surg.* 2009;124:1529–1544.

Scalise A, Tartaglione C, Bolletta E, et al. Profunda femoris artery perforator propeller flap: a valid method to cover complicated ischiatic pressure sores. *Plast Reconstr Surg.* 2015;3:e487.

Schaverien M, Saint-Cyr M. Perforators of the lower leg: analysis of perforator locations and clinical application for pedicled perforator flaps. *Plast Reconstr Surg.* 2008;122:161–170.

Sur Y-J, Morsy M, Mohan AT, et al. Three-dimensional computed tomographic angiographic study of the inter-perforator flow of the lower leg. *Plast Reconstr Surg.* 2016;137(5):1615–1628.

Taylor GI, Palmer JH. The vascular territories (angiosomes) of the body: experimental study and clinical applications. *Br J Plast Surg.* 1987;40:113–141.

Teo TC. The propeller flap concept. *Clin Plast Surg.* 2010;37:615–626.

Wong C, Nagarkar P, Teotia S, et al. The profunda artery perforator flap: investigating the Perforasome using three-dimensional computed tomographic angiography. *Plast Reconstr Surg.* 2015;136:915–919.

34 Fasciotomies of the Lower Extremity

Christopher J. Salgado, Yasmina Zoghbi, Harvey Chim,
Emily A. Borsting, Jimmy H. Chim, and Handel R. Robinson

INDICATIONS/CONTRAINDICATIONS

Compartment syndrome is the most common indication for fasciotomy. Compartment syndrome is a clinical condition with elevated tissue pressure within a closed anatomic compartment. In the extremities, muscles are contained within an osseofascial compartment that has a limited capacity to expand. The causes of compartment syndrome can be divided into two major categories: decreased compartment size and increased compartment volume. Decreases in compartment size can be due to extrinsic factors such as tight dressings or casts or due to intrinsic causes such as bleeding into a compartment after injury or a postoperative coagulopathy. Increased compartment volume can occur at the macroscopic or microscopic level. Bleeding and iatrogenic infiltration of intravenous fluid into a closed compartment are both common causes of compartment syndrome. At the microscopic level, compartment volume can be increased in proportion to either increased capillary permeability or capillary pressure. Conditions associated with tissue damage such as burns, ischemia/reperfusion, and trauma can all lead to increased capillary permeability. Increased capillary pressure is the underlying cause of compartment syndrome due to venous obstruction or exercise.

The underlying pathologic condition leading to compartment syndrome is an elevated tissue pressure that leads to decreased arteriolar perfusion. At this point shunting occurs, bypassing the capillary circulation, which then worsens the tissue ischemia, and in turn, increases the capillary permeability and interstitial tissue pressure. This vicious cycle can quickly lead to permanent tissue damage if not treated expediently. Persistent sustained elevated intracompartmental pressures greater than 6 to 8 hours result in irreversible soft tissue damage. The tissues most at risk in compartment syndrome are the nerves and muscles. If untreated, compartment syndrome can lead to Volkmann contracture, a permanent paralysis of muscles in the compartment due to scarring in a shortened position and fibrosis. Assessment of an injured lower extremity must include a thorough evaluation of factors that can contribute either directly or indirectly to compartment syndrome. A list of such factors is given in Table 34-1. The treatment of compartment syndrome is the correction of the underlying pathologic state and the performance of a fasciotomy. Fasciotomy involves the incision of fascial compartments in order to expand the size of the compartment and to restore perfusion to the contents of the compartment.

PREOPERATIVE PLANNING

Patient Assessment

Preoperative planning for a fasciotomy is based on an accurate and timely diagnosis of compartment syndrome. The most important data guiding this decision is the clinical examination. In the setting of an awake, unsedated patient, the diagnosis can commonly be made based on clinical grounds. The classical clinical signs of compartment syndrome are the six P's: pain, pressure, paresthesia, paralysis, pallor, and pulselessness. Significant muscle damage can occur prior to the onset of pallor, pulselessness, and paralysis, and these are late findings of a missed compartment syndrome. The most sensitive initial clinical sign of compartment syndrome is pain. This is often described as being out of proportion to the injury. In the author's experience, the variability of pain threshold among patients can make the assessment of "expected level of pain" somewhat arbitrary. The presence

TABLE 34-1	Compartment Syndrome Risk Factors	
History	**Injury**	**Treatment**
Crush injury	Open and closed fractures	Fluid administration
Entrapment	Arterial injury	Tourniquets
Ischemia	Venous injury	Positioning
Shock/hypotension	Gunshot wounds to extremity	MAST
Overdose/unconsciousness	Coagulopathy	Arthroscopy pumps
Tight ski boots	Shock	Jet lavage
Coumadin	Deep vein thrombosis	Revascularization
Weightlifting/overuse	Burns	Vein ligation
Knee arthroscopy	Muscle tear	Fracture tables
Prolonged surgery	Snake envenomation	Tight wound closures
Soft tissue filler injections	Ruptured Baker cyst	Constrictive dressings
		Regional anesthesia

MAST, military antishock trousers.

of a greater than expected level of pain does not indicate definitive compartment syndrome, and the absence of pain does not rule out the diagnosis, particularly in the setting of a possible neurologic injury. The use of sedatives and analgesics, a history of central nervous system trauma, and the possibility of peripheral nerve injury highlight the need for a high index of suspicion and the need for early intracompartmental pressure measurements. Passive stretching of muscles within the compartment leads to elevated pressures and increased pain, another valuable tool in establishing a clinical diagnosis. Other signs of compartment syndrome include paresthesias and paralysis. Paresthesias are due to ischemic damage to the peripheral nerves running in the compartment. Decreased two-point discrimination is the most consistent early finding. Correlation has also been reported between diminished vibration sense (256 cycles per second) and increasing compartment pressure. On deep palpation, a firm woody feeling is a specific sign when present. Bullae may also be observed. In later stages, the paresthesias can progress to complete anesthesia in the distribution of the peripheral nerve.

Paralysis can be due to muscle ischemia, nerve ischemia, or direct injury to these structures or secondary to pain inhibition. Pulselessness is uncommon in an isolated compartment syndrome and heralds a probable vascular injury. Laboratory testing revealing a creatine kinase (CK) of 1,000 to 5,000 U/mL or higher or the presence of myoglobinuria may alert the physician to the occurrence of compartment syndrome. When the clinical picture is borderline, compartment pressure measurements must be performed as soon as possible. Ideally, in patients at risk of developing acute compartment syndrome, intramuscular pressure (IMP) measurements should be monitored continuously and single readings should be avoided.

Compartment Pressures

A number of techniques have been employed to determine compartment pressures. At our institution, all compartment measurements are performed with a side-port needle attached to a commercially available pressure monitor (Stryker, Kalamazoo, MI) or a standard arterial line pressure transduction line (Fig. 34-1). The Stryker pressure tonometer is widely used, and pressure measurements from the

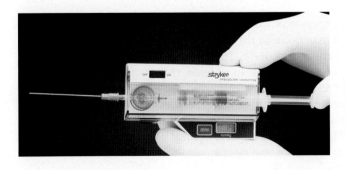

FIGURE 34-1

Stryker pressure monitor with side-port needle. (Courtesy of Stryker, Kalamazoo, MI.)

Stryker device are within 5 mm Hg of the slit catheter for 95% of all readings. Measurements with a standard 18-gauge needle are not accurate and are not recommended. Pressure measurements should be performed within all compartments and at multiple sites. However, when using the needle-insertion technique, catheter patency must be maintained throughout the measurements of IMP. This requires saline flushing/infusion to keep the catheter patent and runs the risk of unnecessarily increasing the IMP by the added volume in the compartment and should preferably be avoided. This may also bias the IMP measurements. An alternative for measuring the IMP has recently been described and involves the use of a forward sensing fiberoptic pressure transducer (Samba 420 LP, Samba Sensors AB, Gothenburg, Sweden). This technique does not require injections and thus inherently lacks hydrostatic biased readings. Its dynamic properties also allow for recordings of pulse-synchronous IMP oscillations, which indicate a reduction in muscle compliance and may therefore be beneficial in diagnosing both acute and chronic compartment syndrome patients.

The compartment pressure data can be viewed in isolation or in relation to the patient's diastolic blood pressure. Although there is no absolute minimum compartment pressure value, most current literature indicates that the ΔP value from measured compartment pressure to diastolic blood pressure is a more valuable guide in performance of a fasciotomy. Some authors still advocate absolute compartment pressure as an indication to perform fasciotomy (over 30 mm Hg for normotensive patients, over 20 mm Hg in hypotensive patients). Studies suggest that the ischemic threshold of muscle is a perfusion pressure of at least 20 mm Hg between the compartment pressure and the diastolic pressure. The ΔP is a direct measure of the pressure gradient between diastolic blood pressure and the tissue pressure within the compartment, indicating the presence of shunting. At our institution, a ΔP of 30 mm Hg combined with increased palpable pressure is a strong indication and a ΔP of 20 mm Hg an absolute indication for fasciotomy. If compartment pressures are not elevated but clinical signs suggest compartment syndrome, surgical decompression should still be performed.

Preoperative Management

Therapy is begun for the treatment of compartment syndrome while preparations are made for actual surgical decompression. The affected limbs are placed at the level of the heart. Elevation is contraindicated because it decreases arterial inflow and narrows the arterial-venous pressure gradient and thus worsens the ischemia. If a cast is on the affected extremity, releasing one side of the plaster cast can reduce compartment pressure by 30%; bivalving can produce an additional 35% reduction; and cutting the cast padding may further decrease compartmental pressure by 10% to 20%. In cases of snake envenomation, administration of antivenom may reverse a developing compartment syndrome. Hypoperfusion may be corrected with crystalloid and blood products, and mannitol may reduce compartment pressures and lessen reperfusion injury.

Three stages of compartment syndrome have been described: the suspected stage, the impending stage, and the established stage. At the suspected stage, frequent neurocirculatory checks should be performed to detect potential progression to the next stage. If the edema-ischemia cycle continues, the condition may advance to the impending stage, in which patients may experience increasing pain, hypesthesias, muscle weakness, discomfort with passive stretch, and/or tenseness in the compartment. In the presence of any of the above signs, pressure measurements should be made. In the established stage of compartment syndrome, immediate fasciotomy must be performed.

SURGERY

Fasciotomy of the Thigh

Anatomy

Thigh compartment syndrome is rare because of the large volume required to cause a pathologic increase in the interstitial pressure. It may occur in the setting of high-energy thigh trauma such as femur fractures with an associated crush component. These patients often have pain and swelling after fixation, which may confound the diagnosis. In addition, these trauma patients are often obtunded and require substantial fluid resuscitation, increasing the risk of compartment issues. The fascial compartments in the thigh blend anatomically with muscles of the hip, potentially allowing extravasation of blood outside these compartments. Anticoagulation can be a major risk factor leading to bleeding into the thigh compartments and the development of a compartment syndrome. There are three compartments: anterior, posterior, and medial.

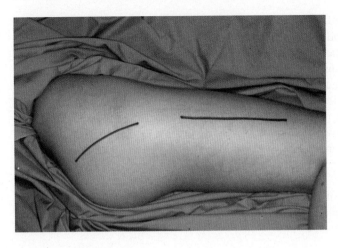

FIGURE 34-2

Skin markings for gluteal and thigh (anterior and posterior) compartment release.

Patient Positioning

The approach to thigh compartments may be medial or lateral depending on the area of injury or suspected hematoma. The thigh should be prepared from the iliac crest to the knee joint with the patient in either the lateral decubitus position or supine.

Technique

For lateral and posterior compartment syndromes, the skin and subcutaneous tissues are incised beginning just distal to the intertrochanteric line and extending to the lateral epicondyle of the femur to expose the iliotibial band or fascia lata (Fig. 34-2). The iliotibial band is incised for the length of the incision. The vastus lateralis muscle is reflected medially to expose the lateral intermuscular septum, which is incised for the length of the incision, thus freeing the posterior compartment (Fig. 34-3). After the anterior and posterior compartments have been released, measure the pressure

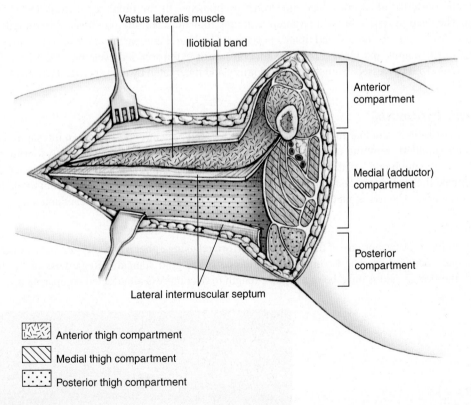

FIGURE 34-3

Schematic lateral view showing decompression of anterior compartment performed by incising the fasciae latae longitudinally. The vastus lateralis is retracted medially to expose the lateral intermuscular septum, which is incised to decompress the posterior compartment.

---

of the medial compartment. If elevated, the compartment can then be approached through a separate medial incision. The incision is carried along the course of the saphenous vein. The sartorius should then be reflected superiorly, and the medial intermuscular septum incised. Intramuscular hematomas may require release through gentle muscle splitting. The wounds are packed open and a large bulky dressing applied or, alternatively, a vacuum-assisted closure (VAC) device is applied.

Two to three days later, the patient is returned to the operating room for debridement of any nonviable tissue. If there is no evidence of necrotic tissue, the skin is loosely closed, packed once again for closure at a later date, or again covered with a VAC device. Often a medial thigh fasciotomy is not needed once a lateral release is performed.

Results

Because this diagnosis is not always obvious, the surgeon must maintain a high index of suspicion. Early treatment by operative compartment release follows anatomic tracts and produces good results.

Fasciotomy of the Leg

Anatomy

The framework of the lower leg is composed of two long bones, the fibula and tibia, which are arranged in parallel and connected along their length by a fibrous membrane termed the interosseous membrane (Fig. 34-4). There are four compartments—anterior, lateral, superficial posterior, and deep posterior.

The anterior compartment has four muscles, the extensor digitorum longus, the extensor hallucis longus, the peroneus tertius, and the tibialis anterior. These muscles are supplied by the anterior tibial vessels and are innervated by the deep peroneal nerve, all traveling deep to the muscles along the interosseous membrane. The posterior compartment is divided into superficial and deep compartments by the transverse intermuscular septum. Three muscles are located in the superficial compartment: the gastrocnemius, soleus, and plantaris. All of these muscles flex the foot in a plantar direction with slight inversion. The muscles are vascularized by branches from the popliteal and posterior tibial artery and innervated by branches of the tibial nerve from the popliteal fossa. The deep posterior leg compartment contains four muscles: the popliteus, flexor digitorum longus, flexor hallucis longus, and tibialis posterior. The lateral compartment contains two muscles, the peroneus longus and brevis. Their action consists of extension and eversion of the foot. They are vascularized by vessels from the peroneal artery and innervated by the superficial peroneal nerve (Fig. 34-5).

Patient Positioning

In cases of isolated compartment syndrome of the leg, the patient is positioned in the supine position on a standard operating table. A general anesthetic is employed in most cases. A tourniquet is applied to the thigh and isolated with broad tape or a plastic isolation dressing. The leg is prepared and draped in the standard fashion. A stockinette or isolation sheet is applied to the foot to maintain the sterile field. The tourniquet is not inflated unless active arterial bleeding is encountered.

Technique

The technique for fasciotomy of the leg can be performed using either a one-incision or two-incision technique (Table 34-2). The two-incision technique is the gold standard. Regardless of the technique, the skin incisions must be of adequate length to decompress all affected compartments.

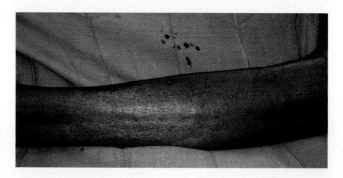

FIGURE 34-4

Left lower extremity prefasciotomy with easily discernible raphe, which separates the anterior and posterior compartments of the lower leg.

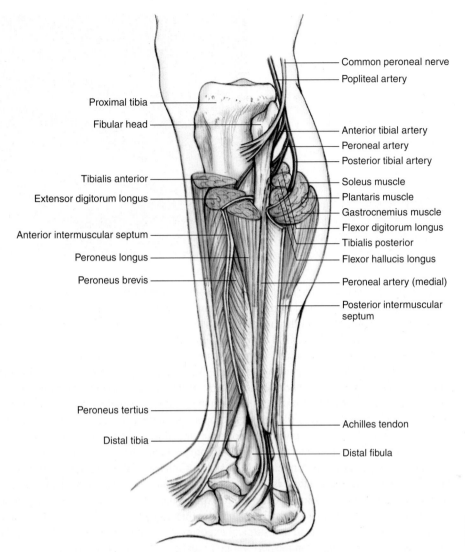

Proximal tibia

Fibular head

Tibialis anterior

Extensor digitorum longus

Anterior intermuscular septum

Peroneus longus

Peroneus brevis

Peroneus tertius

Distal tibia

Common peroneal nerve

Popliteal artery

Anterior tibial artery

Peroneal artery

Posterior tibial artery

Soleus muscle

Plantaris muscle

Gastrocnemius muscle

Flexor digitorum longus

Tibialis posterior

Flexor hallucis longus

Peroneal artery (medial)

Posterior intermuscular septum

Achilles tendon

Distal fibula

FIGURE 34-5

Lateral leg anatomy.

TABLE 34-2   Pearls for Fasciotomy of the Leg

- Check intracompartmental pressures at multiple levels within each compartment.
- Threshold for fasciotomy is intracompartmental pressure within 20 mm Hg of the diastolic blood pressure.
- Beware of compartment syndrome secondary to intraoperative positioning of uninjured extremities.
- Pulselessness is NOT a common finding in compartment syndrome unless a concurrent vascular injury exists.
- Fasciotomy should not be performed more than 12 h after a compartment syndrome is established.
- Compartment syndrome can occur with a late onset 2–4 d after the underlying event.
- Compartment pressure measurements with a standard 18-gauge needle are consistently higher than those obtained with specialized needles with a side-port needle or slit catheter.
- Compartment pressures can vary among several different points in each compartment at risk.
- In any patient at risk, baseline compartment pressures are necessary in the case of a suspicion of compartment syndrome in the future.

Two Incision Leg Fasciotomy (Gold Standard)
- Mark both incisions before making the first surgical incision.
- Beware of the superficial peroneal nerve as it emerges anteriorly within the lateral compartment at the junction of the middle and distal one-third of the fibula.
- Beware of the use of vessel loops or other elastic forms of skin tension applied at the time of fasciotomy, as these may lead to recurrence of the compartment syndrome if excessively tight.
- Close medial wound before the lateral wound to avoid need for soft tissue coverage.

One Incision Leg Fasciotomy
- Obtain complete visualization of the release of the deep posterior compartment, as extensive bleeding can occur secondary to perforating vessels on the posterior aspect of the fibula.
- Extend incision to within 5 cm of either end of the fibula on the anterolateral leg.
- Beware of the superficial peroneal nerve at the junction of the middle and distal one-third of the leg.

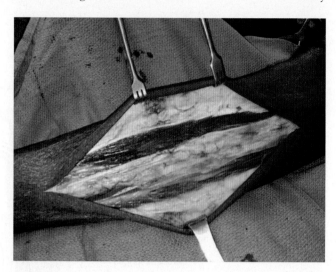

FIGURE 34-6

Intraoperative view showing complete anterior and lateral compartment fasciotomies with separate incisions for each compartment.

ONE-INCISION FASCIOTOMY. The planned incision is marked in line with the fibula extending to 5 cm short of either end of the fibula along the anterolateral septum. Subcutaneous flaps are raised. The initial step is the identification of the lateral intermuscular septum separating the lateral and anterior compartments. The superficial peroneal nerve is identified just deep to the septum. Separate fasciotomies of the compartments are performed with Metzenbaum scissors. The anterior compartment is released proximally by aiming for the patella and distally by aiming for the center of the ankle in line with the tibialis anterior. Then, a longitudinal fasciotomy of the lateral compartment is made in line with the fibular shaft (Fig. 34-6). Extreme care is taken in the distal aspect of the lateral compartment at the junction of the middle and distal thirds, where the superficial peroneal nerve emerges from the lateral compartment. Direct the scissors toward the posterior lateral malleolus to stay posterior to the superficial peroneal nerve. Once the anterior and lateral compartments have been decompressed, the fibula is identified after posterior undermining of the skin for release of the deep posterior compartments. The lateral compartment musculature is elevated off the fibula, demonstrating the posterior intermuscular septum. A longitudinal incision of this septum exposes the superficial posterior compartment. Posterior retraction of the soleus and gastrocnemius muscles then exposes the deep posterior compartment for its decompression. We have found that surgical exposure of the posterior aspect of the fibula is critical in the avoidance of bleeding from the perforating branches of the peroneal artery.

TWO-INCISION FASCIOTOMY. The two-incision fasciotomy is the gold standard treatment for compartment syndrome of the leg, allowing better visualization and release of compartments. The positioning and preparation are identical to that of the one-incision fasciotomy. It is crucial to mark the medial and lateral skin incisions before making the incision to ensure an adequate skin bridge is maintained. After one single incision is made, the skin envelope will retract in the opposite direction resulting in a narrow skin bridge anteriorly, and marking these incisions will avoid this complication. The anterior and lateral compartments are released through a single incision centered along the anterior intermuscular septum. Then, a separate incision is made along the posteromedial leg, 1 to 2 cm posterior to the tibia, measuring at least 15 cm in length (Fig. 34-7).

Skin flaps are elevated in the suprafascial plane. The greater saphenous vein and saphenous nerve are identified and retracted anteriorly. The fasciotomy is extended as far as possible proximally and

FIGURE 34-7

Left lower extremity prefasciotomy. Relative awareness of the GSV while making medial incisions to decompress the posterior compartment is imperative for subsequent revascularizations. Intraoperative view after release of superficial posterior compartment and before release of deep posterior compartment.

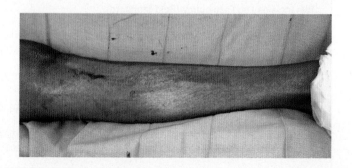

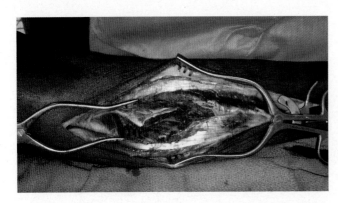

FIGURE 34-8

Medial fasciotomy incisions with decompression of the superficial and deep posterior compartment. Care taken to take down the soleus muscle from its attachment to the tibia, which provides access to the deep compartment. Note the posterior tibial artery and veins in the center of surgical field. Medial approach for four-compartment release of foot compartment syndrome.

distally to the level of the medial malleolus. The soleus is then released from the posteromedial tibia with a concurrent release of the deep posterior compartment, along the course of the flexor digitorum longus muscle (Fig. 34-8). A common pitfall is to not adequately release the soleus muscle insertion thereby not adequately releasing the deep posterior compartment. The posterior tibial neurovascular bundle is just deep to the soleus muscle, which separates the deep from superficial posterior compartments and is therefore in close proximity to the release. The skin incisions can also be slightly staggered, with the lateral more proximal (the anterior and lateral compartments are largely tendinous at their distal extent) and the medial incision more distal. Finally, the fascia and skin are then re-evaluated for adequacy of release.

After either type of fasciotomy, compartment pressures are again checked using a sterile side-port needle attached to the nonsterile pressure monitor held by an unscrubbed assistant or, alternatively, using an arterial pressure monitor setup. The wounds are then copiously irrigated with crystalloid. Devitalized tissue if present is debrided. At our institution, we routinely employ a VAC device over all open fasciotomy wounds to maintain a one-way flow of extravasated fluid, to encourage the formation of granulation tissue and potentially to minimize the area needed for later skin grafting. Definitive closure can be performed subsequently with a split-thickness skin graft. It is imperative to maintain the foot in a neutral position to avoid equinus contracture with either external fixation or external splinting.

Results

A number of studies have demonstrated that the majority of patients have normal leg function if the fasciotomy is performed within 12 hours of the onset of compartment syndrome. In our experience, prompt recognition and early treatment of the compartment syndrome lead to minimal long-term complications. Despite early and aggressive fasciotomy, however, nearly 20% of patients may have persistent motor deficits at 1-year follow-up. Wound complications associated with fasciotomy include numbness and persistent ulceration at the fasciotomy site. The risk of sensory changes has been reported to be as high as 70% in some reports. The use of a VAC dressing may contribute to a lower risk of hematoma and edema and an expeditious granulation of fasciotomy wounds that are not able to be closed. Little or no return of function can be expected when diagnosis and treatment are delayed. Tendon transfers and foot stabilization may be indicated as late treatment, but in most patients, enough scarring and contracture eventually develop in the anterior musculature to prevent footdrop.

Fasciotomy of the Foot

Anatomy

The foot consists of well-demarcated osseofascial spaces that subdivide the foot into discrete compartments. These compartments are filled with muscles, nerves, and tendons and are lined by a tight membrane (the fascia). There are four clinically relevant compartments—the medial, central, lateral, and interosseous (Fig. 34-9). Other anatomic compartments of the foot may be identified with dyes or injection studies but are not clinically relevant. Muscles within the medial compartment are the abductor hallucis and flexor hallucis brevis, and within the central (calcaneal) compartment lie the flexor digitorum brevis, quadratus plantae, and adductor hallucis muscle. There are four dorsal and plantar interosseous muscles between the first and fifth metatarsals, and these constitute the interosseus (intrinsic) compartment. The lateral compartment houses the abductor digiti minimi and flexor digiti minimi brevis muscle.

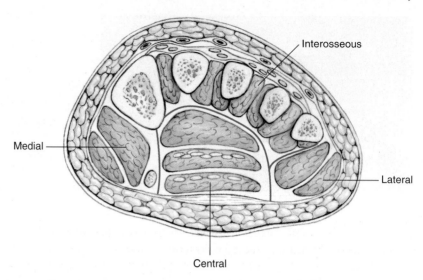

FIGURE 34-9

Schematic coronal section of right foot through base of metatarsals. Medial, central, lateral, and interosseus compartments are shown.

Compartment syndrome in the foot is commonly due to severe local trauma after fairly significant industrial, agricultural, and motor vehicle accidents in which crushing of the foot occurs. Tense tissue bulging may be the most reliable symptom in compartment syndrome of the foot, and in the presence of this massive swelling, pulses are usually not palpable. Increased pain on passive dorsiflexion of metatarsophalangeal joints is another key finding that indicates myoneural ischemia in the foot intrinsic muscles. It is imperative to maintain a high clinical suspicion based on the severity of the traumatic incident. Compartment syndromes of the foot are often associated with compartment syndromes of the deep posterior compartment of the leg.

Patient Positioning

The patient position is supine to allow easy access to the dorsum and medial aspect of the foot. A tourniquet may be used, but is not insufflated unless there is active arterial bleeding. The knee should be included in the preparation to enable better mobility of the limb during the procedure.

Technique

MEDIAL APPROACH. Effective decompression of all four compartments can be accomplished through a medial longitudinal (Henry) approach or through an additional two parallel dorsal incisions along the length of the second and fourth metatarsal bones (more common). The medial approach can be used to decompress the medial and central compartments as well as the remaining foot compartments (lateral and interosseous). The incision on the plantar foot extends from a point below the medial malleolus to the proximal aspect of the first metatarsal (Fig. 34-10). The posterior tibial neurovascular bundle is identified and preserved. This may be very difficult in a massively swollen foot. The fascia overlying the abductor hallucis and flexor hallucis brevis is released. Dissection is continued adjacent and deep to the first metatarsal toward the medial intermuscular septum, separating the medial compartment from the central compartment, which is opened longitudinally. The lateral plantar neurovascular bundle is found between the flexor digitorum brevis and quadratus plantae muscles and preserved. Downward retraction of the flexor digitorum brevis along with lateral dissection will allow access to the lateral intermuscular septum separating the central compartment from the lateral compartment. This septum is divided to release the lateral compartment. Blunt dissection dorsally via the central compartment will release the interosseous compartment. Scissors or sharp instruments are not used during this portion of the dissection, since it is essentially blind to avoid injury to the neurovascular bundle.

DORSAL APPROACH. This approach is more commonly used when there are concomitant metatarsal or Lisfranc fractures. Two parallel dorsal incisions are centered just medial to the second metatarsal and lateral to the fourth metatarsal shafts, maximizing the intervening skin bridge. The dorsal veins and the subcutaneous tissues are elevated laterally and medially to expose the respective interosseous musculature. Injury to the sensory nerves and extensor tendons is avoided. Caution should be used when making the incision between first and second metatarsal to avoid iatrogenic injury to the dorsalis pedis artery. The superficial fascia is incised longitudinally, and the interosseous

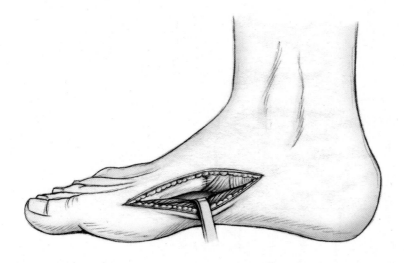

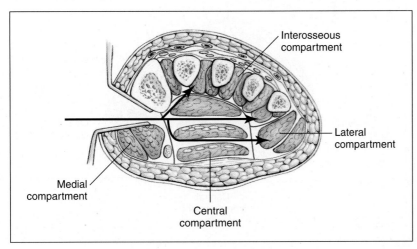

FIGURE 34-10

Medial approach for four-compartment release of foot compartment syndrome.

muscles are elevated off the metatarsals. The first dorsal and plantar interossei are stripped from the medial aspect of the second metatarsal shaft, which is then retracted medially, and the fascia of the central and medial compartment is released longitudinally deep within the inner space. The interosseous musculature is decompressed by releasing the fascia between the second and third metatarsals also through this medial incision. The lateral incision is used to decompress the interosseous muscles between the third and fourth, and fourth and fifth metatarsals, in addition to allowing access to release the central and lateral compartments (Fig. 34-11). More commonly, a separate medial incision as described previously is used to release the medial compartment, since the medial approach only to all four compartments carries an increased risk of damage to the neurovascular bundles in the plantar aspect of the foot.

Results

Controversy exists regarding the sequel of a missed compartment syndrome of the foot. Predominately, patients end up with clawing of the toes that needs to be corrected at a later date. The argument against the release is that it complicates the soft tissue envelope, limits possible incisions for reconstruction, and carries the risk of iatrogenic neurovascular injury.

Treatment of a foot compartment syndrome with "benign neglect" is not advised, and early decompression as in the thigh and leg is recommended. A delay in diagnosis is a potentially devastating occurrence. Early reduction of dislocations and some fractures facilitates reduction in edema in the foot and decreases tissue breakdown due to pressure necrosis. Desire to obtain an early reduction must be weighed heavily against whether the soft tissue envelope of the injured foot will tolerate additional

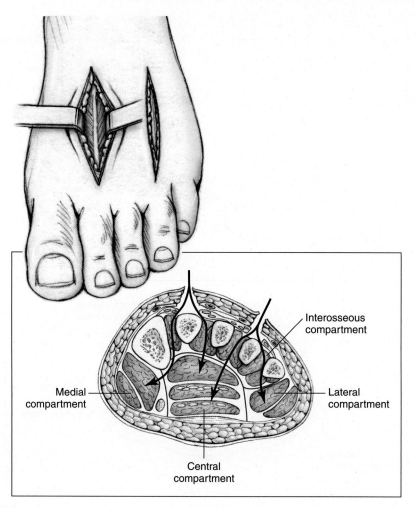

FIGURE 34-11

Dorsal approach for compartment release of foot compartment syndrome.

incisions. The fasciotomy incisions may be used to facilitate reduction and fracture fixation, but caution is warranted to avoid excessive undermining of the soft tissues. Delayed fixation is feasible, but usually not before 7 to 14 days postinjury, due to soft tissue edema. In addition, liberal use of external fixation, particularly in the setting of a mangled foot, is advised for stabilization and edema control.

POSTOPERATIVE MANAGEMENT

Postfasciotomy hyperbaric oxygen therapy is indicated as an adjunct to wound management if one or more of the following findings exist: massive swelling/prolonged ischemia, threatened skin flap or graft, ischemic muscle, residual neuropathy, unclear demarcation of viable and nonviable muscle, and/or markedly impaired host. The best results are obtained when therapy is started early after fasciotomy. Twice-daily treatments at 2.0 ata to 2.4 ata for 90 to 120 minutes for 7 to 10 days, with frequent examinations of the affected area, may be beneficial. This may be more practical in centers familiar with the use of hyperbaric oxygen therapy.

VAC devices have a number of advantages in the treatment of postfasciotomy wounds. They reduce interstitial edema, which improves local blood flow, and provide a one-way flow of bacteria-rich exudate from the wound, while preserving a moist environment for wound healing. Additionally, this therapy increases granulation tissue formation and may lead to an earlier ability to close or skin graft the wound.

Fasciotomy sites are dressed with a wound VAC sponge or wet to dry dressing changes with normal saline solution or silver sulfadiazine depending on the degree of contamination. Alternately, the addition of dilute sodium hypochlorite and boric acid (Dakin solution) may be used and can improve both odor and wound antisepsis. The patient is returned to the operating room several days later to attempt closure. When muscle necrosis ensues, the patient is brought to surgery earlier for debridement. Wound closure should not be performed until all necrotic tissue is debrided. Direct closure can be attempted when the wound approximates without tension. When the wound edges do not approximate easily, the wound is treated conservatively with either dressing changes or a VAC device. The patient is brought back to the operating room at a later date for definitive closure or skin grafting.

Many delayed primary closure techniques have been described. This process of using the skin's elasticity, mechanical and biological creep has been called dermatotraction and is performed in a staged fashion. Gradual approximation techniques may involve crisscrossing nylon sutures, stapling vessel loops in a shoelace manner along both sides of the fasciotomy wound, or the use of any of a variety of commercially available dynamic dermatotraction devices (Sure-Close [Life Medical Sciences, Princeton, NJ], Suture Tension Adjustment Reel [STAR, WoundTEK Inc., Newport, RI], Silver Bullet Wound Closure Device [SBWCD, Boehringer Laboratories, Norristown, PA], Wisebands [Wisebands Company Ltd, Ra'anana, Israel], Dermaclose [Wound Care Technologies Inc., Chanhassen, MN]) that use elastic bands or suture to controllably tension wounds. Case series using these techniques have successfully achieved delayed primary closure in 90% to 100% of cases. Dermatotraction can also be accomplished with the use of Ty-Raps, which are long enough to be applied loosely in the acute setting. They are subsequently tightened every 24 hours once the swelling has subsided. The Ty-Rap cable tie is made of a sturdy nylon tape that is strong enough to prevent secondary retraction of the wound edges, which makes this a preferable alternative over the stitching technique with monofilament sutures or the shoelace technique with Vessel loops.

COMPLICATIONS

Although a fasciotomy incision does result in patient morbidity, the incompletely released compartment, delayed diagnosis, or unrecognized compartment syndrome has substantially higher risks. Systemic complications including acute renal failure, sepsis, and acute respiratory distress syndrome (ARDS) have been reported in some cases. Rising serum creatinine kinase (CK; above 5,000 U/L) suggests risk of kidney injury. Renal failure may be prevented with aggressive administration of normal saline (beginning with 1 to 2 L/h) and should be continued until CK declines and urine is negative for myoglobin. Mannitol and bicarbonate are often used, but their utility is under debate. Most fatalities are due to prolonged intensive care admissions with sepsis and multisystem organ failure. If fasciotomy is done within 12 hours after the onset of compartment syndrome, the prognosis is typically good. Despite early intervention, approximately 1% to 10% of all cases of compartment syndrome develop Volkmann contracture. Little or no return of function can be expected when the diagnosis and treatment are delayed. In no instance was benefit from fasciotomy reported after 2 or 3 days. In cases in which the diagnosis of acute compartment syndrome is delayed or missed and the procedure is done late, severe infections have been shown to develop in the necrotic tissues of many patients, and much higher complication rates have been reported including a twofold increase in amputation rate and four-fold increase in mortality. In these situations, clinically evident by complete absence of demonstrable muscle function in any segment of the involved limb, the extremity should be splinted to maintain a functional position as muscle fibrosis and contracture develop.

PEARLS AND PITFALLS

- Compartment syndrome is a surgical emergency! Fasciotomies are limb saving.
- Check intracompartmental pressures at multiple levels within each compartment.
- Threshold for fasciotomy is intracompartmental pressure within 20 mm Hg of the diastolic blood pressure.
- Beware of compartment syndrome secondary to intraoperative positioning of uninjured extremities.
- Pulselessness in not a common finding in compartment syndrome unless a concurrent vascular injury exists.
- Compartment syndrome can occur with a late onset 2 to 4 days after the underlying event.
- For leg fasciotomies, the two-incision technique is preferable for easier access.
- For leg fasciotomies, ensure the deep posterior compartment is decompressed; this compartment is the first to develop compartment syndrome and the compartment most often missed during decompression.

ACKNOWLEDGMENTS

The authors express their gratitude to the Department of Orthopaedics at the University of Maryland Shock Trauma and the Surgery Audio Visual Department at Cooper University Hospital (Paul Rogers) for their assistance and efforts in the preparation of this chapter.

RECOMMENDED READING

Azar FM, Pickering RM. Traumatic disorders. In: Canale ST, ed. *Campbell's Operative Orthopaedics*. 10th ed. St. Louis, MO: Mosby; 2003:1405–1411.

Boody AR, Wongworawat MD. Accuracy in the measurement of compartment pressures: a comparison of three commonly used devices. *J Bone Joint Surg Am*. 2005;87:2415–2422.

Cohen MS, Garfin SR, Hargens AR, et al. Acute compartment syndrome: effect of dermotomy on fascial decompression in the leg. *J Bone Joint Surg Br*. 1991;73:287–290.

Finkelstein JA, Hunter GA, Hu RW. Lower limb compartment syndrome: course after delayed fasciotomy. *J Trauma*. 1996;40:342–344.

Fitzgerald AM, Gaston P, Wilson Y, et al. Long-term sequelae of fasciotomy wounds. *Br J Plast Surg*. 2000;53:690–693.

Garcia-Covarrubias L, McSwain NE Jr, Van Meter K, et al. Adjuvant hyperbaric oxygen therapy in the management of crush injury and traumatic ischemia: an evidence-based approach. *Am Surg*. 2005;71:144–151.

Goldsmith AL, McCallum MI. Compartment syndrome as a complication of the prolonged use of the Lloyd-Davies position. *Anaesthesia*. 1996;51:1048–1052.

Gulli B, Templeman D. Compartment syndrome of the lower extremity. *Orthop Clin North Am*. 1994;25:677–684.

Heckman MM, Whitesides TE Jr, Grewe SR, et al. Compartment pressure in association with closed tibial fractures: the relationship between tissue pressure, compartment, and the distance from the site of the fracture. *J Bone Joint Surg Am*. 1994;76:1285–1292.

McQueen MM, Court-Brown CM. Compartment monitoring in tibial fractures: the pressure threshold for decompression. *J Bone Joint Surg Br*. 1996;78:99–104.

McQueen MM, Gaston P, Court-Brown CM. Acute compartment syndrome: who is at risk? *J Bone Joint Surg Br*. 2000;82:200–203.

Meyer RS, White KK, Smith JM, et al. Intramuscular and blood pressures in legs positioned in the hemilithotomy position: clarification of risk factors for well-leg acute compartment syndrome. *J Bone Joint Surg Am*. 2002;84-A:1829–1835.

Myerson MM. Soft tissue trauma: acute and chronic management. In: Coughlin MJ, Mann RA, eds. *Surgery of the Foot and Ankle*. St. Louis, MO: Mosby; 1999:1340–1344.

Olson SA, Glasgow RR. Acute compartment syndrome in lower extremity musculoskeletal trauma. *J Am Acad Orthop Surg*. 2005;13:436–444.

Schwartz JT Jr, Brumback RJ, Lakatos R, et al. Acute compartment syndrome of the thigh: a spectrum of injury. *J Bone Joint Surg Am*. 1989;71:392–400.

Sheridan GW, Matsen FA III. Fasciotomy in the treatment of the acute compartment syndrome. *J Bone Joint Surg Am*. 1976;58:112–115.

Slater RR Jr, Weiner TM, Koruda MJ. Bilateral leg compartment syndrome complicating prolonged lithotomy position. *Orthopedics*. 1994;17:954–959.

Strecker WB, Wood MB, Bieber EJ. Compartment syndrome masked by epidural anesthesia for postoperative pain: report of a case. *J Bone Joint Surg Am*. 1986;68:1447–1448.

Templeman D, Lange R, Harms B. Lower-extremity compartment syndromes associated with use of pneumatic antishock garments. *J Trauma*. 1987;27:79–81.

Wiger P, Tkaczuk P, Styf J. Secondary wound closure following fasciotomy for acute compartment syndrome increases intramuscular pressure. *J Orthop Trauma*. 1998;12:117–121.

35 Amputation and Stump Management

Norman S. Turner and Thomas C. Shives

INDICATIONS/CONTRADICTIONS

Amputation is one of the oldest surgical procedures. Early amputations consisted of severing the extremity, and hemostasis was obtained by dipping the stump in hot oil. Techniques have dramatically improved, and most of the advances have occurred during war time. Prosthetic technology now allows for amputees to run, jump, ski, swim, and be involved in competitive sports.

The indications for above- and below-knee amputation include life-threatening infections, malignant tumors, burns, extensive frostbite, congenital anomalies, ischemic pain, osteomyelitis, extensive trauma (including a tibial nerve laceration or unreconstructable vascular injury), and chronic pain. The most common indications for a below- or above-knee amputation are complications of diabetes. Functionally, the patients with below-knee amputation are able to walk with prosthesis, with most patients walking within 3 months after surgery. Amputation should not be viewed as a limb salvage failure but as a reconstructive procedure to improve function.

There are few contraindications to amputations; however, a contraindication to a below-knee amputation is a nonambulatory patient. A nonambulating patient with a below-knee amputation is at high risk for flexion contracture, which can result in increased pressure on the stump and cause ulceration. Therefore, when a patient is wheelchair bound and is not a candidate for prosthetic fitting, an above-knee amputation should be considered.

PREOPERATIVE PLANNING

It is imperative that these patients be evaluated preoperatively to determine the vascular status of the limb. Most patients undergoing a below- or above-knee amputation have diabetes and have some component of peripheral vascular disease. Preoperative noninvasive vascular studies, including ankle-brachial indexes (ABIs), are important to determine the level of amputation. An ABI is determined by measuring the ankle systolic pressure and dividing it by the brachial systolic pressure using Doppler detection of the pulses. The severity of the arterial disease is related to decreased value of the ABI, and a value of less than 0.5 is considered abnormal in people with diabetes. Also, noninvasive vascular studies using transcutaneous oxygen tension measurement ($TcPO_2$) are useful in assisting with amputation levels. Amputations are likely to heal if the $TcPO_2$ measurements are greater than 40 mm Hg. Patients with $TcPO_2$ values below 20 mm Hg are at higher risk for not healing and should be evaluated with further vascular testing and possibly an angiogram before surgical intervention. A vascular surgery consult is almost always indicated before performing an amputation. With the advances in distal bypass surgery and invasive radiologic procedures, certain patients can be successfully treated with limb salvage after vascular reconstruction.

Imaging studies are important in determining the underlying pathology. Imaging of the tibia or femur is important if there is a question regarding extension of tumor or infection into the tissues or bone adjacent to the intended level of amputation or if there is a prosthetic device such as a total knee arthroplasty or internal fixation device in place, which may alter the surgical procedure.

If amputation is contemplated, optimizing the patient's medical condition before surgery is recommended. Literature has shown that patients with a serum albumin less than 3.5 g/dL or true lymphocyte count less than 1,500 cells per mL are at high risk for wound healing difficulties. Patients with diabetes undergoing elective amputation should be evaluated by their medical team with the goal of a hemoglobin A1C less than 7.0.

Determination of the amputation level is important for both healing and function. The more distal the amputation level, the less energy required to ambulate. In elderly patients, a more proximal amputation may not allow for ambulation secondary to energy requirements. If a patient has good cognitive function, balance, and strength, then the most distal level with a realistic chance of healing should be attempted.

SURGERY

For a below-knee amputation to be performed correctly, proper attention to detail is important to improve the quality of the result. Gentle handling of the soft tissues, especially in diabetic patients, is important to minimize wound complications. The level of the amputation is determined by the extent of the infection, tumor, or the level that would provide optimal function with prosthesis. In general, the patient is positioned in the supine position for above- or below-knee amputations.

Full-thickness flaps should be used to minimize skin edge necrosis. Meticulous hemostasis and use of a drain is imperative to decrease the risk of a hematoma. The nerves should be divided sharply under tension to minimize the risk of a symptomatic neuroma. Also, the bone ends are rasped until smooth to prevent bony prominences.

An open amputation is performed in patients with grossly contaminated wounds or in patients with extensive infection. These patients will require further surgeries to optimize the soft tissues around the stump, and then, a definitive closure can be performed once this is accomplished.

Below-Knee Amputation

Below-knee amputation is the most commonly performed lower extremity amputation. A long posterior flap is used and brought anteriorly to cover the distal stump of the tibia, which should be 8.5 to 12.5 cm in length. The flaps, if planned properly, will have minimal redundant skin in the corners, or "dog ears." This will provide a good prosthetic fit.

Patient Positioning

The patient is placed supine on the operating room table. A nonsterile tourniquet is used and the leg is prepared and draped in the usual fashion.

Technique

A skin marker is used to plan the flaps (Fig. 35-1), and the flaps are drawn so that the posterior flap begins two-thirds of the way posterior to the anterior aspect of the tibia and then extends distally and posteriorly so that the distance will be long enough to cover the tibia (Fig. 35-2). A tourniquet can be used at the discretion of the surgeon. The incision is then made through the skin and subcutaneous tissues down to the fascia. The subcutaneous nerves including the saphenous and sural nerve can be identified and divided under tension. The fascia is then incised. The anterior compartment musculature is cut with a cautery (Fig. 35-3) down to the deep peroneal nerve, which is identified and cut under tension (Fig. 35-4), and the anterior tibial artery is identified and tied with silk suture (Fig. 35-5). The superficial peroneal nerve is identified and cut under tension.

The periosteum is reflected off the tibia (Fig. 35-6), and the tibia is cut 1 cm proximal from the skin incision (Fig. 35-7). A segment of the fibula is then resected 1 cm proximal to the tibial bone cut (Figs. 35-8 to 35-10). Traction is applied, and an amputation knife is used to perform the remaining portion of the amputation (Fig. 35-11). Dissection is carried deep until blood from the posterior tibial artery and vein is identified, and then, the cut is beveled distally until the fascia is cut (Fig. 35-12).

The anterior aspect of the tibia is beveled (Fig. 35-13). The remaining edges are rasped until smooth. The tibial nerve is identified and transected under traction (Fig. 35-14). The tibial artery and vein are identified and tied with silk sutures (Fig. 35-15). The wound is then copiously irrigated.

If a tourniquet is used, it is deflated at this time. Hemostasis is obtained. The wound is then closed in layers over a drain with sutures in the fascia (Fig. 35-16). The subcutaneous layer is closed with monofilament suture, and the skin is then closed with nylon sutures in a vertical mattress fashion (Fig. 35-17). A sterile dressing is applied, and then, a compressive Robert Jones dressing is applied with plaster in full extension (Fig. 35-18).

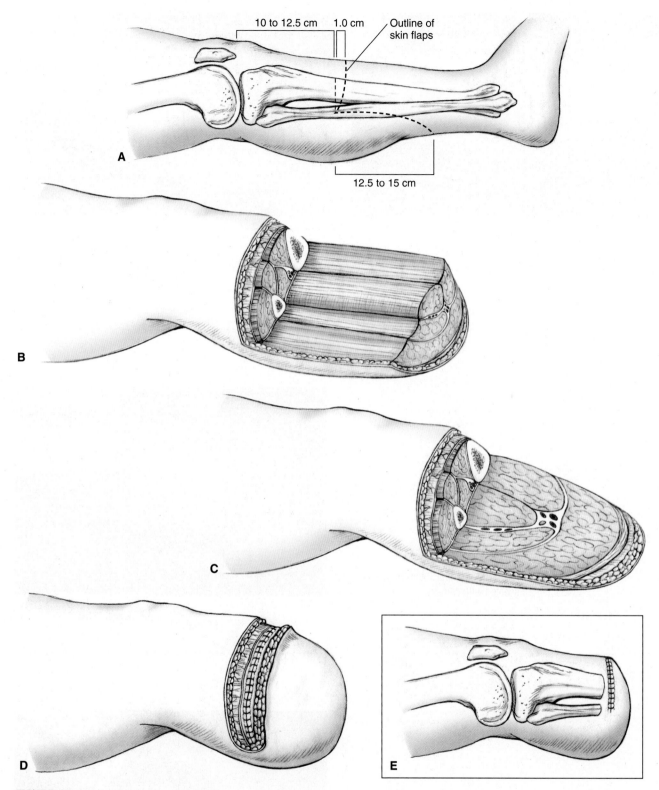

FIGURE 35-1

Below-knee amputation. **A:** Planning of short anterior and long posterior skin flaps. **B:** Amputation of the distal leg. **C:** Tailoring of posterior muscle to form flaps. **D:** Closure of flap to deep fascia. **E:** Closure of skin flaps. (Redrawn after Burgess EM, Zettl JH. Amputations below the knee. *Artif Limbs.* 1969;13:1.)

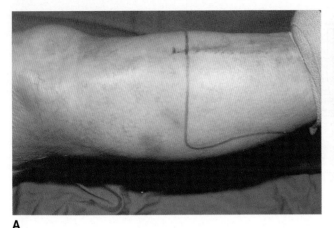

A   **B**

FIGURE 35-2

A and B: The long posterior flap is planned.

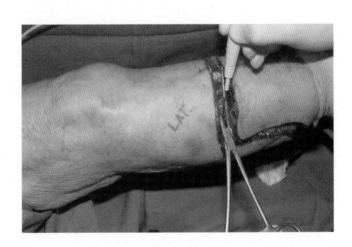

FIGURE 35-3

The anterior compartment muscle is dissected with cautery.

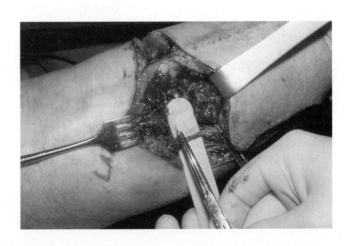

FIGURE 35-4

The deep peroneal nerve is identified and sharply transected.

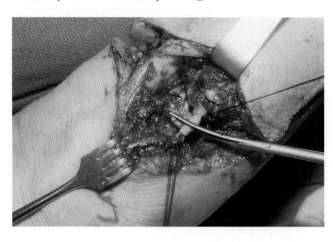

FIGURE 35-5
The anterior tibial artery and vein are ligated.

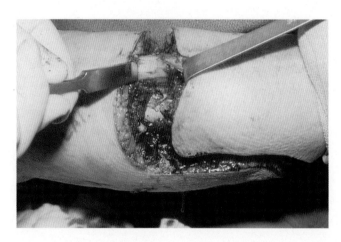

FIGURE 35-6
The periosteum is reflected off the tibia.

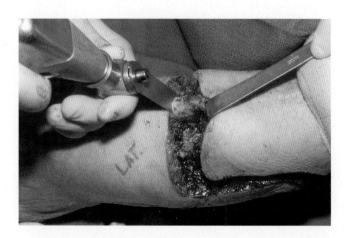

FIGURE 35-7
The tibia is osteotomized 1 cm proximal to skin incision.

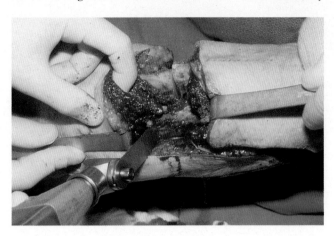

FIGURE 35-8

The fibula is identified and osteotomized 1 cm proximal to tibia osteotomy.

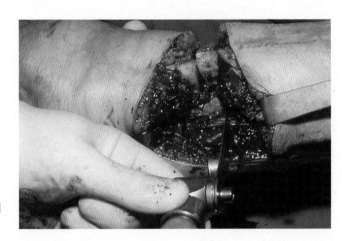

FIGURE 35-9

A second fibula osteotomy is performed 2 to 3 cm distal.

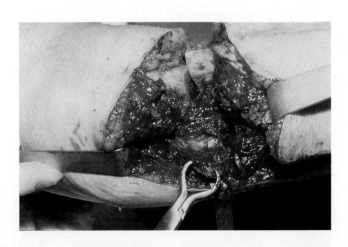

FIGURE 35-10

The segment of the fibula is removed.

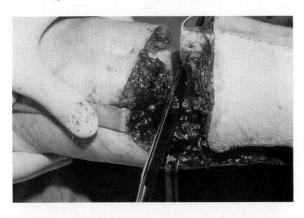

FIGURE 35-11

The amputation knife is used to sharply dissect the posterior compartment muscle.

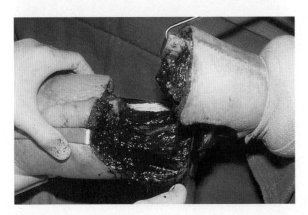

FIGURE 35-12

The posterior compartment muscle is beveled to minimize bulk.

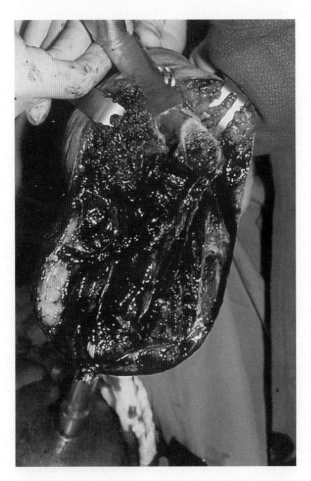

FIGURE 35-13

The saw is used to bevel the anterior tibia.

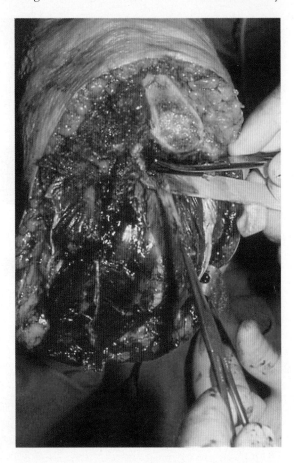

FIGURE 35-14
The tibial nerve is identified and sharply removed.

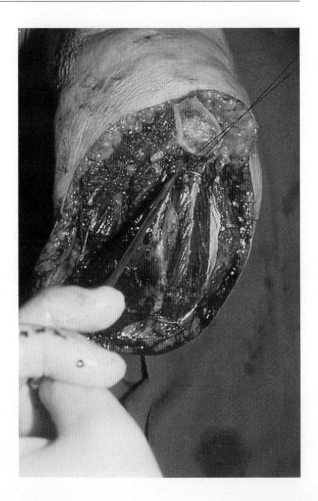

FIGURE 35-15
The tibial artery and vein are ligated.

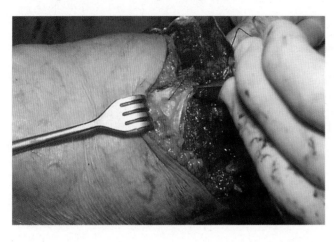

FIGURE 35-16

The fascia is closed with interrupted suture.

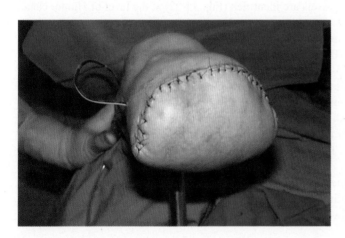

FIGURE 35-17

The skin is closed with interrupted vertical mattress suture.

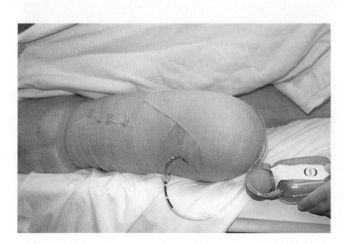

FIGURE 35-18

A compressive bulky dressing with plaster is applied with the knee in full extension.

Above-Knee Amputation

Above-knee amputation is the second most frequently performed lower extremity amputation. Stump length is important for the lever arm control of the prosthesis. Too long of a femoral stump, however, can lead to difficulty with fitting the prosthetic knee joint. Therefore, the bone cut should be 10 to 12 cm proximal to distal femoral articular surface.

For nonambulatory patients with ischemic disease, above-knee amputations are performed with equal anterior and posterior flaps, and myodesis is not performed to prevent further vascular compromise. For patients with adequate vascular supply and the potential to ambulate, a myodesis is performed.

Patient Positioning

Above-knee amputation is performed with the patient in a supine position. A sterile tourniquet can be used at the discretion of the surgeon.

Technique

Skin flaps are marked with a long medial flap and a shorter lateral flap (Fig. 35-19). Dissection is carried through the skin and subcutaneous tissues and down to the muscle. The muscles are then identified. The quadriceps is detached proximal to the patella, retaining some of its tendinous portion (Fig. 35-20). The vastus medialis is reflected off of the intermuscular septum, and the adductor magnus (Fig. 35-21) is detached from the adductor tubercle by sharp dissection and reflected medially, exposing the femoral shaft. The vessels are identified (Fig. 35-22) at the level of Hunter canal, and the artery and vein are ligated.

The femur is then exposed proximally 12 to 14 cm above the condylar level and is cut with an oscillating saw approximately 10 to 12 cm above the joint line. The remaining edges are smoothed with a saw or rasp (Fig. 35-23). Small drill holes through the remaining distal femoral cortex are made with a 2.5-mm drill (Fig. 35-24). The adductor magnus tendon is then sutured with nonabsorbable suture to the lateral femur through the drill holes (Fig. 35-25). The femur is held in maximum adduction while this is being sutured to the bone as a myodesis (Fig. 35-26). The quadriceps is then brought over the bone and anchored to the posterior aspect of the femur through the drill holes (Fig. 35-27). The hip is in extension when this is done to try to minimize hip flexion.

The fascia lata is then sutured to the medial fascia. Subcutaneous tissue is closed with monofilament suture, and the skin is closed with nylon suture (Fig. 35-28). Sterile dressing is applied, as well as a compressive wrap to minimize swelling.

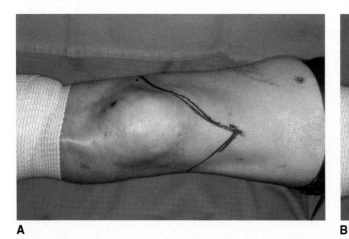
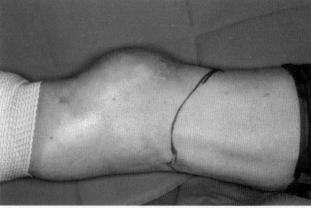

A   **B**

FIGURE 35-19

Skin flaps are marked with a long medial **(A)** and shorter lateral **(B)** flap.

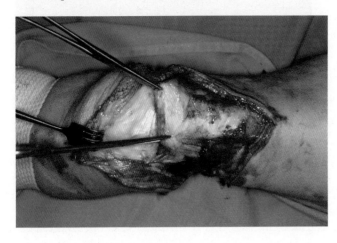

FIGURE 35-20

The quadriceps muscle is detached proximally to the patella, preserving some of the tendinous insertion.

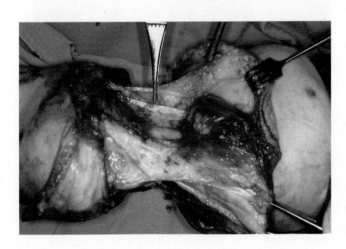

FIGURE 35-21

The adductor magnus is identified and reflected off the femur.

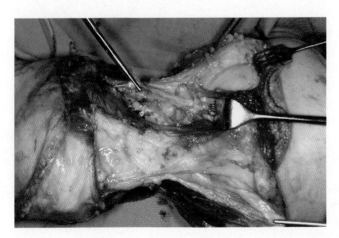

FIGURE 35-22

The femoral vessels at the level of Hunter canal are identified and ligated.

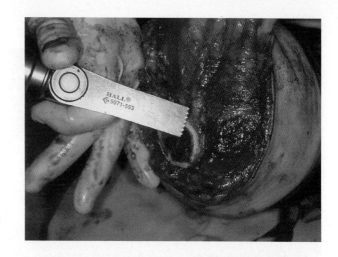

FIGURE 35-23

The femur is osteotomized, and the end is rasped until smooth.

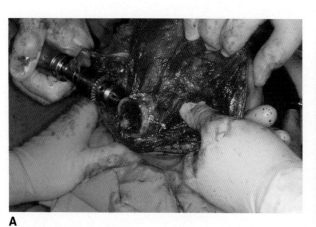

A

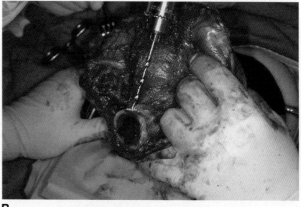

B

FIGURE 35-24

A and B: Four drill holes are made in the femoral stump for the myodesis.

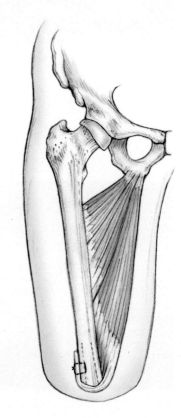

FIGURE 35-25

Attachment of adductor magnus to the lateral femur. (Redrawn from Gottschalk F. Transfemoral amputations. In: Bowker JH, Michael JW, eds. *Atlas of Limb Prosthetics: Surgical, Prosthetic, and Rehabilitation Principles.* 2nd ed. St. Louis, MO: Mosby; 1992.)

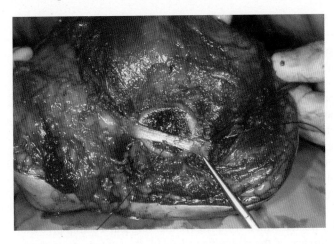

FIGURE 35-26

The adductor magnus tendon is sutured to the femur through the drill holes.

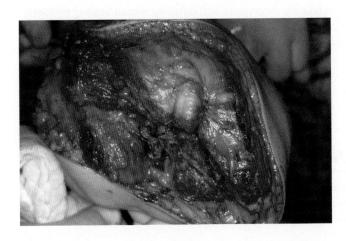

FIGURE 35-27

The quadriceps tendon is brought over the femoral stump and sutured through the drill holes.

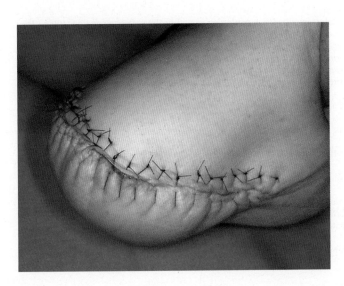

FIGURE 35-28

The skin is closed with interrupted vertical mattress suture.

POSTOPERATIVE MANAGEMENT

For both below- and above-knee amputation, a compressive dressing is used to minimize swelling. The patient is kept in bed for 24 hours. The suction drain is kept in for at least 24 hours or until the drainage has decreased to minimal output. For a below-knee amputation, a compressive Robert Jones dressing is removed approximately 48 hours after the surgery. If the swelling is well controlled and the wounds are in good condition, a pilon cast can be applied with a temporary prosthetic foot. The patient is restricted to minimal weight bearing but is allowed to be up and ambulating with gait aids. The pilon cast is removed at 2 weeks after surgery and another one can be placed. At 4 weeks after surgery, the pilon cast is removed completely. Sutures are removed at 2 to 4 weeks depending on the healing of the wound. A stump protector is used between 4 and 6 weeks. Shrinker socks are used to shrink the stump, and once the stump volumes have stabilized, a permanent prosthesis can be fitted.

Above-knee amputations are initially treated with a compressive dressing and a stump protector. At approximately 2 to 3 weeks after surgery, if the wounds are healed, the sutures are removed. These patients also use shrinker socks as well as a protector. Once their stump volume has stabilized, they can be fitted for their prosthesis.

COMPLICATIONS/RESULTS

The most common complications of amputation surgery are soft tissue or wound healing problems. These can lead to superficial infections that can ultimately cause deep infection and possibly progress to osteomyelitis. Such complications may result in more proximal amputations.

The treatment of wound complication initially begins with dressing changes, and frequently, these patients will heal with local wound care. Occasionally, a vacuum-assisted closure device can be helpful in increasing the granulation tissue to improve the healing in a more timely fashion. Long-term complications include difficulty with prosthetic fitting, which usually can be managed by an experienced prosthetist.

PEARLS AND PITFALLS

- Vascular workup prior to amputation to optimize level of amputation and improve healing.
- Optimize patients medically prior to surgery to minimize complications.
- Develop full-thickness flaps to preserve blood flow.
- Meticulous soft tissue handling.
  - Use a drain to minimize hematomas.
  - Close with suture and make sure the skin edges are well approximated.
- Involve the prosthetist early to assist with getting patients into prosthesis when stump is ready.

RECOMMENDED READING

Dickhaut SC, DeLee JC, Page CP. Nutritional status: importance in predicting wound-healing after amputation. *J Bone Joint Surg*. 1984;66A:71.

Gottschalk F. Transfemoral amputation: surgical procedures. In: Bowker JH, Michael JW, eds. *Atlas of Limb Prosthetics: Surgical, Prosthetic, and Rehabilitation Principles*. 2nd ed. St. Louis, MO: Mosby; 1992.

Gottschalk F. Transfemoral amputation: biomechanics and surgery. *Clin Orthop*. 1999;361:15.

Harris IE, Leff AR, Gitelis S, et al. Function after amputation, arthrodesis, or arthroplasty for tumors about the knee. *J Bone Joint Surg*. 1990;72A:1477.

Heck RK Jr, Carnesale PG. General principles of amputations. In: Canale ST, ed. *Campbell's Operative Orthopaedics*. 10th ed. St. Louis, MO: Mosby; 2003.

Morris CD, Potter BK, Athanasian EA, et al. Extremity amputations: principles, techniques and recent advances. *Instr Course Lect*. 2015;64:105–117.

Pinzur MS. Amputations and prosthetics. In: Beaty JH, ed. *Orthopaedic Knowledge Update 6*. Rosemont, IL: American Academy of Orthopaedic Surgeons, 1999.

Pinzur MS, Bowker JH, Smith DG, et al. Amputation surgery in peripheral vascular disease. *AAOS Instr Course Lect*. 1999;48:687.

Pinzur MS, Gottschalk F, Smith D, et al. Functional outcome of below-knee amputation in peripheral vascular insufficiency: a multicenter review. *Clin Orthop*. 1993;286:247.

Smith DG, Ehde DM, Legro MW, et al. Phantom limb, residual limb, and back pain after lower extremity amputations. *Clin Orthop*. 1999;361:29.

Smith DG, Fergason JR. Transtibial amputations. *Clin Orthop*. 1999;361:108.

Terrell DB. Above-knee amputation. In: Wiesel SW, ed. *Operative Techniques in Orthopaedic Surgery*. Vol. 2. Philadelphia, PA: Lippincott Williams & Wilkins; 2011:2060–2066.

Terrell DB. Below-knee amputation. In: Wiesel SW, ed. *Operative Techniques in Orthopaedic Surgery*. Vol. 2. Philadelphia, PA: Lippincott Williams & Wilkins; 2011:2067–2071.

Waters RL, Perry J, Antonelli D, et al. Energy cost of walking amputees: the influence of level of amputation. *J Bone Joint Surg*. 1976;58A:42.

Wyss CR, Harrington RM, Burgess EM, et al. Transcutaneous oxygen tension as a predictor of success after an amputation. *J Bone Joint Surg*. 1988;70A:203.

PART VI
SOFT TISSUE MANAGEMENT AROUND THE FOOT AND ANKLE

36 Soft Tissue Management of Ankle Fractures and Use of the Gracilis Muscle Flap

S. Andrew Sems and Steven L. Moran

Soft tissue management of injuries around the distal tibia and ankle region will often dictate and drive the timing and methods of definitive fixation. Injuries in this region vary from low-energy ankle fractures to high-energy tibial pilon fractures. The soft tissue injuries often reflect the amount of energy that was involved in creating the bony injury. Regardless of the radiographic appearance of the fractures, certain initial treatment principles hold true for both low- and high-energy injuries, and these include early fracture reduction in combination with adequate soft tissue coverage. Early fracture reduction will restore limb alignment, rotation, and appropriate limb length. Reliable soft tissue coverage allows the surgeon to utilize internal fixation to provide fracture immobilization that will allow for a more rapid resolution of soft tissue swelling and impairment.

ANKLE FRACTURES

Indications/Contraindications

Operative treatment is generally recommended for all unstable ankle fractures in which the talus is unable to be maintained in a position beneath the tibial plafond by closed reduction. Nonoperative management is appropriate for stable ankle fractures where there is no lateral subluxation of the talus within the ankle mortise.

Comorbidities

Open reduction and internal fixation can generally be safely performed on most patients regardless of associated comorbidities. In patients with severe peripheral vascular disease, preoperative transcutaneous pressure oximetry measurements should be obtained to assess the likelihood of the patient healing the surgical wounds. TcPO$_2$ below 30 mm Hg is associated with a higher risk of wound failure and fracture nonunion. Involving vascular medicine professionals to assist with maximizing lower-extremity perfusion is reasonable if vascular disease is a concern. The implications of insulin-dependent diabetes mellitus and peripheral neuropathy should also be considered when determining operative versus nonoperative treatment but are not contraindications to surgery. Postoperative soft tissue management should be modified in patients with high risks of developing wound complications. Longer periods of cast immobilization and protected weight bearing may be indicated for patients with these comorbidities.

Nonoperative management of fractures in the nonambulatory patient is reasonable provided the fracture does not cause deformity that would result in subsequent skin breakdown. Modified techniques of internal fixation in patients who are nonambulatory may be utilized in order to maintain the anatomy around the ankle joint to prevent soft tissue compromise.

Preoperative Planning

Plain radiographs should be obtained in all patients with unstable ankle fractures prior to surgical intervention. Anteroposterior (AP), mortise, and lateral views are necessary to assess the fracture orientation. Ankle fractures tend to include the medial malleolus, lateral malleolus, and, occasionally, the posterior malleolus. Recognition of the three-dimensional plane in which each fracture occurs is important so that surgical incisions are placed appropriately and the correct internal fixation is selected. While computed tomography is used more often for pilon-type tibial fractures, it may be used if there is not a clear understanding of the fracture pattern.

Surgical approach selection for treatment of ankle fractures depends on the location of the fractures and the quality of the surrounding tissues. Fractures of the medial malleolus are typically approached with an anteromedial incision overlying the medial malleolus. This incision can be adjusted anteriorly or posteriorly depending on the size and orientation of the medial malleolar fragment. Fractures that include both the anterior and posterior caliculus may require slight posterior adjustment of the incision, while fractures that only involve the anterior caliculus may be approached through a more anteromedial incision. Fibular fractures are typically treated with a direct lateral approach, although a posterolateral approach is useful for fibula fractures that occur in the coronal plane or in cases of associated posterior malleolus fragments that may be addressed through this same incision.

The timing of surgery is dictated by the state of the soft tissue envelope. For ankle fractures, immediate fixation within the first 24 to 48 hours is feasible so long as the swelling will not compromise wound healing. Patients who present to the clinic or emergency department with ankle fractures within 48 hours from injury can often be treated with immediate open reduction and internal fixation prior to the onset of the maximal amount of soft tissue swelling. Surgery should be delayed when soft issue is so edematous that the surgeon is unable to create skin wrinkles by gently pinching the skin over both the medial and lateral malleolus. Open fractures require immediate surgical intervention for debridement of all contaminated soft tissues. Antibiotic cement bead pouches or vacuum-assisted closure (VAC) devices may be used until definitive fixation or final wound closure. External fixation may be necessary to restore length, alignment, and rotation of both the soft tissues and the bone prior to definitive internal fixation.

Ankle fractures should ideally be treated within 3 weeks of injury, before early callus formation, which can create significant difficulty in fracture reduction. Patients who present in the first week following an ankle fracture and whose soft tissues are not amenable to immediate surgical fixation should be treated with a Robert Jones–type compressive dressing with plaster immobilization. These patients should be encouraged to maintain strict elevation of their limb at all times. They are then seen back in the clinic or preoperative area approximately 7 to 10 days after their injury for soft tissue evaluation prior to surgical intervention. This dressing should be taken down, and the skin should be evaluated prior to any type of anesthetic administration. In patients who are admitted to the hospital, sequential compression boots can be applied to the foot prior to the application of the Robert Jones dressing. These pneumatic boots are usually well tolerated so long as they do not extend up past the ankle.

SURGERY

Medial/Lateral Approaches

Patient Positioning

The patient is positioned supine on a radiolucent table with a thigh-high pneumatic tourniquet and a small bump (towel) placed under the ipsilateral hip to prevent excessive external rotation of the limb. The bump placed underneath the hip area should be adjusted so that the foot points vertically when in its resting position. A foam block or bump of towels can be utilized underneath the leg and ankle area so as to elevate the operative limb from the nonoperative limb. This facilitates obtaining lateral radiographs without manipulation of the operative leg. The intraoperative fluoroscopy unit is brought in from the contralateral side, and it is positioned perpendicular to the long axis of the patient.

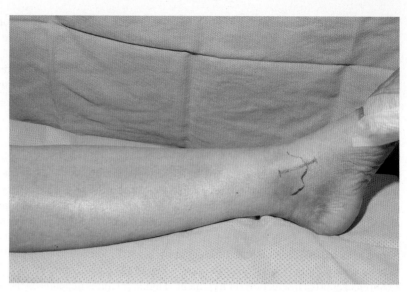

FIGURE 36-1

The incision is made along the midlateral axis of the distal tibia, curving anteriorly beyond the tip of the medial malleolus.

Prophylactic antibiotics are utilized for internal fixation of ankle fractures. They should be administered prior to inflation of the tourniquet. Once the tourniquet is inflated, it should be maintained as long as necessary, but not for more than 2 hours. If it is impossible to complete the procedure in the allotted 2 hours, the tourniquet should be deflated and hemostasis should be obtained, and the procedure should be completed without the aid of a tourniquet. If small vessel bleeding continues to be an issue, consider moving the operative bed into a Trendelenburg position and asking the anesthesiologist to decrease the systolic blood pressure within safe limits.

Technique

ANATOMIC LANDMARKS FOR MEDIAL APPROACH. Palpate the medial malleolus to define the location of the anterior aspect of the anterior caliculus, the posterior aspect of the posterior caliculus, as well as the fracture location. The leg should be palpated to determine the longitudinal axis of the tibia.

INCISION AND SURGICAL APPROACH. The incision is made along the midlateral axis of the distal tibia. Beyond the tip of the medial malleolus, the incision may be slightly curved anteriorly (Fig. 36-1). Be aware that excessive curvature of the incision may create difficulties in placing internal fixation in the medial malleolar fragment. Dissection should be carried through the skin and subcutaneous and hemostasis obtained as this is performed (Fig. 36-2). Care should be taken to preserve and protect the saphenous vein and nerve throughout the case. In this location, the saphenous vein is often very subcutaneous, and an aggressive skin incision may lacerate the vein. With the saphenous vein and nerve protected, the medial malleolar fragment can be retracted distally with sharp bone hooks to allow inspection of the ankle joint (Fig. 36-3). A no. 15 blade, used to elevate the periosteum along the fracture edges, can be utilized to ensure that the fracture is reduced in an anatomic position. Preservation of the soft tissue and minimal periosteal stripping is recommended. Following internal

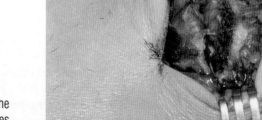

FIGURE 36-2

Exposure of the medial malleolar fracture line prior to elevation of the periosteum along the fracture edges.

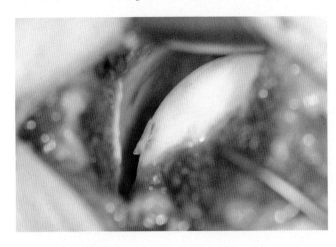

FIGURE 36-3
Retraction of the medial malleolus allows exposure of the talus and ankle joint.

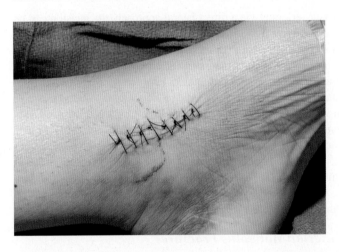

FIGURE 36-4
Skin closure is performed using a nonabsorbable monofilament suture.

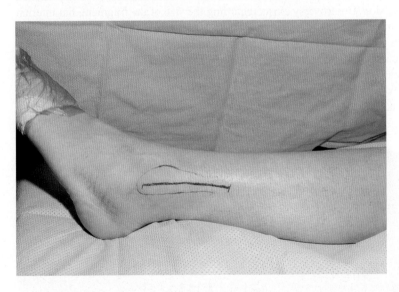

FIGURE 36-5
The incision is positioned in line with the longitudinal axis of the fibula, curving anteriorly at the distal end to allow access for reduction of a Chaput-Tillaux fragment.

fixation, the subcutaneous tissue can be closed using a 2-0 absorbable suture, and the skin closed with a nonabsorbable monofilament suture (Fig. 36-4).

Lateral Approach for Lateral Malleolar Fixation

The direct lateral approach to the fibula allows placement of fixation along the lateral aspect of the fibula. This incision is positioned in line with the longitudinal axis of the fibula and may be curved anterior distally to allow access for reduction of a Chaput-Tillaux fragment (Fig. 36-5). If plate fixation along the posterior aspect of the fibula is desired, such as in a situation when an antiglide plate is used,

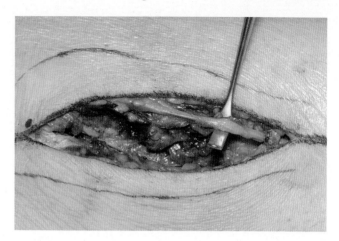

FIGURE 36-6

The superficial peroneal nerve may cross the incision, and care should be taken to identify and protect this structure.

rather than committing excessive soft tissue stripping via a direct lateral approach, the incision can be adjusted posteriorly. The superficial peroneal nerve may cross the surgical approach in a subcutaneous location; therefore, the skin incision should go no deeper than the skin (Fig. 36-6). Dissection through the subcutaneous tissues should be performed using combinations of sharp and blunt dissection with care to identify and protect the superficial peroneal nerve if encountered. Periosteal elevation at the fracture edges with a no. 15 blade is recommended to ensure an anatomic reduction of the fibular fracture.

For long spiral oblique fractures in which lag screw only fixation of the fibula is to be used, this incision can be altered with an apex anterior curve along the midportion of the incision. This "wave" in the incision will allow anterior retraction of the soft tissues and appropriate directional placement of lag screws across the fracture site. The same concerns remain with regard to protection of the superficial peroneal nerve when this modification is performed.

Following internal fixation, closure is performed with interrupted 2-0 absorbable sutures in the subcutaneous tissue followed by nonabsorbable monofilament sutures in the skin (Fig. 36-7).

Posterolateral Approach for Posterior Malleolus Fractures

PATIENT POSITIONING. Fractures that require fixation of the posterior malleolus can be approached through a posterolateral incision. Controversy exists regarding the size of the fragment, but internal fixation is typically recommended for fractures that include 20% to 30% of the articular surface. This approach requires the patient to be in either a lateral or prone position (Fig. 36-8). The prone position allows direct visualization and better stabilization of the limb during the approach and is therefore preferred. The patient should be placed on a well-padded radiolucent table with care to be taken to prevent hyperextension of the shoulders and neck. If the arms are placed in an abducted position, care should be taken to avoid direct compression of the ulnar nerve at the cubital tunnel.

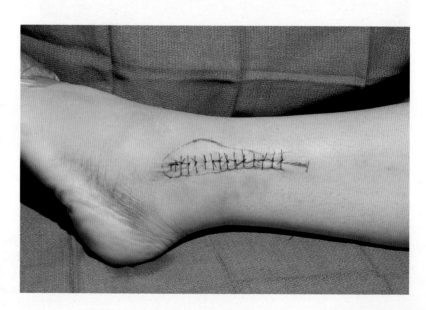

FIGURE 36-7

Skin closure is performed using a nonabsorbable monofilament suture.

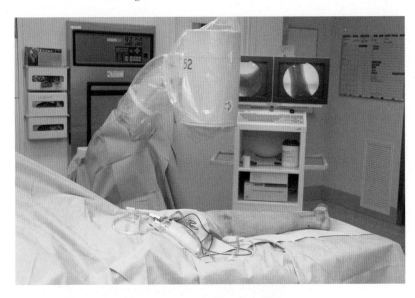

A thigh-high tourniquet is used and can be placed prior to prone positioning. Once the patient is in the prone position, they are translated toward the foot of the bed so that the hindfoot is slightly hanging off the end of the bed to aid with reduction and fixation. The C-arm fluoroscopy unit is placed perpendicular to the longitudinal axis of the patient, and intraoperative films can be used on the patient's uninjured side to guarantee symmetry following reduction.

TECHNIQUE. Palpation of the fibula and Achilles tendon is possible due to the subcutaneous location of these structures. The incision is made midway between the posterior border of the lateral malleolus and the lateral border of the Achilles tendon and will need to extend to the tip of the fibula distally and as far proximally as necessary to obtain visualization of the fibular fracture and the posterior malleolar fracture (Fig. 36-9). The short saphenous vein and sural nerve are located immediately

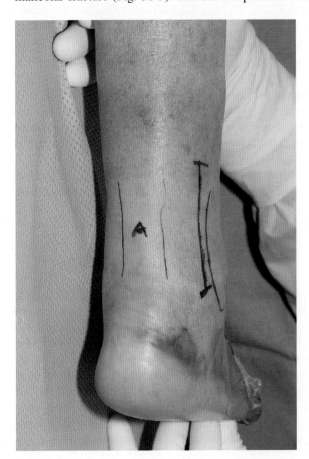

FIGURE 36-9

The incision is made midway between the posterior border of the lateral malleolus and the lateral border of the Achilles tendon.

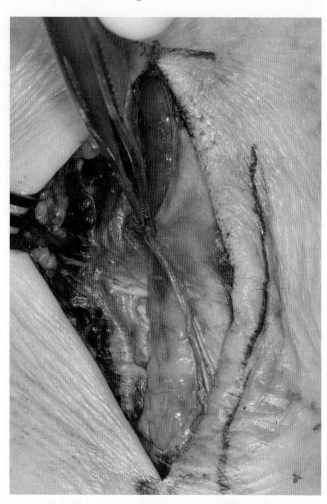

FIGURE 36-10

The deep fascia of the leg is split in line with the incision, and the peroneal retinaculum is incised to release the peroneus longus and brevis.

behind the lateral malleolus, and the incision is placed posterior and medial to these structures. The deep fascia of the leg is split in line with the incision, and the peroneal retinaculum is incised to release the peroneus longus and brevis (Fig. 36-10). The peroneal tendons and muscles are retracted laterally, and the flexor hallucis longus is elevated from its origin on the fibula and retracted medially (Fig. 36-11). This allows access to the posterior aspect of the tibia for reduction and fixation (Fig. 36-12). The peroneal tendons are retracted medial or lateral depending on the location of the fracture. For fibular fractures, which require a more proximal exposure, dissection to the lateral aspect of the peroneal tendons and muscles is necessary.

Following internal fixation of the posterior malleolus fragment and/or lateral malleolar fracture through the posterolateral approach, the peroneal retinaculum is repaired using a 2-0 absorbable suture (Fig. 36-13). If possible, the deep fascia of the leg is also reapproximated using the same absorbable suture. Subcutaneous tissues are closed with a 2-0 absorbable suture, and the skin is closed in interrupted fashion using a 3-0 or 4-0 nylon suture (Fig. 36-14).

Postoperative Management

Following internal fixation, the patient is placed in a well-padded Robert Jones splint to provide further postoperative immobilization (Fig. 36-15). The splint is applied with the knee flexed to allow dorsiflexion of the ankle to a neutral position and avoidance of equinus positioning. This splint is maintained for the first 10 days to allow for postoperative swelling. The patient is then converted to either a short-leg cast or a fracture boot following this initial Robert Jones dressing. The sutures are removed 2 to 3 weeks from the date of surgery; however, they should remain in place if there is any concern of delayed wound healing. Weight-bearing restrictions are tailored to the individual fracture pattern and in patients with excellent bony quality, and excellent healing potential weightbearing may be started at 6 weeks. In patients with multiple comorbidities, poor bone quality, or concerns for delayed fracture healing, weightbearing may be limited for up to 3 months postoperatively.

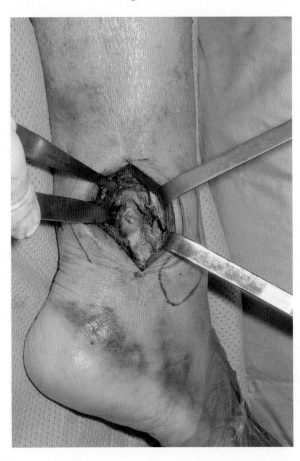

FIGURE 36-11

The peroneal tendons and muscles are retracted laterally, and the flexor hallucis longus is elevated from its origin on the fibula and retracted medially.

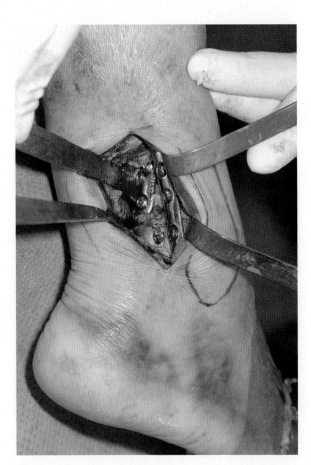

FIGURE 36-12

Following exposure, the reduction and fixation of the posterior malleolar fragment may be completed.

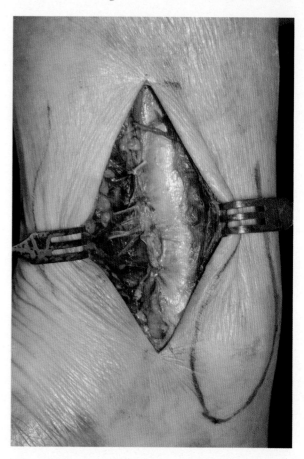

FIGURE 36-13

The peroneal retinaculum is repaired using an absorbable suture.

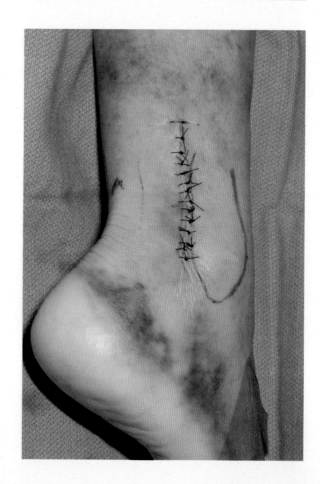

FIGURE 36-14

The skin is closed using a nonabsorbable monofilament suture.

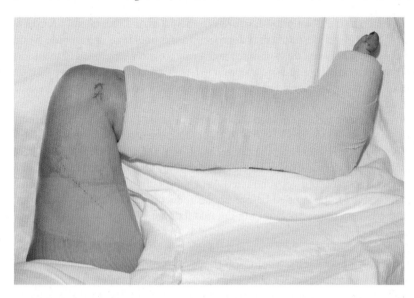

Complications

With appropriate soft tissue management and timing of internal fixation of ankle fractures, post-operative wound dehiscence should be a relatively infrequent complication. Due to the relatively subcutaneous location of the internal fixation, any wound complication involving full-thickness skin dehiscence or necrosis should be considered to communicate with the hardware, and appropriate aggressive surgical intervention involving debridement and dressing changes should be performed.

Patients with partial skin necrosis or minor wound dehiscence that is located away from the hardware, particularly on the medial side, can be treated with local wound care including wet-to-dry dressing changes. If this is noted prior to suture removal, the sutures should be kept in place during these dressing changes, particularly near the portion of the wound adjacent to the dehiscence. Surrounding cellulitis should be treated with appropriate antibiotics.

TIBIAL PILON FRACTURES

The "personality" of tibial pilon fractures is much different from that of ankle fractures. Tibial pilon fractures usually represent a much higher-energy injury with more involvement of the surrounding soft tissues. While immediate open reduction and internal fixation of some ankle fractures is feasible, the same is not true for pilon fractures. The skin around the distal tibia is not very tolerant of excessive swelling with early operative fixation, and therefore, allowing sufficient time for solution of swelling is necessary. Initial series of tibial pilon fractures treated with immediate open reduction and internal fixation had significantly higher rates of postoperative wound complications compared with later series in which a staged protocol was utilized. Initial management of pilon fractures is with limited internal fixation of the fibula and spanning external fixation to gain appropriate limb alignment and length. This will provide appropriate soft tissue stabilization to allow for resolution of the swelling that will inevitably occur following tibial pilon fractures.

Preoperative Planning

Initial evaluation of tibial pilon fractures consists of AP and lateral x-rays of the tibia as well as AP, lateral, and mortise radiographs of the ankle. When a pilon fracture has an associated fibula fracture, there is often shortening of the limb. After appropriate soft tissue evaluation, management consists of initial open reduction and internal fixation of the fibular fracture through a lateral or posterolateral approach in addition to application of an external fixator from the tibia to the calcaneus. This external fixator should be positioned so that the limb length is restored and the tibiotalar joint is reduced. Distraction of the joint may be necessary to prevent "cartilage necrosis" if the articular surface is comminuted and irregular. Preoperative planning is important because the incision for fibular fixation should be tailored to the anticipated approach for the tibial internal fixation. A posterolateral approach to the fibula may be utilized when a future anterolateral approach to the tibia is planned.

When an anteromedial approach to the tibial pilon fracture is anticipated, a direct lateral approach to the fibula is appropriate. By using a posterolateral approach to the fibula, an appropriate 5- or 6-mm skin bridge can be preserved between this approach and an anterolateral approach to the tibia. A direct lateral approach to the fibula should not be combined with an anterolateral approach to the tibia because the proximity of the incisions and resultant narrow skin bridge may result in skin necrosis between the incisions.

Once careful preoperative planning has determined the initial approaches for fibular stabilization, the patient should be positioned on a radiolucent table. A thigh-high pneumatic tourniquet can be used during the initial fibular reduction and stabilization. Fixation of the fibula is generally performed prior to application of the external fixator. In the acute setting, fibular reduction is usually easily obtainable as the soft tissues have not yet contracted. When difficulty is encountered gaining fibular length, the external fixator can be applied before fibular reduction. Careful construction of the external fixator will allow access to the fibula during internal fixation.

If the initial stabilization is performed within 24 hours, there is frequently minimal to moderate soft tissue swelling, and fibular fixation can be performed. In the polytrauma setting, when fibular fixation may not be performed within 48 hours, careful soft tissue evaluation should be made before planning internal fixation. If the skin does not wrinkle when performing the pinch test, then fibular fixation should be delayed; however, spanning external fixation from the tibial to the calcaneus should not be delayed and this should be performed at the first possible time following injury. The external fixator improves length, angulation, and rotation of the fracture, but more importantly, it restores the appropriate soft tissue tension and can prevent further soft tissue compromise and development of fracture blisters. Tibial pin placement should be proximal enough that anticipated tibial plate fixation will not be contaminated by the pin tracts. A calcaneal transfixion pin is frequently used, but pins may also be placed in the talar neck or metatarsals to provide further support to the foot to prevent equinus positioning of the foot.

Following initial spanning external fixation, the patient's lower extremity should be elevated at all times to decrease soft tissue swelling. Deep venous thrombosis prophylaxis should be utilized for these now relatively immobile patients who have joint spanning external fixators in place. Repeat clinical evaluation should be performed on a weekly basis to monitor progression of a soft tissue injury. Once the swelling has subsided to the point that soft tissue wrinkles are attainable over the planned surgical incisions, internal fixation may be performed. There is frequently a 2- to 3-week interval between initial injury and resolution of soft tissue swelling. Once the soft tissues are amenable to surgical intervention, a duplex ultrasound screening examination should be performed on the injured extremity prior to removal of the external fixator and planned internal fixation. Avoidance of tourniquet should be considered in patients who have developed deep venous thrombosis in the injured extremity.

Once the soft tissue swelling has subsided, careful preoperative planning is required to determine appropriate patient positioning, operative approach, and implant choice for internal fixation. Planning consists of reviewing imaging studies, which should include a postreduction CT scan once limb length has been restored with the use of the external fixator and/or fibular fixation. Operative approaches should be selected that allow access to the fracture segment that requires anatomic reduction. Pilon fractures with an associated medial malleolar fracture or coronal split that extends to the fibula are often best approached through a medial or anteromedial approach. Pilon fractures with significant articular comminution, particularly in the anterolateral area, can be approached through an anterolateral approach. Fractures with significant posterior comminution are best approached through a posterolateral approach as previously described for ankle fracture fixation. Two incisions are often necessary, and preoperative planning is required to ensure that there is a minimum 6-cm skin bridge between the incisions to prevent skin necrosis.

Posterolateral Approach to the Distal Tibia and Fibula

The patient is positioned in a prone position on a radiolucent operative table. The patient should be translated toward the foot of the bed so that the midfoot and toes are hanging off the bed so the foot is free. A well-padded pneumatic tourniquet may be placed around the thigh and should be placed prior to placing the patient in a prone position. The landmarks of the lateral malleolus and Achilles tendon are identified by palpation. A longitudinal skin incision is made halfway between the lateral border over the Achilles tendon and the posterior border of the lateral malleolus. The incision should extend distally until it reaches the level of the tip of the lateral malleolus. The deep fascia of the leg is incised in line with the incision, and the peroneal musculature and tendons are identified and retracted laterally. The peroneal retinaculum is incised distally to allow lateral retraction of these tendons. The flexor hallucis longus is elevated from its origin on the fibula and retracted medially to gain access to the posterior aspect of the tibia. Once reduction and fixation have been completed, the peroneal retinaculum and deep fascia of the leg are closed using an absorbable suture. The subcutaneous tissue is closed with a 2-0 resorbable suture, and the skin is then closed using either 3-0 or 4-0 nonabsorbable monofilament sutures such as nylon.

Anterolateral Approach to the Distal Tibia

Patient Positioning

The patient is positioned supine on a radiolucent operating table, and a well-padded pneumatic tourniquet is placed around the thigh. A bump is placed under the operative hip so that the foot rests vertically in the neutral position. The intraoperative C-arm is positioned on the uninjured side perpendicular to the long axis of the patient. A foam block or several folded towels can be used to elevate the operative limb higher than the nonoperative limb to provide a clear image with fluoroscopy. This also minimizes frequent manipulation of the leg that could potentially compromise the reduction.

Surgical Technique

For the anterolateral approach, a longitudinal skin incision is made in line with the fourth metatarsal. The incision is extended proximally as far as necessary to expose the tibia for application of a plate of the appropriate length and distally will end over the talus. The superficial peroneal nerve should be protected and retracted laterally in the wound. The subcutaneous nature of the superficial peroneal nerve requires careful skin dissection and blunt dissection once the skin has been incised. The fascia and extensor retinaculum are incised in line with the skin incisions with care taken to avoid undermining the skin flaps. The extensor digitorum longus is retracted medially, and the peroneal muscles are retracted laterally. During medial dissection, avoid injury to the deep peroneal nerve and anterior tibial artery as they cross the ankle joint.

Following reduction and fixation through the anterolateral approach, the superior and inferior extensor retinaculum is repaired using absorbable suture. Once the retinaculum and fascia have been reapproximated, the wound is closed with 2-0 absorbable subcutaneous sutures followed by interrupted vertical mattress nylon sutures in the skin.

Anteromedial Approach to the Distal Tibia

Preoperative Planning

The patient is positioned supine on a radiolucent operating room table, and a thigh-high pneumatic tourniquet is used. A foam block or set of folded towels is put under the operative leg to elevate it higher than the nonoperative leg for lateral intraoperative fluoroscopic imaging. The foot should rest in a slightly externally rotated position; therefore; placement of bumps underneath the ipsilateral hip is unnecessary. Preoperative templating to select the appropriate implant and length prevents miscalculation and unnecessary delays in the operating room.

Technique

The skin incision parallels the tibialis anterior tendons and extends proximal enough to allow application of an appropriate length of plate. Distally, the incision curves slightly medially over the ankle joint toward the talonavicular joint. The extensor retinaculum over the tibialis anterior is incised in line with the incision, and the tibialis anterior is retracted laterally. Dissection should continue beneath the tibialis anterior on the anterior aspect of the tibia, elevating the hallucis longus and extensor digitorum tendons, which are retracted laterally with the tibialis anterior. The dissection may also be carried medially toward the medial malleolus to expose fractures that extend into this region. Following open reduction and internal fixation, repair the extensor retinaculum over the tibialis anterior using an absorbable size 0 suture. The subcutaneous tissue is closed using a 2-0 resorbable suture, and the skin is then closed using an interrupted vertical mattress nylon suture.

Postoperative Management

Following sterile dressing application, a bulky Robert Jones–type dressing using both a posterior splint as well as a stirrup-type splint, provides added stability. The patient is hospitalized until adequate pain control has been achieved. Careful postoperative evaluation should be performed to monitor for development of possible compartment syndromes in the leg following internal fixation of pilon fractures. The patient is maintained in the initial postoperative dressing for the first 7 to 10 days, which can then be exchanged for a short leg cast for further protection of both the bony and soft tissue elements. Sutures may be removed approximately 2 to 3 weeks postoperatively once the wound has healed. Depending on the bone quality and the quality of fixation, the patient is transitioned into a fracture boot or cast when rigid fixation is a concern. Once the soft tissues have healed, the patient should be encouraged to remove the walking boot multiple times per day to begin range of motion of the ankle. Weightbearing is not permitted until radiographic evidence of healing is seen, usually at 12 weeks from surgery. Initial weightbearing begins in a walking boot, and once the patient is comfortable in the boot, they wean into a regular shoe over a several week period. After progression of weightbearing, radiographs should be obtained in 3 to 4 weeks to assure there is no displacement of the fractures.

Complications

Soft tissue complications can be minimized when an appropriate protocol of external fixation followed by delayed internal fixation is respected. In the event that delayed wound healing with dehiscence occurs, sutures should be left in place if it is a superficial skin dehiscence. Often, these can be treated often with dressing changes and occasionally oral antibiotics if there is surrounding cellulitis. In the event that there is deep or full-thickness necrosis of either the posterolateral or anterolateral approaches, careful clinical inspection should be performed to determine whether the infection communicates with the deep hardware. Because of the relatively subcutaneous nature of the anteromedial approach, full-thickness breakdown should be treated as a deep infection with formal irrigation, debridement, and antibiotic treatment. Full-thickness dehiscence of the anterolateral or posterolateral exposures should be inspected to determine if there is communication with the deep hardware. In the event that the subcutaneous and retinacular layers appear intact, appropriate treatment methods include local debridement and dressing changes. Any infection that communicates deep with the hardware needs to be treated aggressively with formal surgical debridement and postoperative dressing changes to obtain closure. Alternatively, VAC devices may be used in open wounds to help gain granulation tissue prior to an impending soft tissue coverage operation. With any type of wound dehiscence, range-of-motion exercises should be halted until resolution of the wound complication. While a cast boot is convenient for inspection of the wounds, a formal cast application with window cutouts is more effective at immobilizing the limb and allows resolution of the soft tissue complications. In the event of early deep infections, repeat serial irrigation and debridements are necessary with intravenous antibiotic treatment to obtain suppression of the infection until union has occurred. If the infection persists following fracture union, then the hardware may be removed and further soft tissue coverage provided as necessary.

GRACILIS FREE MUSCLE FLAP FOR EXTENSIVE TISSUE LOSS FOLLOWING ANKLE INJURIES

Despite the best attempts at atraumatic tissue handling during the surgical exposure, soft tissue defects surrounding the ankle may still occur. Whether due to the initial trauma, or due to tissue devitalization following fixation, soft tissue deficits surrounding the ankle often require urgent coverage to avoid the complications of hardware infection, nonunion, and osteomyelitis.

For soft tissue closure of ankle defects, there are many options, including the reversed soleus flap, the sural artery flap, and free latissimus dorsi muscle flap. Our preference however, in these situations, is the use of the gracilis free muscle flap. This flap provides a great deal of versatility, contours well to the ankle, and produces minimal donor site morbidity.

Indications/Contraindications

The gracilis muscle free flap can be considered for any soft tissue defect surrounding the foot and ankle with exposed vital structures. The flap is limited in terms of its size and surface area and is not well suited if circumferential coverage of the entire anterior and posterior ankle is necessary. Also the pedicle length can be short; thus, if a wide zone of injury requires the use of recipient vessels higher than the midcalf, there may be inadequate muscle available for distal defect coverage in the ankle or foot.

Patient factors that may increase the risk of flap failure include atherosclerosis, smoking status, and renal failure, but these are not considered absolute contraindications to surgery. Absence of adequate recipient vessels is the only absolute contraindication for flap transfer.

Preoperative Planning

Often following significant lower-extremity trauma, a CT angiogram is obtained to evaluate the arterial inflow to the ankle. In severe ankle trauma, the posterior or anterior tibial arteries may be occluded or transected, limiting recipient vessel options: either vessel may be used as a recipient vessel for successful flap transfer. If an angiogram is not to be performed prior to surgery, a careful assessment of the posterior and anterior tibial vessels must be performed with the use of a handheld Doppler probe.

SURGERY

Patient Positioning

The patient is placed supine on the operating room table with the leg in mild abduction and the knee slightly bent. Depending on the extent of the concomitant trauma, either the ipsilateral or contralateral gracilis may be used. If possible, we prefer to harvest the gracilis from the same leg as the original ankle trauma.

Technique

The gracilis receives its blood supply from the medial femoral circumflex artery, which originates from the profunda femoral artery. The major pedicle can be identified approximately 8 to 10 cm inferior to the pubic tubercle. The flap also has a minor arterial pedicle that enters the muscle at the level of the midthigh. This artery originates from the superficial femoral artery. The muscle receives its nervous innervation from the anterior branch of the obturator nerve. This branch of the obturator nerve can be harvested with the muscle if there are requirements for functional muscle transfer (Fig. 36-16).

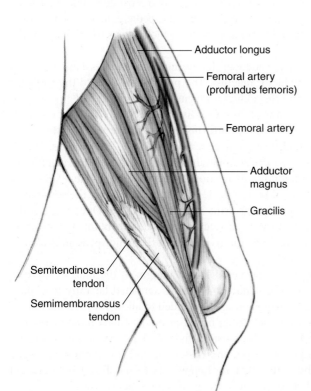

Adductor longus

Femoral artery
(profundus femoris)

Femoral artery

Adductor
magnus

Gracilis

Semitendinosus
tendon

Semimembranosus
tendon

FIGURE 36-16

The gracilis muscle lies in the medial thigh. Its major pedicle is a branch of the medial femoral cutaneous artery, which is a branch of the profunda femoris artery. The major pedicle can be identified entering the muscle 8 to 10 cm inferior to the pubic tubercle.

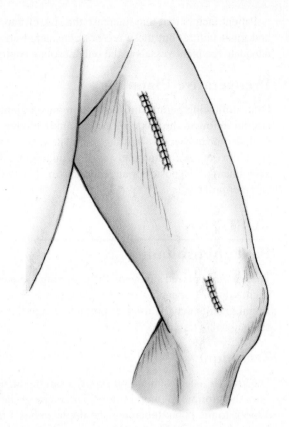

FIGURE 36-17

The muscle may be harvested through a long medial incision or alternatively through two smaller incisions; a 10- to 12-cm incision may be created over the area of the vascular pedicle, and a second 5-cm incision can be created at the level of the medial femoral condyle, which allows for division of the muscle insertion.

The muscle is exposed through a medial thigh incision. The incision is made 3 cm posterior to a line connecting the pubic tubercle and the medial condyle of the femur. A single long incision provides the most expedient means of identification of the gracilis muscles; however, the resultant scar can be unsightly. Alternatively, the muscle may be harvested through two separate smaller incisions; a 10- to 12-cm incision may be created over the area of the vascular pedicle, and a second 5-cm incision can be created at the level of the medial femoral condyle, which allows for division of the muscle insertion (Fig. 36-17).

Proximally, the gracilis muscle lies between the adductor longus medially and the semitendinosus muscle inferiorly. It lies superficial to the adductor magnus. The pedicle lies deep to the adductor longus but runs along the superficial surface of the adductor magnus.

Once the skin incision has been made, the muscle is carefully identified inferiorly at the level of the knee. Inferiorly, the muscle lies posterior to the sartorius muscle and anterior to the insertion of the semimembranosus and semitendinosus muscles (Fig. 36-18). The gracilis can be confused with the sartorius muscle. It may be differentiated from the sartorius and semimembranosus tendon by looking for the musculotendinous portion of the gracilis. At the level of the medial femoral condyle, the gracilis consists of both muscle and terminal tendon, the semimembranosus is entirely composed of tendon, and the sartorius is entirely muscle. Once the gracilis is identified, it may be rapidly separated from the surrounding tissue with blunt dissection to the level of the minor pedicle. The minor pedicle is not divided until the major pedicle is clearly visualized (Fig. 36-19).

The major pedicle is identified running at the proximal lateral margin of the muscle approximately 8 to 10 cm from the pubic tubercle. The adductor longus is retracted laterally to expose the major pedicle. The fascia of the adductor magnus must be divided to allow for mobilization of the pedicle significantly. The pedicle is traced back to its origin at the profunda femoris vessels. Multiple perforating branches to the adductor muscles must be divided to gain exposure to the profundus artery, thus maximizing pedicle length of up to 6 cm. Dissection and visualization are aided with the use of lighted retractors; alternatively, the adductor longus may be mobilized and retracted medially allowing visualization of the pedicle origin deep to the muscle (Fig. 36-20).

Once the major pedicle is identified and determined to be adequate for microvascular anastomosis, the secondary pedicle is divided. The origin of the muscle and branch of the obturator nerve is

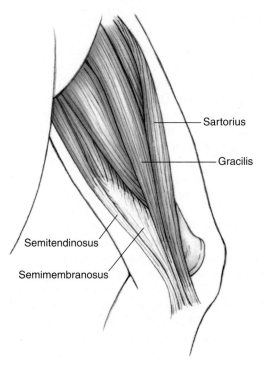

Sartorius

Gracilis

Semitendinosus

Semimembranosus

FIGURE 36-18

Inferiorly, the muscle lies posterior to the sartorius muscle and anterior to the insertion of the semimembranosus and semitendinosus muscles. The gracilis can be confused with the sartorius muscle. It may be differentiated from the sartorius and semimembranosus tendon by looking for the musculotendinous portion of the gracilis. At the level of the medial femoral condyle, the gracilis consists of both muscle and terminal tendon, the semimembranosus is entirely composed of tendon, and the sartorius is entirely muscle.

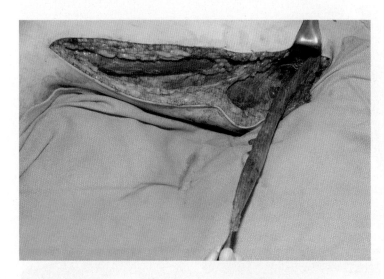

FIGURE 36-19

The muscle may be rapidly elevated back to the major pedicle. The pedicle can be seen inferior to the soft tissue retractor. The saphenous vein has been preserved as it crosses the incision midway down the thigh.

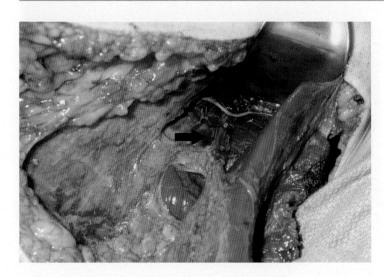

FIGURE 36-20

The pedicle (*black arrow*) is dissected back to its origin at the profunda femoris. This allows for a significant improvement in pedicle length. A branch of the obturator nerve can be seen running on top of pedicle and the adductor magnus muscle.

now divided. The muscle is left to perfuse on its major pedicle until the recipient vessels have been prepared for microvascular anastomosis.

Prior to muscle transfer, a final definitive debridement of the defect site is performed. The recipient vessels are then exposed away from the original zone of injury (Fig. 36-21). Donor vessel preparation is performed with the use of high-power operative loop magnification or the microscope to verify that the vessels are adequate for microvascular anastomosis. The anterior tibial artery is used as a recipient vessel for lateral malleolar defects, while the posterior tibial artery is preferentially used for medial defects (Fig. 36-22). End-to-side anastomosis to the artery is preferred, while an end-to-end anastomosis to the venous comitantes is performed in most settings. If two veins are present within the arterial pedicle, both of the venous comitantes to the gracilis muscle are anastomosed to minimize the chances of postoperative venous insufficiency.

Once the anastomosis is complete, the muscle is allowed to reperfuse for 20 minutes as the donor site is closed. An implantable Doppler probe is placed circumferentially around one of the two veins to allow for evaluation of anastomotic patency postoperatively. Donor site closure is performed with deep dermal sutures and an absorbable subcutaneous monofilament suture. A closed suction drain is also used to prevent postoperative seroma or hematoma formation. Flap insetting is then performed. Muscle insetting is facilitated with the use of half-buried absorbable sutures placed within the muscle and pulled beneath the native skin. The epimysium of the muscle is often excised to allow for expansion of the muscle's surface area. This allows for improved contouring over the malleolus. At the completion of insetting, the muscle is covered with a meshed split-thickness skin graft. The flap is covered with a Xeroform, and the patient's leg is then loosely wrapped in sterile

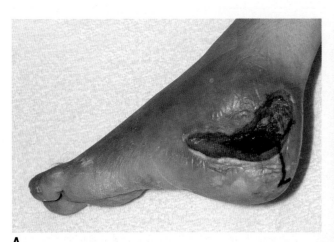

A

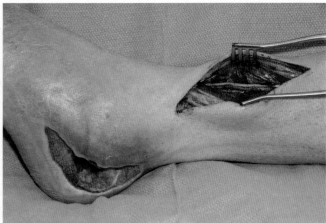

B

FIGURE 36-21

A: A lateral malleolar defect developed in a 48-year-old man after stabilization of a complex malleolar and calcaneal fracture. **B:** The anterior tibial vessels are exposed away from the zone of injury in preparation for free tissue transfer. **C:** The anterior vessels are identified just lateral and deep to the anterior tibialis muscle. The perineal nerve is surrounded with a vessel loop and gently freed from the underlying vessels.

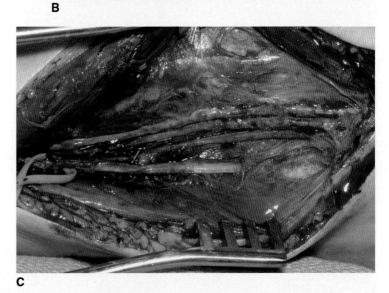

C

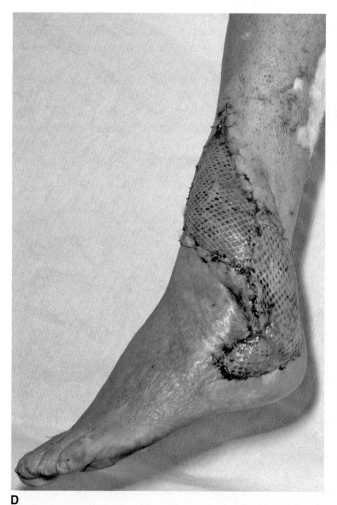
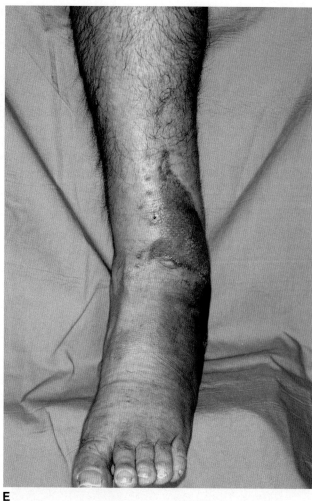

D   E

FIGURE 36-21 (*Continued*)
D: The flap at 1 week shows good take of the skin graft. **E:** Four-month view shows excellent contouring of the flap with stable wound coverage allowing for normal shoewear.

cotton and placed into a posterior splint for postoperative comfort. A large window is created in the dressing for postoperative flap monitoring. A single suture is placed superficially within the muscle over the pedicle so that anastomotic patency can be evaluated postoperatively with the use of a handheld Doppler device.

Postoperative Management

Flap monitoring may be performed with either the use of an implantable Doppler probe or with the use of a handheld Doppler probe at the bedside. Evaluation of perfusion is performed every hour for the first 24 hours by a skilled microsurgical nursing staff who are familiar and knows the signs of arterial insufficiency and venous thrombosis.

On postoperative day 4 or 5, the entire dressing is removed, and skin graft survival is assessed. At this point, the patient may be placed into a loose Robert Jones dressing or a removal posterior splint. The donor site drain is removed once output is less than 30 cc a day.

Complications and Results

The most devastating complication following any free tissue transfer include partial flap loss and total flap loss. If arterial insufficiency or venous insufficiency occurs postoperatively, immediate reexploration is recommended. At the time of surgical exploration, thrombosis may be identified at the anastomotic site. In such cases, early revision of the anastomosis will often allow for flap salvage. If the flap is unsalvageable and flap loss occurs, an additional flap will be required. In such cases, a secondary free flap, pedicled flap, or cross-leg flap can be considered. In cases of partial flap loss, occasionally, the flap may be advanced distally to cover critical structures. Alternatively, small areas of distal necrosis may be managed with dressing changes, skin grafting, or pedicle flap coverage.

In an examination of 50 acute traumatic and posttraumatic wounds, Redett and colleagues found the gracilis muscle effective for covering defects up to 165 cm^2. Successful free tissue transfer was performed in 93% of patients, and limb salvage was possible in 96%. Studies by Hallock have shown that the vascular pedicle is of adequate length for reconstruction of defects extending over the calcaneus and lateral malleolus (Fig. 36-21). For defects that exceed the limits of a gracilis transfer, a latissimus free muscle flap can be considered. We have found the gracilis to contour nicely over time allowing for normal shoewear following reconstruction.

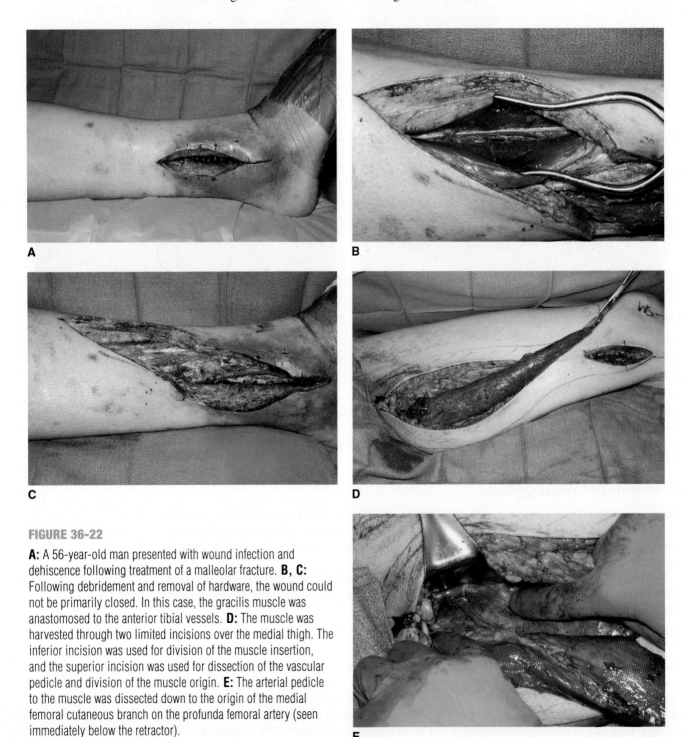

FIGURE 36-22

A: A 56-year-old man presented with wound infection and dehiscence following treatment of a malleolar fracture. **B, C:** Following debridement and removal of hardware, the wound could not be primarily closed. In this case, the gracilis muscle was anastomosed to the anterior tibial vessels. **D:** The muscle was harvested through two limited incisions over the medial thigh. The inferior incision was used for division of the muscle insertion, and the superior incision was used for dissection of the vascular pedicle and division of the muscle origin. **E:** The arterial pedicle to the muscle was dissected down to the origin of the medial femoral cutaneous branch on the profunda femoral artery (seen immediately below the retractor).

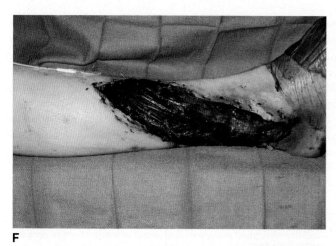

F

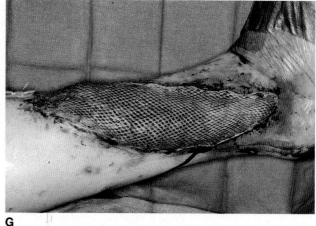

G

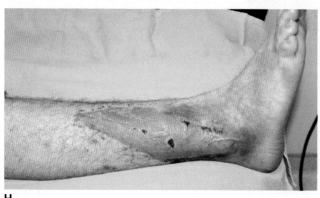

H

FIGURE 36-22 (*Continued*)
F: The epimysium was opened over the muscle to improve contour and allow for a larger surface area to be covered with the muscle. An implantable Doppler was used to monitor flow within the flap (blue cord at anterior margin of leg). **G:** The muscle was immediately covered with a split-thickness skin graft. **H:** The wound was stable at 4 months with no further drainage or signs of ongoing infection.

PEARLS AND PITFALLS

- When using either the medial or lateral approach to the ankle, one can use a foam block or bump of towels to elevate the operative limb away from the nonoperative limb. This facilitates obtaining lateral radiographs without having to manipulate of the operative leg during fracture fixation. The intraoperative fluoroscopy unit is brought in from the contralateral side, and it is positioned perpendicular to the long axis of the patient.
- Fractures that require fixation of the posterior malleolus can be approached through a posterolateral incision. This approach requires the patient to be in either a lateral or prone position. The prone position allows direct visualization and better stabilization of the limb during the approach and is therefore preferred.
- Immediate open reduction and internal fixation is not possible for many pilon fractures. The skin around the distal tibia is not very tolerant of excessive swelling with early operative fixation and therefore one should allow time for resolution of soft tissue swelling prior to definitive fixation.
- A direct lateral approach to the fibula should not be combined with an anterolateral approach to the tibia because the proximity of the incisions and resultant narrow skin bridge may result in skin necrosis between the incisions.
- Because of the relatively subcutaneous nature of the anteromedial approach, full-thickness breakdown should be treated as a deep infection with formal irrigation, debridement, and antibiotic treatment, as hardware is directly below the skin.
- While a cast boot is convenient for inspection of the wounds following soft tissue dehiscence following open reduction and internal fixation of ankle fractures, we prefer a formal cast with window cutouts. We feel this is a more effective means of immobilizing the limb and allows for quicker resolution of edema and improves the outcomes of soft tissue complications.
- If soft tissue flap coverage is needed, a CT angiogram is obtained to evaluate the arterial inflow to the ankle.
- If a gracilis muscle is going to be used for flap coverage, remember that the gracilis can be confused with the sartorius muscle during the dissection in the distal thigh. It may be differentiated

from the sartorius and semimembranosus tendon by looking for the musculotendinous portion of the gracilis. At the level of the medial femoral condyle, the gracilis consists of both muscle and terminal tendon, the semimembranosus is entirely composed of tendon, and the sartorius is entirely muscle.

- An implantable Doppler probe is placed circumferentially around one of the two veins of the flap to allow for evaluation of anastomotic patency postoperatively.
- The epimysium of the muscle is often excised to allow for expansion of the muscle's surface area. This allows for improved contouring over the malleolus. At the completion of insetting, the muscle is covered with a meshed split-thickness skin graft.

RECOMMENDED READING

Blauth M, Bastian L, Krettek C, et al. Surgical options for the treatment of severe tibial pilon fractures: a study of three techniques. *J Orthop Trauma*. 2001;15(3):153–160.

Gopal S, Majumder S, Batchelor AG, et al. Fix and flap: the radical orthopaedic and plastic treatment of severe open fractures of the tibia. *J Bone Joint Surg Br*. 2000;82(7):959–966.

Hallock GG, Arangio GA. Free-flap salvage of soft tissue complications following the lateral approach to the calcaneus. *Ann Plast Surg*. 2007;58(2):179–181.

Redett RJ, Robertson BC, Chang B, et al. Limb salvage of lower-extremity wounds using free gracilis muscle reconstruction. *Plast Reconstr Surg*. 2000;106(7):1507–1513.

Sirkin M, Sanders R, DiPasquale T, et al. A staged protocol for soft tissue management in the treatment of complex pilon fractures. *J Orthop Trauma*. 1999;13(2):78–84.

37 Calcaneal Fractures/Talar Neck Fractures

Hassan R. Mir and Roy W. Sanders

Fractures of the calcaneus and talus are among the most complex and challenging of fractures for the orthopedic surgeon to effectively manage. Both structures are three-dimensionally unique with highly specialized biomechanical function and a distinctly limited surrounding soft tissue envelope. Fractures of the calcaneus and talus are generally the result of high-energy trauma, such as a motor vehicle accident or a fall from a height, and as such, the severity of fracture displacement and the extent of soft tissue disruption are directly proportional to the amount of force and energy absorbed by the limb.

FRACTURES OF THE CALCANEUS

Indications/Contraindications

General Considerations

Operative treatment is generally indicated for displaced intra-articular fractures involving the posterior facet as demonstrated on computed tomography (CT) scanning. Nonoperative treatment is best reserved for non- or minimally displaced extra-articular calcaneal fractures and truly nondisplaced intra-articular fractures as determined on CT scan.

Comorbidities

While nicotine use/dependence is not a contraindication to operative treatment, all patients who are smokers are counseled at length as to the associated risks and encouraged to discontinue tobacco use. We consider heavy smoking ($\geq$2 packs per day) as a relative contraindication to surgery. Specific contraindications for operative treatment include fractures in patients with insulin-dependent diabetes mellitus, severe peripheral vascular disease, or other major medical comorbidities precluding surgery, as well as fractures in elderly patients who are minimal (household) ambulators. Because many older patients are healthy and active, chronologic age itself is not necessarily a contraindication to surgical treatment.

Delayed Treatment by Necessity

Operative treatment may also be contraindicated if initial evaluation has been delayed beyond 3 or 4 weeks from the date of injury or in certain situations in which injury severity prohibits early surgical intervention, including fractures associated with severe fracture blisters or prolonged edema, fractures with large open wounds, and fractures in patients with life-threatening injuries. Operative treatment following a prolonged delay (greater than 4 weeks) from initial injury to definitive treatment is complicated by the fact that early consolidation of the fracture has occurred, making the fracture fragments increasingly difficult to separate to obtain an adequate reduction, and the articular cartilage may delaminate away from the underlying subchondral bone. In these instances, delayed treatment by necessity is used whereby the fracture is allowed to heal and is later managed as a calcaneal malunion following resolution of the prohibitive factors.

Preoperative Planning

In completing preparations for surgery, the surgeon should thoroughly review the plain radiographs and CT scans to gain a preliminary understanding of the fracture pattern, which then allows for planning of patient position and surgical approach, as well as anticipation of specific technical steps in

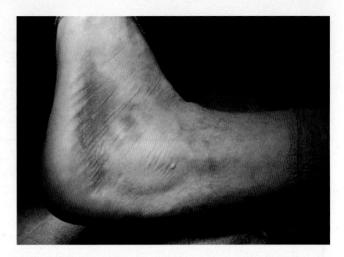

FIGURE 37-1

Preoperative "wrinkle" test. Note presence of skin creases indicating that surgery may now be safely undertaken.

obtaining fracture reduction, and the necessary implants for definitive stabilization. While multiple surgical approaches have been described, the extensile lateral approach can be utilized for most displaced intra-articular calcaneal fractures, with select cases managed via the sinus tarsi approach. Percutaneous reduction techniques, such as the Essex-Lopresti maneuver, are particularly ideal for certain tongue-type fracture (Sanders type II-C) patterns.

Surgery is ideally completed within the first 3 weeks of injury before early fracture consolidation; however, surgery should not be attempted until the associated soft tissue swelling has sufficiently dissipated as demonstrated by a positive wrinkle test. The test involves assessment of the lateral calcaneal skin with passive dorsiflexion and eversion of the injured foot. A positive test is confirmed by the presence of skin wrinkling without residual pitting edema and indicates that surgical intervention may be safely undertaken (Fig. 37-1). A variety of modalities may used to decrease swelling in the affected extremity. We prefer initial elevation and immobilization in a bulky Jones dressing and supportive splint as the acute swelling begins to dissipate in the ensuing days. For patients with marked deformity, or those with fracture-dislocation patterns, the use of acute reduction and either percutaneous pinning or medially based external fixation allows for staged definitive fixation with restoration of bony and soft tissue length and alignment (Fig. 37-2).

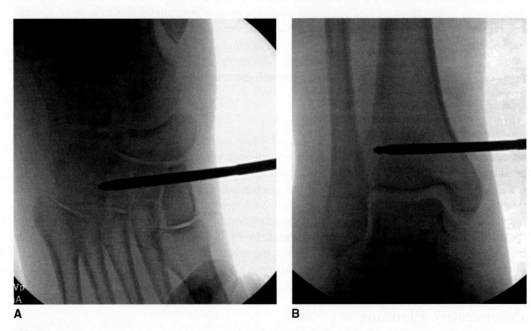

A   **B**

FIGURE 37-2

Calcaneus medial spanning external fixation. Schanz pins are placed into the cuneiforms, distal tibia, and calcaneal tuberosity **(A–C)**. Bony and soft tissue alignment and length are restored, allowing for staged definitive internal fixation at a later date when edema has subsided **(D, E)**.

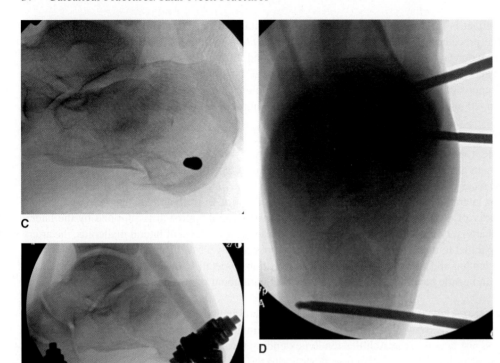

C

E

D

FIGURE 37-2 (*Continued*)

EXTENSILE LATERAL APPROACH

Surgery

Patient Positioning/General Considerations

The procedure requires use of a radiolucent table and a standard C-arm. For isolated injuries, we prefer placing the patient in the lateral decubitus position on a beanbag. The lower extremities are positioned in a scissor configuration, whereby the operative ("up") limb is flexed at the knee and angles toward the posterior, distal corner of the operating table, and the nonoperative ("down") limb is extended at the knee and positioned away from the surgical field to facilitate intraoperative fluoroscopy. Protective padding is placed beneath the contralateral limb for protection of the peroneal nerve, and an operating "platform" is created with blankets or foam padding to elevate the operative limb (Fig. 37-3). The prone position may alternatively be used in the event of bilateral injuries.

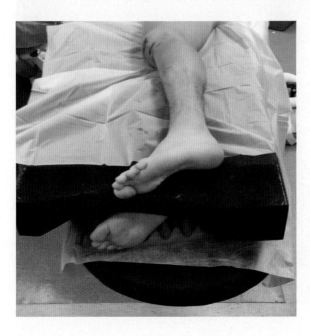

FIGURE 37-3

Lateral decubitus position. Note scissor-like limb configuration to facilitate intraoperative fluoroscopy.

The patient is given prophylactic preoperative antibiotics, and a pneumatic thigh tourniquet is used. The procedure should be completed within 120 to 130 minutes of tourniquet time, so as to minimize wound complications. If the procedure extends beyond that time, the tourniquet should be released and the remainder of the procedure performed without it. In allocating tourniquet time, the surgical approach should be completed within 20 minutes, allowing up to 60 minutes for fracture reduction, 20 minutes for implant placement, and 20 minutes for wound closure.

Technique

ANATOMIC LANDMARKS. Wound complications following surgical management of calcaneal fractures remain a major source of morbidity with these injuries. The soft tissues overlying the lateral hindfoot receive blood supply from a confluence of three arterial branches: the lateral calcaneal artery, the lateral malleolar artery, and the lateral tarsal artery. Borrelli and Lashgari determined that the majority of the full-thickness flap with an extensile lateral approach is supplied by the lateral calcaneal artery, typically a branch of the peroneal artery. At the level of lateral malleolus, the artery courses parallel to the Achilles tendon and lies approximately 11 to 15 mm anterior to the terminal Achilles tendon and its insertion. Thus, strict attention to detail with respect to placement of the incision and gentle handling of the soft tissues is of paramount importance.

INCISION AND SURGICAL APPROACH. The extensile lateral incision is then outlined on the skin with a marking pen (Fig. 37-4). The incision begins approximately 2 cm proximal to the tip of the lateral malleolus, just lateral to the Achilles tendon extending toward the plantar foot. In this manner, the vertical limb of the incision will course posterior to the sural nerve and the lateral calcaneal artery, thereby avoiding devascularization of the lateral calcaneal flap. The horizontal limb of the incision is drawn along the junction of the skin of the lateral foot and heel pad, the demarcation of which can be identified by compressing the heel. We prefer to substitute a gentle curve where these two lines intersect to form a right angle, primarily to avoid necrosis of the apical skin. The terminal portion of the horizontal limb includes a gentle curve anteriorly along the skin creases, extending over the calcaneocuboid articulation.

With a sterile bolster placed beneath the medial ankle, the incision begins at the proximal portion of the vertical limb, becoming full thickness at the level of the calcaneal tuberosity; dissection is specifically taken from "skin to bone" at this level while avoiding any beveling of the skin. Scalpel

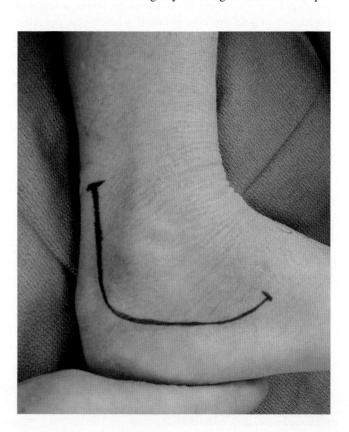

FIGURE 37-4
Planned extensile lateral incision.

499

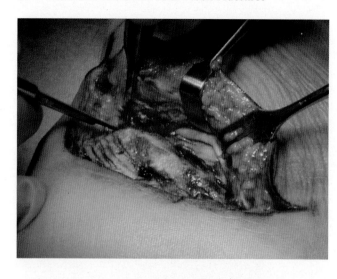

FIGURE 37-5
Full-thickness subperiosteal flap.
Note peroneal tendons contained within
the flap.

pressure is again lessened beyond the apical curve, roughly at the midpoint of the horizontal limb, at which point a layered incision is again developed.

A full-thickness subperiosteal flap is then developed starting at the apex. Any use of retractors should be avoided until a sizeable flap has been raised, so as to avoid separation of the skin from the subcutaneous tissues and periosteum. The calcaneofibular ligament and inferior peroneal retinaculum are released sharply, thus exposing the peroneal tendons. Both tendons are identified and released from the peroneal tubercle through the cartilaginous pulley and further gently mobilized distally with a periosteal elevator, thereby exposing the anterolateral calcaneus and calcaneocuboid joint. In this manner, the peroneal tendons and sural nerve are contained entirely within the subperiosteal flap (Fig. 37-5).

Deep dissection continues anteriorly to the sinus tarsi and anterior process and posteriorly to the superior-most portion of the calcaneal tuberosity for "window visualization" of the posterior facet, so as to prevent rotational malalignment of the posterior facet articular surface in the sagittal plane. Three 1.6-mm Kirschner wires are then placed for retraction of the subperiosteal flap using the "no touch" technique. In this technique, one wire is placed into the distal fibula as the peroneal tendons are slightly subluxated anteriorly; a second wire is placed in the talar neck; a third wire is placed in the cuboid as the peroneal tendons are levered away from the anterolateral surface of the calcaneus with a periosteal elevator. Thus, each Kirschner wire retracts its respective portion of the peroneal tendons and subperiosteal flap (Fig. 37-6). A small Bennett-type retractor may additionally be used at the distal margin of the sinus tarsi for further exposure of the anterolateral calcaneus.

ASSESSMENT OF THE PERONEAL TENDONS. Following fracture reduction, definitive stabilization, and final fluoroscopic images, the wound is copiously irrigated. As the previously placed Kirschner wires are manually removed, the peroneal tendons should easily reduce into the peroneal groove at the posterior border of the lateral malleolus. A Freer elevator is introduced into the tendon sheath, advanced proximally to the level of the lateral malleolus, and levered anteriorly to assess the stability of the peroneal tendon sheath and superior peroneal retinaculum. If the tendon sheath is detached from the lateral malleolus and therefore incompetent, the elevator will easily advance anterior to the lateral malleolus, indicating that a retinacular repair is required. A 3-cm incision is then made along the posterior margin of the lateral malleolus, exposing the tendon sheath and retinaculum. With the peroneal tendons held reduced in the peroneal groove, one to two suture anchors are placed in the lateral malleolus to secure the detached tendon sheath and retinaculum. Tendon stability is then reassessed with a Freer elevator in the same manner.

CLOSURE TECHNIQUE. A deep drain may be placed exiting proximally in line with the vertical limb of the incision. Deep No. 0 absorbable sutures are then passed in interrupted, inverted fashion starting with the apex of the incision. Sutures are placed thereafter at the proximal and distal ends of the incision, and progressing toward the apex of the incision, while attempting to advance the flap toward the apex. The suture ends are temporarily clamped until all sutures have been passed.

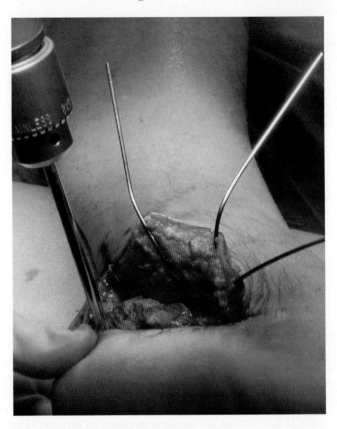

FIGURE 37-6

"No touch" technique: K-wire placement for retraction of the full-thickness flap.

The sutures are then hand tied in sequential fashion, starting at the ends proximally and distally, progressing toward the apex of the incision to minimize tension at the apex.

ALLGÖWER-DONATI SUTURE. The skin layer is closed with 3-0 monofilament suture using the modified Allgöwer-Donati technique, again starting at the ends and working toward the apex (Fig. 37-7). The suture technique is a modified vertical mattress stitch, whereby the far end passes subcutaneous to the skin edge to minimize tension on the skin margin. Alternatively, the sutures may be passed in modified horizontal mattress fashion. In the context of an extensile lateral approach, the knots are placed along the periphery of the incision, avoiding violation of the skin margin of the subperiosteal flap. Following completion of wound closure, the tourniquet is deflated and sterile dressings are applied, followed by a Jones-type bulky cotton dressing and Weber splint.

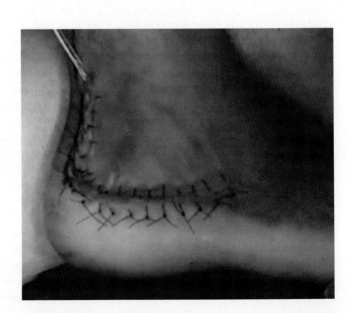

FIGURE 37-7

Skin closure using modified Allgöwer-Donati technique.

Postoperative Management

The patient is converted back into an elastic compression stocking and fracture brace at 2 to 3 weeks postoperatively, and subtalar range-of-motion exercises are initiated. The sutures are removed once the incision is fully sealed and completely dry, typically at 3 to 4 weeks; however, they should not be removed until the wound is fully healed. We prefer that the patient sleep in the fracture brace at night until weight bearing is begun to prevent an equinus contracture. Weight bearing is not permitted until 10 to 12 weeks postoperatively, at which point the fracture should be radiographically healed. The patient is then advanced to a walking boot and gradually transitioned to a regular shoe, and activities are advanced. In our experience, the patient should be able to return to a moderately active job at approximately 4 to 6 months postoperatively.

Complications

Delayed Wound Healing/Wound Dehiscence

Delayed wound healing or wound dehiscence is the most common complication following surgical management of a calcaneal fracture and may occur in up to 25% of cases. Risk factors for wound complications include smoking, diabetes mellitus, open fractures, high body mass index, and a single-layered wound closure. While the extensile lateral incision approximates relatively easily at the time of initial closure, wound separation may later occur—typically at the apex of the incision and even up to 4 weeks postoperatively. The vast majority of wounds, however, will ultimately heal; deep infection and osteomyelitis develop in only 1% to 4% of closed fractures.

In the event of a wound dehiscence, all range-of-motion activities are discontinued to prevent further dehiscence of the wound. We prefer a fairly aggressive approach to the wound, with a management regimen of daily damp-to-dry dressing changes and oral antibiotics. Other granulation-promoting wound agents may also be beneficial in this instance. Alternatively, the limb may be immobilized in a short leg cast, with a window overlying the wound for access for dressing changes. These treatment regimens will typically prove successful, so long as the wound necrosis is limited to partial thickness of the skin layer. Range-of-motion exercises are reinitiated once the wound seals and remains dry with the patient off antibiotics.

We prefer use of a negative pressure device (Vacuum-Assisted Closure, KCI, Inc., San Antonio, TX) to promote healing in the event of a recalcitrant wound; if all other treatment methods fail, a low-profile fasciocutaneous flap such as a lateral arm flap may be required for wound coverage.

Peroneal Tendon Adhesions

Peroneal tendon adhesions and scarring may develop in up to 18% of cases, either from the extensile lateral exposure itself or from prominent screwheads adjacent to the tendons, particularly surrounding the anterior process of the calcaneus. Nonoperative treatment includes tendon massage, stretching, strengthening, and other local modalities. Peroneal tenolysis or removal of the symptomatic hardware may be required in refractory cases.

Cutaneous Nerve Injury

The most common neurologic complication with surgical treatment of calcaneal fractures is iatrogenic injury to a sensory cutaneous nerve, particularly the sural nerve. Sural nerve injury occurs in up to 15% of cases and ranges from a stretch neurapraxia, which can be transient or permanent, to complete laceration of the nerve. Clinically, the patient may experience decreased or complete loss of sensation in the lateral hindfoot or perhaps even a painful neuroma. Initial treatment includes gabapentin or amitriptyline, shoe modifications or soft accommodative inserts, and physical therapy modalities. In the event of a painful neuroma refractory to these measures, surgical neurolysis and resection may be considered, including burial of the proximal stump into deep tissues.

SINUS TARSI APPROACH

Surgery

Patient Positioning/General Considerations

Simple fracture patterns that do not result in comminution of the posterior facet (Sanders type II and Sanders type III) or in comminution of the posterior tuberosity may be amenable to fixation via a sinus tarsi approach. This approach provides excellent exposure of the posterior facet for articular reduction, but the surgeon must be familiar with the complex three-dimensional anatomy of the calcaneus to properly restore the overall morphology. Since the exposure is more limited, it is easier to perform when the fracture is more mobile and is usually done within the first 3 to 7 days after injury if the soft tissues are amenable.

For isolated injuries, we prefer placing the patient in the supine position with a nonsterile bolster beneath the ipsilateral hip and pelvis on a radiolucent table with a standard C-arm. The patient is given prophylactic preoperative antibiotics, and a pneumatic thigh tourniquet is used. The procedure should be completed within 120 to 130 minutes of tourniquet time, so as to minimize wound complications.

Technique

ANATOMIC LANDMARKS. As described previously, the course of the lateral calcaneal artery must be considered in all lateral surgical approaches to the calcaneus. Although less frequently reported, wound complications following surgical management of calcaneal fractures remain a source of morbidity with these injuries even with the sinus tarsi approach. Thus, strict attention to detail with respect to placement of the incision and gentle handling of the soft tissues is of paramount importance, in particular when the approach is extended posteriorly.

INCISION AND SURGICAL APPROACH. The sinus tarsi incision is outlined on the skin with a marking pen (Fig. 37-8). The incision begins approximately 1 cm distal to the tip of the lateral malleolus and extends to the level of the calcaneocuboid joint in line with the fourth metatarsal. This incision is between the superficial peroneal and sural nerves, but occasionally, small branches may cross the field and need to be retracted or sharply transected. The sinus tarsi fat pad is mobilized dorsally. The inferior extensor retinaculum is released and the extensor digitorum brevis muscle is sharply elevated off of the anterior process and reflected dorsally and distally.

The peroneal tendons are mobilized and the inferior peroneal retinaculum is released to expose the lateral calcaneal wall down to the anterior process. The subcutaneous tissues overlying the peroneal tendons are left untouched, which also preserves the sural nerve and the lateral calcaneal artery more posteriorly. Following exposure of the anterior calcaneus and sinus tarsi, the peroneal tendons are retracted and sharp dissection is used for subperiosteal elevation of the soft tissues off of the lateral calcaneus to the tuberosity. Care is taken to make sure that plane of dissection is lateral to the lateral wall fragment. The superior peroneal retinaculum is inspected and repaired if warranted as in the extensile approach. The lateral calcaneal artery passes deep to and just along the proximal border of the superior peroneal retinaculum and must be considered when extending the approach more posteriorly.

Excellent direct visualization of the articular surface of the posterior facet is possible (Fig. 37-9). A percutaneous Schanz pin placed laterally or posteriorly can be used for traction and control of the tuberosity. A lateral plate can be placed beneath the elevated soft tissue flap and directly fixed to the

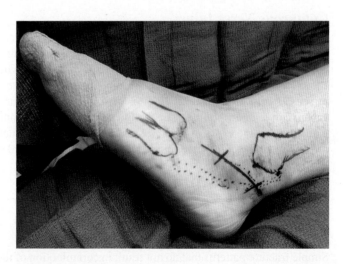

FIGURE 37-8
Planned sinus tarsi approach incision.

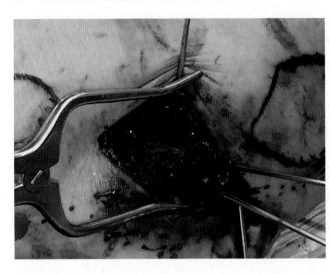

FIGURE 37-9

Sinus tarsi approach. Note visualization of posterior facet.

anterior calcaneus and the articular fragments through the surgical exposure, with additional screws for fixation to the posterior tuberosity placed percutaneously.

CLOSURE TECHNIQUE. After fixation is complete and final fluoroscopic or x-ray images obtained, the wound is thoroughly irrigated and the extensor digitorum brevis and sinus tarsi fat pad are reduced and secured with absorbable sutures. The calcaneofibular can be repaired if desired. The skin is closed in two layers with 2-0 absorbable sutures and the skin with 3-0 monofilament sutures (Fig. 37-10). The monofilament sutures are placed with the Allgöwer-Donati technique. Following completion of wound closure, the tourniquet is deflated and sterile dressings are applied, followed by a Jones-type bulky cotton dressing and Weber splint.

Postoperative Management

Postoperative management is the same as described for the extensile lateral approach. The patient is converted back into an elastic compression stocking and fracture brace at 2 to 3 weeks postoperatively, and subtalar range-of-motion exercises are initiated. The sutures are removed once the incision is fully sealed and completely dry, typically at 3 to 4 weeks; however, they should not be removed until the wound is fully healed. We prefer that the patient sleep in the fracture brace at night until weight bearing is begun to prevent an equinus contracture. Weight bearing is not permitted until 10 to 12 weeks postoperatively, at which point the fracture should be radiographically healed. The patient is then advanced to a walking boot and gradually transitioned to a regular shoe, and

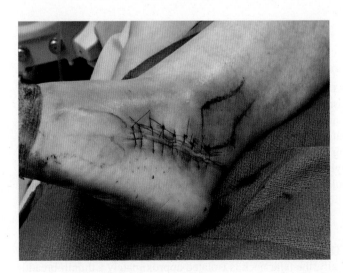

FIGURE 37-10

Skin closure using modified Allgöwer-Donati technique.

activities are advanced. In our experience, the patient should be able to return to a moderately active job at approximately 4 to 6 months postoperatively.

Complications

Although less commonly reported than with the extensile lateral approach, delayed wound healing or wound dehiscence is still the most common complication following surgical management of a calcaneal fracture with the sinus tarsi approach and may occur in up to 15% of cases. However, in properly selected patients, the time to surgery may be shorter with equal quality of reduction and outcome scores to the extensile lateral approach.

FRACTURES OF THE TALAR NECK

Indications/Contraindications

Operative treatment is generally indicated for all displaced fractures of the talar neck, and these fractures had traditionally been considered a surgical emergency, due to the high incidence of osteo-necrosis associated with displaced fractures. More recent studies have indicated that a delay in surgical management from the time of injury does not necessarily increase the risk of osteonecrosis, such that definitive stabilization based upon patient and soft tissue optimization following injury is now accepted as standard of care.

Severely displaced fractures or fracture-dislocations, however, may produce sufficient tension and pressure on the surrounding skin acutely to impair local circulation and result in skin necrosis and slough, potentially leading to a catastrophic deep infection and/or osteomyelitis. Thus, a timely attempt at closed reduction of the involved fracture fragment or dislocation is of paramount importance in minimizing soft tissue complications associated with these injuries, particularly if a delay in definitive stabilization is anticipated.

Nonoperative management is reserved for truly nondisplaced fractures as confirmed on CT scan. Because of the high-energy nature of these injuries, displaced talar neck fractures occur most commonly in young adults. Thus, in the majority of cases, the primary contraindication to surgery is the presence of severe life-threatening injuries where the patient is too medically unstable to tolerate surgery. In this instance, however, an attempt at closed reduction or manipulation of any dislocated fragments should be made in the emergency room to minimize the risk of skin necrosis.

Preoperative Planning

The surgeon should thoroughly review the plain radiographs and CT scans to gain an initial understanding of the fracture pattern, which then allows for appropriate preoperative planning, including the surgical approach, anticipation of specific technical steps in obtaining fracture reduction, and the necessary implants for definitive stabilization. In general, we prefer dual anteromedial and anterolateral approaches for talar neck fractures.

Surgery

Patient Positioning/General Considerations

DUAL ANTEROMEDIAL AND ANTEROLATERAL APPROACHES. The procedure requires use of a radiolucent table and a standard C-arm. For isolated injuries, we prefer placing a nonsterile bolster beneath the ipsilateral hip and pelvis to allow sufficient limb exposure both medially and laterally. Protective padding is placed beneath the contralateral limb for protection of the peroneal nerve, and the contralateral limb is secured to the operating table to allow for axial plane rotation as needed for surgical exposure. The patient is given prophylactic preoperative antibiotics, and a pneumatic thigh tourniquet is employed. The procedure should be completed within 120 to 130 minutes of tourniquet time to minimize wound complications.

Technique

INCISION AND SURGICAL APPROACH. The dual anteromedial and anterolateral incisions are outlined on the skin with a marking pen. Medially, the talar neck is isolated approximately a thumb-breadth distal to the anterior tip of the medial malleolus or midway between the medial malleolus and

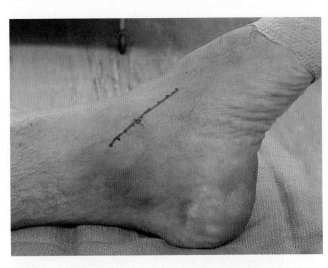

FIGURE 37-11
Planned anteromedial incision.

navicular tubercle. Thus, the anteromedial incision extends from the tip of the medial malleolus in line with the medial column of the foot to a point approximately 1 cm beyond the navicular tubercle (Fig. 37-11). In this manner, the deep dissection will course through the "soft spot" between the anterior and posterior tibial tendons and posterior to the saphenous nerve and vein. The approach is potentially extensile, as it can be extended proximally to allow for a medial malleolar osteotomy for talar neck fractures extending into the talar body or posteromedial process, as well as distally for access to the entire medial column of the foot as necessary.

Laterally, the talar neck is found immediately dorsal to the sinus tarsi in line with the extensor digitorum longus and peroneus tertius tendons. The anterolateral incision actually consists of the Böhler approach, coursing from the anterolateral corner of the ankle joint in line with the extensor digitorum longus and peroneus tertius tendons toward the base of the fourth metatarsal (Fig. 37-12). This approach is also considered extensile, as it can be extended proximally to allow for exposure of the lateral talar dome, with or without a lateral malleolar osteotomy, and distally for exposure of the entire lateral column of the foot as necessary.

We prefer completing the anterolateral approach first because the majority of the comminution is typically found medially; thus, the most accurate initial indication of the extent of fracture displacement or rotational malalignment is found laterally. With sterile bolsters placed beneath the knee and

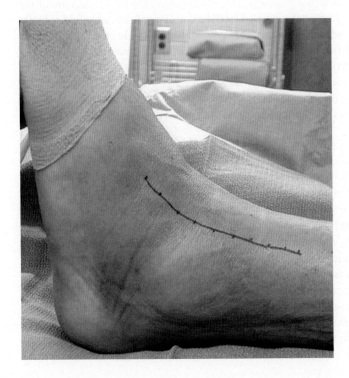

FIGURE 37-12
Planned anterolateral incision.

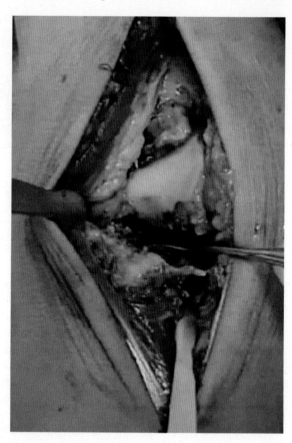

FIGURE 37-13

Anterolateral approach. Note full-thickness flap with simultaneous exposure of ankle, subtalar, and talonavicular joints.

ankle, the anterolateral approach is initiated, and superficial dissection continues to the extensor retinaculum and tendon sheath of the extensor digitorum longus and peroneus tertius tendons. Care is taken to avoid violation of the superficial peroneal nerve proximally.

The tendon sheath is incised at the lateral margin of the tendons, and deep dissection is continued to the deep capsule of the ankle and subtalar joints proximally and the extensor digitorum brevis muscle distally. The extensor brevis muscle is then traced to its origin beneath the tendons working dorsally, and subsequently reflected plantarly, thereby exposing the lateral capsule of the talonavicular joint and distal portion of the talar neck. The deep capsules of the ankle and subtalar joints are then released in line with and including the talonavicular joint capsule extending dorsally and plantarly, thereby completing a full-thickness flap (Fig. 37-13). In this manner, the foot may be adducted to expose the lateral portion of the talar head, thereby facilitating eventual placement of screws, which may be countersunk within the talar head. We make a conscious effort to limit the extent of subperiosteal dissection into the sinus tarsi, exposing only what is necessary to obtain an anatomic reduction, to minimize further compromise of the already precarious blood supply to the talar body.

The anteromedial approach is then initiated, and superficial dissection continues to the extensor retinaculum and deep capsules of the ankle and subtalar joints proximally and dorsal margin of the posterior tibial tendon sheath distally. The extensor retinaculum and deep capsules are longitudinally incised, continuing along the dorsal edge of the posterior tibial tendon through the underlying talonavicular joint capsule and spring ligament. Care is taken to avoid violation of the deltoid ligament fibers at the proximal margin of the incision.

The talonavicular joint capsule is then elevated in subperiosteal fashion off of the navicular tubercle, extending roughly to the midpoint of the navicular dorsally. The dorsal-most portion of the posterior tibial tendon insertion may also be reflected plantarly to ease soft tissue tension as necessary (Fig. 37-14). In this manner, the foot may be abducted to expose the medial portion of the talar head, again facilitating eventual screw placement. We again limit the extent of subperiosteal dissection along the undersurface of the talar neck medially in an attempt to preserve the vascular anastomoses extending into the tarsal canal. At the completion of the anterolateral and

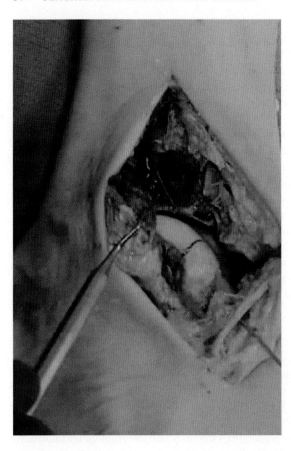

FIGURE 37-14

Medial malleolar osteotomy: anteromedial approach extended proximally for exposure of talar body.

anteromedial approaches, the fracture patterns traversing the dorsal portion of talar neck should be easily visualized.

CLOSURE TECHNIQUE. Following fracture reduction, definitive stabilization, and final fluoroscopic imaging, the wound is copiously irrigated. The deep capsular layers are closed medially and laterally with interrupted No. 0 absorbable sutures placed in figure-of-eight fashion. Laterally, the extensor digitorum brevis muscle is gently approximated distally with interrupted 2-0 absorbable sutures in similar fashion, as is the extensor retinaculum and extensor digitorum longus and peroneus tertius tendon sheath more proximally. Medially, the extensor retinaculum and posterior tibial tendon sheath are closed in identical fashion with interrupted 2-0 absorbable sutures. The subcutaneous and subcuticular layers are closed with inverted, interrupted 2-0 absorbable sutures. The tourniquet is then deflated, and the skin layers are approximated with interrupted 3-0 monofilament suture, again using the modified Allgöwer-Donati technique. Sterile dressings are applied, followed by a Jones-type bulky cotton dressing and Weber splint with the ankle in neutral dorsiflexion-plantar flexion.

Postoperative Management

The patient is converted into an elastic compression stocking and fracture brace at 2 to 3 weeks postoperatively, and ankle and subtalar range-of-motion exercises are initiated. The sutures are removed once the incision is fully sealed and completely dry, typically at 3 to 4 weeks; however, they should not be removed until the wound is fully healed. We prefer that the patient sleep in the fracture brace at night until weight bearing is begun to prevent an equinus contracture.

Weight bearing is not permitted until 10 to 12 weeks postoperatively, and the patient is gradually transitioned from a walking boot to a regular shoe, and activities are advanced. Postoperative radiographs are carefully scrutinized beginning at 6 weeks following surgery for the presence of a Hawkins sign, suggesting revascularization of the talar body. The absence of a Hawkins sign at that time, however, does not necessarily indicate osteonecrosis, as revascularization of the talar body may not occur for up to 2 years following surgery.

Complications

Delayed Wound Healing/Wound Dehiscence/Infection

Delayed wound healing or wound dehiscence following open reduction and internal fixation occurs in a relatively small percentage of patients, ranging from 0% to 4%. In the event of a wound dehiscence, all range-of-motion activities are discontinued to prevent further dehiscence of the wound. We prefer a fairly aggressive approach to the wound, with management regimen of daily damp-to-dry dressing changes and oral antibiotics. Other granulation-promoting wound agents or use of a negative pressure device may also be beneficial in this instance. Alternatively, the limb may be immobilized in a short leg cast, with a window overlying the wound for access for dressing changes. These treatment regimens typically are successful, as long as the wound necrosis is limited to partial thickness of the skin layer. Range-of-motion exercises are reinitiated once the wound seals and remains dry with the patient off antibiotics.

Deep infection and osteomyelitis rates are similarly low, occurring in up to 5% of closed fractures. Open injuries, however, are associated with markedly higher rates of deep infection and osteomyelitis, up to 38% in some series. Deep infection and osteomyelitis may also result from skin necrosis and slough from an unreduced closed fracture or fracture-dislocation due to excessive tension on the surrounding soft tissue envelope. Management of a deep infection includes serial surgical debridements, with local or flap coverage as needed, and long-term intravenous antibiotics. In the event of osteomyelitis, partial or complete talectomy with staged salvage arthrodesis is usually required.

OSTEONECROSIS. Osteonecrosis of the talar body is a frequent complication following a displaced talar neck fracture, owing to the inherently tenuous blood supply. Historically, osteonecrosis rates for displaced fractures (Hawkins type II, III, and IV fractures) treated with closed reduction and casting or pinning have ranged from 70% to 100%. Because of these factors, treatment of a displaced talar neck fracture has traditionally been considered a surgical emergency. Despite modern advances in internal fixation techniques and implants, osteonecrosis still develops in up to 30% to 50% of displaced fractures. It is well established in the literature that osteonecrosis is most related to the extent of initial fracture displacement; recent reports have suggested that the timing of definitive fixation has little influence on the risk of osteonecrosis.

PEARLS AND PITFALLS

Extensile Lateral Approach

- Await for resolution of edema (positive "wrinkle test") for definitive surgery.
- Acute percutaneous pins or medial external fixation can be helpful for patients with marked deformity or those with fracture-dislocation patterns to allow for staged definitive fixation with restoration of bony and soft tissue length and alignment.
- Use full-thickness flaps for dissection.
- Use K-wires to aid with retraction ("no touch technique").
- Avoid tension at the corner of the wound during closure by tying in a sequential fashion from the ends and progressing toward the apex.
- The skin layer is closed with 3-0 monofilament suture using the modified Allgöwer-Donati technique.
- Do not remove the sutures until the wound is fully healed (3 to 4 weeks).
- Discontinue range-of-motion activities in the event of a wound dehiscence and manage aggressively with daily damp-to-dry dressing changes and oral antibiotics.

Sinus Tarsi Approach

- Simple fracture patterns (Sanders type II and Sanders type III) may be amenable to fixation via a sinus tarsi approach.
- Reduction is easier to perform when the fracture is more mobile (3 to 7 days postinjury) if the soft tissues are amenable.
- When dissecting the posterior soft tissue flap, make sure that the plane of dissection is lateral to the lateral wall fragment.

- If extending the approach posteriorly, remember that the lateral calcaneal artery passes deep to and just along the proximal border of the superior peroneal retinaculum.
- A percutaneous Schanz pin placed laterally or posteriorly can be used for traction and control of the tuberosity.
- A lateral plate can be placed beneath the elevated posterior soft tissue flap and directly fixed to the anterior calcaneus and the articular fragments through the surgical exposure, with additional screws for fixation to the posterior tuberosity placed percutaneously.
- Delayed wound healing or wound dehiscence is still the most common complication following surgical management of a calcaneal fracture with the sinus tarsi approach.

Fractures of the Talar Neck

- Definitive fixation of talar neck fractures based upon patient and soft tissue optimization following injury is now accepted as standard of care.
- However, severely displaced fractures or fracture-dislocations may impair local circulation and result in skin necrosis and slough and therefore must be acutely reduced with closed/percutaneous/open methods to minimize soft tissue complications.
- Dual anteromedial and anterolateral approaches provide optimal visualization for reduction and implant placement.
- Make a conscious effort to limit the extent of subperiosteal dissection, exposing only what is necessary to obtain an anatomic reduction, to minimize further compromise of the already precarious blood supply to the talar body.

RECOMMENDED READING

Abidi NA, Dhawan S, Gruen GS, et al. Wound-healing risk factors after open reduction and internal fixation of calcaneal fractures. *Foot Ankle Int.* 1998;12:856–861.

Basile A, Albo F, Via AG. Comparison between sinus tarsi approach and extensile lateral approach for treatment of closed displaced intra-articular calcaneal fractures: a multicenter prospective study. *J Foot Ankle Surg.* 2016;S1067-2516(15)00520-7.

Benirschke SK, Kramer PA. Wound healing complications in closed and open calcaneal fractures. *J Orthop Trauma.* 2004;18:1–6.

Benirschke SK, Sangeorzan BJ. Extensive intraarticular fractures of the foot. Surgical management of calcaneal fractures. *Clin Orthop.* 1993;291:128–134.

Böhler L. Diagnosis, pathology and treatment of fractures of the os calcis. *J Bone Joint Surg.* 1931;13:75–89.

Borrelli J Jr, Lashgari C. Vascularity of the lateral calcaneal flap: a cadaveric injection study. *J Orthop Trauma.* 1999;13:73–77.

Canale ST, Kelly FB Jr. Fractures of the neck of the talus: long-term evaluation of seventy-one cases. *J Bone Joint Surg Am.* 1978;60:143–156.

Carr JB, Hamilton JJ, Bear LS. Experimental intra-articular calcaneal fractures: anatomic basis for a new classification. *Foot Ankle.* 1989;10:81–87.

Clare MP, Lee WE III, Sanders RW. Intermediate to long-term results of a treatment protocol for calcaneal fracture malunions. *J Bone Joint Surg Am.* 2005;87:963–973.

Crosby LA, Fitzgibbons T. Computerized tomography scanning of acute intra-articular fractures of the calcaneus. *J Bone Joint Surg Am.* 1990;72:852–859.

Dodd A, Lefaivre KA. Outcomes of talar neck fractures: a systematic review and meta-analysis. *J Orthop Trauma.* 2015;29(5):210–215.

Ebraheim NA, Elgafy H, Sabry FF, et al. Sinus tarsi approach with trans-articular fixation for displaced intra-articular fractures of the calcaneus. *Foot Ankle Int.* 2000;21(2):105–113.

Essex-Lopresti P. The mechanism, reduction technique, and results in fractures of the os calcis. *Br J Surg.* 1952;39:395–419.

Farrell BM, Lin CA, Moon CN. Temporising external fixation of calcaneus fractures prior to definitive plate fixation: a case series. *Injury.* 2015;46(suppl 3):S19–S22.

Folk JW, Starr AJ, Early JS. Early wound complications of operative treatment of calcaneus fractures: analysis of 190 fractures. *J Orthop Trauma.* 1999;13:369–372.

Gould N. Lateral approach to the os calcis. *Foot Ankle.* 1984;4:218–220.

Haliburton RA, Sullivan CR, Kelly PJ, et al. The extra-osseous and intra-osseous blood supply of the talus. *J Bone Joint Surg Am.* 1958;40:1115–1120.

Harvey EJ, Grujic L, Early JS, et al. Morbidity associated with ORIF of intra-articular calcaneus fractures using a lateral approach. *Foot Ankle Int.* 2001;22:868–873.

Hawkins LG. Fractures of the neck of the talus. *J Bone Joint Surg Am.* 1970;52:991–1002.

Herscovici D Jr, Sanders RW, Infante A, et al. Bohler incision: an extensile anterolateral approach to the foot and ankle. *J Orthop Trauma.* 2000;14:429–432.

Herscovici D Jr, Sanders RW, Scatudo JM, et al. Vacuum-assisted wound closure (VAC therapy) for the management of patients with high-energy soft tissue injuries. *J Orthop Trauma.* 2003;17:683–688.

Herscovici D Jr, Widmaier J, Scaduto JM, et al. Operative treatment of calcaneal fractures in elderly patients. *J Bone Joint Surg Am.* 2005;87:1260–1264.

Howard JL, Buckley R, McCormack R, et al. Complications following management of displaced intra-articular calcaneal fractures: a prospective randomized trial comparing open reduction internal fixation with nonoperative management. *J Orthop Trauma.* 2003;17:241–249.

Kikuchi C, Charlton TP, Thordarson DB. Limited sinus tarsi approach for intra-articular calcaneus fractures. *Foot Ankle Int.* 2013;34(12):1689–1694.

Levin LS, Nunley JA. The management of soft-tissue problems associated with calcaneal fractures. *Clin Orthop.* 1993;290:151–160.

Lim EV, Leung JP. Complications of intraarticular calcaneal fractures. *Clin Orthop.* 2001;391:7–16.

Lindvall E, Haidukewych G, Dipasquale T, et al. Open reduction and stable fixation of isolated, displaced talar neck and body fractures. *J Bone Joint Surg Am.* 2004;86:2229–2234.

Marsh JL, Saltzman CL, Iverson M, et al. Major open injuries of the talus. *J Orthop Trauma.* 1995;9:371–376.

Mulfinger GL, Trueta J. The blood supply of the talus. *J Bone Joint Surg Br.* 1970;52:160–167.

Nosewicz T, Knupp M, Barg A, et al. Mini-open sinus tarsi approach with percutaneous screw fixation of displaced calcaneal fractures: a prospective computed tomography-based study. *Foot Ankle Int.* 2012;33(11):925–933.

Palmer I. The mechanism and treatment of fractures of the calcaneus. *J Bone Joint Surg Am.* 1948;30:2–8.

Sanders R. Intra-articular fractures of the calcaneus: present state of the art. *J Orthop Trauma.* 1992;6:252–265.

Sanders R. Fractures and fracture-dislocations of the calcaneus. In: Coughlin MJ, Mann RA, eds. *Surgery of the Foot and Ankle.* 7th ed. St. Louis, MO: Mosby; 1999:1422–1464.

Sanders R. Fractures and fracture-dislocations of the talus. In: Coughlin MJ, Mann RA, eds. *Surgery of the Foot and Ankle.* 7th ed. St. Louis, MO: Mosby; 1999:1465–1518.

Sanders R. Displaced intra-articular fractures of the calcaneus. *J Bone Joint Surg Am.* 2000;82:225–250.

Sanders R, Fortin P, DiPasquale T, et al. Operative treatment in 120 displaced intraarticular calcaneal fractures. Results using a prognostic computed tomography scan classification. *Clin Orthop.* 1993;290:87–95.

Stephens HM, Sanders R. Calcaneal malunions: results of a prognostic computed tomography classification system. *Foot Ankle Int.* 1996;17:395–401.

Thordarson DB, Krieger LE. Operative vs. nonoperative treatment of intra-articular fractures of the calcaneus: a prospective randomized trial. *Foot Ankle Int.* 1996;17:2–9.

Tornetta P III. The Essex-Lopresti reduction for calcaneal fractures revisited. *J Orthop Trauma.* 1998;12:469–473.

Vallier HA. Fractures of the talus: state of the art. *J Orthop Trauma.* 2015;29(9):385–392.

Vallier HA, Nork SE, Barei DP, et al. Talar neck fractures: results and outcomes. *J Bone Joint Surg Am.* 2004;86:1616–1624.

Vallier HA, Reichard SG, Boyd AJ, et al. A new look at the Hawkins classification for talar neck fractures: which features of injury and treatment are predictive of osteonecrosis? *J Bone Joint Surg Am.* 2014;96(3):192–197.

White RR, Babikian GM. Tibia: shaft. In: Reudi TP, Murphy WM, eds. *AO Principles of Fracture Management.* New York: Thieme; 2000:525–526.

Yeo JH, Cho HJ, Lee KB. Comparison of two surgical approaches for displaced intra-articular calcaneal fractures: sinus tarsi versus extensile lateral approach. *BMC Musculoskelet Disord.* 2015;16:63.

38 Flap Coverage for the Foot

L. Scott Levin and William C. Pederson

The goals of soft tissue reconstruction for the foot and ankle region are satisfactory wound coverage and restoration of function. Ancillary considerations include acceptable appearance and minimal donor site morbidity. For soft tissue coverage alone, muscle and axial fasciocutaneous flaps remain primary choices in the lower extremity. Random pattern cutaneous flaps and musculocutaneous flaps usually have more limited applications, but should be considered. Free flaps are generally the soft tissue coverage of choice for most extensive defects of the foot and of the lower third of the leg. Amputations and fillet flaps always represent a fourth possible option when the limb cannot be preserved in its entirety. Finally, procedures such as osteotomies and/or ostectomies for the production of soft tissue "gain" and resultant coverage of the defect is becoming more common.

INDICATIONS

Each anatomic region of the foot has certain characteristics that will influence selection of the flap to be transferred for reconstruction. The foot has special requirements for shoeing and ambulation. The reconstructive ladder for injury to the foot is based on whether there is a fracture, what part of the foot is exposed, and whether the area is weightbearing or nonweightbearing. The ankle and the dorsum of the foot require thin, pliable soft tissue coverage for exposed tendons, bones, or joints. The plantar skin is thick and heavily keratinized, designed to resist high stress and anchored to underlying bones and ligaments by thick fibrous connective tissue.

Topographically, the forefoot includes the dorsal areas of the metatarsals and toes. The plantar aspect includes the metatarsal heads and the instep. The hindfoot can be divided into the plantar aspect, instep, and lateral aspect of the calcaneus. The ankle can be divided into the area of the Achilles tendon and the anterior aspect of the tibiotalar joint. In the forefoot, the dorsum and the area over the toes are primarily skin and subcutaneous tissue, making the exposure of tendons and joints more probable with high-energy injury. The plantar forefoot is prone to avulsion because of the vertically oriented septa that bridge from the plantar fascia to the dermal elements of the skin. The heel pad is a unique structure that contains cushion-like shock-absorbing chambers of fat that are not easily replaced if loss is due to such an avulsion injury.

Achilles Tendon Area

The Achilles tendon area is characterized by thin skin with little or no subcutaneous layer. Among local flaps, we consider the sural fasciocutaneous flap one of the best options for covering this area. Other flap options include lateral supramalleolar and lateral calcaneal artery.

Ankle and Foot Dorsum

Most shallow wounds on the foot dorsum may be safely closed with a split-thickness skin graft. If necessary, exposed extensor tendons may be resected, and the skin graft may be applied to the underlying periosteum, providing a simple and quick solution to the clinical problem. For management of larger wounds with bone or tendon exposure, flaps may be required. The most common local flaps used for coverage of this area are AH–ADM muscle flaps, extensor digitorum brevis (EDB) muscle flap, lateral supramalleolar flap, and sural fasciocutaneous flap.

Plantar Forefoot

Local flaps play a major role in the management of deep wounds of the distal third of the foot. Severe injury or infection to a single toe may be best managed by toe or ray amputation and subsequent closure by means of a plantar or of a dorsal skin flap. If additional skin is required, an adjacent toe may be filleted and transposed for closure. Ray amputation may be necessary if the metatarsal bone is infected, injured, or devascularized. Metatarsal head ulceration is the most frequent lesion occurring in this area, especially in patients presenting with peripheral neuropathy and associated arthropathy. Many local flaps have been described to treat plantar forefoot defects. The most commonly used are neurovascular island flap (Moberg's flap), toe fillet flap, V-Y plantar flap, and suprafascial flaps medially or laterally based.

Transmetatarsal amputation provides a functional option when three or more rays have been seriously damaged, especially in posttraumatic, ischemic, or neuropathic patients. No prosthetic or orthotic device would be necessary, and the patient may be able to wear normal shoes. Achilles tendon lengthening should be performed in conjunction with transmetatarsal amputation to avoid equinus deformity and stump ulceration.

Plantar Midfoot

The midfoot is defined as the region between the midshaft of the metatarsals and the proximal tarsal row. It comprises the medial non–weight-bearing arch as well as the more lateral weight-bearing area. Small wounds in this region may be reconstructed with a variety of reconstructive options. Split-thickness skin grafts may provide adequate coverage if the transverse arch of the foot has been maintained, thus allowing the midfoot to remain a largely non–weight-bearing region. Local flap options for reconstruction of defects in this area include neurovascular island flap, V-Y advancement flap, and medially or laterally based suprafascial flaps.

Wounds larger than 4 to 6 cm generally require either free flap reconstruction or midfoot amputation to achieve a stable coverage. Clearly amputation would represent the second option if foot salvage is not indicated or possible with free tissue transfer. The two most common forms of midfoot amputation are the Lisfranc amputation and the Chopart amputation. The Lisfranc amputation is the amputation at the tarsometatarsal joint and is associated with a high rate of equinovarus deformity. The Chopart procedure requires an intertarsal resection, just distal to the cuboid and navicular bone. Both types of midfoot amputations will affect the patient's ability to dorsiflex and evert the residual limb because of disruption of the insertions of the peroneal and tibialis anterior tendons.

Plantar Hindfoot

Hindfoot soft tissue repair is the most challenging to the reconstructive surgeon. Reconstruction should provide durable soft tissue for safe weightbearing, while permitting a normal ankle motion. The dualism of form and function represents a mandatory principle to be considered in the management of wounds in this area. Damage to the neurovascular and tendinous structures beneath the flexor retinaculum is an event that may impair permanently the patient's gait, mandating a below-knee amputation.

Many local flaps have been described to restore healing in the hindfoot area. The most common are intrinsic muscle flaps (abductor hallucis [AH], flexor digitorum brevis [FDB], abductor digiti minimi [ADM]), medial plantar artery flap, heel pad flaps, and sural fasciocutaneous flap. With the only exception being the sural artery fasciocutaneous flap, all the regional flaps listed require antegrade blood flow through the posterior tibial artery and its branches. Those procedures are therefore often not possible in patients affected by peripheral vascular disease.

Large hindfoot defects greater than 5 to 6 cm in patients devoid of the posterior tibial vessels should be considered for microsurgical reconstruction. Many neurosensory flaps have been described for microvascular transplantation in an effort to provide sensation to the plantar reconstruction. Lateral arm and deltoid represent two useful donor sites because of their reliable neurovascular anatomy, the ability to recover protective sensation, and because of their thickness; however, a correlation between the presence of flap sensation and the success of hindfoot reconstruction has never been established. Microvascular transplantation of muscle with skin graft

Foot Region	Locoregional Flaps	Free Flaps	Amputation and Ancillary Procedures
Achilles tendon region	Sural fasciocutaneous	Fasciocutaneous	Syme
	Lateral calcaneal artery		Below knee
Ankle and dorsum	Intrinsic muscle flaps (AH, ADM, EDB)	Fasciocutaneous	Syme
	Sural fasciocutaneous	Myocutaneous	Below knee
	Lateral supramalleolar		
Plantar forefoot	Toe fillet flap	Fasciocutaneous	Ray
	Neurovascular island flap	Myocutaneous	Transmetatarsal
	V-Y advancement	Muscle	
	Suprafascial flaps		
Plantar midfoot	Neurovascular island flap	Fasciocutaneous	Lisfranc
	V-Y advancement	Myocutaneous	Chopart
	Suprafascial flaps	Muscle	
Plantar hindfoot	Intrinsic muscle flaps (AH, FDB, ADM)	Fasciocutaneous	Syme
	Medial plantar artery flap	Myocutaneous	Calcanectomy
	Sural fasciocutaneous	Muscle	
	Suprafascial flaps (heel pad flaps)		

TABLE 38-1   Surgical Reconstructive Options

coverage can provide successful outcomes if the surgeon remembers to remove the underlying bone prominences, educates the patient on proper shoe wear, and performs frequent follow-up. We believe the use of muscle to obliterate dead space and aid in delivering antibiotics to the region is important for successful outcomes in cases of osteomyelitis. Because of its proximity to the wound margin, the posterior tibial artery is usually the preferred recipient vessel in hindfoot reconstruction. For hindfoot coverage, it is important to avoid scarring around the posterior tibial nerve and around the posterior tibial tendon, which may become exposed or trapped during the healing process.

Syme's amputation has a well-established role in the management of complex hindfoot deformities, especially in diabetic patients. The procedure involves the use of the heel pad as a soft tissue cover over the distal end of the residual tibia and fibula. Table 38-1 summarizes the main surgical reconstructive options for each region of the foot.

PREOPERATIVE PLANNING

Evaluation of the patient with soft tissue injury should include determination of the time of injury, mechanism, energy absorption, fracture configuration, systemic injuries, damage to the soft tissue envelope, vascularity of the extremity, sensibility, ultimate ability to salvage the foot (which is both functional and sensate), and underlying medical conditions of the patient. The principles of evaluation of orthopedic trauma are the same for any basic medical evaluation. These principles apply whether in the outpatient clinic, emergency room, or trauma unit. An evaluation of the perfusion of the traumatized limb is of paramount importance, and if vascular (arterial) injury is suspected, a vascular surgery or microsurgery consultation should be obtained. Compartment syndrome should be considered and ruled out in any injured extremity, particularly after crush injuries. A general motor examination including the active and passive range of motion as well as a detailed sensory examination should be performed. A nerve deficit may be secondary to a spinal cord injury, nerve laceration, compartment syndrome, traction injury, or entrapment between bony fragments. The radiologic evaluation starts with standard plain radiographic examination. Computed tomography (CT) is indicated in complex foot injuries and may give valuable information regarding soft tissue damage as well.

The wound should be inspected once and the wound pattern and contamination noted. The next inspection of the wound should then be in the operating room under sterile conditions. Repetitive examination of open wounds in the emergency room has led to higher rates of wound infections and osteomyelitis and should be avoided. In cases of open fractures in polytrauma patients, workup of other injuries may take several hours, not to mention the need for emergent lifesaving visceral surgery that may precede definitive care for open fractures. Prophylactic antibiotics are administered and given on a regular basis until definitive wound debridement and fracture stabilization can be performed.

Recipient Vessels

If free tissue transfer is required for wound coverage, then the last point of consideration prior to surgery should be the selection of recipient vessels for microvascular transfer as this will influence patient positioning within the operating room. A general agreement on which vessels to use has not yet been reached. Conflicting data have been reported on the survival and outcome of the transferred flaps, depending on the vessel used or the location of anastomosis proximal or distal to the zone of injury. For example, the anterior tibial vessels may be preferred for their easy accessibility, whereas the posterior tibial vessels are strongly advocated by others due to their larger diameter.

The most important factors influencing the site of recipient vessel are the site of the injury and the vascular status of the lower extremity; it is best to ensure adequate arterial inflow and adequate venous outflow before surgery. Intraoperatively, it is imperative that the anastomosis be performed outside the zone of injury. The type of flap used, method, and type of microvascular anastomosis represent less important factors in determining the recipient vessels.

SURGERY

Locoregional Flaps

Toe Fillet Flap

The flap is based on the medial and lateral neurovascular bundles of the toe to be amputated. The toe adjacent to the wound is outlined. This island flap is better dissected with the patient in supine position under tourniquet control.

TECHNIQUE. The flap is elevated beginning distally, off the distal phalanges and flexor tendons. The medial and lateral bundles are identified in the associated web spaces. A connecting incision to the wound is made. The toe is thus disarticulated at the metatarsophalangeal joint, and the dorsal skin is used for donor site closure. The flap is then rotated to the defect, ensuring a safe placement of the neurovascular structures (Fig. 38-1).

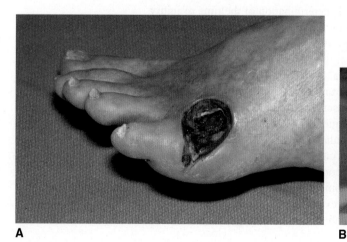
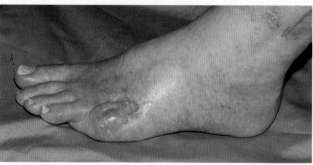

A   **B**

FIGURE 38-1

Dorsal forefoot diabetic ulcer covered with fifth toe fillet flap shown before **(A)** and after **(B)** surgery.

Neurovascular Island Flap

The flap is designed on the fibular side of the great toe, centered over the area of the neurovascular bundle. These flaps may cover wounds up to 2 to 3 cm in diameter. The use of a tourniquet facilitates a safe dissection. The donor site often requires a skin graft closure.

TECHNIQUE. The flap is elevated on the lateral plantar aspect of the great toe at the level of the phalangeal periosteum. The vascular bundle can be proximally dissected in the web space to allow a longer arc of rotation. An incision is made to connect the web space to the wound, and the flap is thus transposed to the defect.

V-Y Advancement Plantar Flaps

These flaps are based on vertical perforating vessels throughout the plantar aspect of the foot. Many V-Y advancement flaps may be designed with different orientation on the plantar foot. The use of a tourniquet facilitates a safer dissection.

TECHNIQUE. The skin adjacent to the defect is incised in a V fashion (Fig. 38-2). The plantar fascia about the circumference of the flap must be incised as well. Septal attachments to the underlying metatarsal may be divided to provide further advancement. Two V-Y opposing flaps may be combined in the management of a larger wound.

Suprafascial Flaps

Medially or laterally based flaps of plantar skin and fat may be advanced, rotated, or transposed to cover plantar defects. Although popular in the 1970s as random flaps, they have been largely

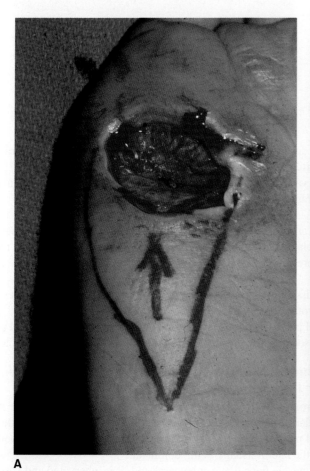
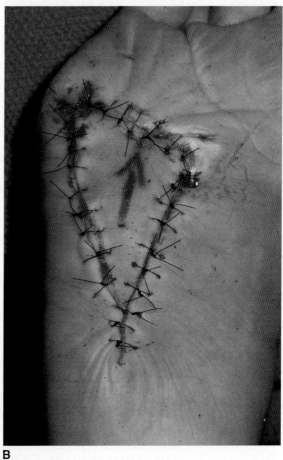

A   B

FIGURE 38-2

Plantar forefoot pressure sore in a myelodysplastic patient treated with a V-Y advancement flap shown before **(A)** and after **(B)** surgery.

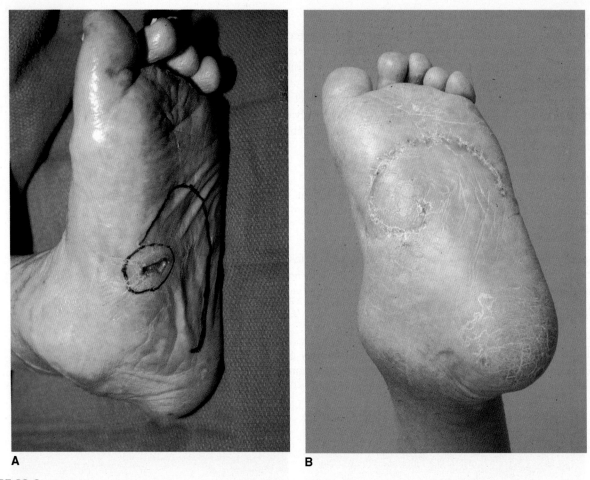

FIGURE 38-3

Plantar midfoot diabetic ulcer covered with a suprafascial rotation flap medially based shown before **(A)** and after **(B)** surgery.

supplanted by the other techniques described. Their vascularization is based on cutaneous branches from the medial or lateral plantar arteries (Fig. 38-3).

The design of a suprafascial flap varies largely according to location of the defect. The donor site often requires a skin graft for coverage.

TECHNIQUE. Medially based flaps are raised by incising laterally and elevating the subcutaneous tissues off the ADM muscle and plantar fascia from lateral to medial. Branches from the medial plantar nerve and artery should be preserved as they emerge from the cleft between the plantar fascia and the AH muscle.

For the laterally based flap, the dissection is similar but requires the sacrifice of the branches from the medial plantar artery, to allow rotation or transposition.

If the flap is designed on the heel pad to cover a small wound over the weight-bearing and posterior heel, a calcanectomy may be associated to remove bone prominences and to simplify the closure.

Intrinsic Muscle Flaps: Abductor Hallucis, Flexor Digitorum Brevis, Abductor Digiti Minimi, and Extensor Digitorum Brevis

The AH muscle is vascularized proximally by branches of the medial plantar artery. The flexor hallucis brevis (FHB) is also vascularized by analogue branches. The FDB is the largest of the foot muscles and is very useful for heel pad reconstructions. It is vascularized by branches of both the medial and lateral plantar arteries, the lateral usually being dominant.

The ADM is the smallest of the muscle flaps that can be harvested. It is innervated and vascularized by the lateral plantar neurovascular bundle through branches entering its proximal portion.

The EDB is a dorsal muscle. It is vascularized by the lateral tarsal artery, which is a branch of the dorsalis pedis artery, at the level of the distal edge of the extensor retinaculum.

The AH muscle with or without the medial head of the FHB and the ADM can be used to close small proximal dorsal foot wounds, but it is better qualified in the management of plantar hindfoot defects. The use of an ADM flap alone is not recommended because of its small dimensions and its short arc of rotation. The FDB is especially qualified in heel pad reconstruction. The EDB muscle is usually transposed proximally to cover the ankle, the dorsal foot, and the malleoli provided that the anterior tibial artery has antegrade blood flow.

TECHNIQUE. When harvesting the AH, a medial foot incision is placed on the non–weight-bearing surface. The tendon is divided distally, and the muscle is separated from the medial head of the FHB, if the latter component is not required to enhance the flap dimensions. If an increase in the arc of rotation is needed, the medial plantar artery is ligated and divided distal to the branches to the abductor, and a more proximal dissection of the medial plantar artery to its origin can be accomplished.

When harvesting the FDB, a midline plantar foot incision is used to expose the muscle. The skin is elevated laterally and medially and detached from the plantar fascia. The fascia is usually elevated with the muscle to add bulk. The four tendons are divided distally, and the muscle is turned on itself, after detaching it from the quadratus plantae. The lateral plantar artery may be ligated after it passes beneath the muscle, if further mobilization is required to reach the defect. The division of the origin of the AH also increases the arc of rotation of this flap.

When harvesting the ADM, a lateral foot incision is made onto the non–weight-bearing skin. The muscle is detached from the fifth metatarsal, and the tendinous insertion is divided, allowing posterior rotation of the flap. Further rotation is obtained ligating the lateral plantar artery distal to the branches to the muscle and dissecting the pedicle proximally after dividing the FDB and the AH.

When harvesting the EDB, a curvilinear incision is made on the dorsum of the foot, in continuity to the defect to be repaired. The entire dorsalis pedis pedicle is divided distally to the origin of the lateral tarsal vessels to provide the needed arc of rotation for muscle transposition. The long extensors are then dissected off the underlying short extensor muscle slips. The dissection proceeds proximally ligating the medial tarsal branches. The lateral tarsal vessels are elevated with the muscle while the origin and the tendinous extensions of the muscle are divided. The muscle may thus be rotated to the defect.

Lateral Supramalleolar Flap

This flap is vascularized by a perforating branch of the peroneal artery as it pierces the interosseus membrane 5 cm proximal to the tip of the lateral malleolus. Cutaneous vessels then course upward, anterior to the fibula, and anastomose with the vascular network that accompanies the superficial peroneal nerve.

The flap is qualified in the coverage of defects over the lateral malleolus and anterior ankle. The flap should be distally based, with the pedicle centered onto the perforator artery. Flap width includes the tissue between the fibula and tibia. The length should be 6 to 8 cm or more according to the defect. Often the flap is harvested only in its fascial component then turned over to the defect in a book page fashion then skin grafted. If designed in this way, the donor site can be closed directly.

TECHNIQUE. The skin incision is made so that skin flaps may be elevated off the underlying fascia. The fascia is then incised anteriorly and reflected until the perforating branch is visualized. Branches of the superficial peroneal nerve are divided to allow elevation. The posterior margin is eventually incised and released from the septum between the anterior and lateral compartment of the leg.

Medial Plantar Artery Flap

This is a true neurosensory type A fasciocutaneous flap supplied by cutaneous fascicles from the medial and lateral plantar nerves. It is vascularized by the medial plantar artery and its vena comitans. The flap provides an invaluable amount of specialized skin that configures its chief value in heel reconstruction, because of its nonshearing, well-padded, adherent qualities.

Patency of anterior and posterior tibial arteries should be assessed prior to surgery. The presence of a Charcot deformity with midfoot collapse contraindicates the flap harvest. In this deformity, the instep area should remain covered by specialized plantar skin. For heel reconstruction, the flap is designed as an island centered on the medial plantar artery. It has to be outlined 2 to 3 cm proximal to the metatarsal heads, distal to the heel and medial to the lateral midsole weight-bearing area. The donor site is usually closed with a split-thickness skin graft.

TECHNIQUE. The flap is incised distally, exposing the medial plantar artery and nerves. After ligation of the artery, the dissection continues proximally beneath the plantar aponeurosis, including the medial plantar artery and the neurovascular bundles to the overlying fascia and skin. This requires an intraneural dissection of the midsole cutaneous branches from those fascicles supplying three and one-half digits. Often, the second common digital nerve is included with the branches to the flap because of difficulties encountered in separation. The flap is thus elevated in a distal to proximal direction in the plane between the plantar fascia and the first layer of muscles. Fascial communications to the clefts between the underlying muscles (AH, FDB, and ADM) are cut.

Fascicles from the lateral plantar nerve may also be included in the flap following an intraneural dissection. The medial plantar artery and the fascicles from the medial plantar nerve are traced proximally to the AH muscle, which may be cut if a longer pedicle is required.

Sural Artery Fasciocutaneous Flap

This type A fasciocutaneous flap is innervated by the medial sural cutaneous nerve (S1-2). Its dominant vascular supply is a direct cutaneous sural artery branch that arises in the distal popliteal fossa between the two heads of the gastrocnemius muscle and minor musculocutaneous perforators from the gastrocnemius muscle. In most patients, the arterial supply will not be an identifiable vessel, but a "vascular network" that also anastomoses with the peroneal artery. The most relevant of these connections is located approximately 5 cm cephalad to the lateral malleolus. The lesser saphenous vein and its branches provide venous drainage.

The flap is centered between the popliteal fossa and the midposterior leg with a width up to 12 cm, but the length can be extended 20 cm to the Achilles tendon. The donor site is usually closed with a split-thickness skin graft.

TECHNIQUE. The flap is raised from distal to proximal in the plane beneath the deep fascia and the above gastrocnemius muscle. The sural nerve and the lesser saphenous vein are divided distally and elevated with the flap. The pedicle is carefully dissected proximally, leaving abundant fascio-subcutaneous tissues around the neurovascular structures. It can be dissected up to 7 to 9 cm from the lateral malleolus, according to the location of the defect to be reached. After flap rotation to the defect, the skin over the pedicle is usually not sutured to avoid compression, and a skin graft is usually applied to provide coverage. Flap delay procedures and/or venous supercharging should be evaluated to avoid congestion, which commonly complicates the postoperatory course (Fig. 38-4).

Heel Reconstruction with Neurosensory Medial Plantar Artery Flap

The weight-bearing heel represents one of the most difficult areas to reconstruct on the foot. This area must bear the weight of the entire body with ambulation. The ideal flap for heel reconstruction

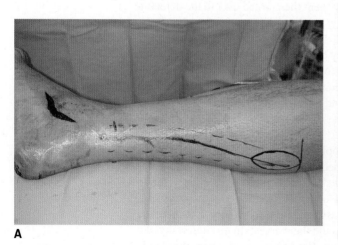
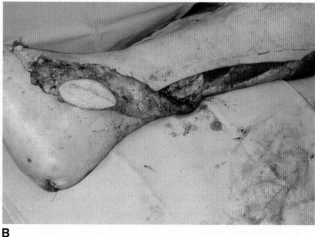

A   **B**

FIGURE 38-4

Wound dehiscence post–triple-ankle arthrodesis covered with a distally based sural flap. **A:** Preoperative view and flap design. **B:** The flap is transposed to the defect.

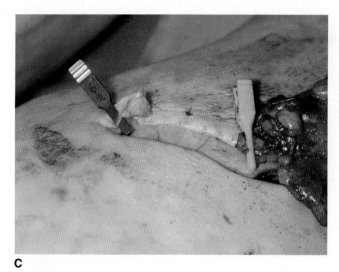

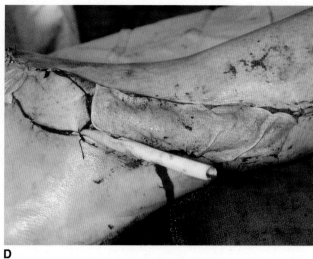

C

D

FIGURE 38-4 *(Continued)*

C: The flap will be turbo-charged to improve the venous outflow (lesser saphenous vein to superficial dorsal vein). **D:** The pedicles are protected with split-thickness skin grafts.

must be sensate and resist shear forces during ambulation. Studies have shown that with special shoeing and attention, patients may successfully ambulate following the placement of a nonsensate flap over the heel, but we have found that these reconstructions are prone to breakdown. The one flap that fulfills all the criteria for successful stable coverage of the heel is the medial plantar artery flap.

The medial plantar artery flap is indicated primarily for defects of the weight-bearing heel, but the flap may also be utilized to cover wounds of the lateral foot as well. The flap is based on the medial geniculate artery, which is a terminal branch of the posterior tibial artery. The patency of the posterior tibial artery must be verified prior to using this flap, particularly in diabetics and patients with peripheral vascular disease. If pulses are absent, a vascular study may be required. If there has been damage to the posterior tibial artery at the level of the ankle and the flap is to be utilized, it must then be used as a free flap.

TECHNIQUE. The flap is raised from the non–weight-bearing surface of the instep and is based on the medial plantar artery and vein. The flap receives sensation from branches of the medial plantar nerve, which accompanies the vessels. Design of the flap should avoid including areas of the weight-bearing surface of the metatarsal heads or lateral foot. Most surgeons prefer to elevate this flap with the plantar fascia, which lies superficial to the medial plantar artery. We feel that inclusion of the fascia within the flap provides a reconstruction that is more resistant to sheer stress as the septa from the plantar fascia to the dermis are left intact.

The flap is dissected under tourniquet control. The flap is elevated from distal to proximal (Fig. 38-5A). The pedicle runs deep to the plantar fascia, and perforators to the flap can be visualized crossing through the fascia in the septum between the FDB muscle and AH muscle. The nerve branches entering the flap may require intraneural dissection from the proximal tibial nerve in order to increase the length of the pedicle. Once the pedicle is dissected, an incision can be made to allow rotation of the flap into the heel defect as necessary. The donor site is covered with a meshed split-thickness skin graft, which is usually managed with a bolster of some type for 2 to 3 weeks (Fig. 38-5B–E).

This flap provides excellent coverage of the heel, and the donor site is very well tolerated. Breakdown at the incision line can occur but is uncommon. Hyperkeratosis at the margins of the skin graft can also occur.

Free Flaps

Latissimus Dorsi

This flap is based on the thoracodorsal artery as the major pedicle and on branches of the intercostals and lumbar arteries as secondary segmental branches. The pedicle length is 8 to 10 cm. The

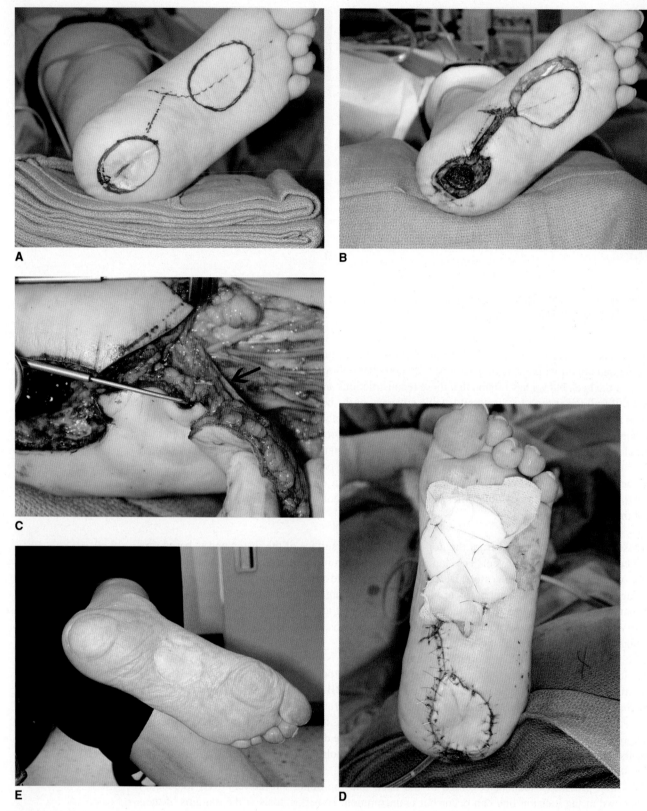

FIGURE 38-5

A: View of plantar foot in 24-year-old patient with spina bifida and long-term heel ulceration and osteomyelitis. Medial plantar artery flap is marked in instep of foot centered over the medial geniculate artery. **B:** View after flap has been elevated and ulcer excised along with sequestrum of osteomyelitis in calcaneus. **C:** View of pedicle of flap, *arrow* points out branch of medial plantar nerve going into flap. **D:** Image of the inset flap. The donor site is covered with a split-thickness skin graft, a bolster placed over the skin graft. **E:** View of foot at 2 years. There has been no further breakdown, and the donor site is well healed.

latissimus is innervated by the thoracodorsal nerve, which is a direct branch of the brachial plexus and enters the muscle 10 cm from the apex of the axilla. This flap's consistent anatomy and long vascular pedicle make it a common flap choice for larger defects of the foot and Achilles tendon region. Some of the technical problems associated with this flap for lower extremity reconstruction include difficulty in positioning the patient to allow for flap elevation and simultaneous recipient site preparation. If the anterior tibial system is to be used as a recipient vessel, the ipsilateral latissimus is usually harvested; if the posterior tibial system is to be used, the contralateral latissimus should be harvested to allow for simultaneous flap elevation and recipient site exposure. In addition, in obese patients, the musculocutaneous flap may be excessively thick for smooth contour over the foot (Fig. 38-6).

Rectus Abdominis

The rectus abdominis can be harvested with the patient in a supine position. This vertically oriented muscle extends between the costal margin and the pubic region and is enclosed by the anterior and posterior rectus sheaths. It is a type 3 muscle (two dominant pedicles) based on the superior epigastric artery and vein and inferior epigastric artery and vein. The pedicle length is 5 to 7 cm superiorly and 8 to 10 cm inferiorly.

Each of the dominant pedicles supplies just over half the muscle. There is an anastomosis between these vessels that is usually sufficient to support the nondominant half if one of the two pedicles is ligated. Because of the larger size and easier dissection of the inferior epigastric vessel, it is usually used for free tissue transfer.

The motor innervation is supplied by segmental motor nerves from the seventh through twelfth intercostal nerves that enter the deep surface of the muscle at its middle to lateral aspects. The lateral cutaneous nerves from the seventh through twelfth intercostal nerves provide sensation to the skin territory of the rectus abdominis muscle. The size of the muscle is up to 25×6 cm^2. The skin territory that can be harvested is 21×14 cm^2 and is based on musculocutaneous perforator (Fig. 38-7).

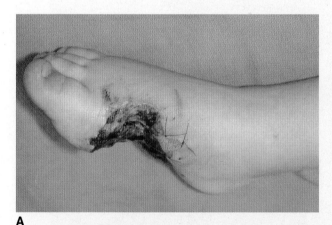

A

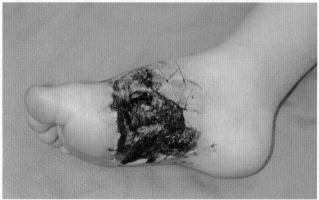

B

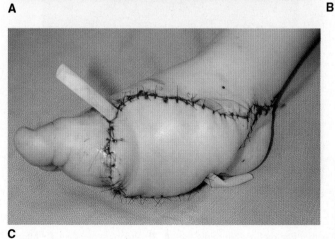

C

FIGURE 38-6

Medial plantar midfoot traumatic defect in a pediatric patient after a lawnmower injury. The defect is reconstructed with a free latissimus dorsi flap shown before **(A)** and after **(B)** surgery. **C:** The flap is revascularized and sutured to the defect.

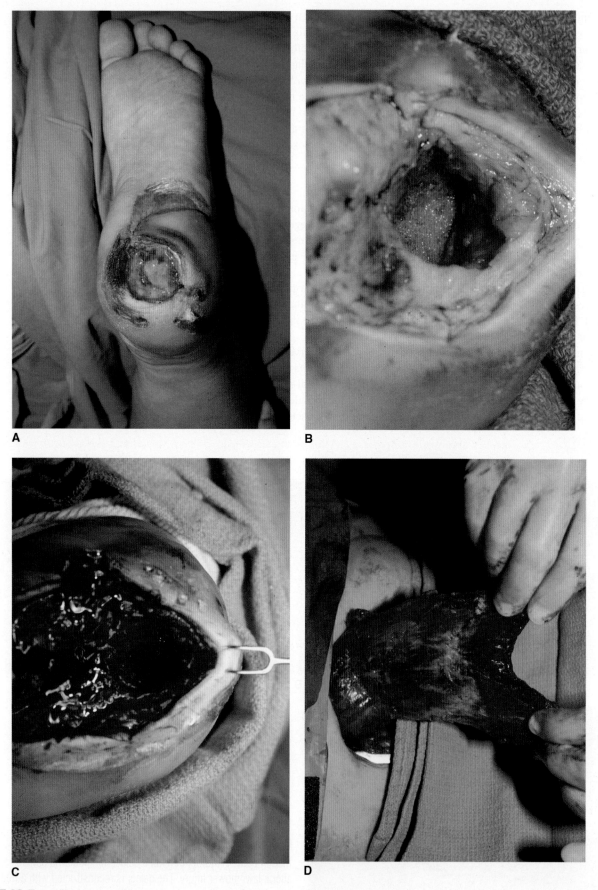

FIGURE 38-7

Calcaneal osteomyelitis on a diabetic foot. The defect was reconstructed with a free rectus abdominis flap. **A, B:** Preoperative view. **C:** After debridement. **D:** The rectus muscle is harvested from the abdomen.

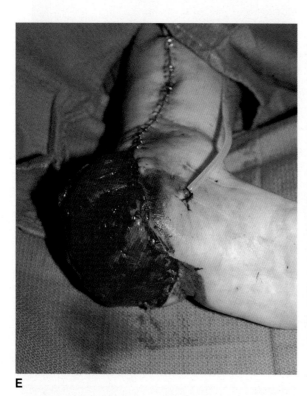

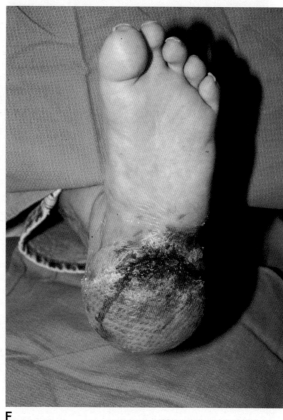

E   F

FIGURE 38-7 (*Continued*)

E: The flap is tailored to the defect and revascularized. **F:** Late postoperative view showing calcaneal salvage.

Gracilis

The gracilis is a smaller transplant and is useful for defects requiring less bulk than the latissimus or rectus. The gracilis muscle is a type 2 muscle (with a dominant pedicle and several minor pedicles). It is a thin, flat muscle that lies between the adductor longus and sartorius muscle anteriorly and the semimembranosus posteriorly. The dominant pedicle is the ascending branch of medial circumflex femoral artery and venae comitantes. The length of the pedicle is 6 cm, and the diameter of the artery is 1.6 mm. The minor pedicles are one or two branches of the superficial femoral artery and venae comitantes. Their length is 2 cm, and their diameter is 0.5 mm.

Motor innervation is via the anterior branch of the obturator nerve, which is located between the abductor longus and magnus muscles, and it usually enters the muscle above the level of the dominant vascular pedicle. The anterior femoral cutaneous nerve (L2–3) provides sensory innervation to the majority of the anterior medial thigh.

This muscle functions as a thigh adductor. The presence of the adductor longus and magnus makes it an expendable muscle.

The size of the muscle is 6×24 cm². The skin territory is 16×18 cm², but the skin over the distal half of the muscle is not reliable when the flap is based on its dominant vascular pedicle with division of the minor vascular pedicles. In obese patients, the musculocutaneous flap may be too bulky, necessitating use of a skin graft placed on the muscle (Fig. 38-8).

Radial Forearm Flap

This is a thin, well-vascularized fasciocutaneous flap on the ventral aspect of the forearm that was widely used in China before it was popularized in the Western literature. The flap is based on the radial artery, which can achieve a 20-cm pedicle and has a diameter of 2.5 mm. This length of the pedicle facilitates the microsurgical anastomosis out of the zone of injury. The venous drainage is through the venae comitantes of the radial artery, but the flap can include the cephalic vein, the

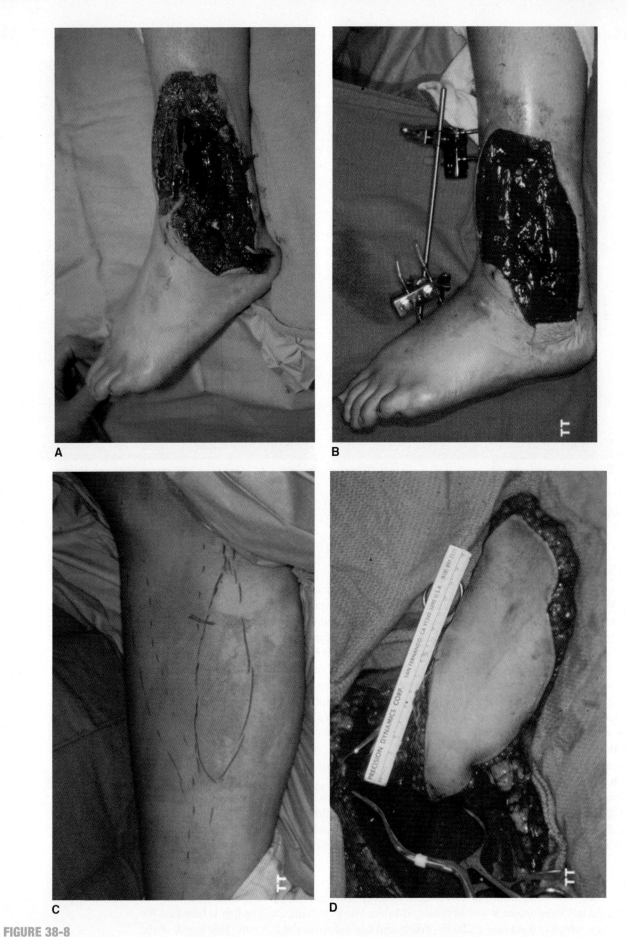

FIGURE 38-8

Gunshot wound to the distal leg-hindfoot. The defect is reconstructed with a free gracilis flap. **A:** Significant soft tissue and bony defects are present. **B:** Debridement and external fixation. **C:** A myocutaneous free gracilis flap is planned. **D:** The free flap is harvested.

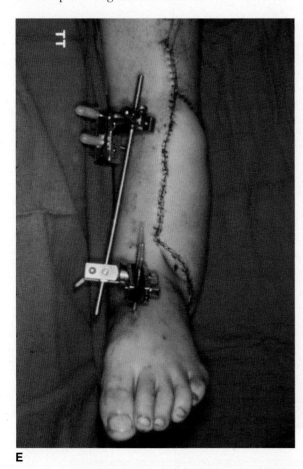

E

FIGURE 38-8 (*Continued*)
E: The flap is inset to the defect and revascularized.

basilic vein, or both. The flap can contain the lateral antebrachial cutaneous nerve or the medial antebrachial cutaneous nerve and then serve as a neurosensory flap. The size of the flap can be 10×40 cm^2.

A portion of the radius can be included as a vascularized bone with this flap. The advantages of this flap are a long pedicle and potential sensory innervation. The quality of the bone from the radius is mainly cortical and not of any substantial volume. Including the bone in the radial forearm flap may lead to stress fracture of the donor radius. Preliminary tissue expansion will increase the flap dimensions, and more importantly, it will allow direct closure of the donor defect (Fig. 38-9).

Scapular and Parascapular Flap

The scapular flap remains the workhorse of skin flaps. It is a thin, usually hairless, skin flap from the posterior chest and can be de-epithelialized and used as subcutaneous fascial flap, pedicled or free.

The flap is perfused by the cutaneous branches of the circumflex scapular artery (CSA) and drained by its venae comitantes. The CSA is the main branch of the subscapular artery and the main blood supply to the scapula, the muscles that attach to the scapula, and the overlying skin. The length of the pedicle is 5 cm, and the diameter of the artery is 2.5 mm. The vascular pattern of this territory makes it possible to raise multiple skin flaps on a single vascular pedicle or to harvest the lateral border of the scapula as an osteocutaneous flap for a complex reconstruction.

The cutaneous territory can be 20×7 cm^2 and can be divided in two components—a horizontal territory (horizontal scapular flap) and a vertical territory (parascapular flap)—based on the branches of the CSA after the vessel courses through the triangular space. Preliminary expansion of the territory of the scapular flap will increase the flap dimensions and permit direct donor site closure. This flap can be combined with other flaps based on subscapular blood supply and may greatly facilitate certain complex reconstructions. These include the latissimus dorsi and serratus anterior flaps, which can supply additional skin, muscle, and bone (rib) if necessary. The primary indication for the scapular flap is a defect requiring a relatively thin, large cutaneous flap. These kinds of defects

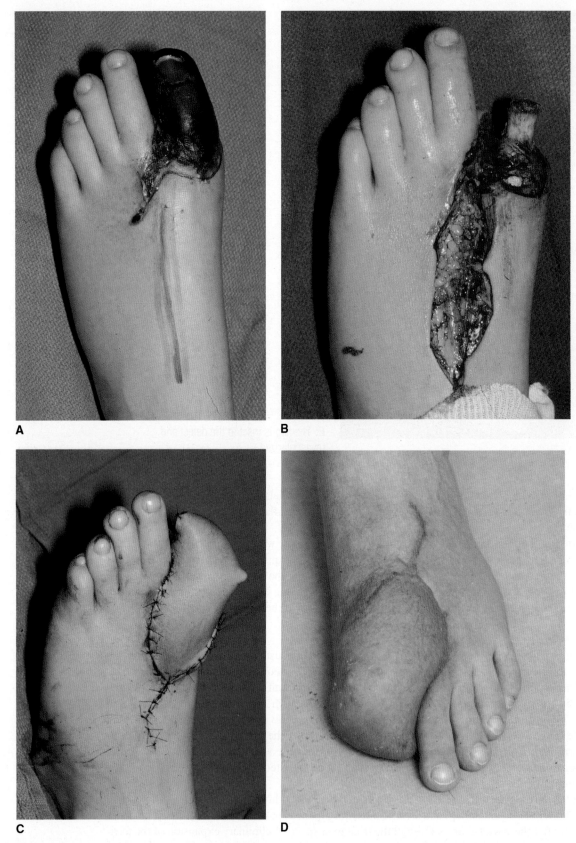

FIGURE 38-9

Posttraumatic left great toe necrosis. After debridement, the soft tissue defect is restored with a free radial forearm flap. **A:** Preoperative view. **B:** After debridement. **C:** Radial forearm flap is tailored to cover the exposed phalanx. **D, E:** Four weeks postoperative showing toe salvage and flap donor site.

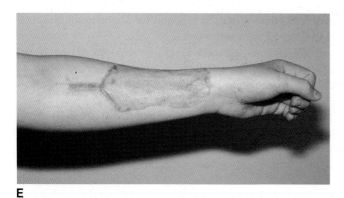

E   FIGURE 38-9 *(Continued)*

are often found in the foot. The osteoseptocutaneous free scapular flap reconstruction has been described in the lower extremity (Fig. 38-10).

Medial Geniculate Artery Flap

This flap is extremely versatile and has great application in foot and ankle surgery. In cases where there is need for small vascularized bone grafts, this flap is ideal. It can be harvested as a periosteal flap, corticocancellous flap, osteocutaneous flap, myo-oseteocutaneous flap, or an osteotendocutaneous flap. The skin paddle can be based on the saphenous artery system or as a perforator emanating

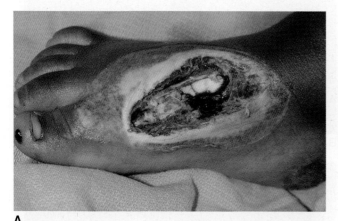

A

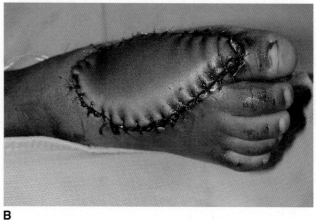

B

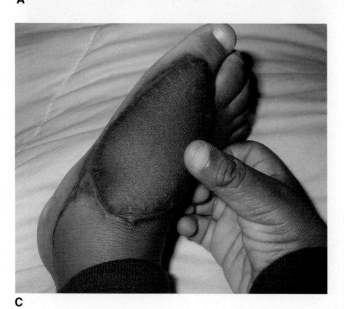

C

FIGURE 38-10

Dorsal foot avulsion injury in a pediatric patient after go-cart trauma. The dorsal aspect of the foot is reconstructed with a free scapular-parascapular flap. **A:** After debridement. **B:** Free scapular-parascapular flap is inset to the defect and revascularized. **C:** Two months postoperative view.

from the descending branch of the medial geniculate system. It is useful for treatment of avascular necrosis, subtalar nonunions, and failed or delayed ankle arthrodesis.

The vascularized bone, skin, muscle, and tendon (adductor longus tendon) are based on the descending medial geniculate system emanating from the deep femoral artery and femoral vein. On occasion, the blood supply for the vascularized bone originates from the superior geniculate artery posterior to the femoral condyle.

The flap is based on the specific soft tissue and bone needs of the reconstructive defect. It is best to harvest this as a "free-style" flap, that is, selection of bone and skin or other tissues is performed once the descending geniculate system is identified and the periosteal perforators to the medial femoral condyle have been identified. Subsequently, custom bone segments and skin islands can be harvested.

The flap is harvested under tourniquet control. The knee should be flexed and the medial collateral ligament is palpated at the level of the medial joint line. The medial femoral condyle is also palpated, as well as the patella medial border. For orientation, it is helpful to draw topical landmarks of the aforementioned structures (Fig. 38-11A). An incision is made over the midpoint of the medial femoral condyle and carried proximally over the vastus medialis muscle. The dissection is carried to the level of the vastus medialis fascia (Fig. 38-11B). The fascia is then divided over

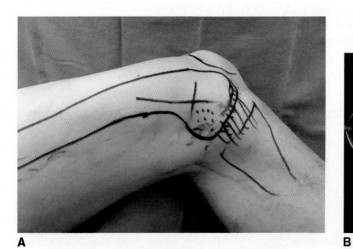

A

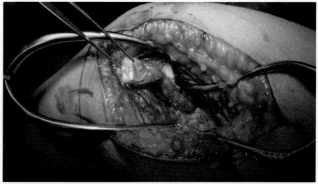

B

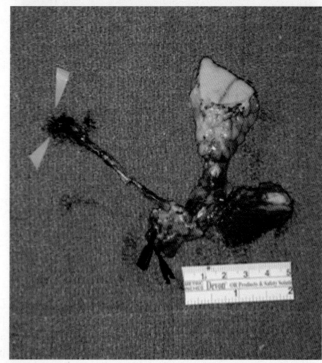

C

FIGURE 38-11

Medial geniculate artery flap. **A:** Anatomic landmarks. **B:** Surgical dissection. **C:** Artery and vein are included to maintain blood supply to the bone segment.

the condyle, and the muscle is reflected anteriorly. The adductor tendon is an important landmark. The descending geniculate artery travels within the sheath of the adductor tendon or just superior to it. The fascia over the medial femoral condyle is incised, and the perforating periosteal vessels are identified. It is easy to be confused by the looser fascia layer over the condyle and its rich blood supply, but this layer does not supply the bone to the medial femoral condyle. Once the condylar arcade is identified, the descending geniculate artery is traced from distal to proximal, taking care to preserve perforators to the anterior or posterior skin. A large diaphyseal vessel is identified approximately 6 to 10 cm proximal to the posterior femoral condyle. This branch must be divided in order to lengthen the pedicle. Dissection is carried proximally to the takeoff of the descending geniculate artery and vena comitantes from the femoral and artery and vein. The saphenous branch to the posterior thigh skin can be traced distally, and a separate skin paddle can be fabricated if required for soft tissue closure.

Removal of the bone can be done with osteotomes or a small power saw. The periosteum is cauterized several millimeters away from the bone. Osteotomes or a saw is then used to cut the bone based on defect dimensions. It is advisable to harvest a periosteal cuff proximally with the artery and vein to maintain blood supply to the bone segment (Fig. 38-11C). The bony defect is packed with gel foam or surgical and the overlying fascia closed. A drain is used during closure of the thigh.

POSTOPERATIVE MANAGEMENT

The success of a reconstructive foot surgery importantly relies on well-planned multidisciplinary postoperative management and rehabilitation. A non–weight-bearing regimen for at least 3 weeks is mandatory for every patient carrying plantar sutures. Elevation is required for 3 to 8 days after a local flap or a skin graft and for 2 to 3 weeks after a free flap. Heparin regimen is advisable while the patient is in the aforementioned bed rest phase. Elastic wraps may be useful in controlling edema once the patient's limb is permitted in a dependent position. Clinical findings should dictate the use of antibiotics.

The L'Enard splint (Fig. 38-12) is a useful tool to provide immobilization of the foot and ankle and in keeping the posterior heel off the bed. It is also useful when the patient begins non–weight-bearing ambulation with crutches. Local care of all weight-bearing surfaces is also recommended after suture removal, together with a frequent multidisciplinary follow-up that involves the plastic surgeon, the orthopedic surgeon, the podiatrist, and, if required, the prosthetist.

Postoperative care of free tissue transfer patients requires the patients to be adequately hydrated. Maintenance of proper body temperature and hematocrit is also important. Routine heparinization and anticoagulation are not used.

Flaps are usually monitored for a minimum of 5 days with a laser Doppler in addition to clinical observation. While the immediate postoperative period of 24 to 48 hours is critical, there have been occasional late failures; thus, laser Doppler monitoring should be continued for 4 or 5 days.

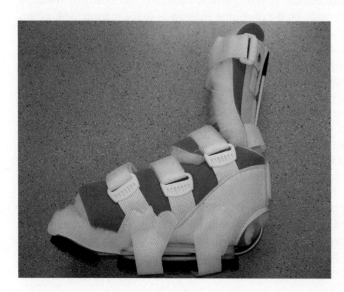

FIGURE 38-12
L'Enard splint.

COMPLICATIONS

Any flap failure requires a new detailed evaluation of the patient's local and general conditions before undertaking a new reconstruction. If a locoregional flap fails, and no other local option is available, the next step on the reconstructive ladder would be a free flap.

The success of free tissue transfer should be on the order of 95% to 99%. Acute complications usually occur in the first 48 hours and include venous thrombosis, arterial thrombosis, hematoma, hemorrhage, and excessive flap edema. Arterial insufficiency can be recognized by decreased capillary refill, pallor, reduced temperature, and the absence of bleeding after pinprick. This complication can be caused by arterial spasm, vessel plaque, torsion of the pedicle, pressure on the flap, technical error with injury to the pedicle, a flap harvested that is too large for its blood supply, or small vessel disease (due to smoking or diabetes). Management of arterial compromise requires prompt surgical intervention to restore the blood flow. Pharmacologic intervention at the time of exploration includes use of vasodilators, calcium channel blockers, and systemic anticoagulants for flap salvage presenting with arterial insufficiency. Ultimately, if these pharmacologic agents do not relieve spasm at the level of the arterial inflow, the anastomosis should be redone to rule out intra-arterial thrombus.

Venous outflow obstruction can be suspected when the flap has a violaceous color, brisk capillary refill, normal or elevated temperature, and production of dark blood after pinprick. Venous insufficiency can occur due to torsion of the pedicle, flap edema, hematoma, or tight closure of the tissue over the pedicle. The venous outflow obstruction can result in extravasation of red blood cells, endothelial breakdown, microvascular collapse, thrombosis in the microcirculation, and finally flap death. Given the irreversible nature of the microcirculatory changes in venous congestion that occur even after short periods of time, the surgeon must recognize venous compromise as early as possible.

These complications can occur alone or in any combination. The clinical observation and the monitoring of the patient (such as with laser Doppler) should alert the surgeon who has to decide between conservative and operative intervention. Conservative treatment may include drainage of the hematoma at the bedside with release of a few sutures to decrease pressure. In cases of venous congestion, leeches may be helpful if insufficient venous outflow cannot be established despite a patent venous anastomosis. The leeches inject a salivary component (hirudin) that inhibits both platelet aggregation and the coagulation cascade. The flap is decongested initially as the leech extracts blood and is further decongested as the bite wound oozes after the leech detaches.

The donor site should be given the same attention as the recipient site during the postoperative period. Complications of the donor site include hematoma, seroma, sensory nerve dysfunction, and scar formation.

Occasionally, free flaps, despite early return to the operating room for vascular compromise, do fail. Options for management include the performance of a second free tissue transfer, noting the technical or physiologic details that led to initial failure. Most of the time, free tissue transfers that fail are due to technical errors in judgment, whether they be flap harvest, compromise of the pedicle during the harvest, improper microvascular technique during anastomosis, improper insetting resulting in increased tissue tension and edema, or postoperative motion of the extremity resulting in pedicle avulsion. The next decision made by the operating surgeon as to the management of this patient is based on several factors. If a patient required a free flap in the first place, a second free flap should be considered. If a decision is made not to redo the flap, it could be left in place using the Crane principle to see if underlying granulation will be sufficient such that skin grafting can be performed once the necrotic flap is removed.

The Crane principle can be applied to cases where a local flap or free tissue transfer that necrotizes in part or totally acts as a biologic dressing or eschar over a wound bed. If there is no infection, the eschar can be left on the wound bed to see if some healing in the form of granulation occurs underneath it. Ultimately, the eschar is removed and the granulation bed skin grafted, obviating another free tissue transfer. If wound observation shows that such a bed is not produced, then a second flap must be considered.

It is usually our preference not to follow this course, as the flap can become a source of sepsis and further compromise local tissues. Necrotic nonviable flaps should be removed, and a temporary wound dressing such as an antibiotic bead pouch or wound vacuum-assisted closure (VAC) should be used. Occasionally, when flaps fail in a severely compromised extremity, consideration should be given to amputation. If a second free flap is considered, errors that lead to flap compromise need to be recognized and avoided. It may be prudent to obtain an arteriogram, evaluate the coagulation profile, and research other issues that might have led to failure.

PEARLS AND PITFALLS

- With any lower extremity reconstruction, three basic principles are of great importance and should therefore be carefully optimized before undertaking any reconstructive effort:
  - Evaluation of underlying skeletal architecture, stabilization, and management of associated orthopedic injuries
  - Adequate wound preparation, which includes full debridement and control of any local infection prior to coverage
  - Overall assessment of the patient's suitability for reconstruction and rehabilitation, including the opportunity of restoring some degree of protective sensation to the limb
- The majority of free tissue transfers require debulking and reinsetting for optimal shoewear. Patients should be informed about this phenomenon. An average of two or three additional outpatient procedures may be required.
- Diabetic and dysvascular patients are good candidates for limb salvage with local and free flaps. Complications and delayed wound healing may occur around flaps. Flap reconstruction requires adjunctive orthotics and possible bracing following soft tissue reconstruction. Failure to compensate for plantar resurfacing with inserts results in a higher breakdown of flaps despite successful transfer.
- Often a failure to recognize problems with wounds early results in the need for more complex salvage procedures, especially in Achilles repairs and calcaneal fracture ORIF through a lateral approach.
- Failed ankle arthrodesis is ideally treated with vascularized bone grafting as a salvage. Repeat fixation and nonvascularized graft have a high rate of failure in these cases.
- Salvage of exposed hardware is possible if treated early, and there is no evidence of gram-negative organisms in the wound cultures.

RECOMMENDED READING

Arnold PG, Yugueros P, Hanssen AD. Muscle flaps in osteomyelitis of the lower extremity: a 20-year account. *Plast Reconstr Surg.* 1999;104:107.

Attinger CE, Ducic I, Zelen C. The use of local muscle flaps in foot and ankle reconstruction. *Clin Podiatr Med Surg.* 2000;17(4):681.

Colen L, Uroskie T. Foot reconstruction. In: Mathes SJ, ed. *Plastic Surgery.* 2nd ed. Vol. 6. Philadelphia, PA: Elsevier; 2006.

Follmar KE, Baccarani A, Levin LS, et al. The distally based sural flap. *Plast Reconstr Surg.* 2007;119(6):138e–148e.

Fraccalvieri M, Verna G, Dolcet M. The distally based superficial sural flap: our experience in reconstructing the lower leg and the foot. *Ann Plast Surg.* 2000;45:132.

Heller L, Levin LS. Lower extremity microsurgical reconstruction. *Plast Reconstr Surg.* 2001;108:1029.

Koshima I, Narushima M, Mihara M, et al. Island medial plantar artery perforator flap for reconstruction of plantar defects. *Ann Plast Surg.* 2007;59(5):558–562.

Kuran I, Turgut G, Bas L, et al. Comparison between sensitive and nonsensitive free flaps in reconstruction of the heel and plantar area. *Plast Reconstr Surg.* 2000;105(2):574–580.

Levin LS. Foot and ankle soft-tissue deficiencies: who needs a flap? *Am J Orthop.* 2006;1:11–19.

Mourougayan V. Medial plantar artery (instep flap) flap. *Ann Plast Surg.* 2006;56(2):160–163.

Paget JT, Izadi D, Haj-Basheer M, et al. Donor site morbidity of the medial plantar artery flap studied with gait and pressure analysis. *Foot Ankle Surg.* 2015;21(1):60–66.

39 Soft Tissue Coverage of the Cervical and Thoracic Spine

Harvey Chim and Christopher J. Salgado

Soft tissue defects over the cervical and thoracic spine are difficult problems for the reconstructive surgeon. These wounds most often result following spinal surgery. They can also develop from other etiologies such as pressure ulcers or trauma. Conditions such as osteomyelitis, radiation therapy, and previous spinal surgery can all predispose the patient to wound dehiscence and breakdown. These cases are often surgical emergencies as spinal hardware and the spinal cord can all be exposed at the base of the wound; in these cases, urgent soft tissue coverage is required to prevent infection and loss of neurologic function.

INDICATIONS/CONTRAINDICATIONS

Risk factors for wound dehiscence include smoking, alcohol abuse, advanced age, diabetes, obesity, malnutrition, radiation to the spine, use of corticosteroids, and prolonged hospitalization. In these cases, prophylactic coverage of the spinal and paraspinal incisions with a well-vascularized flap has been shown to result in a lower incidence of major wound complications. Providing prophylactic soft tissue coverage can aid in healing and minimize major complications when difficult wound closure is anticipated. This is particularly useful in patients who have had previous radiation therapy, chemotherapy, or previous failed surgeries. While not a strong indication, patient with comorbidities such as diabetes who are at increased risk of infection may also be considered for prophylactic wound coverage. In cases where there has been extensive resection of bone or soft tissue, muscle flaps may be useful to fill the space and decrease risk of seroma and infection. A systematic review of the literature by Chieng et al. showed that patients who had undergone placement of extensive spinal instrumentation or had prior radiation exposure, positive smoking history, or diabetes mellitus were all at risk for spinal wound complications requiring flap coverage. The mean time interval from the index spine surgery to flap reconstruction was 4.7 months.

In the cervical and thoracic spine, the most common reconstructive options are local muscle or musculocutaneous flaps. Muscle flaps have been shown to actively inhibit bacterial growth in both moderate and minimally contaminated wounds. Calderon and colleagues demonstrated that obliteration of dead space contributed to a marked decrease in the bacterial concentration within wounds;

this was a result of higher collagen and hydroxyproline content within the wound bed, ultimately decreasing the space in which bacteria could proliferate.

PREOPERATIVE PLANNING

Patient Optimization

Before initial surgery and after the index surgery, several measures can be taken to decrease the likelihood of wound complications:

- Waiting the appropriate amount of time (3 to 4 weeks) between the index surgery and postoperative radiation therapy. The importance of wound healing before starting radiation therapy cannot be overemphasized.
- Maximizing the patient's nutritional status. Albumin and prealbumin should be routinely checked to monitor for signs of a positive protein balance.
- Use of vitamin A to help counteract the detrimental effects of steroid use on wound healing.
- Use of minimally invasive techniques for spinal reconstruction, such as percutaneous pedicle screws or minimally invasive lateral approaches for corpectomy, can decrease the need for long incisions in high-risk patients.
- Prophylactic antibiotics should be given to patients who carry high risk of developing infection.

Vacuum-assisted closure (VAC) technology can play a role in closure of an open wound by reducing dead space and hence reducing complications such as seroma or hematoma. A VAC dressing placed over the incision of a closed wound up to postoperative day 3 has been shown to improve outcomes by removing excess subcutaneous fluid, improving blood flow, and increasing granulation formation. Other postoperative preventative measures in high-risk patients include hyperbaric oxygen therapy, which may be employed to increase oxygen tension at the surgical site, augmenting bactericidal activity, and stimulation of angiogenesis in irradiated tissue. A reduction in the infection rate of complex wounds following scoliosis surgery has been shown through the use of hyperbaric oxygen prophylaxis. Finally, intraoperative local administration of vancomycin powder before closure has proved to be protective in decreasing incidence of surgical site infection (SSI). A meta-analysis of 5,102 patients by Khan et al. demonstrated robust relative risk reduction of 68% in developing SSI, especially in the instrumentation group following vancomycin administration.

In patients where there is no alternative to flap reconstruction, patients should have their nutrition optimized and comorbidities, such as smoking and diabetes mellitus, under control before undergoing reconstruction. Albumin should be greater than 2.0 and prealbumin greater than 20. Ideally, the wound bed should be clean and granulating, with no evidence of active infection. Exposed hardware that may harbor biofilm may be switched out for new hardware at the time of flap coverage if possible.

Wound Preparation

Optimization of the wound is vital before definitive soft tissue coverage. Stahl et al. described a four-pillar concept of debridement in which four columns of support need to preserved, with loss of two or more pillars resulting in spinal deformity. These columns are defined as the paravertebral musculature, posterior elements and their related ligaments, the facet joints and their surrounding ligaments, and finally the anterior vertebral column. Preservation of columnar support influences the decision to retain or remove exposed hardware. In different studies, hardware removal rates following wound complications have ranged from 0% to 41.9%. Reasons for removal of hardware included development of severe hematoma, infection, seroma, and dehiscence. In addition to removal of grossly loose or infected hardware, the wound should be debrided of any necrotic material. This may require multiple operative debridements with removal of all marginal tissue. Cultures should be obtained to optimize coverage with broad-spectrum antibiotics, which may be required for infected wounds, even after flap coverage.

SURGICAL ALGORITHM AND FLAP OPTIONS

Small defects over the spine may be covered with the paraspinal muscle, which may be used in either an advancement or a turnover fashion. Alternatively, for small defects with no exposed hardware, local fasciocutaneous flaps can also be used for wound coverage. For larger defects in the cervical spine, the trapezius muscle flap is a useful option. Alternatively, an ante grade latissimus dorsi muscle flap based on the thoracodorsal vessels can be used for coverage of defects in the lower cervical and upper thoracic spine. For defects in the mid to lower thoracic spine, a turnover latissimus dorsi flap based on paraspinal segmental perforators from the intercostal arteries provides adequate tissue to cover exposed hardware. For defects in the thoracic and lumbar spine where other options are not available, an omental flap passed through the abdominal wall or free flaps are also options for reconstruction.

TRAPEZIUS FLAP

Anatomy

The trapezius is a large broad and flat triangular muscle in the upper back. It is particularly useful for coverage of cervical spine defects. Its dominant pedicle is the transverse cervical artery. This arises from the thyrocervical trunk or occasionally directly from the subclavian artery. The dorsal scapular artery or deep branch or the transverse cervical artery is a minor pedicle that perforates the rhomboid muscle and enters the distal segment of the trapezius muscle. Preservation of this branch is important if a large skin paddle is harvested extending caudally beyond the boundary of the trapezius muscle. The muscle measures 34 × 18 cm, and a skin paddle up to 10 cm in width can be harvested and still allow primary closure.

Patient Positioning

The patient is positioned in the prone position. Flap harvest is performed under general anesthesia.

Technique

The trapezius can be harvested as a muscle-only flap or a myocutaneous flap. For a muscle-only flap (Fig. 39-1), surgical access is made either through the previous midline spinal wound or through a paramedian incision centered directly over the muscle. A line from T12 to the acromion marks the lateral boundary of the trapezius muscle. After the incision is made, wide undermining of skin and subcutaneous tissue is performed over the trapezius, which is the most superficial muscle in the medial upper back. The origin of the trapezius is released off the spinous processes in a caudal to cephalic direction. Then the muscle is divided lateral to its pedicle, which runs inferiorly on the undersurface of the muscle. This allows the trapezius to be either flipped over or rotated to cover a cervical spine defect.

For a myocutaneous flap, a skin paddle measuring up to 10 cm in width can be harvested and still allow primary skin closure. After incision is made around the skin paddle, elevation of the flap proceeds in a caudal to cephalic direction. If an extended skin paddle is design reaching beyond the caudal border of the trapezius muscle, the dorsal scapular artery perforator, which penetrates through the rhomboid muscle to supply the trapezius, should be included in the flap and preserved.

Preservation of the superior fibers of the trapezius helps to minimize functional impairment from shoulder weakness.

ANTEGRADE LATISSIMUS DORSI FLAP

Anatomy

The latissimus dorsi is a large flat muscle covering most of the posterior trunk. It originates from the spinous processes of the lower six thoracic and lumbar vertebrae, thoracolumbar fascia, iliac crest, inferior three ribs and inferior angle of the scapula, and inserts onto the medial lip of the bicipital groove of the humerus. Its dominant pedicle is the thoracodorsal artery (Fig. 39-2), which arises from the subscapular artery. Minor pedicles arise from the segmental paraspinal perforators from the posterior intercostal arteries and perforators from the lumbar arteries. As it is a type V muscle, the flap can be based off its dominant pedicle or minor pedicles as a turnover flap. A flap based in antegrade fashion off the thoracodorsal artery is useful for covering lower cervical and upper thoracic spine wounds.

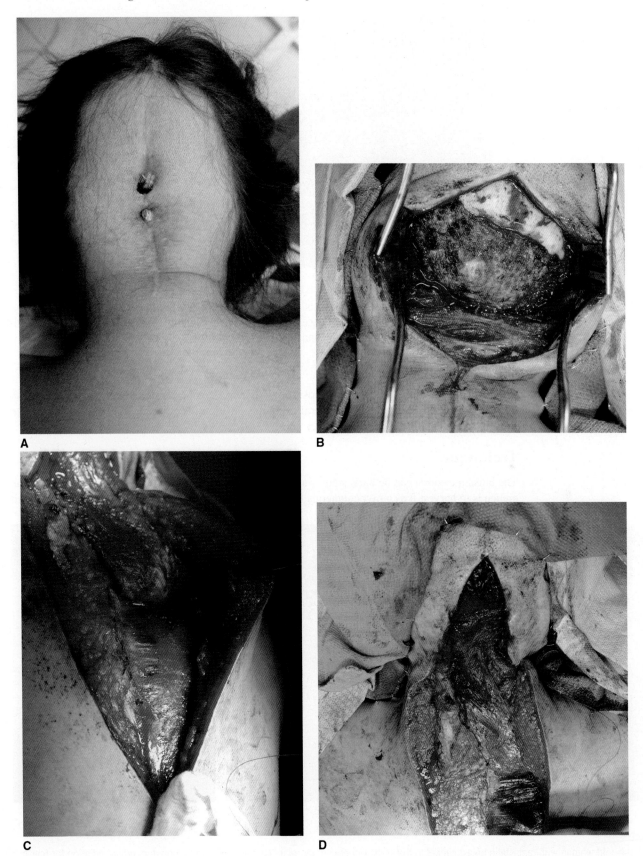

FIGURE 39-1

A: A 28-year-old woman presented with a nonhealing wound and draining sinus after an occipital craniectomy and coverage with titanium mesh. **B:** Removal of titanium mesh resulted in an area of exposed dura. **C, D:** A muscle-only trapezius flap was elevated through a midline incision and turned over to cover the exposed dura.

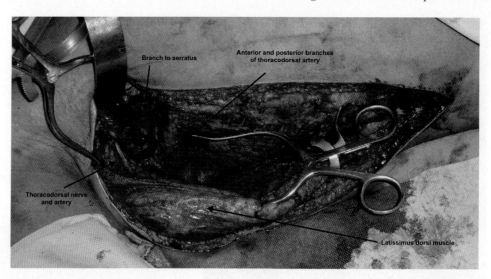

FIGURE 39-2

The latissimus dorsi muscle has been exposed through an anterior approach. The thoracodorsal artery and nerve can be seen running on the deep surface of the latissimus dorsi muscle, before giving off a branch to the serratus anterior and dividing into anterior and posterior branches.

Patient Positioning

The patient is positioned in the prone position. Flap harvest is performed under general anesthesia. The flap can also be harvested in a lateral decubitus position for other indications, but this is often not conducive to spinal wound coverage.

Technique

The latissimus dorsi can be harvested as a muscle-only or myocutaneous flap (Fig. 39-3). Our preference is to harvest it as a myocutaneous flap. In this fashion, a skin paddle prevents tension on the

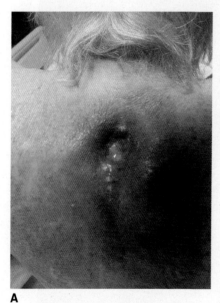
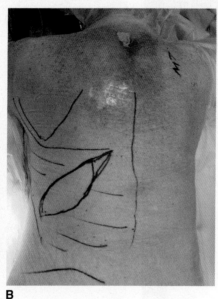
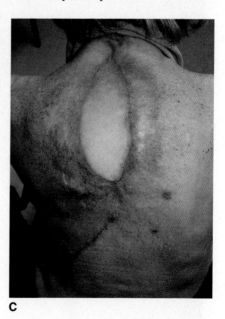

A   B   C

FIGURE 39-3

A 70-year-old woman with metastatic breast cancer to the spine underwent thoracic laminectomy and had postoperative radiation for 5 weeks. **A:** She developed progressive thoracic kyphosis and a nonhealing infected open wound over the lower cervical and upper thoracic spine with extensive radiation dermatitis around the wound. Six months after the initial surgery, she underwent revision C7-T4 laminectomy and a C7 to T7 fusion. Coverage was performed with a pedicled myocutaneous latissimus dorsi flap based on the thoracodorsal vessels. **B:** An oblique skin paddle was designed to facilitate rotation into the spinal wound. **C:** Eight weeks postoperatively, the wound is well healed.

posterior midline closure and also provides additional padding for spinal instrumentation, if present. The skin paddle is designed obliquely to allow rotation over the defect.

Incision is made around the skin island. Then dissection is carried over the muscle circumferentially, raising skin and subcutaneous fat flaps until the boundaries of the muscle are reached. The flap is then divided from its attachments circumferentially. This can be done in a number of ways. Our preference is to identify the superior border of the latissimus muscle below the angle of the scapula first, as this area is always well defined. Then the superomedial tendinous origin of the latissimus muscle is identified, which is typically under the inferior trapezius muscle fibers, which are preserved. Dissection then continues caudally, detaching the trapezius from its medial and then caudal attachments to the iliac crest before proceeding anteriorly to elevate the latissimus muscle from a caudal to cephalic direction. Care should be taken to separate the latissimus from the serratus posterior inferolaterally and the serratus anterior laterally, where it is very easy to enter the wrong plane deep to the serratus.

Dissection then proceeds cephalically to the axilla until the muscle is completely free of all attachments except its insertion into the humerus. It is not usually necessary to identify the thoracodorsal artery and nerve or to disinsert the latissimus from its insertion into the humerus for pedicled flap coverage of spinal wounds. However, disinserting the latissimus can increase the arc of rotation if this is required. A subcutaneous tunnel is then created between the donor site and the spinal wound to pass the flap to the midline. The donor site is closed in layers over closed suction drainage.

TURNOVER LATISSIMUS DORSI FLAP

Anatomy

The latissimus dorsi can also be harvested as a turnover flap based on perforators from the posterior intercostal arteries and lumbar arteries. These arise within 4 to 6 cm from the midline. The turnover latissimus dorsi flap can be used to cover mid to lower thoracic and upper lumbar spine defects.

Patient Positioning

The patient is positioned in the prone position. Flap harvest is performed under general anesthesia.

Technique

The flap can be harvested as a muscle-only or myocutaneous flap. If a skin paddle is included with the flap, this is positioned over the superior third of the muscle. A muscle-only flap allows more reach and flexibility in insetting of the flaps in the spinal wound. The latissimus muscle can be approached medially through the spinal wound. For access to the thoracodorsal pedicle, an anterior counter incision (Fig. 39-4) is needed. Alternatively, transverse incisions can be made, extending laterally from the midline wound (Fig. 39-5).

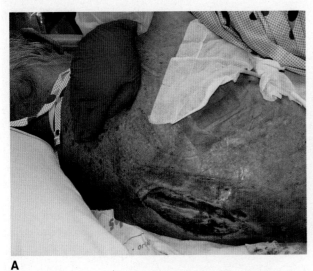
A

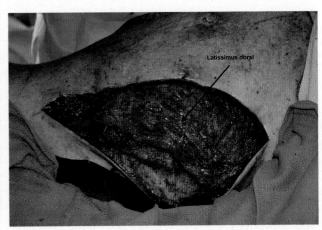
B

FIGURE 39-4

A: A 69-year-old man developed complications following abdominal surgery, with a pressure ulcer over the mid to lower thoracic spine and exposed spinous processes. **B:** The latissimus dorsi muscle was elevated through the midline wound, with an anterior counterincision.

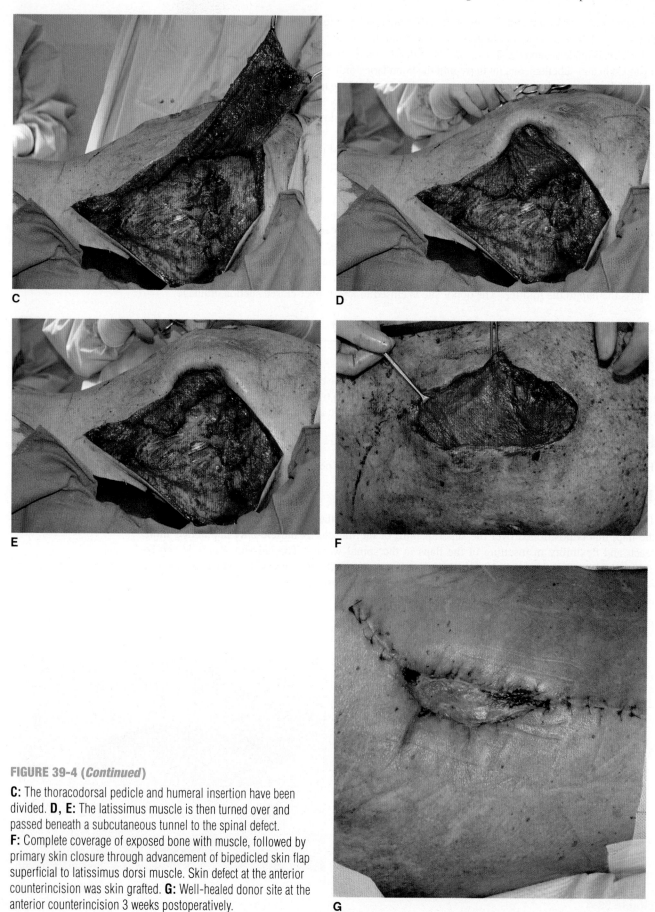

FIGURE 39-4 (Continued)

C: The thoracodorsal pedicle and humeral insertion have been divided. **D, E:** The latissimus muscle is then turned over and passed beneath a subcutaneous tunnel to the spinal defect.
F: Complete coverage of exposed bone with muscle, followed by primary skin closure through advancement of bipedicled skin flap superficial to latissimus dorsi muscle. Skin defect at the anterior counterincision was skin grafted. **G:** Well-healed donor site at the anterior counterincision 3 weeks postoperatively.

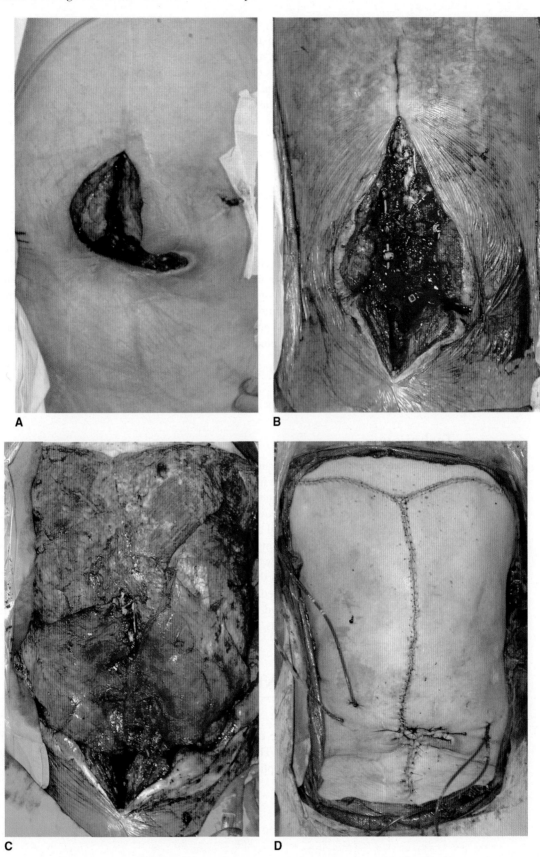

FIGURE 39-5

A: A 54-year-old male paraplegic developed an open wound and exposed hardware in the lower thoracic and upper lumbar region following T12 to L4 fusion. He was brought to the operating room for a T10 to iliac crest fusion after developing spinal dislocation at the L2 to L3 level. **B:** Wound after placement of hardware. Transverse incisions were made extending laterally from the cephalic margin of the spinal wound for access to the latissimus dorsi muscles bilaterally. **C:** These were turned over to cover exposed hardware. **D:** Skin closed primarily.

Unilateral or bilateral latissimus dorsi turnover flaps can be elevated, based on the extent of the spinal defect. Dissection is carried over the muscle circumferentially, raising skin and subcutaneous fat flaps until the boundaries of the muscle are reached. Then the thoracodorsal pedicle and nerve are identified and divided, as well as the insertion of the latissimus into the humerus. The muscle is then elevated from a lateral to medial direction, care taken to preserve perforators near the midline. Elevation of the muscle should stop at a distance of 6 cm from the midline or when large perforators are identified. This will maximize perfusion to the muscle. The muscle is then turned over and inset into the spinal wound. Skin can be closed primarily or by advancing a bipedicle advancement flap and back grafting the donor site (see Fig. 39-4G).

PARASPINAL MUSCLE FLAPS

Anatomy

The paraspinal muscles consist of a complex of muscles on either side of the spinous processes extending from the occiput to the sacrum. They consist of the semispinalis and longissimus muscles in the cervical, thoracic, and lumbar areas and the multifidus in the lower thoracic and lumbar areas. Blood supply to these muscles is segmental, with the dominant pedicles being segmental medial perforators arising from the posterior intercostal arteries and minor pedicles consisting of a lateral row of perforators arising from the posterior intercostal arteries. Paraspinal muscle flaps are useful for closing narrow midline spine defects with minimal skin deficit.

Patient Positioning

The patient is positioned in the prone position. Flap harvest is performed under general anesthesia.

Technique

The paraspinal muscles can be elevated bilaterally to cover exposed hardware in the spine. Access is typically through an open midline incision, which has broken down or been used for spinal instrumentation. The incision can be extended cephalically or caudally as needed to provide more muscle exposure beyond the wound. Dissection is carried superficial to the paraspinal muscles for a distance of 6 to 8 cm laterally. In the cervical and thoracic regions, the trapezius and latissimus muscles can be elevated together with the overlying skin, superficial to the paraspinal muscles, to preserve perfusion from perforators and facilitate wound healing.

The fascia is incised 6 cm from the midline to allow access to the lateral border of the paraspinal muscles, which are mobilized. The paraspinal muscles can then be advanced and brought together in the midline and sutured to cover exposed hardware. Our preference is to use interrupted figure of eight 0 PDS sutures. The skin can usually be closed primarily over the paraspinal muscles.

LOCAL FASCIOCUTANEOUS FLAPS

Anatomy

Local fasciocutaneous flaps can be elevated either as random flaps or based on perforators in a keystone or propeller-type fashion. These types of flaps should be limited to small wounds with no exposed hardware or where other options are not available.

Patient Positioning

The patient is positioned in the prone position. Flap harvest is performed under general anesthesia.

Technique

Local flaps are elevated in a subfascial plane and used to cover a defect anywhere along the spine. Small superficial wounds are the ideal indication for this technique. An example is a Z-plasty (Fig. 39-6).

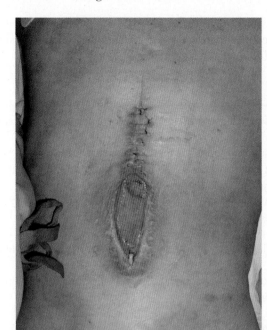
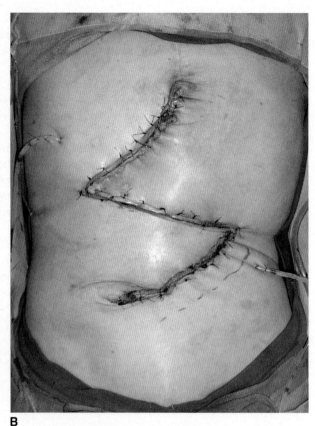

A   **B**

FIGURE 39-6

A: Lower thoracic wound with osteomyelitis of a spinous process and otherwise well-granulating wound. **B:** Coverage with Z-plasty.

POSTOPERATIVE MANAGEMENT

Perhaps the most important measure to prevent wound healing problems is to avoid pressure on the flap and wound after soft tissue coverage. Nursing care is vital to ensure that patients are turned from side to side to avoid pressure on the spine wound. A low-air-loss mattress is very useful to prevent pressure on the wound during the first 3 to 4 weeks following surgery. Nutritional optimization is also important, to help with wound healing. Finally, long-term antibiotics may be required if intraoperative cultures are positive for bacterial or fungal growth.

RESULTS

In a systematic review of the literature on flap coverage after spinal surgery by Chieng and colleagues noted that the most common flaps used for spinal coverage were the paraspinal muscle flaps in 56% of cases, followed by the latissimus muscle (19%) and trapezius muscle (15%) flaps. Forty-five percent of the flaps were used for coverage of defects within the thoracic spine, while the 36% and 19% were used for coverage of the lumbar and cervical levels, respectively. For defects involving the lumbosacral region, gluteal flaps were most commonly used followed by paraspinal muscle flaps. At the thoracic level, the latissimus dorsi flap and paraspinal muscle flaps were most commonly used. At the cervical level, paraspinal muscle flaps were most commonly used, followed by latissimus and trapezius flaps. Within this series, spinal hardware was successfully salvaged with flap coverage in the majority of patients, with the rate of hardware removal ranging from 0% to 41.9% in patients with instrumentation.

COMPLICATIONS

In a study by Chieng, complications following flap placement for coverage of spinal hardware included wound infection, wound dehiscence, reoperation, seroma, hematoma, hardware exposure, and cerebrospinal fluid (CSF) leak; however, these complications were not directly related to flap placement. Skin necrosis has been reported after paraspinal flap or latissimus dorsi flap coverage; however, all wounds were treated successfully with skin grafting.

PEARLS AND PITFALLS

- Elevation of the trapezius should preserve the superior fibers to minimize morbidity from shoulder weakness.
- During dissection of the latissimus muscle, care must be taken to separate the trapezius from the latissimus medially and to separate the latissimus from the serratus anterior laterally. It is very easy to carry dissection in the wrong plane deep to the serratus.
- Seromas in the back following latissimus harvest are common. These can be prevented by placing two large drains in the back and leaving these in place until there is minimal drainage or by using quilting sutures.
- Secure suturing of paraspinal muscle flaps in the midline is essential for complete coverage of exposed hardware.
- Avoidance of pressure on spinal wounds after flap coverage may be the single most important preventable measure to avoid wound complications.

RECOMMENDED READING

Adogwa O, Fatemi P, Perez E, et al. Negative pressure wound therapy reduces incidence of postoperative wound infection and dehiscence after long-segment thoracolumbar spinal fusion: a single institutional experience. *Spine J.* 2014:14;2911–2917.
Calderon W, Chang N, Mathes SJ. Comparison of the effect of bacterial inoculation in musculocutaneous and fasciocutaneous flaps. *Plast Reconstr Surg.* 1986;77:785–794.
Chieng LO, Hubbard Z, Salgado CJ, et al. Reconstruction of open wounds as a complication of spinal surgery with flaps: a systematic review. *Neurosurg Focus.* 2015;39(4):E17.
Chun JK, Lynch MJ, Poultsides GA. Distal trapezius musculocutaneous flap for upper thoracic back wounds associated with spinal instrumentation and radiation. *Ann Plast Surg.* 2003;51:17–22.
Garvey PB, Rhines LD, Dong W, Chang DW. Immediate soft-tissue reconstruction for complex defects of the spine following surgery for spinal neoplasms. *Plast Reconstr Surg.* 2010;125:1460–1466.
Hultman CS, Jones GE, Losken A, et al. Salvage of infected spinal hardware with paraspinous muscle flaps: anatomic considerations with clinical correlation. *Ann Plast Surg.* 2006;57:521–528.
Inanmaz ME, Kose KC, Isik C, et al. Can hyperbaric oxygen be used to prevent deep infections in neuro-muscular scoliosis surgery? *BMC Surg.* 2014;14:85.
Khan NR, Thompson CJ, DeCuypere M, et al. A meta-analysis of spinal surgical site infection and vancomycin powder. *J Neurosurg Spine.* 2014;21:974–983.
Mericli AF, Tarola NA, Moore JH Jr, et al. Paraspinous muscle flap reconstruction of complex midline back wounds: risk factors and postreconstruction complications. *Ann Plast Surg.* 2010;65:219–224.
O'Shaughnessy BA, Dumanian GA, Liu JC, et al. Pedicled omental flaps as an adjunct in the closure of complex spinal wounds. *Spine (Phila Pa 1976).* 2007;32:3074–3080.
Stahl RS, Burstein FD, Lieponis JV, et al. Extensive wounds of the spine: a comprehensive approach to debridement and reconstruction. *Plast Reconstr Surg.* 1990;85:747–753.

40 Soft Tissue Coverage of the Pelvis and Sacrum: Hemipelvectomy and Pedicled Flap Coverage

Matt T. Houdek, Peter S. Rose, Franklin H. Sim, and Steven L. Moran

Extensive defects of the pelvis and sacrum can result from tumors, ablation, and severe trauma. Because of the limited amounts and relative immobility of the pelvic soft tissue, these defects may pose a serious reconstructive challenge. Until the late 1970s, most large pelvic tumors were treated with external hemipelvectomy. Advances in imaging, chemotherapy, and radiation therapy, as well as improvements in resection and reconstructive techniques, have greatly reduced the need for radical lower extremity amputations, allowing limb preservation in a majority of cases.

Historically, buttock tumors were not amenable to a classic hemipelvectomy and just a few decades ago were considered unresectable. Likewise, extensive buttock defects inflicted by trauma, infection, or end-stage pressure ulcers in paraplegics could not be effectively reconstructed. Secondary intention healing frequently resulted in protracted hospital course, extensive scarring, contractures, and unstable soft tissue coverage. Many of these patients were bound to years of ongoing wound care and immobility.

External hemipelvectomy denotes removal of the hemipelvis with affected lower extremity by disarticulation of the pubic symphysis and the sacroiliac joint. Because external hemipelvectomy resulted in major functional impairment, limb-sparing procedures removing part or all innominate bone with preservation of the extremity have been advocated. These pelvic resections are referred to as internal hemipelvectomies.

Large, composite pelvic defects associated with internal hemipelvectomies are more challenging to reconstruct than the soft tissue defect typically created in external hemipelvectomy patients for two main reasons. First, following removal of the bony hemipelvis in external hemipelvectomy, a large amount of soft tissue of the buttock or proximal thigh becomes available for reconstruction. Second, a decrease of the pelvic volume obliterates the dead space.

Sacral resections may be performed as a part of extended external hemipelvectomy for musculoskeletal sarcomas and, as such, reconstructed as a part of hemipelvectomy closure. Isolated sacral defects result from composite pelvic resections for locally advanced anal and rectal malignancies or tumors intrinsic to the sacrum such as sacral chordomas and sarcomas.

INDICATIONS/CONTRAINDICATIONS

When embarking on treatment of pelvic sarcomas, three important questions should be borne in mind.

1. Is this patient operable, that is, can the individual medically withstand a major oncologic resection?
2. Is this tumor resectable, that is, can this patient be rendered disease-free surgically?
3. Can the residual defect or deformity from the proposed resection be reconstructed in a functionally satisfactorily manner with stable soft tissue coverage?

TABLE 40-1   Basic Tumor Flap Principles
● Safe oncologic margins are the primary requirement ● Reconstruction does not take precedence over adequate, safe resection ● Adequate soft tissue coverage of bony reconstruction/prosthesis and neurovascular structures ● Healed surgical wound ● Durable ● Minimal donor morbidity ● Appropriate function, contour

The answers to these questions have to be determined during preoperative evaluation by the surgical oncologist, reconstructive surgeon, and anesthesiologist. Resection of the tumor with negative margins is the only reliable means of obtaining a cure in cases of tumor.

Internal hemipelvectomy is indicated in cases of localized tumor where margin negative resection of the tumor is possible with preservation of the lower extremity with function greater than the patient would experience with an amputation. The three critical structures that define lower extremity function are the hip joint, the lumbosacral plexus/sciatic nerve, and the external iliac vessels/femoral nerve. In practice, if two of these three structures can be saved and the tumor removed with a negative margin, the patient will generally experience greater ultimate function (and equivalent survival) with an internal hemipelvectomy. If two or three of these structures require resection, limb salvage function is generally inferior to function following amputation, and external hemipelvectomy is indicated. As well, tumors large enough to involve two or three of these critical structures usually are so large that the bulk of an amputation flap is needed for proper closure. If clean margins cannot be achieved, external hemipelvectomy should be performed. Main indications for external hemipelvectomy are large tumors involving multiple compartments unresponsive to neoadjuvant therapies, contamination of compartments from pathologic fracture, or failed previous resection, a nonviable extremity. Nononcologic external hemipelvectomy may be performed in the cases of uncontrolled pelvic osteomyelitis, traumatic hemorrhage, and failed aortofemoral revascularizations (Table 40-1).

Wound complication rates following hemipelvectomy are notoriously high and have been reported to range from 20% to 80%. Proper technical execution of the procedure and the use of well-designed skin and muscle flaps can minimize postoperative wound morbidity.

Although infrequently, pelvic and sacral resections are performed en bloc with pelvic visceral structures for locally advanced rectal and gynecologic malignancies eroding or invading the skeletal pelvis. When such pelvic resection involves removal of a part of the pelvis or sacrum, it is referred to as *composite resection*. Any type of external hemipelvectomy performed in continuity with visceral structures is known as *compound hemipelvectomy*. Due to the aggressive nature of these tumors, the disease has to be limited to the pelvis, and extensive imaging is required to select the patients who can benefit from these extensive operations.

Primary sacral tumors such as chordomas and sarcomas are relatively uncommon. These tumors generally will pose progressive symptoms of pelvic outlet obstruction with rectal and urinary obstruction as well as venous thrombosis without local control. Reconstruction of these defects with flaps facilitates optimal postoperative wound healing.

PREOPERATIVE PLANNING

Prior to surgical resection, patients should undergo local and systemic staging studies. Musculoskeletal malignancies have a propensity to pulmonary spread. Therefore, a chest CT is mandatory to screen for systemic disease. An MRI (and plain radiographs for primary bone tumors) is sufficient for gauging the local extent of disease and response to treatment. A CT of the pelvis is often useful to complement the MRI as this area is difficult to image; a useful protocol is to give a bolus of IV contrast and then image in the arterial, venous, and excretory phases to allow full imaging of the vascular structures and ureters prior to resection. This will also help detect any regional lymphadenopathy. Likewise, MRI is useful to determine if there is vascular invasion or if the tumor abuts vascular structures, which would need to be sacrificed. Surgical planning relies on MRI images taken before and after neoadjuvant therapies. Pretreatment MRI images may be helpful in distinguishing radiation-induced reactive changes from actual tumor tissue.

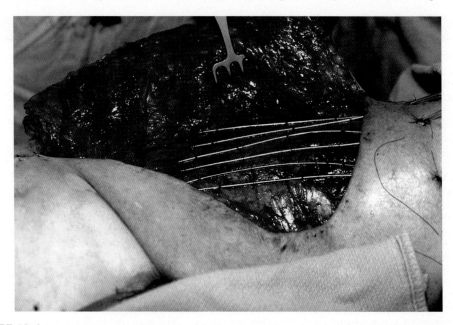

FIGURE 40-1

Placement of afterloading brachytherapy catheters under inferiorly based TRAM flap in treatment of recurrent sarcoma of the thigh.

Most patients with high-grade bone malignancies will undergo some form of neoadjuvant treatment, including chemotherapy and/or radiation therapy prior to tumor resection. Typically, primary bone sarcomas such as osteosarcoma are treated with several cycles of preoperative chemotherapy, surgery, and then several additional cycles of chemotherapy. Radiation therapy also has an established role in treatment of soft tissue sarcomas. Note that the time to resumption of postoperative chemotherapy has prognostic significance for patient survival in some malignancies, highlighting the importance of good initial flap coverage to minimize healing delays.

The treatment team must choose between pre- and postoperative radiation therapy. Both approaches have advantages and shortcomings. Preoperative treatment requires a smaller area of treatment, creation of a fibrous rind around the tumor, and often causes tumor shrinkage, leading to an improved ability to obtain wide margins without sacrificing vital structures. Preoperative radiation's disadvantages include a higher rate of wound problems and less viable tumors available for pathologic examination. Postoperative radiation has the advantage of earlier surgery, viable tumors for pathologic study, and fewer wound complications. Treatment volumes, however, are increased, and there is a delay in administering treatment to allow time for adequate healing of operative wounds. We prefer preoperative radiation for most pelvic and retroperitoneal sarcomas.

Brachytherapy requires proper reconstruction planning so that flaps do not interfere with catheter placement (Fig. 40-1). After loading, catheters should be evenly spaced and sutured in place to the tumor bed with fast absorbable sutures to prevent their displacement during postoperative therapy. Alternatively, VAC dressing can be used as a temporary coverage of brachytherapy catheters, followed by delayed primary reconstruction of the defect after completion of brachytherapy. Intraoperative radiation therapy is another means of augmenting a preoperative radiation therapy regimen, allowing for directed treatment at close intraoperative margins.

Preoperatively, the patients with large pelvic tumor undergo mechanical bowel preparation and intravenous antibiotic coverage. Ostomy sites must be preoperatively marked in accordance with anticipated flap use because inappropriate colostomy or ileostomy placement may burn an important reconstructive bridge and prevent rectus abdominis flap elevation. Involvement of several surgical services such as urological, colorectal, vascular, spine, and plastic surgery is common. Large-bore intravenous access is established in an event of rapid blood loss. We liberally use ureteral stents that facilitate intraoperative identification of the ureters. After placement of the stents and Foley catheter, the patient is placed in the rolling lateral decubitus position; this allows access to full abdominal compartment in a nearly supine orientation as well as access to the posterior pelvis and sacrum. This position is preferred for internal or external hemipelvectomy because it permits a wide

TABLE 40-2 Principles of Pelvic Reconstruction
● Routine use of preoperatively placed ureteral stents aids in the identification of ureters intraoperatively.
● Patients should receive both antibiotic and mechanical bowel prep.
● Standard hemipelvectomy flaps provide adequate soft tissue coverage, and there is no difference in postoperative wound complications related to flap design.
● Abdominal and pelvic wall reconstruction is not necessary if the muscle with its investing fascia is a component of an external hemipelvectomy flap, but the abdominal wall should be reconstructed in cases of internal hemipelvectomy.
● Omentum should be interposed between the intestine and hemipelvectomy flap whenever possible to wall off intra-abdominal contents in the event of hemipelvectomy flap necrosis.
● Precise surgical technique, thorough hemostasis throughout the entire hemipelvectomy wound, wide drainage with multiple closed-suction drains, debridement of all nonviable tissue off hemipelvectomy flap, and meticulous layered closure of the operative wound are the keys to successful postoperative healing.
● Hemipelvectomy wound complications are common and related to the extensive nature of the procedure and the level of vascular ligation. Infected wounds have to be aggressively debrided until control of the wound is achieved.
● Secondary intention healing with wet-to-moist dressing changes, and VAC® therapy is the most common approach to complicated hemipelvectomy wounds.
● Tertiary closure is reserved for the patients with healthy granulating wounds and extensive defects who are otherwise good operative candidates.
● Local tissue rearrangement by advancement of the skin flaps is the most common form of tertiary intention closure.
● Contralateral inferiorly based rectus abdominis muscle or musculocutaneous flap is the flap of choice for tertiary closure of large hemipelvectomy wounds. To preserve contralateral rectus abdominis muscle, contralateral ostomies should be avoided by careful preoperative planning and communication between different surgical specialties involved in this procedures.
● Hemipelvectomy reconstruction with a microvascular fillet flap obtained by ex vivo anatomic exploration of an amputated extremity is an underutilized reconstructive option and should be considered in the cases of paucity or poor quality of local tissues and vascular ligation above the bifurcation of common iliac vessels that is plagued with the high rate of flap necrosis rate.

skin preparation and an easy access to the abdomen, buttock, and perineal regions. If additional procedures on the spine, sacrum, or rectum need to be performed, intraoperative repositioning of the patient will be required (Table 40-2).

Low sacral resection can also be performed in the "sloppy" lateral decubitus position (abdominolateral sacral portion) or a full lateral position with the hip and knee joints in 90-degree flexion. When combined abdominal exploration may be required to deal with the intrapelvic anterior component of the tumor, we start the abdominal portion of the operation supine and later reposition the patient for the posterior, sacral stage of the procedure. Plastic surgeon performs an initial marking and flap dissection as dictated by an anticipated defect.

SURGERY

External Hemipelvectomy Reconstruction

Pelvic reconstruction following external hemipelvectomy is principally accomplished with three pedicled flap designs: posterior, long anterior, and total thigh fillet flaps. For oncologic indications, posteriorly based tumors (which involve the internal iliac vessels) are closed using an anterior thigh flap pedicled off the external iliac vessels; anterior tumors (which involve the external iliac or femoral vessels) are closed using a posterior flap pedicled off the internal iliac vessels. Total thigh flaps are accessible for nononcologic hemipelvectomies in which pelvic vessels do not require sacrifice for oncologic margins.

The vast majority of hemipelvectomy defects can be closed with these flaps, which constitute the *first choice for hemipelvectomy flap reconstructions*. If these standard hemipelvectomy flaps are unusable due to very proximal vascular ligation, causing flap ischemia, division of the flap origin during tumor resection or previous procedure, or extensive radiation damage, then alternative flaps must be used for coverage. These *second-line reconstructive options* include contralateral inferiorly based vertical rectus abdominis musculocutaneous (VRAM) flaps, microvascular lower extremity fillet flaps, or standard free flaps depending on the defect configuration. The most common secondary flap in our practice is a free flap using the calf of the amputated leg. Likewise, the second-line

TABLE 40-3 Purpose of Soft Tissue Flaps in Tumor Surgery
• Covers exposed neurovascular structures
• Coverage for endoprostheses or allografts
• Addresses functional deficits (neurotized flaps)
• Obliterates dead space
• Enhances healing of irradiated wounds

reconstructive options are useful for closure of hemipelvectomy wounds in the setting of postoperative wound complications (Table 40-3).

Posterior Hemipelvectomy Flap

The classic hemipelvectomy technique relies on pelvic exploration, ligation of the common iliac vessels, division of the pelvic rim by disarticulation of the pubic symphysis and the sacroiliac joint, and creation of the posterior fasciocutaneous flap to achieve soft tissue closure. It was initially recommended that gluteal muscles be left with the specimen. This fasciocutaneous hemipelvectomy flap was based on relatively poor random blood supply due to ipsilateral ligation of the common iliac vessels and was further compromised by removal of the gluteal muscles that greatly increased wound complication rates.

Three modifications of this classic technique aimed to decrease high wound complication rates:

• Incorporation of gluteus maximus muscle in the hemipelvectomy flap
• Whenever oncologically appropriate, ligation at the level of external iliac vessels with preservation of the internal iliac vessels to improve the flap blood supply
• Limited resection of the bony pelvis that allows preservation of the sacral perforators

With these modifications, the posterior hemipelvectomy flap is designed as a musculocutaneous flap based on the superior and inferior gluteal vessels (Fig. 40-2). Preservation of the gluteal muscle decreases posterior flap necrosis rates and makes the construction of a long, viable posterior flap that would reach up to or above the level of umbilicus possible. Impact of the level of vascular ligation on hemipelvectomy wound outcomes has been a point of controversy. Several reports from Karakousis et al. suggested that the level of vascular ligation does not affect the posterior hemipelvectomy flap viability and the rate of postoperative wound complications. These authors believed that there was an adequate blood supply of the gluteal muscle through small arterial branches along its sacral origin, which was sufficient to sustain the viability of the flap unless resection of the edge of the sacrum was oncologically necessary. In our experience, we found 2.7-fold higher rates of posterior hemipelvectomy flap necrosis in the patients that had ligation at the level of common iliac vessels. This finding was independent from sacral resection performed during extended hemipelvectomy in some of these patients.

Long Anterior and Total Thigh Fillet Hemipelvectomy Flaps

One of the major limitations of the posterior flap external hemipelvectomy is its inability to deal with the advanced tumors of the buttock and posterior pelvis in an oncologically sound manner. In 1953, Bowden et al. described utilization of the skin of the femoral triangle based on the preserved segment of the superficial femoral artery for closure of the hemipelvectomy performed for the sarcoma of the buttock. However, it was the critical need for soft tissue reconstruction of the advanced decubiti and the infection of the bony pelvis in paraplegic patients that led to increased utilization of the soft tissue obtained from high amputations. The total thigh flap was proposed by Georgiade et al. as a last-resort reconstructive option for such patients in the 1950s and subsequently gained widespread use. This principle was subsequently applied for coverage of the hemipelvectomy defects whereby a musculocutaneous flap of the anterior thigh compartment was elevated based on the superficial femoral artery. The technique was further refined by Sugarbaker et al., who also demonstrated that the anterior flap can be used as a sensate island flap based on the superficial femoral vessels and saphenous nerve.

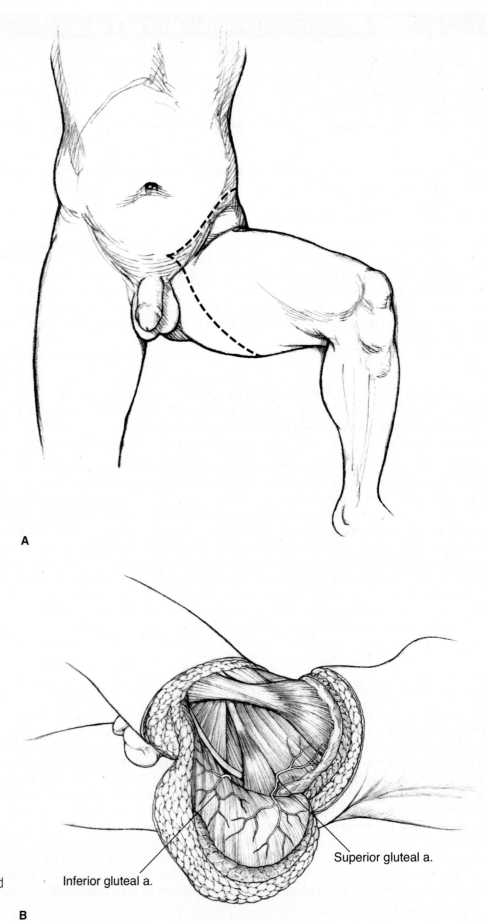

A

B

FIGURE 40-2

A: Skin markings of external hemipelvectomy with utilization of the posterior flap.
B: Musculocutaneous design of the posterior hemipelvectomy flap based on the superior and inferior gluteal vessels.

Inferior gluteal a.

Superior gluteal a.

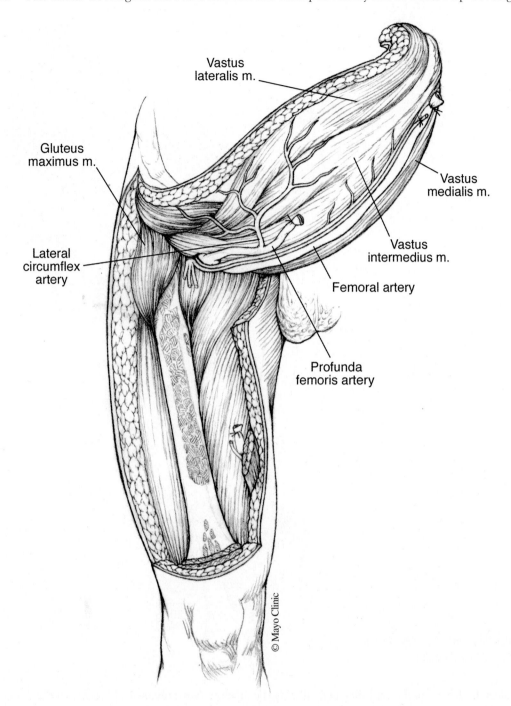

Vastus
lateralis m.

Gluteus
maximus m.

Vastus
medialis m.

Lateral
circumflex
artery

Vastus
intermedius m.

Femoral artery

Profunda
femoris artery

© Mayo Clinic

FIGURE 40-3

Long anterior hemipelvectomy flap based on the branches of profunda femoris and superficial femoris vessels.

Standard long anterior flap hemipelvectomy includes the bulk of quadriceps femoris muscle (Fig. 40-3). A total thigh fillet flap utilizing the majority of the thigh musculature can also be designed as a variation of the anterior hemipelvectomy flap technique (Fig. 40-4). Anterior hemipelvectomy flap is an axial-pattern musculocutaneous flap based on the branches of femoral vessels, including lateral and medial circumflex arteries, which arise from branches from the profundus femoris artery. In preparing this flap, care should be taken to preserve the proximal profundus vessel to maintain these branches. The latter perforate the adductor magnus muscle to the posterior and lateral compartments of the thigh and play a role in supporting a total thigh fillet flap.

The skin of the anterior thigh down to the knee is innervated by the lateral and anterior femoral cutaneous nerves. These nerves can be preserved to provide sensory flap coverage of the hemipelvectomy

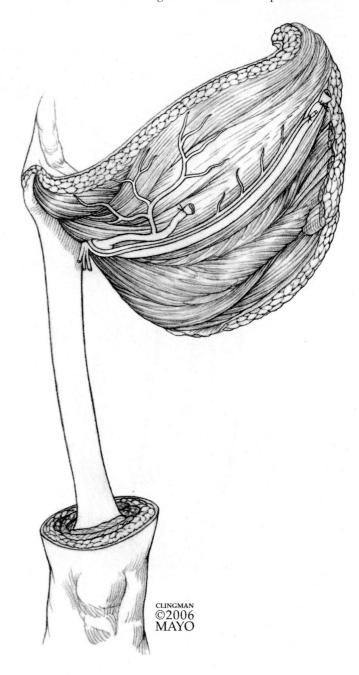

FIGURE 40-4

Total thigh fillet flap uses most of the thigh musculature.

defect. Both anterior flap and total thigh fillet flap hemipelvectomy provide well-vascularized and sensate immediate coverage of the hemipelvectomy defect. An effort should be made to preserve innervation of this flap by protecting sensory nerves during the dissection (Fig. 40-5). Both long anterior and total thigh fillet hemipelvectomy flaps are sufficient to cover even very extensive hemipelvectomy defects (as well as spinopelvic resections) with tissues that have rich axial-pattern blood supply.

Second-Line Hemipelvectomy Reconstructions

Standard hemipelvectomy flaps either posteriorly or anteriorly based provide reliable reconstruction in a vast majority of the cases because removal of the hemipelvis creates relative soft tissue excess for three reasons:

1. Reduction of pelvic volume decreases requirement for the size of soft tissue envelops.
2. Skeletal resection eliminates the issue of the dead space.
3. Tissues or the proximal part of the amputated lower extremity can be used for hemipelvectomy defect reconstruction.

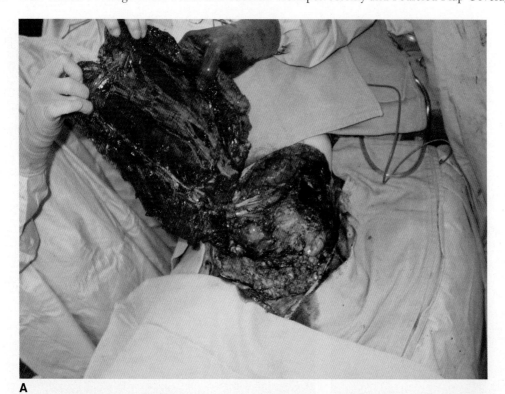

A

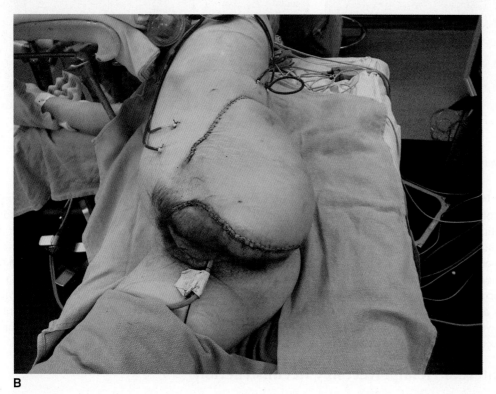

B

FIGURE 40-5

A: Total thigh fillet flap provides abundance of well-vascularized soft tissue. **B:** The flap provides excellent contour and adequate posterior reach.

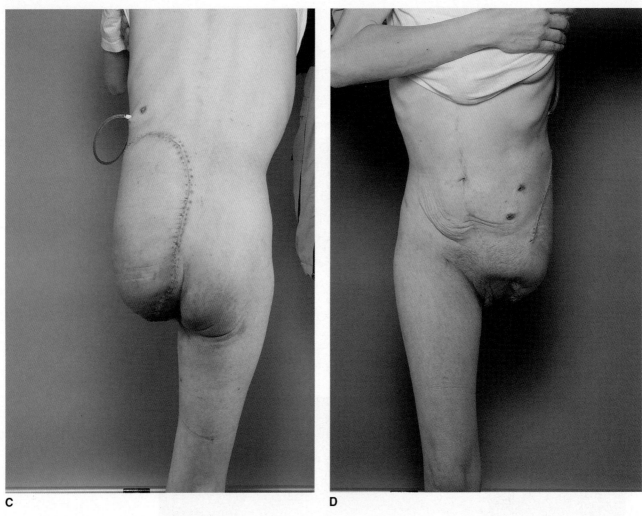

C   D

FIGURE 40-5 (Continued)

C, D: Postoperative result following extended hemipelvectomy for the tumor of the buttock.

For these reasons, external hemipelvectomy itself is the ultimate solution to soft tissue coverage problems. The difficulty arises when common iliac vessels have to be ligated for oncologic reasons, which precludes creation of the anterior hemipelvectomy flap, and, at the same time, tissues of the buttock are not suitable for posterior flap design due to tumor involvement or sequela of previous operations or radiation therapy. In the past, such patients were considered unresectable. With the advent of microvascular tissue transfer, however, a suitable and tumor-free block of tissue can be recovered by ex vivo anatomic exploration of an amputated extremity and transferred as a free flap to achieve coverage of the hemipelvectomy defect. Note that free flap reconstructions generally develop lymphedema and are insensate; these factors complicate prosthetic fitting if this option is needed for wound closure.

Internal Hemipelvectomy Reconstruction

Internal hemipelvectomy involves total or partial removal of the innominate bone with preservation of the lower extremity. This operation provides local tumor control and acceptable functional outcome. Several types of internal hemipelvectomy as proposed by Enneking and Dunham exist based on the part of innominate bone resected: type 1—ileum; type 2—periacetabular region; type 3—pubic bone; and, described by some, type 4—ileum and sacral ala (Fig. 40-6). This classification provides the basis for the surgical oncologic approaches to malignant tumors of the nonvisceral pelvis.

Introduction of internal hemipelvectomies increases requirements for soft tissue reconstruction since the pelvic volume is not reduced and lower extremity cannot be filleted. Additionally, a large amount of the dead space is created and often requires obliteration with a flap, especially in the

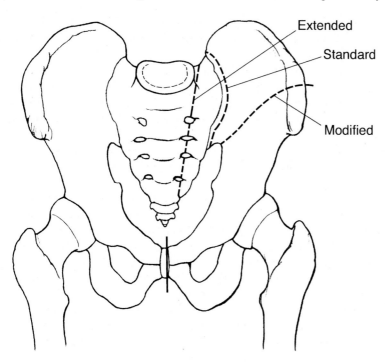

FIGURE 40-6

Osteotomy lines for standard modified and extended hemipelvectomies.

settings of preoperative radiation. Several regional pedicled flap options for filling these defects exist (Table 40-4). Muscle flaps and de-epithelialized musculocutaneous flaps can be used effectively for dead space obliteration. De-epithelialized flaps create more bulk and are used for filling larger defects. Because fat is a part of the skin paddle, the flap retains volume long term. In addition to dead space obliteration, these flaps bring blood supply into relatively ischemic radiated tissues of the operative site and thus enhance stable coverage and promote wound healing. Although flap demands for bony sarcomas without soft tissue extension are not high, however, in the cases of soft tissue sarcomas or soft tissue involvement from the bony sarcomas, flap reconstruction becomes critical for the coverage of exposed skeletal structures. Musculocutaneous, muscle pedicled, or free flaps can be used. When the skin is not part of such a flap, a split-thickness skin graft can be used for coverage of exposed muscle of the flap.

Sacral Reconstruction

Primary sacral tumors are often low-grade lesions such as chordoma. They usually metastasize late in the disease process but have a tenacious local course. Chordomas and locally advanced rectal cancers are the two most commonly encountered sacral tumors. Sacral surgery presents a major challenge due to regional anatomic complexity, technical difficulty in obtaining clear margins, functional impairment, and an often prolonged postoperative course due to poor wound healing. Sacrectomy is a procedure that is uncommon outside of specialized cancer centers. Although distal sacral resections are safely performed through the posterior approach, larger tumors, tumors of rectal origin, and resections proximal to S2 require an initial abdominal exploration to dissect visceral

---

TABLE 40-4   Flap Options for Internal Hemipelvectomy Defect Reconstruction

- Rectus abdominis muscle based are inferiorly based ipsilateral or contralateral:
  - Vertical rectus abdominis musculocutaneous (VRAM) flap
  - Transverse rectus abdominis musculocutaneous (TRAM) flap
  - Rectus abdominis muscle flap with or without skin graft
- Rectus femoris muscle flap
- Latissimus dorsi muscle or musculocutaneous flap
- Vastus lateralis muscle flap
- Tensor fascia lata muscle or musculocutaneous flap
- Anterolateral thigh flap

and neurovascular structures, perform formal visceral resection when required, assure hemostasis, and complete anterior sacrectomy dissection. Following the anterior procedure, the sacrectomy is completed through the posterior approach.

Soft tissue reconstruction becomes important in preventing postoperative wound complications following a sacrectomy. Two flaps are commonly utilized: pedicled omentum and rectus abdominis muscle/musculocutaneous flaps. *Omentum* is preferred for smaller defects (the defects smaller than the surgeon's fist), and the rectus flap is used for larger ones. Inferiorly based VRAM flap is the most commonly used reconstructive technique.

The flap accomplishes two main objectives: it obliterates large dead space and provides tension-free closure of the sacrectomy wound. In the cases of preoperative radiation, well-vascularized tissue of the flap enhances local circulation and further promotes wound healing. Implementation of this practice in our institution led to a marked decrease in sacrectomy wound complication rates. Careful preoperative planning and communication between different services is critical in executing these operations. VRAM flap as a reconstructive option must always be borne in mind in the light of previous abdominal incisions as well as ostomies, drains, and feeding tube placements. The VRAM flap represents a very important surgical technique in oncologic pelvic reconstruction.

If soft tissue defect is too large for sole VRAM coverage, fasciocutaneous V-to-Y advancement flap provides additional recruitment of the local tissues. If aforementioned techniques are not sufficient to achieve an immediate coverage of sacrectomy-buttockectomy defect, microvascular tissue transfer should be performed with a free flap of appropriate dimensions. Finally, anterior flap external hemipelvectomy is reserved as a last-resort reconstructive operation.

Technical Elements of Pelvic Flap Surgery

Omentum Pedicled Flap

Omentum is readily available during laparotomy although it can also be harvested laparoscopically. Its blood supply is based on the right or left gastroepiploic artery. Significant mobilization and extent of reach can be gained by basing the flap on left gastroepiploic vessels, dividing the short gastric vessels along the greater curvature of the stomach, and further dividing middle omental artery to release a long vascular pedicle (Fig. 40-7). The latter maneuver releases omentum to its fullest length, which may be important for the reconstruction of the larger pelvic defects in the event that the VRAM flap is unavailable.

Rectus Abdominis Muscle and Musculocutaneous Flaps

The rectus abdominis muscle can be elevated alone or with a skin paddle. The skin paddle may be oriented transversely or vertically. The transverse rectus abdominis musculocutaneous (TRAM) or VRAM flaps can be utilized as either pedicled or microvascular free flaps. The rectus abdominis muscle has a dual blood supply from the superior and inferior epigastric vessels. For the purposes of pelvic soft tissue reconstruction, the rectus abdominis muscle flaps are based on the deep inferior epigastric vessels when pedicled to cover the pelvis or sacrum.

Several key elements of preoperative planning are important in preparation for this procedure. A detailed history of previous intra-abdominal surgery needs to be obtained, because the inferior epigastric vessels may be divided during operations such as appendectomy, inguinal hernia repair, C-section, and colostomy creation. The pedicle may also be damaged by radiation therapy. If there is any question about the integrity of the vascular pedicle, duplex evaluation should be performed.

Flap elevation is performed prior to abdominal exploration. We open the rectus sheath close to midline and dissect it off the rectus abdominis muscle (Fig. 40-8A–C). In this part of procedure, care should be taken to dissect inscriptions due to their proximity to the underlying vessels that run on the undersurface of the muscle. Once the flap has been dissected for coverage of the sacrum and posterior defects, the flap is placed in a plastic bag or wrapped with towels and placed over the anterior portion of the lumbar spine and sacrum. The abdominal portion of the procedure is then completed, and the abdomen is closed. If a large fascial defect remains following VRAM harvest, this is reconstructed with synthetic mesh or allograft fascia. Following abdominal closure, the patient is placed in the prone jackknife position for the sacral portion of the operation, and the flap is easily visualized after removal of the specimen (Fig. 40-8D–F). Inset should ideally be performed with no tension to prevent sacral closure breakdown when the patient starts to sit.

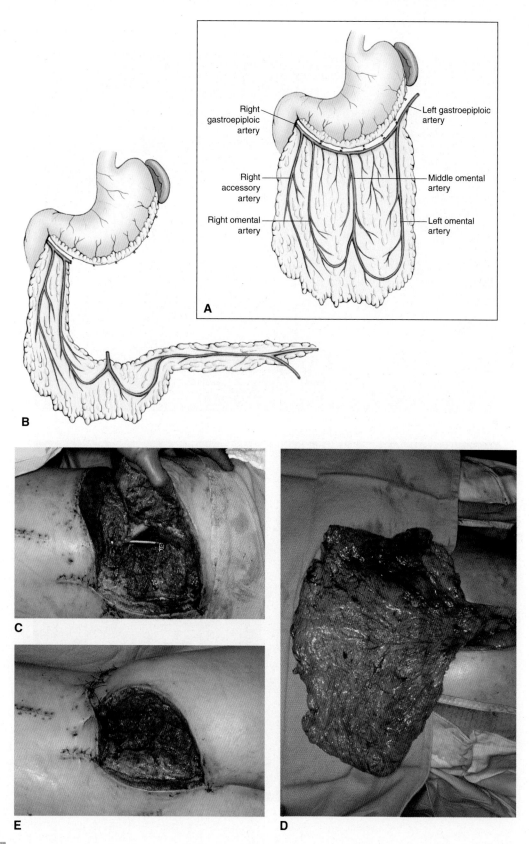

FIGURE 40-7

A: Omentum can be used for coverage in difficult situations following pelvic resection and soft tissue deficit. While the omentum lacks significant structural strength, it provides a well-vascularized bed, which can support skin grafting. The division of the left gastroepiploic arch allows the omentum to be mobilized off the greater curvature of the stomach. The right gastroepiploic vessels are preserved to supply the flap. **B:** The omentum may be lengthened by dividing the omental arcade along the lines within the illustration, creating a long vascularized pedicle. **C–E:** Clinical example of a 16-year-old woman with exposed spinal hardware **(C)** following sacrectomy. The omentum was harvested through a midline anterior incision **(D)**, lengthened as shown in **(B),** and then passed through the back to provide coverage for the spinal hardware.

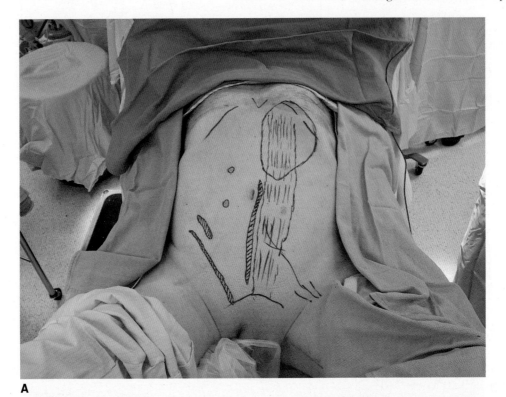

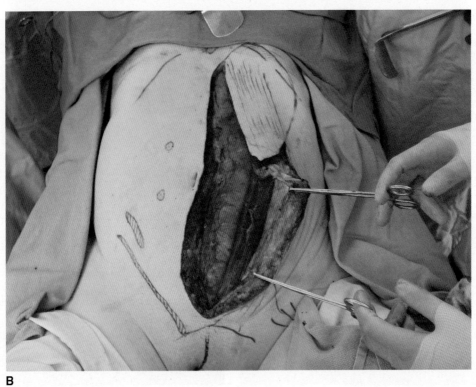

FIGURE 40-8

A: VRAM flap is planned for reconstruction of the defect from en bloc abdominoperineal resection with sacrectomy. Skin paddle is designed to overlie rectus abdominis muscle. **B:** The rectus sheath is open and the rectus abdominis muscle is exposed. The anterior fascia is preserved with the skin paddle.

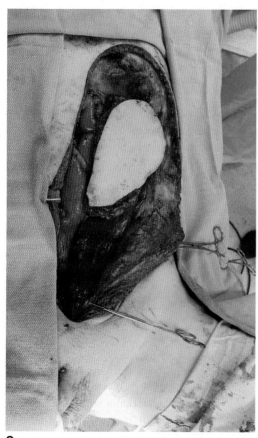

C

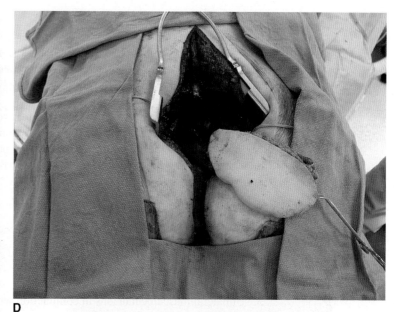

D

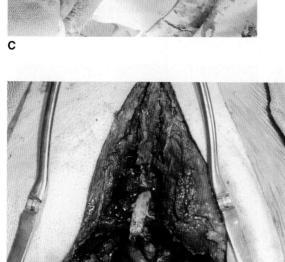

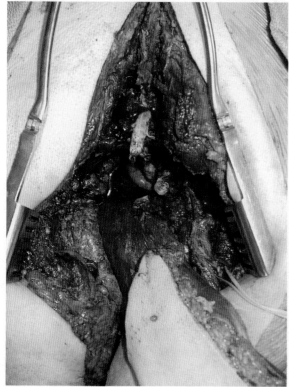

E

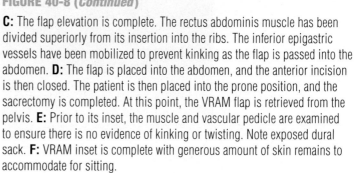

F

FIGURE 40-8 (*Continued*)

C: The flap elevation is complete. The rectus abdominis muscle has been divided superiorly from its insertion into the ribs. The inferior epigastric vessels have been mobilized to prevent kinking as the flap is passed into the abdomen. **D:** The flap is placed into the abdomen, and the anterior incision is then closed. The patient is then placed into the prone position, and the sacrectomy is completed. At this point, the VRAM flap is retrieved from the pelvis. **E:** Prior to its inset, the muscle and vascular pedicle are examined to ensure there is no evidence of kinking or twisting. Note exposed dural sack. **F:** VRAM inset is complete with generous amount of skin remains to accommodate for sitting.

Other Flap Options

In many instances, the safest approach to patients with pelvic sarcomas is a laparotomy, and, when it is performed, omentum becomes a valuable reconstructive material. Omentum, if present, should always be interposed between hemipelvectomy flap and intra-abdominal viscera. This provides an additional protective layer in the event of hemipelvectomy wound problems. Omental flaps can be effectively used for dead space obliteration.

Although omentum and VRAM are truly the workhorses of pelvic reconstruction, several other flaps may become important as second-line reconstructive options. Rectus femoris, tensor fascia lata, and anterolateral thigh flap can be used as pedicled flaps. Latissimus dorsi and anterolateral thigh flaps can be transferred as microvascular flaps depending on soft tissue requirements and availability of recipient vessels.

V-to-Y Advancement Gluteal Flaps

This versatile reconstructive technique can be performed in escalating complexity and is usually tried in the following sequence:

1. Unilateral fasciocutaneous
2. Bilateral fasciocutaneous
3. Unilateral musculocutaneous in conjunction with contralateral fasciocutaneous
4. Bilateral musculocutaneous
5. VRAM and bilateral fascio- or musculocutaneous advancement flaps (Fig. 40-9)

The surgeon must be careful in utilizing this flap in an ambulatory patient as it may affect functional performance. It is safer to reserve musculocutaneous gluteal flaps for paraplegic individuals. As well, high sacral resections often require division of the internal iliac vessels, limiting the vascularity of V-to-Y advancement flaps. For large buttock defects, lateral donor sites of the V-to-Y advancement flaps sometimes may need to be temporarily covered with vacuum-assisted closure

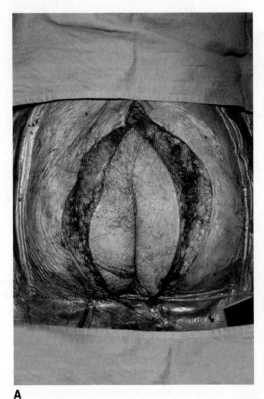 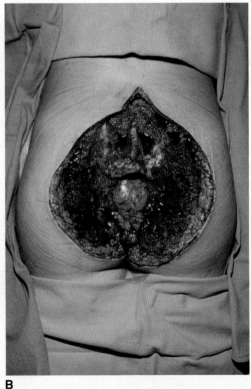

A B

FIGURE 40-9

A, B: Combination of inferiorly based pedicled VRAM flap and bilateral fasciocutaneous V-to-Y advancement flaps for closure of a large sacral defect after wide local excision of the sacral sarcoma.

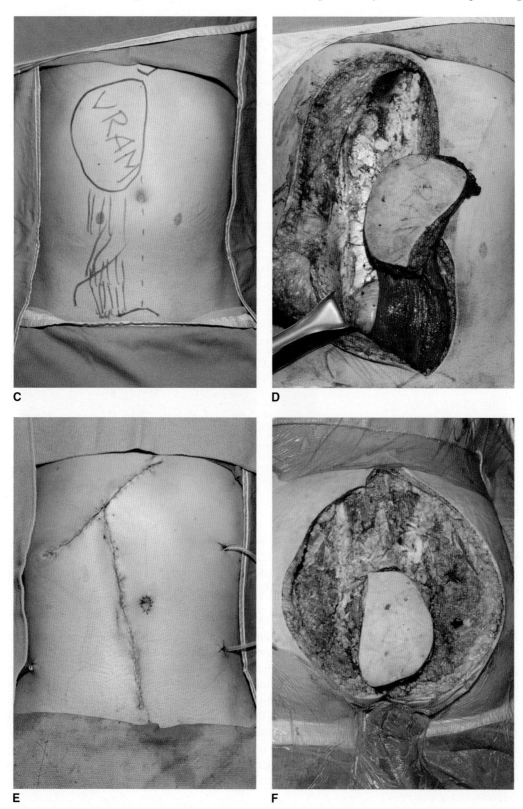

FIGURE 40-9 (*Continued*)

C–E: Inferiorly based VRAM is elevated with large skin island based over superior portion of rectus abdominis muscle. The abdomen is closed with the aid of extensive undermining. The umbilicus is repositioned beneath the skin flaps to lie in the midline. **F:** VRAM flap allows for soft tissue coverage over sacrectomy defect and allows for reconstruction of pelvic floor; however, large soft tissue defect remains at margins of sacrectomy incision.

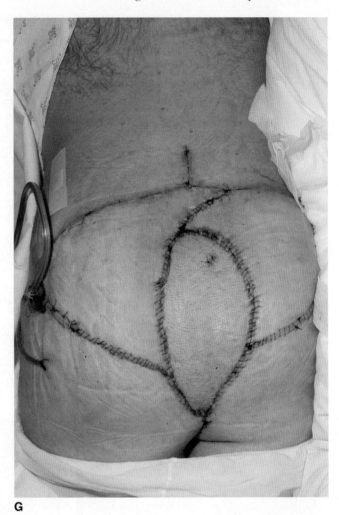

FIGURE 40-9 (*Continued*)

G: Remaining portion of sacral wound is closed with use of bilateral fasciocutaneous flaps. Flaps are elevated with fascia only to avoid injury to gluteus muscles to maximize postoperative ambulatory ability.

G

(VAC) dressings to be closed later when the edema subsides, skin is grafted, or allowed to heal by secondary intention (Fig. 40-10).

In the face of insufficient amounts of local tissues, the donor part of the V-to-Y advancement flap can be skin grafted or covered with a wound VAC to allow healing by secondary intention.

Abdominal Wall Reconstruction in Pelvic Surgery

Integrity of the abdominal wall has to be maintained to prevent postoperative hernias. For a standard external hemipelvectomy defect without extensive resection of the abdominal wall, in the patients with musculocutaneous design of hemipelvectomy flap, no specific reconstruction of the abdominal wall is necessary other than meticulous layered closure of the hemipelvectomy wound. We did not observe postoperative hemipelvectomy hernias under these circumstances because sturdy fascia of the anterior compartment of the thigh or gluteus muscle along with muscular bulk of the flap effectively withstands pressure of the intra-abdominal viscera. Conversely, abdominal wall reconstruction becomes important for internal hemipelvectomy defects and sacrectomy defects because frequently in these patients, there is a very clear area of weakness in the lower abdominal wall. This situation is also aggravated by higher functional level of the internal hemipelvectomy patients.

Reconstructive efforts are guided by the extent of the abdominal wall deficit and degree of operative contamination. Time-tested surgery principles of ventral hernia repair apply. Hernia repair should be tension free with liberal use of prosthetic mesh materials or acellular dermal matrix (ADM). Well-incorporated prosthetic mesh is superior to nonneurotized autologous options because it secures the dimensions of the abdominal wall and prevents postoperative bulge and recurrent hernia formation. The downside of prosthetic mesh reconstruction is its propensity to infection in the presence of intraoperative contamination. Although prosthetic mesh can be used in clean-contaminated cases,

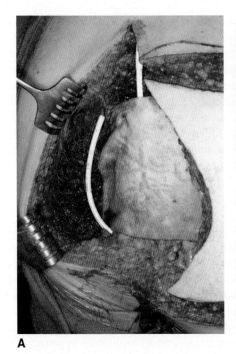
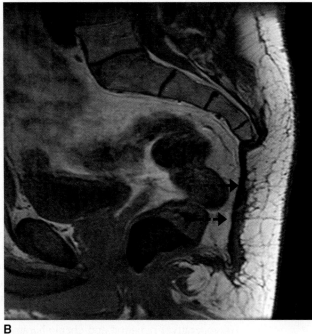

FIGURE 40-10

ADM is useful for restoration of posterior abdominal domain. The use of ADM has been found to significantly decrease the incidence of intra-abdominal hernia formation and intra-abdominal complications. **A:** ADM inset at base of wound. **B:** MRI of a patient after tumor resection and partial sacrectomy with *arrows* pointing to layer of ADM (*dark line*). Notice how it prevents bowel from communicating with reconstruction site.

most surgeons are reluctant to use nonabsorbable mesh in this setting and prefer either absorbable mesh such as Vicryl or a biologic substitute (ADMM) such as AlloDerm, processed cadaveric human acellular dermis (Life Cell Corporation, Branchburg, NJ), or Surgisis, a product obtained by the processing of porcine small intestine submucosa (Cook Surgical, Bloomington, IN). Vicryl mesh is a temporary abdominal reconstruction solution that permits a conversion of the contaminated situation into a clean one at the time of the second procedure. The latter aims for definitive reconstruction, but requires utilization of costly biologic materials and postoperative formation of abdominal wall hernia or bulge continues to be a problem.

POSTOPERATIVE MANAGEMENT

Postoperatively, patients usually require an ICU admission after major pelvic resections or hemipelvectomies. They are commonly kept on mechanical ventilation overnight until intravascular volumes are stabilized and gas exchange is adequate. To optimize postoperative recovery as well as systemic and flap perfusion, the patient needs to be kept well hydrated, and adequate urine output needs to be maintained. The patient with pelvic or sacral flap is usually kept on a Clinitron bed to avoid pressure injury to the flap. Recovery of bowel function, ostomy care, deep venous thrombosis (DVT) prophylaxis, and wound care are similar to that for a general surgery patient undergoing abdominal procedures.

Physical and occupational therapy services are involved early in the care of these patients. Even when the patients are on bed rest, range of motion exercises on nonoperated extremities and activities of daily living should be started. When it is safe, from a surgical perspective, to resume ambulation, the patients are evaluated for short-term rehabilitation placement.

RESULTS

Our experience shows that the outcome of external hemipelvectomy wounds was not dependent on hemipelvectomy flap selection. Reliability of its blood supply determines the success of the reconstruction. Historically, classic hemipelvectomy flaps that are based on the random circulation are exceedingly prone to necrosis. Preservation of the gluteal muscle as a part of the flap decreased, but did not solve, the problem of hemipelvectomy flap necrosis. We also observed that preservation of the branches of the internal iliac vessels providing direct blood supply to the gluteus maximus muscle further decreased hemipelvectomy flap necrosis rates. Hemipelvectomy wound outcomes therefore can be improved by increased utilization of microvascular fillet flap transfer that provides superb blood flow to the transferred tissue, not comparable with the periphery of a random hemipelvectomy following common iliac vessel ligation. Finally, we have recently shown that the use of ADM for reconstructing the posterior abdominal wall provides a barrier between the intra-abdominal contents and the flap reconstruction, preventing bowel adhesions/obstruction and fistulas as well as prevents sacroperineal hernia.

COMPLICATIONS

Wound complications such as surgical site infection and skin flap necrosis are the most common postoperative complications in musculoskeletal oncology. There are multiple reasons for the high rate of wound complications following major resections of musculoskeletal malignancies. Despite the fact that the vast majority of these procedures are clean cases with only occasional visceral resection that is applicable for pelvic tumors, wound complication rates are well beyond what one would expect. In modern musculoskeletal oncology practice, many sarcoma patients undergo neoadjuvant (preoperative) radiation and chemotherapy. Soft tissue complication rates approach 40% to 50% in this group of patients. Moreover, even without neoadjuvant therapy, the duration and operative extent of the procedures significantly influence rates of postoperative wound complications. As noted earlier, wound complications that delay the administration of postoperative adjuvant therapies may have serious oncologic consequences. Rapid, uncomplicated wound healing is essential for patients who require postoperative adjuvant therapy, highlighting the need for early and close collaboration with plastic surgeons.

A hematoma can occur after any oncologic surgery, ranging from incisional biopsy to extensive surgery. All tumor resections should utilize at least one suction drain, although larger resections may require several drains placed deep and in more superficial tissues. The pressure from the collection of blood products in a wound can compromise soft tissue reconstructions and may become infected. Drain sites and tracks are contaminated and usually are resected at the time of definitive tumor removal. For this reason, drains should exit the skin in line with the longitudinal incision used for biopsy. It is important to remember that drain placement can be as important as where one makes an incision. Drains should come out in line and close to an incision.

Hematomas are especially problematic following incisional biopsy, potentially compromising future resection and successful local control of a tumor. A hematoma can spread neoplastic cells beyond the immediate area and even into surrounding compartments if a transverse incision is used. Rigorous attention to hemostasis is therefore essential. Compressive dressings bolstered with plaster can also help minimize hematomas in the immediate postoperative period.

Seromas can occur following tumor resections, again potentially compromising soft tissue reconstructions and wound closures. Most surgeons therefore take a conservative approach to removing drains, allowing output to decrease (to less than 30 mL/day) and remain low before removal; note however that drains following major pelvic resections are often in continuity with the peritoneal space. These drains will commonly have a high serous output and serve as a means for third spaced fluid to leave the patient. Drains usually remain in place for a minimum of several days, but often are left in for much longer in large or irradiated wound beds. As with other facets of patient care, good communication with plastic surgery is important regarding the timing of drain removal. It is recommended that patients going home with suction drains remain on oral antibiotics.

Oncology patients often have a compromised nutritional status, making them prone to wound infections. Moreover, these patients are subject to the immunosuppressive actions of chemotherapy agents and the local wound effects from radiation. As many oncologic reconstructions rely on allografts, endoprostheses, or combinations of the two, surgeons should approach wound infections extremely aggressively. This approach entails a low threshold for surgical debridement. As with all surgical procedures, orthopedic oncology patients should receive pre- and perioperative intravenous antibiotics as well as postoperative coverage when appropriate.

Sacrectomy is prone to wound complications that are related to the extent of the procedure, intra-operative contamination, use of preoperative radiation therapy, local tissue ischemia, hematoma, positional pressure, dead space, and tight closure. In the setting of preoperative radiation, wound complication rates are as high as 50%. These factors can be minimized by meticulous surgical technique, obliteration of the dead space with a flap, and postoperative use of a Clinitron bed.

Between 1985 and 2005, 160 external hemipelvectomies were performed in our institution. External hemipelvectomy has been associated with high morbidity but low mortality (5% to 7%). Overall, 54% of patients had at least one complication. Hemipelvectomy wound morbidity was the most common postoperative complication. Thirty-nine percent of patients experienced wound infection and 26% had hemipelvectomy flap necrosis. Wound complications were managed with serial debridement until control of the wound was achieved; however, this may result in a sizable defect.

In a delayed reconstruction setting, the amputated extremity is no longer available for tissue procurement, and the contralateral pedicled VRAM flap becomes critical in closure of such defects. This flap provides a superb reconstruction and in fact is the flap of choice for postoperative hemipelvectomy wounds. In a very rare circumstance, when VRAM is unavailable and the hemipelvectomy wound is so large it cannot be closed by local tissue rearrangement or a skin graft, a free flap such as a contralateral anterolateral thigh flap or latissimus dorsi may be required. One has to consider a paucity of recipient vessels and the need for vein grafts or saphenous arteriovenous loop that significantly increase the risk of flap failure.

Oncologic outcomes of musculoskeletal tumors are largely dependent on tumor pathology. Limb salvage is possible in the vast majority of sarcoma patients. In those patients who still require proximal amputations such as external hemipelvectomy, stable soft tissue coverage is almost uniformly achieved. Despite postoperative wound complications related to the operative extent of the resection, intraoperative contamination, and preoperative radiation therapy, the vast majority of the patients heal the surgical wounds. Both successful wound healing and high rates of limb salvage became possible due to advances in reconstructive surgery over the past three decades. In our practice, we emphasize early involvement of a plastic and reconstructive surgeon in care of a sarcoma patient.

PEARLS AND PITFALLS

- Plastic surgery consultation should be obtained in these cases early in the care course.
- Early, durable reconstructions are important for functional recovery and also prevent delays in administration of postoperative chemotherapy and radiation therapy.
- All surgeons should be present in the operating room at the start of a combined case.
- Don't use an Esmarch—exsanguinate, if necessary, by elevating the extremity.
- When performing a posterior thigh flap include incorporate the gluteal muscles in the hemipelvectomy flap. Additionally, whenever oncologically appropriate, preservation of the internal iliac vessels will improve the flap blood supply.
- The VRAM is a reliable flap for posterior coverage in cases of partial and complete sacrectomy.
- In cases of total sacrectomy, the use of ADM for reconstructing the posterior abdominal wall provides a barrier between the intra-abdominal contents and flap, preventing bowel adhesions/obstruction and fistulas as well as prevents sacroperineal hernia.
- The VRAM may be combined with bilateral V-Y fasciocutaneous advancement flaps if the posterior defect dimensions exceed those provided by a VRAM flap.

RECOMMENDED READING

Abramson DL. Single-stage, multimodality treatment of soft-tissue sarcoma of the extremity. *Ann Plast Surg.* 1997;39:454–460.

Apffelstaedt JP, Driscoll DL, Spellman JE, et al. Complications and outcome of external hemipelvectomy in the management of pelvic tumors. *Ann Surg Oncol.* 1996;3(3):304–309.

Butler CE. Reconstruction of an extensive hemipelvectomy defect using a pedicled upper and lower leg in-continuity fillet flap. *Plast Reconstr Surg.* 2002;109:1060–1065.

Dickey ID, Mugate RR, Fuchs B, et al. Reconstruction after total sacrectomy: early experience with a new surgical technique. *Clin Orthop.* 2005;438:42–50.

Enneking WF, Dunham WK. Resection and reconstruction for primary neoplasms involving the innominate bone. *J Bone Joint Surg Am.* 1978;60(6):731–746.

Fuchs B, Dickey ID, Yaszemski MJ, et al. Operative management of sacral chordoma. *J Bone Joint Surg Am.* 2005;87(10):2211–2216.

Ghert MA, Davis AM, Griffin AM, et al. The surgical and functional outcome of limb-salvage surgery with vascular reconstruction for soft tissue sarcoma of the extremity. *Ann Surg Oncol.* 2005;12:1102–1110.

Kane JM, Gibbs JF, McGrath BE, et al. Large, deep high-grade extremity sarcomas: when is a myocutaneous flap reconstruction necessary? *Surg Oncol.* 1999;8:205–210.

Karakousis CP, Emrich LJ, Driscoll DL. Variants of hemipelvectomy and their complications. *Am J Surg.* 1989;158(5):404–408.

Kulaylat MN, Froix A, Karakousis CP. Blood supply of hemipelvectomy flaps: the anterior flap hemipelvectomy. *Arch Surg.* 2001;136(7):828–831.

Lotze MT, Sugarbaker PH. Femoral artery based myocutaneous flap for hemipelvectomy closure: amputation after failed limb-sparing surgery and radiotherapy. *Am J Surg.* 1985;150(5):625–630.

Maricevich M, Maricevich R, Chim H, et al. Reconstruction following partial and total sacrectomy defects: an analysis of outcomes and complications. *J Plast Reconstr Aesthet Surg.* 2014;67(9):1257–1266.

Mugate R Jr, Sim FM. Pelvic reconstruction techniques. *Orthop Clin North Am.* 2006;37(1):85–97.

Senchenkov A, Moran SL, Petty PM, et al. Predictors of complications and outcomes of external hemipelvectomy wound: account of 160 consecutive cases. *Ann Surg Oncol.* 2008;15(1):355–363.

Sugarbaker PH, Chretien PA. Hemipelvectomy for buttock tumors utilizing an anterior myocutaneous flap of quadriceps femoris muscle. *Ann Surg.* 1983;197(1):106–115.

Temple WJ, Mnaymneh W, Ketcham AS. The total thigh and rectus abdominis myocutaneous flap for closure of extensive hemipelvectomy defects. *Cancer.* 1982;50(11):2524–2528.

Yamamoto Y, Minakawa H, Takeda N. Pelvic reconstruction with a free fillet lower leg flap. *Plast Reconstr Surg.* 1997;99:1439–1441.

41 Management of Major Upper Limb Amputations

S. Raja Sabapathy and Hari Venkatramani

INDICATIONS/CONTRAINDICATIONS

Any amputation proximal to the wrist is considered a *major amputation*. If replantation of the limb at this level is unsuccessful, late reconstructive surgical options for such amputations are limited and include toe transfers, hand transplantation, or prosthesis. There are downsides to all these reconstructive options including cost, incomplete functional return, and risks of immunosuppressive drugs. Experience has taught us that the complications associated with major upper limb replants are related to the ischemia time and the ongoing damage seen within the remaining muscle; however, these complications can be minimized by proper technique and sound surgical judgment. In our institution, we still believe that immediate replantation provides the best chance for successful outcome following major upper limb amputation.

Though all amputations proximal to the wrist level are termed major amputations, technical considerations, complications, and outcomes are different for replantation performed at the upper arm compared to replantation performed at the distal forearm. Factors in the recovery of function include the length required for neural reinnervation of muscle and the status of the remaining muscle. The mechanism of upper limb amputation can be guillotine, crush, avulsion, or a combination of crush and avulsion injury. Guillotine amputations have been found to be easier to replant and tend to regain better functional outcomes compared to limbs that are crushed or avulsed. In our experience over the last two decades, we have found that guillotine amputations account for only 10% of major upper limb amputations. If the crush and avulsion amputation are not replanted, there will be a large number of amputees who will need prosthesis or hand transplantation. Experience has shown us that by refining the techniques of upper limb replantation, many crush avulsion amputations can be replanted with gratifying results (Fig. 41-1).

The main determinant for an acceptable outcome is the structural integrity of the hand and keeping ischemia time to a minimum. Secondary procedures like tendon transfer, selective arthrodesis, and free functioning muscle transfer can be used to make major replants more functional when performed as delayed secondary procedures. The basic tenet in replantation surgery is that the ultimate outcome must be better than closure of the amputation stump at that level of injury and fitting the patient with the best available prosthesis. This outcome must be achieved without subjecting the patient to undue risk to life or severe morbidity. This chapter details the technical considerations one must concentrate on to achieve acceptable outcomes.

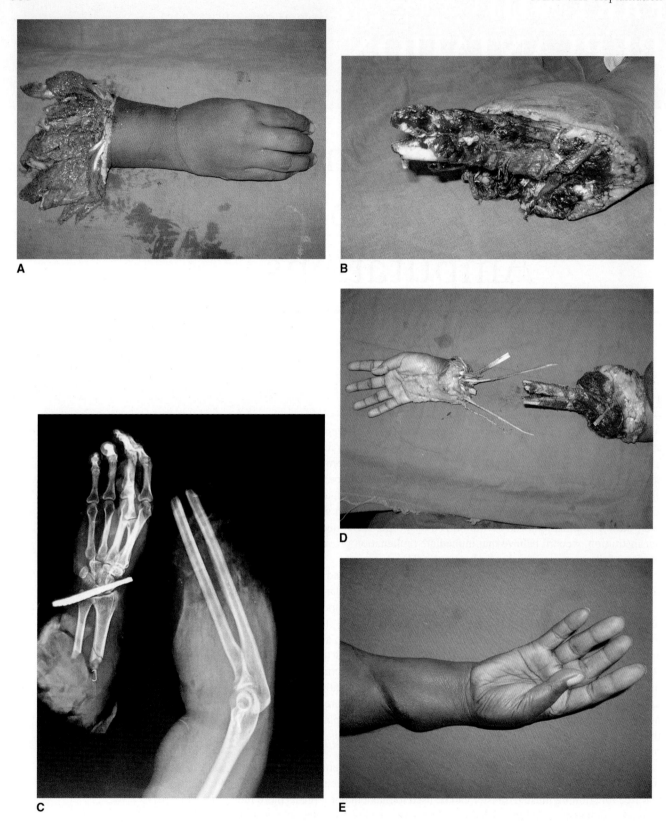

FIGURE 41-1

A, B: Avulsion amputation of the right forearm due to a bangle being caught in a rolling machine. **C:** Radiograph of the proximal and distal segments. **D:** The proximal and distal parts after debridement before bone shortening. **E–G:** Postoperative results at the end of 1 year. Patient is able to pinch and has gross grip. **G:** Primary bone union at the replanted site.

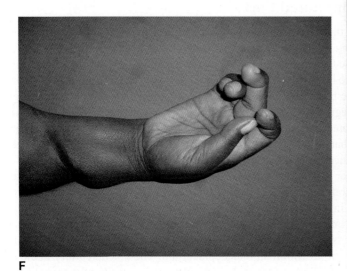

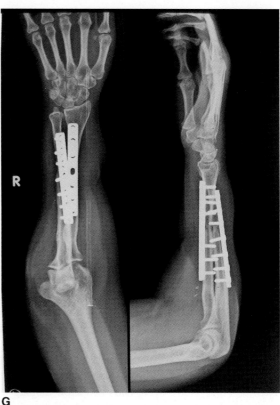

F   **G**

FIGURE 41-1 (*Continued*)

PREOPERATIVE PLANNING

Assessment

The most important consideration in a major replant is to reestablish arterial flow within the amputated part as quickly as possible to reduce muscle necrosis and ischemia. A key step to this goal is getting the patient into the operating theater as quickly as possible. This involves setting up of a protocol for major replantations within your local institution. At Ganga Hospital, major upper limb amputation patients bypass the emergency room and are received in the ante room of the operation theater. The patients are resuscitated as per Advanced Trauma Life Support protocol. If there are any life-threatening associated injuries, these are managed first. When the periods of hypotension, hypoxia, and hypothermia are minimized, the patient will have an improved outcome.

Following resuscitation, a supraclavicular brachial plexus block is placed. This is done immediately after the preliminary patient assessment and as the resuscitation is in progress. This is called the "On Arrival Block." Reduction in the patient's pain enhances the resuscitative efforts. Radiological assessment is done after the patient is in a pain-free state. As this process is being carried out, a team of surgeons does a preliminary examination of the amputated part.

Decision for Replantation

The decision for replantation is dependent on the status of the amputated part. The following factors must be present to proceed with replantation: (1) the hand must essentially be uninjured and (2) muscle ischemia time should be short (less than 4 hours). One needs to look for certain definitive signs of severe ischemia that could cause potential systemic complications to the patient if it is replanted. If the joints are stiff to passive motion, then one should abandon the replant. In above-elbow amputation, the fingers are stretched, and if there is resistance, the part should not be replanted. In below-elbow amputation, this test cannot be applied, so in these cases, we passively move the thumb. If there is stiffness of the thumb, this is a contraindication for replantation.

If the decision is made to proceed with replantation, the patient and the family are briefed about the process of replantation, the possible outcome, and the potential complications and consent is obtained. The patient and the family are unable to understand the time required for rehabilitation and the time required for recovery of function; it is the surgeon's responsibility to explain and help them decide with the interest of the patient in mind.

SURGERY

Debridement of the Amputated Part

At all times during this process, the amputated part is kept covered with ice to continue the cooling of the part. We do this by placing a number of glove bags with ice around the amputated part and wrapping it up (Fig. 41-2). As the team is preparing the patient, the amputated part can be examined and debrided. Debridement has to be radical. The goal is that after revascularization, all tissues present must be well perfused. In the beginning, the main vessels and nerves are identified and tagged. This is done early so that good segments of the vessels and nerves are not excised inadvertently during the process of muscle excision. Debridement is started with skin edge excision and performed in a methodical manner. Muscles that are crushed or avulsed are excised. Muscles attached to distally avulsed tendons are excised, since they will not be perfused after revascularization (Fig. 41-3). When excising muscle, remember to cauterize small vessels as to avoid troublesome bleeding later.

The vessels and nerves are carefully debrided. Even if there is extensive contamination, the vessels can be cleaned by debriding in the thin layer of fascia, which usually encloses the neurovascular structures. The vessel ends are trimmed and then visualized under the microscope to assess the suitability of their repair. The cut ends of the vessels must look clean with no intimal damage. Healthy nerve ends will show bulging fascicles within an intact epineurium. The brachial artery in the arm and the radial and ulnar arteries in the forearm are identified and tagged, as well as the cephalic vein, brachial vein, and venae comitantes. Tagging of the vessels and nerves is important since it will be difficult to identify unmarked vessels and nerves after skeletal fixation.

Contaminated bone ends are debrided and loose fragments without soft tissue attachment are removed. The interior of the marrow is also inspected for contamination. The bone ends are debrided and the extent of final bone shortening is determined according to the status of the surrounding soft tissue injuries. Up to 10 cm of bone shortening is compatible with good functional outcome.

At this stage (prior to reperfusion), fasciotomies are performed. Most forearm replantations will need carpal tunnel release and intrinsic muscle compartment release. Above-elbow replants will need forearm compartment release in addition to carpal tunnel and intrinsic release. Our rationale for performing fasciotomies prior to reperfusion are threefold: (1) fasciotomies may be done more efficiently prior to reperfusion, (2) fasciotomies prior to reperfusion produce less bleeding, and (3) compromised visualization following reperfusion can lead to incomplete releases of fascial compartments.

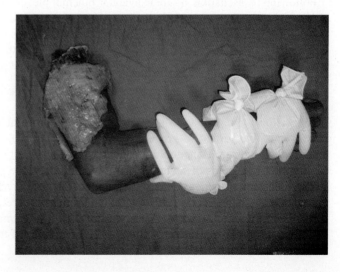

FIGURE 41-2

Technique of keeping the amputated part cool during dissection and later storage. Numerous glove bags with ice are placed all around the hand and wrapped with bandage.

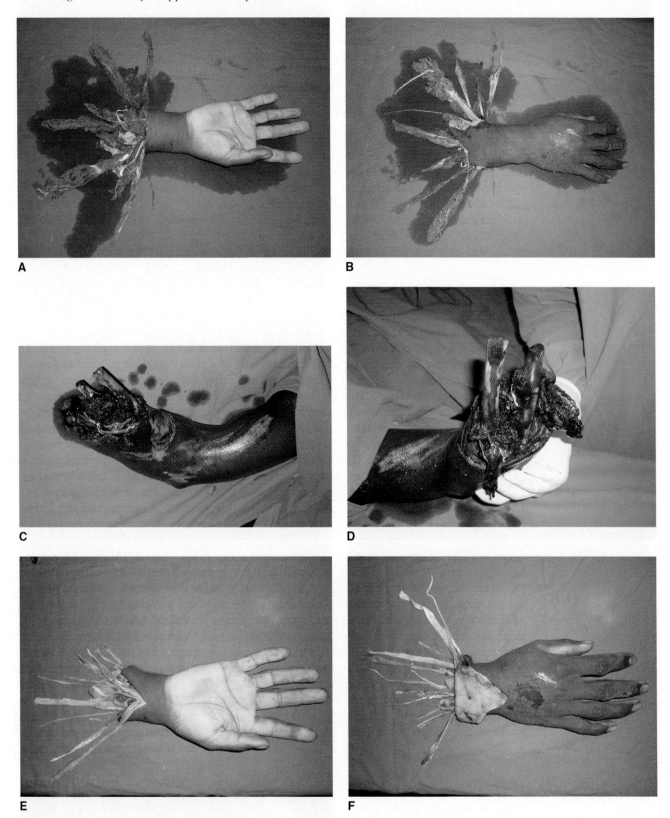

FIGURE 41-3

A–D: Avulsion amputation of the forearm. **E, F:** Postdebridement picture.

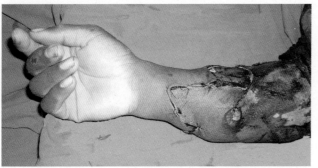

G

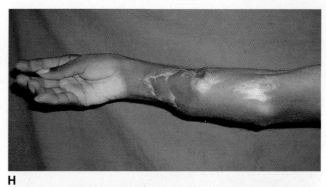

H

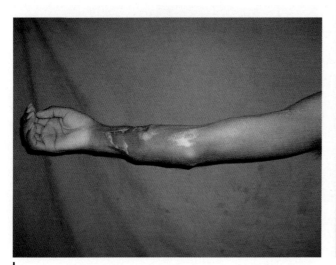

I

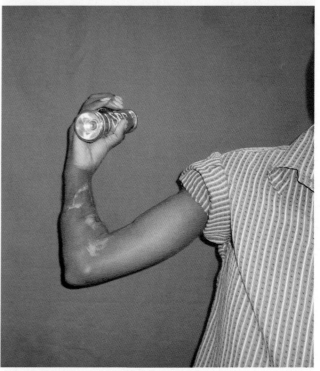

J

FIGURE 41-3 (*Continued*)

G: The tendons in the distal part are weaved into the proximal muscle, sutured and the replantation completed. **H–J:** Patient developed thumb-index side pinch and some flexion at the fingers to allow gross grip. **K:** Postoperative radiograph showing primary bone union.

K

Preliminary Vascular Shunting of the Amputated Part

In very proximal amputations and when the ischemia time approaches 3 to 4 hours, arterial shunting of the amputated part is advisable. The Ganga Hospital guideline for preliminary shunting and the sequence of steps in replantation are given in Table 41-1. This is based on the extent of injury and ischemic time at the time of arrival to the hospital. These guidelines are based on the premise that even in the best of the surgical centers, it will take at least 3 to 4 hours for the completion of the replantation, and this is taken into account while calculating the possible ischemia time of the muscles in the amputated part.

The simplest way of shunting is to keep the amputated part near the proximal stump and then introduce a silicone cannula into the proximal and the distal vessels and perfuse the distal part. A tight knot secures the cannula to the blood vessels and this segment of vessel will be excised during the definitive anastomosis. The limb is perfused for about 15 minutes. Significant blood loss is possible by this maneuver and one must be prepared to rapidly compensate the loss. If shunting is performed, the areas of muscle that do not perfuse are debrided. We do not know the optimum time for perfusion; however, we perfuse for about 10 to 15 minutes and feel that this gives us an hour of extra time for the completion of the replantation. Usually, two units of blood are transfused during the reperfusion process as blood will be lost through unrepaired veins.

Skeletal Fixation

Achieving primary bone union is the desired outcome in major replantation. Nonunion after a major replant is difficult to treat and nonunion will substantially delay rehabilitation. Internal fixation is our favored method of skeletal fixation during replantation. The fixation techniques that are chosen should be simple and quick and must ensure bone union. Skeletal fixation should take no more than 20 to 30 minutes. In many centers, failures in replantation have occurred due to the long time

| TABLE 41-1 Guidelines for Replantation Depending on the Level of Amputation ||||
Level of Amputation	Time from Injury to Arrival at Hospital	Decision to Replant	Technical Considerations
Proximal to midarm level	(i) ≤3 h	Replant	Debride; fix bone; do artery, vein, and nerve repair; and then release clamps (regular sequence).
	(ii) 3–4 h	Replant	Debride, fix bone, do artery first, release artery clamp to perfuse for 5 to 10 min, clamp artery, repair other structures, and then release arterial clamp only initially (venous clamp released after 5 min).
	(iii) 4–5 h	Replant	Use preliminary arterial shunting on arrival and then do the sequence as in (ii). If any delay occurs during procedure, the artery clamp can be released once every 30 min for 5 min.
	(iv) 5–6 h	Gray zone for replanting	Replant only if the fingers are freely passively mobile. Replant and do a proximal below-elbow amputation to gain length for prosthesis fitting.
	(v) >6 h	Do not replant	Consider replanting only if the part is very well preserved and kept cool especially in a child with lesser muscle mass.
Lower third arm and proximal forearm	(i) ≤4 h	Replant	Regular sequence. Preserve the elbow by shortening on nonjoint side.
	(ii) 4–6 h	Replant	Elbow arthrodesis enables more muscle debridement. Do artery first after bone fixation, release clamp for perfusion for 5 to 10 min, clamp artery, and then repair other structures. Then, release arterial clamp only initially (venous clamp released after 5 min).
	(iii) 6–7 h	Replant	Consider preliminary arterial shunting. Do replant only if the thumb is passively mobile and follow sequence as in (ii).
	(iv) >7 h	Do not replant	Consider replanting only if the part is very well preserved and kept cool especially in a child with lesser muscle mass.
Midforearm to wrist level	(i) ≤6 h	Replant	Regular sequence. Ensure excision of muscles attached to tendons in the amputated part.
	(ii) 6–8 h	Replant	Debride, fix bone, do artery first, release clamp, allow perfusion for 5 to 10 min, clamp artery, and then repair other structures.
	(iii) >8 h	Gray zone for replanting	Replant if the thumb is passively mobile.

From Sabapathy SR, Elliot D, Venkatramani H. Major replantation. In: Boyd B, Jones NF, eds. *Operative Microsurgery*. New York: McGraw-Hill; 2015.

taken for applying complex fixation. Rarely do we use external fixation; however, external fixation is occasionally needed in replants near the elbow with severe bone loss. The prime determinant for primary union is that the bone is debrided adequately. This is achieved by bone shortening. Bone ends with circumferential periosteal stripping and bone fragments without significant soft tissue attachments are removed. As a practical guide, bone is shortened to facilitate the repair of blood vessels and nerves. Up to 10 cm of shortening of bone in the arm or the forearm segment still provides acceptable cosmetic and functional outcome. In addition to ensuring good viable bone ends, bone shortening also helps to avoid the need for vein grafts, nerve grafts, and additional procedures for soft tissue cover. This significantly reduces the total operating time. When the amputation is very near the joint, shortening is preferably done in the portion of the limb not containing the joint. In amputation at the wrist, proximal row carpectomy is a good option for facilitating soft tissue closure and provides about 2 cm of shortening. Even in guillotine amputations, where there is minimal to no soft tissue loss, a couple of centimeters of bone shortening allows for easier vessels and nerves repair without any tension.

Bone gaps in segmental fractures and in avulsion amputation pose a particular reconstructive challenge. In such instances, immediate construction of one-bone forearm is a good option and can save substantial time (Fig. 41-4). When creating a one-bone forearm, the surgeon has to be mindful of hand position; the hand should be fixed either in midpronation or in midsupination to allow for accommodation of forearm position by remaining shoulder motion. A forearm that is fixed in full pronation is very difficult to rehabilitate.

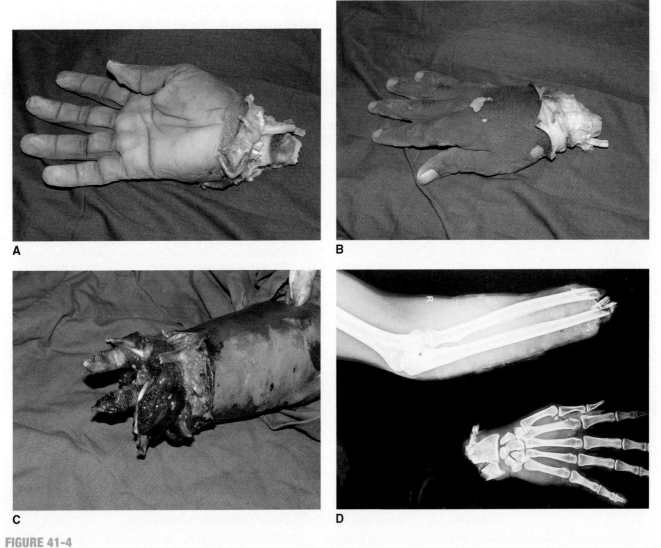

A 　　　　　　　　　　　　　　　　　　　　　　　**B**

C 　　　　　　　　　　　　　　　　　　　　　　　**D**

FIGURE 41-4

A–D: Crush amputation at the distal third of the forearm.

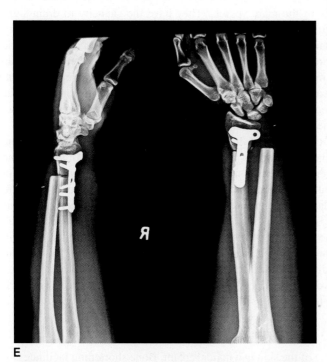

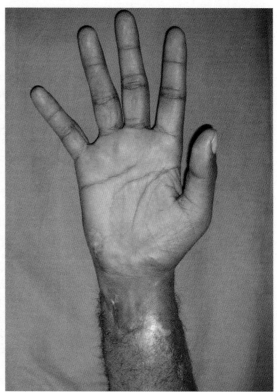

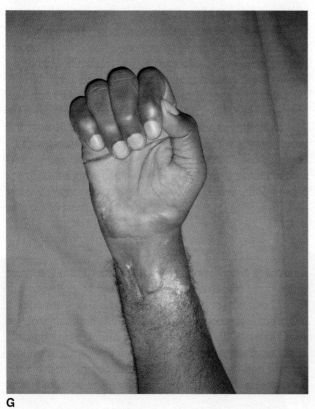

FIGURE 41-4 (*Continued***)**
E: Replantation by creating a one-bone forearm, since after debridement the distal ulna segment was very small.
F, G: Functional outcome at 2 years.

Repair of Vessels, Nerves, and Musculotendinous Units

The sequence of repair will depend upon the ischemia time and the level of amputation. A practical guideline is provided in the table (see Table 41-1). If the ischemia time is on the borderline (3 to 4 hours), it is preferable to repair the artery first. In this way, distal perfusion is established and the effluent blood is drained into the surgical field thus minimizing the amount of toxic metabolites reaching the kidneys once venous drainage is reestablished. If one is comfortable with the ischemia time, the basic musculotendinous units are repaired first to provide a good bed for the vessels and nerves. We repair as many veins as possible. In addition to superficial veins, we always look for and repair the venae comitantes of the main vessels. They have the capacity to drain significant amount of blood and postreperfusion hemorrhage is much less if the venae comitantes are repaired in addition to the major subcutaneous vessels. After circulation is established, the muscle viability is checked and any remaining nonviable muscle is removed. It is unknown if replanted limbs ever recover substantial collateral circulation, so the site of the primary vascular repairs needs to be protected with adequate soft tissue coverage, which will protect it from subsequent daily trauma. In addition, the sites of vascular repair should be carefully documented in the surgical note, so these sites may be avoided in subsequent surgical procedures.

While survival of the replant depends upon the patency of the vessel repairs, the functional outcome depends upon the recovery of the nerves and musculotendinous units. In avulsion amputations, if primary repair of the nerves is not possible, the nerves are banked in an easily acceptable subcutaneous plane and the location is marked on the surface of the skin. At 8 to 12 weeks following the initial surgery, a secondary procedure may be performed to repair the nerves. At this time point, the proximal nerve stumps can be located by a corresponding Tinel sign and the site of the distal nerve end is located by the markings on the skin. The nerve ends are identified through small incisions and nerve grafts are tunneled subcutaneously for repair. This avoids lengthy incisions with the risk of injury to the repaired blood vessels. This technique is useful in forearm replants, where extensive incisions are avoided during secondary reconstruction. In arm replants, incisions can be more liberally performed in the forearm (Fig. 41-5).

Providing Soft Tissue Cover

One must aim for primary healing of the skin in a major replant. Bone shortening facilitates primary skin closure and reduced the need for any additional flap or skin graft procedures. Even in instances where primary closure of skin is not possible, there is often available muscle to cover the repair site of critical structures allowing for subsequent simple skin graft closure. We do not recommend putting skin graft directly over vessels and nerve repair sites, as we are concerned that skin grafting alone does not provide long-term durable coverage. In addition, skin grafts can become infected or fail to take in the initial postoperative period; this could potentially lead to exposure and potential hemorrhage from the anastomotic sites. We have used local flaps, pedicle flaps, or free flaps to cover the critical structures (Fig. 41-6). In forearm replants, one vessel could be used to revascularize the distal part and the other vessel for a free flap to provide soft tissue coverage. "Flow-through" free flaps are preferable since additional arterial input is available. For smaller defects near the wrist, the posterior interosseous island flap is a good option.

The wound is always well drained with wide corrugated drains. The drain tip must be placed away from the vessel anastomosis site and placed such a way that no damage will occur when the drain is withdrawn.

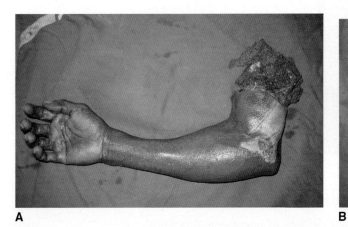
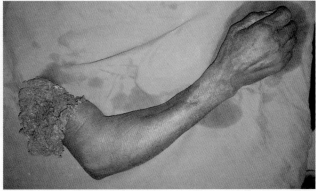

A **B**

FIGURE 41-5

A, B: Crush avulsion amputation at the level of the proximal third arm.

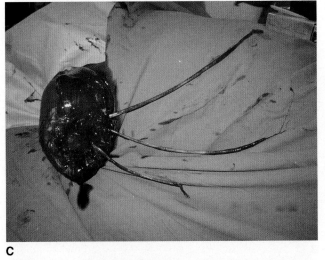

C

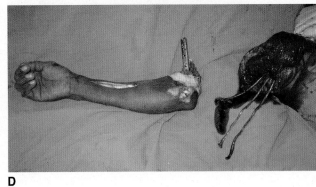

D

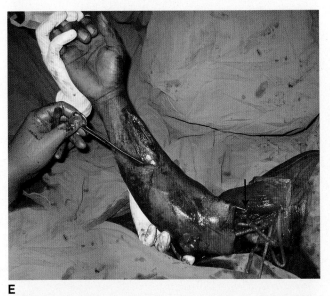

E

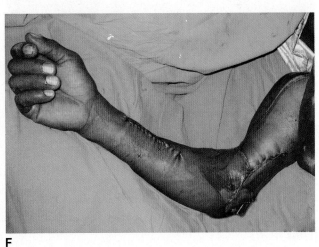

F

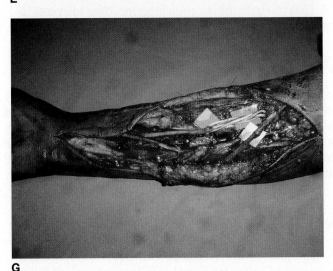

G

FIGURE 41-5 *(Continued)*

C: At debridement, long-segment avulsion of nerves was found. **D:** Proximal and distal segments after debridement before skeletal fixation. Note the fasciotomy incision in the forearm. Through this wound, all compartments are well released. Preplating is done in the distal segment. **E:** After replantation with the help of tendon tunneler, the nerves are tunneled. *Arrow* shows the tunneler picking up the nerve end. **F:** The nerve ends kept in subcutaneous plane and skin site marked. **G:** Secondary procedure for nerve grafting.

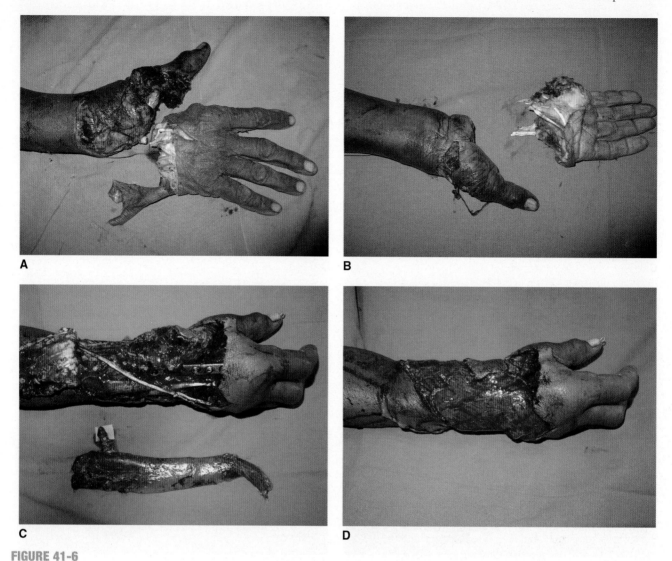

FIGURE 41-6

A: Avulsion amputation at the wrist level. **B:** Picture after debridement. **C:** Long vein grafts used for repair of vessels. Ulnar artery used for revascularization. A free gracilis flap has been harvested and ready for attachment. **D:** The gracilis flap has been attached to the radial artery.

Anticoagulation Regimen after Major Replants

We do not give any additional anticoagulants after major replants. When we perform digital replants, a bolus of heparin is given at the time of clamp release and it is followed up with 5,000 units of heparin given over 24 hours in normal saline. In proximal replants, this sometimes causes significant hemorrhage and hence we avoid it. We do sometimes give it in replants near the wrist level and when vein grafts have been used in avulsion amputations. Within the scientific literature, there is no level 1 or 2 evidence to support or refute the routine use of postoperative anticoagulation in major upper limb replants.

POSTOPERATIVE MANAGEMENT

The limb is immobilized in an above-elbow plaster leaving the fingers visible for observation. After a major replant, one needs to monitor for signs of kidney injury, infection, hypotension, and systemic inflammatory response syndrome (SIRS) as well as limb perfusion. Regular and repeated clinical observation by the same person is the best form of monitoring. After a major replant, the fingertips should have a normal capillary refill time. If the fingers are pale, it denotes arterial insufficiency; if the fingers are blue, it suggests venous insufficiency. If either of these events occur, the dressings need to be removed and the limb further assessed. For any concerns of vascular compromise, the surgeon should return the patient to the OR to better evaluate the limb. We continuously monitor pulse oximetry in the replanted hand. A sudden loss of the pulse oximetry signal should alert the surgeon to an arterial problem and a fall in saturation should arouse the suspicion of a venous thrombosis. Over the past 25 years, the combination of regular clinical observation combined with pulse oximetry has been reliable in alerting us to vascular problems.

COMPLICATIONS

Major replantation surgery shares the same general complications as any major surgical procedure, but reperfusion injury is the most feared complication as it may lead to kidney failure and mortality. Reperfusion injury is due to the by-products of anaerobic metabolism and cell death (myoglobin). These by-products are released into the general circulation following reperfusion and can cause acidosis and hyperkalemia. To avoid reperfusion injury, we keep the patient well hydrated and increase the intravenous fluid rate to 200 mL/h prior to reperfusion and clamp release. A 1 mEq/kg of 8.4% sodium bicarbonate is added to the intravenous fluids 3 minutes before clamp release. Myoglobin crystallizes in acidic urine, and hence, alkalization of urine is useful to prevent kidney damage. Following replantation, patients are placed on continuous electrocardiogram (EKG) monitoring. Signs of reperfusion injury, while under regional anesthesia, include restlessness, tachypnea, and difficulty in breathing. Tented T waves on the EKG are a warning sign for hyperkalemia. The urine dip will be positive for myoglobin, and the urine will be dark brown color in cases of myoglobinuria. If myoglobin is present in the urine, hydration should be increased to produce 100 to 150 mL of urine per hour. In addition, 100 mL of 20% mannitol (0.5 g/kg) is infused over a period of 20 minutes. Sodium bicarbonate infusions can also be repeated. If the myoglobinuria does not improve or if the patient continues to have significant EKG changes, one must consider removing the limb to prevent further kidney damage and the risk of cardiac arrest. If the serum potassium in the venous blood from the amputated part remains above 6.5 mmol/L, it is prudent to remove the replanted part.

If there are no signs of reperfusion injury at the time of clamp release, a close watch is kept in the postoperative period. The procedure could result in significant loss of blood and so hemoglobin levels are checked at the end of the operation and at 24 hours. Transfusion needs to be considered when hemoglobin levels are lesser than 8 gms%. Hemorrhage is another complication that is to be watched for. Hemorrhage in the early postoperative time period is usually due to a subcutaneous vein that has opened up during the rewarming and reperfusion period. Hematoma near the anastomotic sites is dangerous, and hence, we always leave drains following these procedures.

Sepsis and the SIRS are also major concerns following replantation. We have found that tachypnea is one of the initial signs of systemic problems. Usually, these patients are on mask oxygen and they may become tachypneic with fall in oxygen saturation when the oxygen support is removed for brief periods, like when taking food. One needs to reassess the patient in detail for sepsis as even small amounts of retained dead tissue or retained foreign material can be a nidus for infection. The wound is inspected for redness or drainage, and if any doubt exists, the wound is examined under brachial block. The sutures are removed and the status of muscles is inspected. If the superficial compartment muscles are ischemic, it is possible to save the replant by excising the muscles. If the whole of the deep compartment is ischemic, then it is not possible to preserve a functional replant and the arm should be removed. It is important to remember that the skin perfusion can be excellent (with the fingertip pulse oximetry reading 100%), but the underlying muscle may still be necrotic. If on secondary exploration there is ischemia of the deep compartment (particularly in an above-elbow replant), revision amputation is done.

Rehabilitation

Distal transradial amputations can be rehabilitated as one would rehabilitate a zone V tendon repair. For more proximal amputations, finger and wrist motion can begin once the tendon/muscle repairs have had time to heal. At 5 to 7 days, gentle passive motion can start in the fingers and wrist. Since nerve recovery will take many months, the prime responsibility is to keep the joints supple by appropriate splinting and mobilization. All patients will need a claw correction splint as most will develop intrinsic muscle palsy related to ulnar nerve injury. Secondary surgeries for nerve grafting or tenolysis are done between 8 and 12 weeks, when the wound has settled and the suture line is supple.

TABLE 41-2   Chen Criteria for the Evaluation of Function after Extremity Replantation

Grade	Function
I	a. Ability to resume original work with a critical contribution from the reattached parts
	b. Collective range of joint motion exceeds 60% of normal, including the joint immediately proximal to the reattached part
	c. Recovery of sensibility to a high grade without excessive intolerance of cold
	d. Muscular power of 4 to 5 on a scale of 1 to 5
II	a. Ability to resume some gainful work but not original employment
	b. Range of joint motion exceeds 40% of normal
	c. Recovery of near-normal sensibility in the median and ulnar nerve distributions without severe intolerance of cold
	d. Muscular power of grade 3 to 4
III	a. Independence in activities of daily living
	b. Range of motion of the joints exceeds 30% of normal
	c. Poor but useful recovery of sensibility (e.g., only median or ulnar recovery is good or quality is only protective in both median and ulnar areas)
	d. Muscular power of grade 3
IV	a. Tissue survival with no recovery of useful function

From Meyer VE. Hand amputations proximal but close to the wrist joint: prime candidates for reattachment (long-term functional results). *J Hand Surg Am.* 1985;10(6 pt 2):989–991.

RESULTS

We assess replant success according to the Chen Grading Scale (Table 41-2). We recently assessed the outcomes of 21 consecutive major crush (12) and avulsion (9) replantations with at least 2 years of follow-up. Six patients had achieved excellent results (Chen I), six had good results (Chen II), five had fair result (Chen III), and only four had poor results. Even the patients who had poor results used the hand in their day-to-day activities and said that they would advise other patients to have the procedure. Postreplant work status depends upon the type of work patients performed prior to injury. After replantation, patients with forearm guillotine amputations take about 6 months to go back to work, crush amputations 12 months, and avulsion amputations 15 months. In our experience of over two decades, we have found that all the patients use the replanted hand better as time goes on. Until an immunological breakthrough occurs and hand transplantation becomes safer for patients, replantation following major amputation will continue to be the best functional option for reconstruction following a major amputation of the upper limb.

PEARLS AND PITFALLS

- Replantation is the best method of reconstruction following a major upper limb amputation.
- Serious complications following major replants are related to the ischemia time and the extent of the muscle mass in the amputated part. Every effort must be made to revascularize the arm as soon as possible.
- Debridement in a major replant case has to be radical to prevent infection. Muscles attached to the avulsed distal tendons have to be excised. Perfusion status of the muscles is assessed after revascularization and debridement if necessary is done again.
- Bone shortening is a significant part of preparation of the operation. Technically, it makes fixation simpler, facilitates primary bone union, and in most instances avoids the use of vein and nerve grafts and additional soft tissue procedures for cover.
- Primary repair of all structures is encouraged. If primary nerve repair is not possible, the nerve ends are banked subcutaneously in easily accessible sites and a detailed note is kept of the procedure.
- If there are any signs of significant reperfusion injury, the care team must act decisively and remove the replant.
- Regular clinical examination is the best way of monitoring a major replant.
- Secondary procedures in major replants improve the functional status of the replant. Since major replants depend upon the repaired blood vessels for survival for long, injury to the repaired vessels has to be avoided during secondary procedures.

RECOMMENDED READING

Axelrod TS, Buchler U. Severe complex injuries to the upper extremity: revascularization and replantation. *J Hand Surg.* 1991;16(4):574–584.

Beris AE, Soucacos PN, Malizos KN, et al. Major limb replantation in children. *Microsurgery.* 1994;15(7):474–478.

Cavadas PC, Landín L, Ibáñez J. Temporary catheter perfusion and artery-last sequence of repair in macroreplantations. *J Plast Reconstr Aesthet Surg.* 2009;62(10):1321–1325.

Chin KY, Hart AM. Temporary catheter first perfusion during hand replantation with prolonged warm ischaemia. *J Plast Reconstr Aesth Surg.* 2012;65(5):675–677.

Chuang DC, Lai JB, Cheng SL, et al. Traction avulsion amputation of the major upper limb: a proposed new classification, guidelines for acute management, and strategies for secondary reconstruction. *Plast Reconstr Surg.* 2001;108(6):1624–1638.

Daigle JP, Kleinert JM. Major limb replantation in children. *Microsurgery.* 1991;12(3):221–231.

Graham B, Adkins P, Tsai TM, et al. Major replantation versus revision amputation and prosthetic fitting in the upper extremity: a late functional outcomes study. *J Hand Surg.* 1998;23(5):783–791.

Gulgonen A, Ozer K. Long-term results of major upper extremity replantations. *J Hand Surg (Eur).* 2012;37(3):225–232.

Laing TA, Cassell O, O'Donovan D, et al. Long term functional results from major limb replantations. *J Plast Reconstr Aesth Surg.* 2012;65(7):931–934.

Meyer VE. Hand amputations proximal but close to the wrist joint: prime candidates for reattachment (long-term functional results). *J Hand Surg Am.* 1985;10(6 pt 2):989–991.

Pinzur MS, Angelats J, Light TR, et al. Functional outcome following traumatic upper limb amputation and prosthetic limb fitting. *J Hand Surg.* 1994;19(5):836–839.

Russell RC, O'Brien BM, Morrison WA, et al. The late functional results of upper limb revascularization and replantation. *J Hand Surg Am.* 1984;9(5):623–633.

Sabapathy SR. Management of complex tissue injuries and replantation across the world. *Injury.* 2006;37(11):1057–1060.

Sabapathy SR. Secondary procedures in replantation. *Semin Plast Surg.* 2013;27:198–204.

Sabapathy SR, Elliot D, Venkatramani H. Major replantation. In: Boyd B, Jones NF, eds. *Operative Microsurgery.* New York: McGraw Hill; 2015.

Sabapathy SR, Venkatramani H, Bharathi RR, et al. Replantation surgery. *J Hand Surg.* 2011;36(6):1104–1110.

Sabapathy SR, Venkatramani H, Bharathi RR, et al. Technical considerations and functional outcome of 22 major replantations: the BSSH Douglas Lamb Lecture, 2005. *J Hand Surg (Eur).* 2007;32(5):488–501.

Wood MB, Cooney WP. Above elbow limb replantation: functional results. *J Hand Surg.* 1986;11(5):682–687.

Yaffe B, Hutt D, Yaniv Y, et al. Major upper extremity replantations. *J Hand Microsurg.* 2009;1(2):63–67.

42 Replantation of Digits

Sang-Hyun Woo

In traumatic amputation of one or more fingers, the decision of whether to perform microsurgical replantation or revision amputation depends on the condition of the amputation stump, the condition of the amputated parts, the level of injury, and the patients' medical condition. With the advancement of microsurgical techniques and microscope capabilities, the success rate of digital replantation has increased dramatically. Moreover, due to the cultural background of Asian countries, where physical appearance is of great importance, most hand and microsurgeons have tried to perform replantation at all levels and with all types of injury patterns.

Replantation of a digit is defined as the reattachment of all structural tissues following complete amputation. The term *revascularization* is used to refer to the repair of an incompletely amputated finger where there is some tissue still intact, but the digit is without arterial circulation. The term *ring avulsion* refers to cases where there is a circumferential laceration around the digit with intact tendon and bone. These injuries are due to a ring being forcefully pulled distally on the finger and result in the avulsion of the skin and underlying soft tissues. The severity of these injuries can vary from venous injury only to cases where both the artery and vein are avulsed. To help delineate what has been injured in cases of ring avulsion injury, we assess the bleeding pattern of the injured digit through a stab incision or by pricking the remaining skin. Dark brisk bleeding indicates an injury to the venous system, while minimal to no bleeding indicates an arterial injury.

INDICATIONS/CONTRAINDICATIONS

The indications for digital replantation have not changed significantly over the years and these include amputation of the thumb, amputation of more than one digit, and amputations in children. All indications for replantation must take into consideration the status of the amputated part and the mechanism of amputation (such as guillotine, crush, or avulsion), in addition to the overall health. The indications for replantation are not based solely on potential to get the finger to survive but are predicated on the potential for long-term function.

In the case of thumb amputation, replantation probably offers the best option for restoration of normal function. Even with poor motion and sensation, the thumb is useful to the patient as a post for opposition. Although single-finger replantation is generally not performed, replantation distal to the level of the flexor digitorum superficialis (FDS) tendon insertion usually results in good function. However, the replantation of a single digit amputated proximal to the insertion of the FDS should be an indication for revision amputation, as replantation at this level usually leads to a stiff proximal interphalangeal joint (PIPJ) that interferes with overall hand function. In cases of multiple-finger amputations, surgeons should try to reattach as many fingers as possible, as late toe transfer will not provide as good function as the native finger. In cases of multiple-finger amputation, some digits may be damaged severely for replantation. In these cases, the best amputated fingers can be heterotopically replanted to more important functional position such as thumb, index, and middle finger positions, to try to preserve as much hand function as possible.

Amputation of the digits in children is a clear indication for replantation, no matter whether it is single or multiple digits or whether the proximal or distal digit is amputated. Digital replantation in children is no longer a challenging procedure, and survival rates are increasing. With refinement of replantation techniques, the success rate is as high as in adults and the ultimate functional result is shown to be successful in long-term follow-up studies. Regarding the level of digital amputation, a classification suggested by Sebastin and Chung is adopted for description (Fig. 42-1).

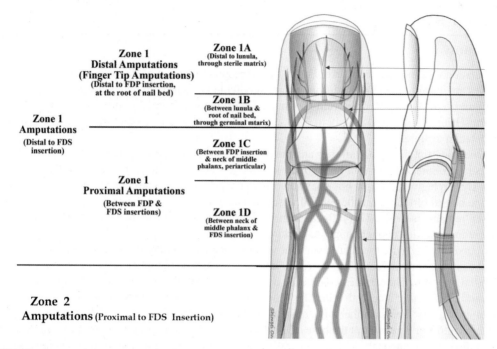

FIGURE 42-1

Amputation level of digit with digital arterial system. FDS(P), flexor digitorum superficialis (profundus).
(From Sebastin SJ, Chung KC. A systematic review of the outcomes of replantation of distal digital amputation.
Plast Reconstr Surg. 2011;128:725, with permission.)

Contraindications of replantation include severe systemic illness, life-threatening injuries, poorly social support system, or reluctance to have replantation surgery. Delayed replantation (after 48 hours of cold ischemia time) can be considered for patients with immediate life-threatening injuries that can be stabilized during the first 24 hours. Injury mechanism and amputation level are not absolute contraindications to replantation. Even in severe crushing injuries or very distal amputation, if the patient is insistent on replantation, the final decision to replant the digit can be made after exploration of the vessels in the operating room using the microscope. One exception to this is the case of multilevel or segmental amputation; in this case, we always recommend revision amputation. A past history of smoking has not been clearly shown to affect survival, but postoperative smoking does negatively affect surgical outcomes. Finally, age is not a contraindication to replantation. There is no difference in perioperative complications or mortality when comparing replantation in patients under and over 65 years of age.

PREOPERATIVE PLANNING

In the emergency room, tetanus prophylaxis and broad-spectrum antibiotic should be given depending on the condition of the wound. The discussion surrounding replantation should include the potential need for 5 to 7 days of hospitalization, the need for blood transfusion, the potential for emergency reexploration should the finger become ischemic, and the need for revision amputation or local flap coverage should the replantation fail. Patients should also be informed that most will require additional surgery in the future to improve the function as well as appearance of the digits.

When the patient arrives in the emergency room, one should rule out concomitant injuries and screen for any medical problems that would preclude an extended operative procedure for replantation. The mechanism of amputation should be obtained. The amputated part should be wrapped in gauze moistened with lactated Ringer's or saline solution and placed inside a watertight vinyl bag, which is then placed on ice or in the refrigerator. *To avoid permanent tissue damage to the amputation stump, it should not be put in direct contact with ice or immersed into ice water.* If the operating room is available, the amputation stump should be explored and prepared in advance under a microscope before the patient comes to the room. This can also determine if the part is suitable for replantation or if it has been damaged beyond what is replantable.

SURGERY

Anatomy

Amputation level is described according to the corresponding zone of flexor tendon injury. Zone 1 injuries are distal to the FDS insertion and are subdivided into proximal and distal according to the insertion site of the flexor digitorum profundus (FDP) tendon. Zone 2 injuries are proximal to the FDS insertion. The arterial supply to each zone is important to understand prior to a discussion of replantation technique.

In the fingertip, the digital arteries and nerves trifurcate near the distal interphalangeal joint. The two palmar digital arteries join in the midline at the level of lunula to form the distal digital palmar arch. This arch gives multiple branches adjacent to the periosteum. The central palmar artery is usually the largest of these branches and of adequate size for end-to-end anastomosis in cases of zone 1 distal replants (see Fig. 42-1). Because these arteries are very tortuous, pulling a tortuous vessel straight may provide enough length to avoid vein grafting.

Around the fingertip, there are abundant venous channels composed of superficial dorsal veins and the palmar central vein. The superficial dorsal veins are the main channels for venous drainage from the fingertip. The venules commence at the sides of the fingernail and converge proximal to the nail bed, forming a central vein. The vein divides into two or three branches after passing 2 to 4 mm proximally. Veins on the palmar aspect of the finger begin as a network at the fingertip and converge into 1 or 3 venules at the base of the distal phalanx. The largest vein runs proximally along the midline subcutaneously and two lateral veins run along the lateral side of the neurovascular bundles. These veins can be used in arteriovenous anastomoses, venocutaneous fistulas, or even delayed venous repairs to increase the likelihood of successful replantation.

An understanding of neurovascular anatomy of the digits in zone 2 is very important to shorten the operation time. To find the digital artery and nerve quickly, the operator should know the location by looking at the surface anatomy. The position of the digital nerve can be easily determined by first fully flexing the finger; when the finger is flexed, the most dorsal aspect of both proximal interphalangeal and distal interphalangeal joint flexion creases should be marked with a dot. Connecting a line between these dots shows the course of the digital nerve. The digital nerve runs with the digital arteries along the sides of each finger. Because the digital nerves are approximately 2 to 3 mm in diameter, they are much easier to identify than the smaller digital artery. Locating the nerve is the easiest way to find the digital artery. The digital artery is always located on the dorsolateral aspect of the digital nerve (Fig. 42-2). Each finger has a dominant digital artery. The dominant artery of each finger is usually located closer to the midline. In the index finger, the ulnar digital artery is dominant, and in the little finger, the radial digital artery is dominant. In the middle and ring fingers, ulnar and radial digital arteries are dominant respectively, but dominance is less obvious.

One should also be familiar with the arterial supply to the thumb as positioning the hand for thumb replantation can often obscure the underlying arterial anatomy. The princeps pollicis artery is present on the ulnar aspect of the thumb at the level of the middle of the thumb metacarpal and

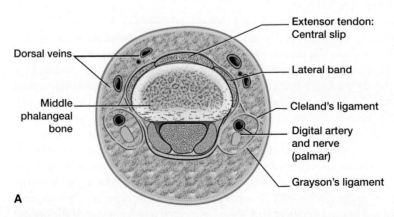

FIGURE 42-2

A: Cross-section of digit and **(B)** midlateral incision for digital artery and nerve exposure.

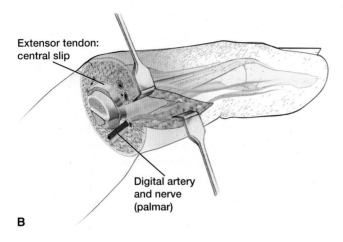

Extensor tendon:
central slip

Digital artery
and nerve
(palmar)

B

FIGURE 42-2 (*Continued*)

is the origin of the radial and ulnar digital arteries. Occasionally, the digital arteries will originate from the palmar metacarpal artery. Dorsally, the dorsal ulnar artery is always present and originates mainly from the princeps pollicis artery. The dorsal radial artery is a direct branch of the radial artery. There are several anastomoses between the radial and ulnar digital arteries and between the dorsal and palmar systems.

Anesthesia and Patient Positioning

For adults or older children, a brachial plexus block placed under ultrasound guidance with sedation is recommended. Long-acting regional anesthesia can maintain pain-free status even after the operation as well as provide vasodilatation of the affected extremity. An axillary nerve block with an infusion mixture of 20 mL 2% lidocaine, 20 mL 0.75% ropivacaine, 10 mL normal saline, and 1 mL epinephrine keeps the patient pain free for 8 to 10 hours. Postoperative use of indwelling pain catheters is not recommended because of concerns about hematoma formation secondary to anticoagulation protocols used following replantation. A pneumatic tourniquet is placed on the upper arm. Preparation and cleansing of the stump and amputated part are performed in the usual manner. In cases of multiple digital amputations, a central venous catheter or large-caliber intravenous line should be placed in case there is a need for blood transfusion. A urine catheter is placed for monitoring of fluid status.

Technique

The sequence of surgery varies slightly among surgeons, but the standard operative sequence for digital replantation is as follows: (1) debridement and identification of structures, (2) bone fixation, (3) extensor tendon repair, (4) flexor tendon repair, (5) anastomosis of artery, (6) digital nerve repair, (7) anastomosis of vein, and (8) closure of the wounds.

Debridement and Identification of Structures

The initial step of the replantation is cleansing and debridement of the wound. Gentle surgical preparation and debridement of obviously devitalized tissue can convert a localized crush injury to a sharp injury. The critical structures are then identified and tagged. At least 1 cm of digital artery should be dissected free. Arteries are then tagged with 6-0 black silk for easy and quick locating after later bone fixation and tendon repair. A longitudinal midlateral incision placed slightly volar to the midaxial line is made on both sides of the severed digit and extended to the next joint. Through this incision, a volar and dorsal flap can be elevated. During dissection of the two dorsal and volar flaps, the thickness should be constant to avoid late necrosis. The longitudinal incisions over the vascular pedicles are sometimes difficult to close without compressing the pedicles. In zone 1 amputation, a straight incision around the end of the dominant vascular pedicle is preferred. During debridement and exploration, intact skin bridges should be maintained as they may contain patent veins.

Technique

Bone Fixation

The importance of stable bone fixation cannot be emphasized enough, as finger stability aids in the subsequent steps of replantation and aids in ability to begin early motion. In guillotine-type injury patterns where the zone of injury is narrow, direct contact between the ends of fractured bone allows easy fixation; however, in most cases, bone shortening is essential. Bone shortening allows one to create two congruent bone ends for fixation and it many times allows for primary artery and nerve repair and skin closure without grafts or flaps. Bone shortening from the amputated segment is preferred in order to maintain the maximum stump length if the replantation fails.

The method of bone fixation depends on the fracture pattern and level of skeletal injury relative to the joints. There are many suggested fixation methods including the use of longitudinal Kirschner wires, interosseous wires, screws and plates, intramedullary wires or bone pegs, absorbable rods, and external fixators (Fig. 42-3). Intraosseous wire fixation is a quick and secure method of bony

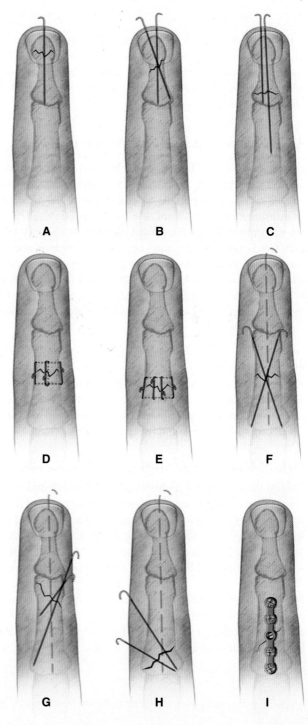

FIGURE 42-3

A–C: Distal phalangeal bone fixation with Kirschner wire dependent on fracture site. **A:** Single longitudinal K-wire at tuft fracture. **B:** Cross two K-wire for shaft fracture. **C:** Double longitudinal K-wire for base fracture. **D–I:** Middle phalangeal bone fixation with Kirschner wire or screw, *dotted line* shows temporary fixation for 2 to 3 weeks after operation. **D:** 90-90 intraosseous wiring. **E:** Three 90-90 intraosseous wiring. **F–H:** Crossed K-wire. **I:** Single-screw fixation.

fixation for digital replantation. Fixation of the diaphyseal fractures is recommended with interosseous wiring, consisting of 2 wires oriented at 90 degrees to each other, with or without the addition of an oblique K-wire. Preparation for this 90-90 wiring technique can begin on the back table where two tunnels, one radial to ulnar and one dorsal to volar, are made with a 21-gauge needle in the amputated finger at the proximal bone end. The 21-gauge needle allows a 26-gauge wire to pass through the tunnel easily. Transarticular amputations are usually fused with two K-wires for the DIP joint. Two intraosseous wires with a lag screw technique or tension band wiring with two parallel Kirschner wires are appropriate for arthrodesis of PIPJ.

Tendon Repair

Before flexor and extensor tendon repair, periosteum repair should be performed when possible. Repaired periosteum can provide a smooth gliding surface for the tendons and also will cover any exposed wires or metal plates following bone fixation. Tendon repair should be as strong as possible to allow early mobilization. In zone 1 and zone 2 injuries, extensor repairs are performed with a running 5-0 Prolene sutures. For zone 3 or 4 extensor tendon repairs, a modified 4-0 Kessler suture is used with 5-0 or 6-0 running epitendinous suture. A Silfverskiöld cross-stitch epitendinous repair may be useful. In amputations at the proximal phalanx, repair of the lateral bands of the extensor tendon is essential to get an appropriate extension of the distal joints. In extensor tendon repair of the thumb, modified Becker suture or Silfverskiöld cross-stitch with braided polyester 4-0 (Ti-Cron) suture is recommended.

For flexor tendon repair, a four-strand or more core suture technique with 4-0 nonabsorbable suture is preferred. In zone 2 injuries, repair of only the FDP tendon may be undertaken to avoid adhesions between the FDS and FDP tendon suture lines; however, we prefer to repair both the FDP and FDS if possible. FDS repair can provide independent PIPJ motion as well as a gliding surface for the FDP. Repairing the proximal profundus to distal superficialis tendon is another option to get flexion in cases of significant injury to the substance of the distal FDP.

Vessel and Nerve Repair

To facilitate successful arterial anastomosis, adventectomy should be performed by pulling the adventitia of the arterial ends horizontally and then removing it with sharp-ended microscissors under an operating microscope. Removal of the adventitia helps prevent arterial spasm and thrombus formation. Adequate resection of the proximal vessel is verified by seeing spurting blood from the cut end. The proximal vessel should be trimmed back until it is free of adventitial bruising and free of intraluminal thrombus. A curling shape to the vessel (also known as the ribbon sign) seen under the microscope indicates vessel injury. Persistent spasm or thrombus indicates a damaged proximal artery and the artery should be resected back further. Before performing the anastomosis, the vessel should be flushed with a dilute heparin solution at a concentration of 100 units/mL.

To overcome arterial gap, undamaged adjacent arteries may be shifted from inside the same finger or another finger. Transposition of vascular pedicles is very useful for replantation of avulsion amputation of the thumb. However, the use of vein grafts is easier, quicker, and more reliable. Depending on the amputation level, selection of donor sites of the vein graft is very important to minimize discrepancy of diameter between the vein graft and the artery. In zone 1 amputation, sections of vein graft shorter than 1 cm can be harvested from volar aspect of the PIPJ crease to digitopalmar crease. Where vein grafts of longer than 1 cm are needed, the harvesting from the thenar area is appropriate (Fig. 42-4).

For zone 2 amputation, vein graft can be harvested from the thenar eminence to volar aspect of the wrist. All vein grafts should be marked and reversed when used for arterial reconstruction because even the smallest digital veins contain valves. To match the arterial defect, measuring the vein graft in situ before division is probably the best way to avoid making it too short or too long. The technique of anastomosis of the proximal end first and filling the graft with blood assures the vein graft is at its natural length. The effect of intravenous injection of heparin is controversial, but it is necessary in cases of severe crush or avulsion amputation.

In the case of thumb replantation, visualizing the palmar arterial repair is very difficult after bone fixation. Occasionally, in these cases, artery repair can precede bone fixation. Temporary fixation of the metacarpophalangeal joint with a K-wire is very helpful to prevent kinking of the repaired artery.

Tension on the anastomosis or excessive handling of the intima can cause arterial thrombosis or spasm. If the proximal arterial anastomosis is patent and blood flow to the finger is absent or weak,

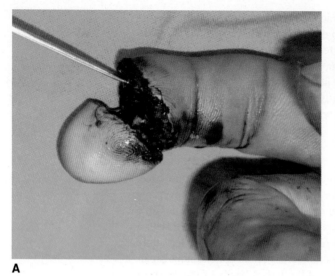

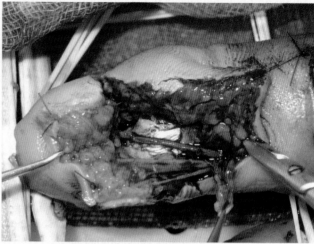

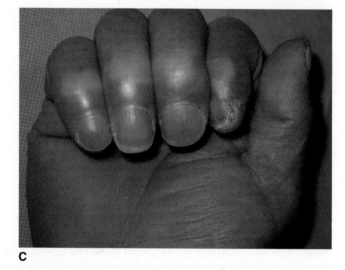

FIGURE 42-4

A: A 50-year-old man suffered a crushing amputation of his right index tip. **B:** Vein graft of about 1.3 cm was harvested from the volar aspect of the thenar area. Ulnar digital artery was anastomosed to central palmar artery with vein graft and one volar vein was repaired. **C:** Six months after revascularization of the index.

one must suspect that there is microvascular occlusion or spasm in the amputated part. One should also remember that there are several factors besides vessel condition that can affect blood flow to the amputated part; these include the patient's temperature, the patient's hydration status, systolic blood pressure, and any more proximal injuries.

After anastomosis of the artery, one or two veins are selected for venous anastomosis. We try to choose the veins that are actively draining the most blood. In zone 2, we prefer to repair at least two veins. If two arteries have been repaired, then we prefer to repair at least three veins. To increase the number of anastomosed veins, it may be necessary to mobilize or harvest adjacent branches of the vein. The biggest mistake in vein anastomosis is attempting to perform the repair under tension, so small vein grafts should be used liberally. Maintaining venous drainage is the key to successful replantation because venous insufficiency is the most common cause of replantation failure. In distal tip amputation, performing venous anastomosis avoids external bleeding and can produce higher survival rates (Fig. 42-5). In zone 1 amputations, dorsal veins as well as volar vein can be used to restore venous outflow.

In very distal replants, it may not be possible to identify veins dorsally. In such cases, delayed venous repair can be attempted. Postoperative venous congestion during the first 48 hours can result in dilatation of distal veins, allowing for easier identification and anastomosis. Delayed venous anastomosis with vein graft increases the success rate of distal phalangeal replantation as well as reducing external bleeding. In cases where vein repair is not possible, the use of medicinal leeches or external bleeding with a topical heparinized saline solution can be used in combination with hyperbaric oxygen therapy to help overcome venous congestion.

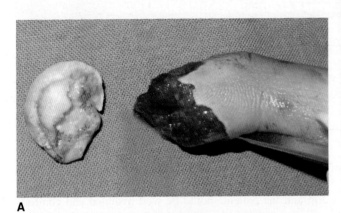

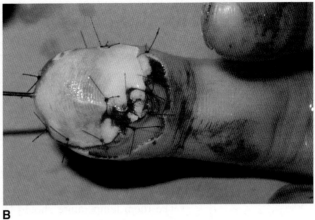

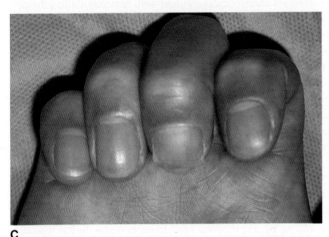

FIGURE 42-5

A: A 45-year-old man suffered a crushing amputation of his right long fingertip. **B:** After longitudinal K-wire fixation, central palmar artery was repaired. External bleeding with medical leech was applied for 5 days. **C:** Twelve months after operation.

In most replants, nerve repair is not difficult because of the amount of bone shortening. Epineurial repair of digital nerve is performed with 8-0, 9-0, or 10-0 nylon sutures. Only two or three sutures are necessary to repair these small nerves. A short defect of the nondominant digital nerve is reconstructed with a vein conduit. We feel this technique is appropriate for defects of less than 2 cm in length. Nerve conduits consisting of collagen or polyglycolide can also be used. When a nerve graft is required, we prefer to use the posterior intraosseous or medial antebrachial cutaneous nerve of the forearm. In multiple-digit amputations, nerve grafts may be taken from the discarded digits.

Soft Tissue Repair

During skin closure, one must be sure not to create pressure over the repaired vessels. One tight stitch can result in venous congestion. When there is an open wound, it may need a skin graft or local flap to cover the vascular pedicles. In the case of a soft tissue defect of the volar aspect with artery or vein, a venous flap can be useful to cover tendons as well as the artery or veins. Furthermore, when there is a composite defect of the tendon, or soft tissue and vessel together in a digit, composite venous free flap with vein or palmaris longus tendon from the ipsilateral volar wrist is recommended.

POSTOPERATIVE MANAGEMENT

Circulation status should be checked frequently (once every hour) in microsurgical intensive care unit by experienced nursing staff. Capillary refill, temperature, and the color of replanted digits are monitored hourly (Table 42-1). When the circulation of the digit is in question, pricking the finger with a needle is the most accurate means of judging perfusion. Normally, there should be rapid light pink bleeding from the pinprick site; however, in arterial insufficiency, there will be a scant amount

TABLE 42-1	Monitoring of Circulation in Replanted Digit		
	Normal	**Arterial Occlusion**	**Venous Insufficiency**
Color	Pink	Pale or white pink	Dark pink or purple
Capillary refilling	Fast	Very slow	Very fast
Temperature	Warm	Cold	Warm-cool
Turgor	Full	Hollow	Swollen
Bleeding	Bright red	Minimal, only serum	Dark red or purple

of dark blood or just serum. In cases of venous congestion, there is rapid dark red or purple bleeding following finger pricking.

The room temperature should be warm and the patient should be well hydrated and comfortable to avoid peripheral vasospasm. Intravenous antibiotics combined with anticoagulation therapy vary according to the conditions of the replant. The use of intravenous heparin does not correlate with higher success rates of replantation but has been associated with a threefold increase in local complications. Despite the risks, heparin therapy may be warranted in cases of intimal damage by crush and avulsion injuries, intraoperative thrombus, or following successful thrombolysis and arteriosclerotic changes.

The rehabilitation protocol is started at the bedside with early protective motion. According to the specific condition of replantation, the surgeon and therapist discuss the regimen schedule with a particular emphasis on maintaining the range of motion in noninjured digits. Psychological support and occupational counseling are important factors in long-term postoperative care.

RESULTS

One prospective replantation series of 1,018 digits reported a survival rate of 92%. A recent report of cases of multiple digital replants showed an 87.5% survival rate. Even in distal digital replantation, survival rates have been reported at 76% to 85%. In a recent meta-analysis of 4,678 amputated digits in 2,641 patients, age, injured hand, injury type, zone, and the method of preservation of the amputated digit were found to significantly influence the survival rate of digital replantation, while delayed replantations demonstrate result that are comparable to immediate replantation in regard to graft survival and clinical outcome.

Functional outcomes following fingertip replantation vary according to the level of injury. PIPJ range of motion averages 35 degrees after the replantation of a single digit proximal to the FDS insertion but averages 82 degrees when replantation is performed distal to the insertion of the FDS tendon. According to Chen's criteria, an excellent result following replantation includes the patient returning to his vocation with more than 60 degrees of active range of motion and almost normal sensation without cold intolerance. Active range of motion of the PIPJ is greater in successful replantation than in patients undergoing amputation through the middle phalanx.

Sensory recovery of digital nerve repair depends on the patient's age, with younger patients obtaining better results. It has been shown that in pediatric cases with no repair of the digital nerves, normal sensation can still return in the distal pulp. The average two-point discrimination after the replantation of sharply amputated fingers in adults averages 8 mm but only averages 15 mm after crush and avulsion cases.

Pediatric Replantation

Compared with digital amputations in adults, the indications for replantation in children is very broad. Crush and avulsion injuries from bicycle and mechanical sports equipment are common mechanisms for amputation in children and should not be considered contraindications for replantation. Bone fixation of finger replants in children is preformed with K-wires rather than plate and screws due to finger size (Fig. 42-6). Sensory recovery is much better than in adults due to improved regenerative capabilities of children. According to the long-term follow-up studies of pediatric replants, the success rate is 88% and the growth rate of the digit is 86% compared to the contralateral digits.

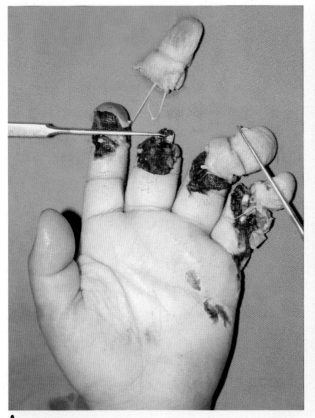

A

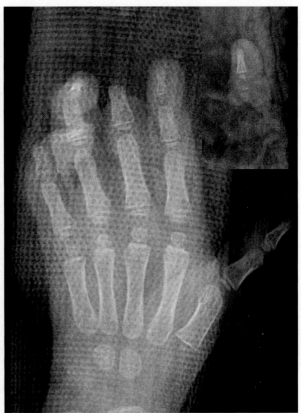

B

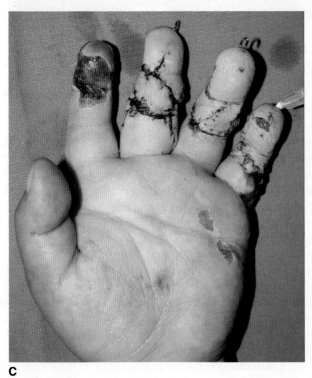

C

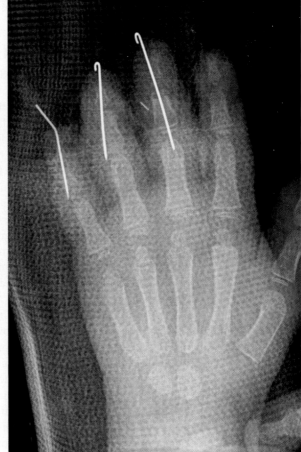

D

FIGURE 42-6

A: A 34-month-old baby sustained amputation by a running machine. The left long finger was completely amputated in zone 1 and the ring and small finger were incompletely amputated at the level of the middle phalanx. **B:** Preoperative radiograph. **C:** Immediate postoperative view after successful replantation and revascularization. **D:** Immediate postoperative radiograph.

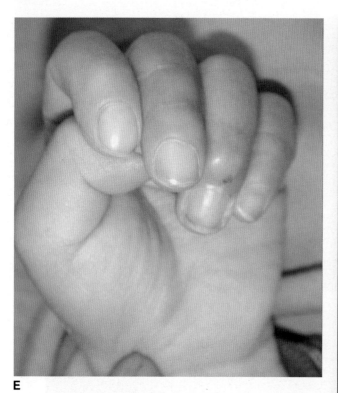

E

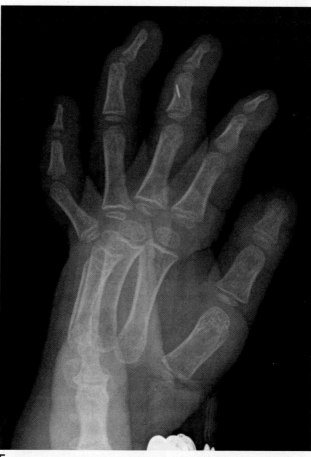

F

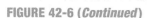

FIGURE 42-6 (*Continued*)
E, F: A 9-month follow-up demonstrating excellent range of motion of fingers.

Thumb Avulsion and Ring Avulsion Amputation

The force applied to soft tissue in avulsion injuries creates a zone of injury that extends beyond the actual skin disruption. Primary anastomosis of blood vessels in these cases is not possible because of the extent of intimal injury to the vessels during the accident. Vein grafting will be required in almost all cases.

In cases of thumb avulsions, a midlateral incision along the side of the thumb is necessary to dissect the vessel proximal until no evidence of intimal injury is seen. Transposition of an artery from the healthy digit or vein grafting will be required to restore blood flow. The stretched, avulsed digital nerve ends are cut back until healthy fascicles are found. Occasionally, a nerve coaptation is carried out in the carpal tunnel at the point of avulsion from the median nerve. If a choice has to be made between repairing one of the digital nerves to the thumb, the ulnar digital nerve should be repaired. In the case of severe stretch damage of both digital nerves, the radial digital nerve should be used as a graft to reconstruct the ulnar digital nerve. In these cases, it is common to find tendons avulsed from their muscle belly in the forearm or avulsed from lumbricals in the hand (Fig. 42-7). Optimal management of the tendon injuries in these cases is challenging; however, there are many options for avulsed tendon reconstruction, including resection alone, reattachment of the tendon, immediate tendon transfers, side-to-side repair, and staged reconstruction. Reattachment of the flexor pollicis longus (FPL) tendon to its muscle belly and direct repair of the extensor pollicis longus tendon (EPL) is most promising in the recovery of function. An immediate tendon transfer of the fourth FDS for FPL and extensor indicis proprius transfer to EPL are our second choice in these cases. The soft tissues are closed without tension wherever they approximate easily. If not, a skin graft is used to cover the exposed dorsal subcutaneous tissues and the venous anastomoses.

In cases of ring avulsion, the best indication for replantation is those cases that occur distal to the insertion of the FDS with a functioning PIPJ. Replantation will require either long reverse venous interposition grafts or transfer of a digital artery from an adjacent digit and at least two dorsal vein repairs. Additional flap coverage is often necessary for the late necrosis of soft tissue on the volar or dorsal aspects of the finger (Fig. 42-8). Both success rate and functional results for replantation

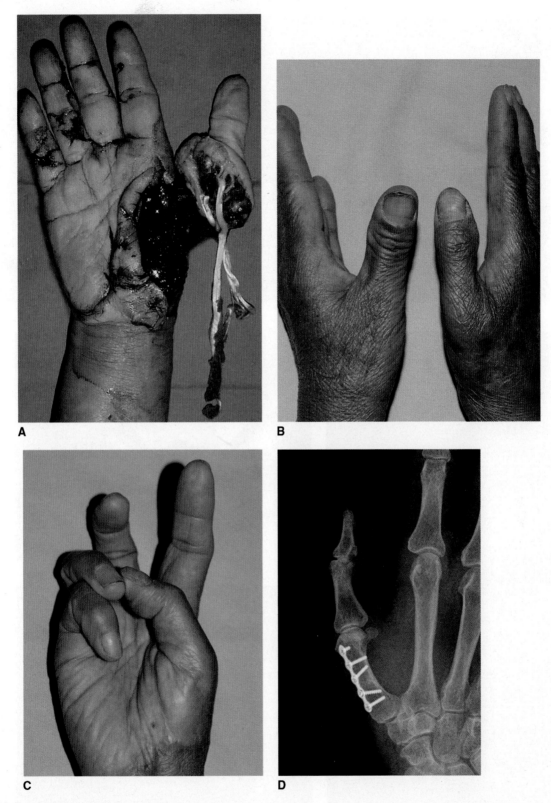

FIGURE 42-7

A: A 58-year-old man suffered an avulsion amputation of his right thumb. The thumb was fractured at the middle shaft of the metacarpal bone. Skin envelope was avulsed proximally near the level of the metacarpal shaft area. Princeps pollicis arteries were avulsed from the superficial radial artery at the snuffbox. The digital nerves were avulsed proximally near the level of the wrist. The FPL tendon was avulsed at the level of the musculotendinous junction. The FPL tendon was reattached to its muscle belly and direct repair of the extensor pollicis longus tendon was carried out by modified Becker technique. Princeps pollicis artery was reconstructed with vein graft from the volar aspect of wrist and two dorsal veins were repaired. **B, C:** Nine months after replantation of the thumb. **D:** Postoperative radiograph showing secure fixation of the metacarpal shaft with plate and screws.

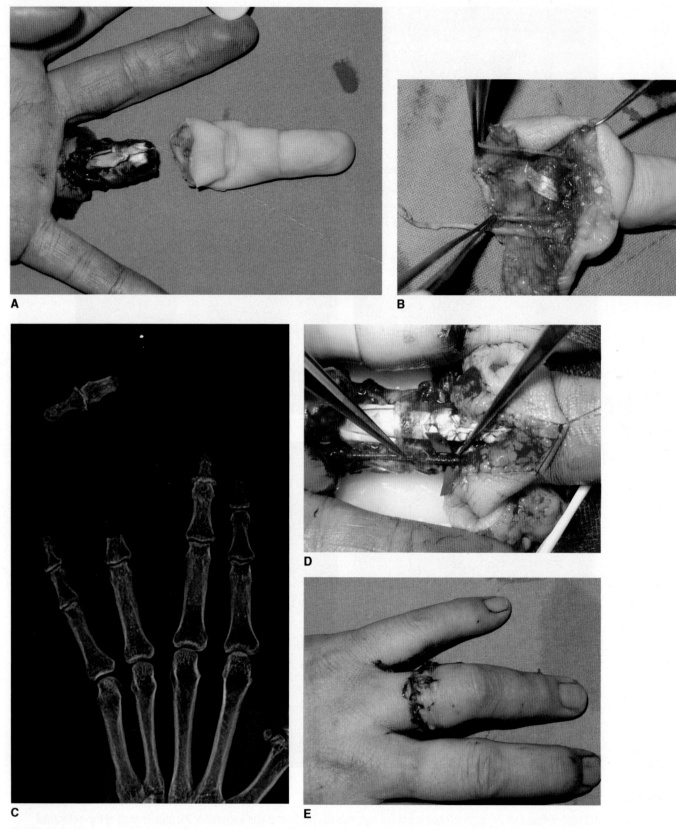

FIGURE 42-8

A: A 43-year-old woman sustained ring avulsion amputation by henhouse chicken wire. The left ring finger was completely avulsed with intact PIPJ. **B:** Both digital artery and nerve were avulsed. **C:** Radiograph showed amputation at the proximal one-third of middle phalangeal bone. **D:** Ulnar digital artery was anastomosed with vein graft about 1.2 cm from the volar aspect of the PIPJ. Proximal radial digital nerve was transposed to the distal ulnar digital nerve. **E:** Immediate after the operation.

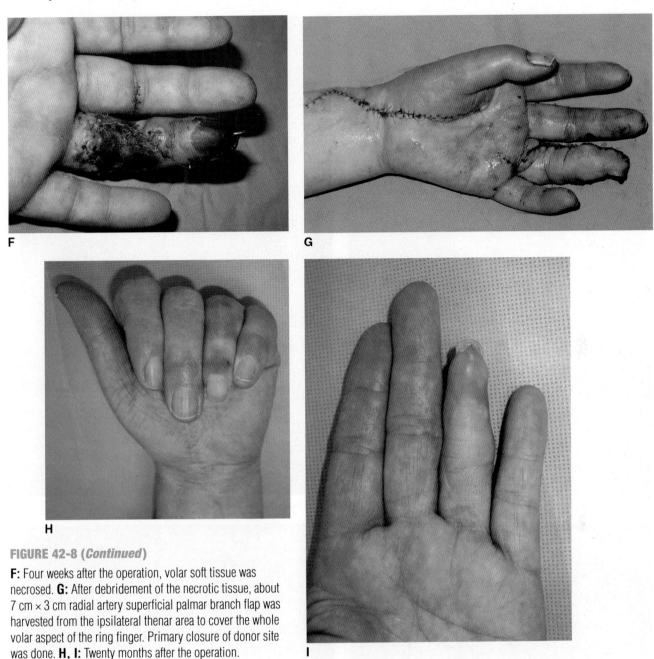

FIGURE 42-8 (*Continued*)

F: Four weeks after the operation, volar soft tissue was necrosed. **G:** After debridement of the necrotic tissue, about 7 cm × 3 cm radial artery superficial palmar branch flap was harvested from the ipsilateral thenar area to cover the whole volar aspect of the ring finger. Primary closure of donor site was done. **H, I:** Twenty months after the operation.

in cases of ring avulsion have been considered unsatisfactory. The mean survival outcome rate in complete avulsion injuries varies from 66% to 78%. Most fingers, if salvaged, will require additional procedures for tenolysis.

Multiple-Digit/Heterotopic Replantation

These cases can be very long and attention needs to be given to managing the patient's fluid status and hemodynamics. To reduce operative time, we prefer to replant all digits simultaneously and perform a structure-by-structure repair during replantation instead of replanting each finger in sequence. Cold ischemic time at this level of amputation does not affect the survival rate and final functional results of the replanted digits. To decrease the amount of blood loss, we utilize the tourniquet intermittently throughout the case (Fig. 42-9). The need for vein grafts, tendon grafts, and skin grafts can also be avoided by the shortening of the phalangeal bone during osteosynthesis. In cases of bilateral amputation, intentionally delayed or suspended replantation is a good option for one hand to allow time for the patient to stabilize hemodynamically and give the surgical team time to rest.

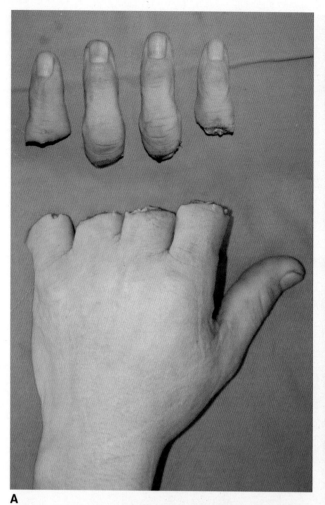

A

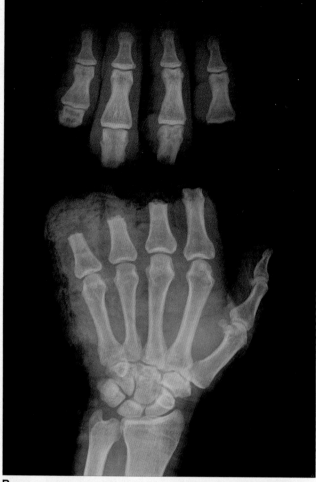

B

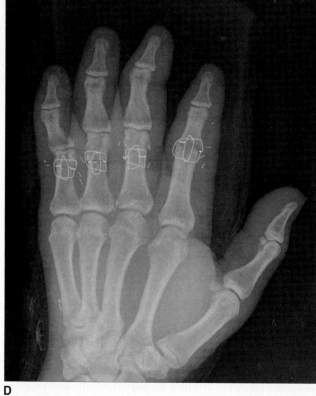

C

D

FIGURE 42-9

A, B: A 38-year-old man suffered from a sharp cutting injury on
the left hand by a machine saw. The left index was amputated at
PIPJ and the long, ring, and small finger were amputated at the
proximal phalanx. **C:** According to the structure-by-structure
sequence of replantation, all amputated stumps were debrided
and digital nerve and artery were tagged with 6-0 black silk.
Perpendicular 90-90 degree intraosseous wires were passed
on the fracture site. Operation time was 7 hours 45 minutes
and total amount of transfusion was 3 points. **D:** Postoperative
radiograph. The PIPJ of the index finger was fused.

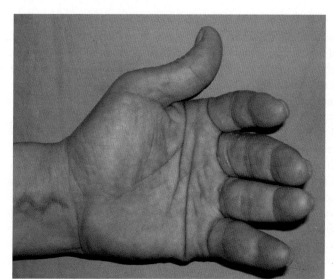

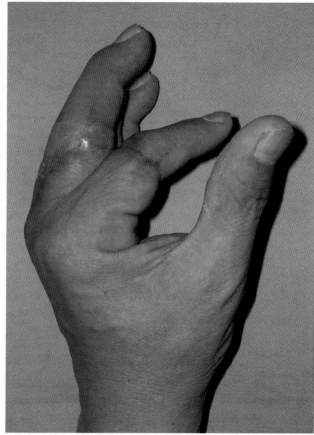

FIGURE 42-9 (Continued)
E, F: At 7 months follow-up, the patient had a limited range of motion, which required secondary tenolysis and wire removal. **F**

To achieve maximal pinch or grasp function in cases of multiple-finger amputation, the technique of heterotopic or transposition replantation is often used. In such cases, the amputated digits with the least damage are chosen for replantation. Function can also be improved when the fingers with the least damage are replanted into the most useful positions. For example, an amputated digit can be used to substitute for a nonreplantable thumb. With index or long finger replantation, emphasis should be placed on achieving stable key pinch, tripod pinch, and opposition grip.

COMPLICATIONS

Early Complications

Early complications include bleeding, infection, and soft tissue necrosis. A significant amount of bleeding suggests venous insufficiency. Bleeding decreasing hemoglobin in cases of pediatric or multidigit replantation can result in hypovolemic shock. Anticoagulation therapy exacerbates this situation. If the blood is seen outside of the dressing as well as concealed inside a bulky dressing, hemoglobin should be checked and anticoagulation should be stopped. To definitively resolve bleeding, the threshold of reexploration should be low.

In cases of postoperative arterial insufficiency, the dressing should be removed and the flaps inspected for hematoma or excessive tension. Return to the operating room is often the best plan as this allows one to inspect the anastomosis directly. In cases of arterial thrombosis, resection of a thrombosed vessel followed by reanastomosis with a healthy artery or vein graft is the best means of restoring blood flow. In cases of venous congestion, loosening of the tight dressing and removal of skin stitches are the first steps to resolve congestion. If there is no improvement after 20 minutes, return to the operating room for reexploration and reanastomosis of the vein will be necessary. Venous oozing or drainage through small minor veins should be controlled with ligation to allow one or two dominant veins to dilate. These dominant veins should be selected for reanastomosis. In distal replantation, salvage by leech therapy or external bleeding through the incision of the nail bed or pulp area is best as there are often few remaining veins for anastomosis. If the venous congestion happens 2 or 3 days after the initial surgery, reexploration may harm the neovascularization of the replanted parts. This is rather common in the case of venous occlusion associated with infection. In these cases, leeches may be needed to support the finger until new venous channels are established. The most feared complication of leech use, however, is an infection from the bacterium *Aeromonas hydrophila*. The incidence of this infection ranges from 2.4% to 20%, with clinical presentations ranging from cellulitis or abscess to extensive soft tissue infections causing tissue loss and systemic sepsis. Routine antimicrobial prophylaxis with a fluoroquinolone should be used for cases of leech therapy.

The long-term patency of the microanastomosed digital arteries after successful replantation varies. In spite of successful replantation, the pulsation of Doppler and angiography reveals occlusion of the arteries in 37% of vessels after an average of 15 postoperative days. Therefore, early wound healing of the soft tissue is critical to allow for neovascularization of the replanted finger. In crush amputation cases, neovascularization of the replanted part occurs slowly. In these cases, we have seen replantation failures after 1 week to 10 days postoperatively. Radical debridement of the soft tissue, as well as apposition between fresh tissues, is essential at the completion of the case. In cases of soft tissue defects following replantation, local or free flaps are necessary.

The worst complication in the early postoperative period is replantation failure. Failed distal replants can be allowed to mummify and be left in situ to act as a dressing for the underlying stump. In children, in young women, and in multiple-digit amputation, preservation of middle phalangeal bone length at the time of revision amputation is important to preserve hand competence and prevent objects from slipping through the hand. Later, secondary reconstruction with toe-to-hand transfer is possible only where at least 1 cm of the middle phalangeal bone remains.

Late Complications

Thirty percent to 40% of patients need one or two secondary procedures after replantation. In our opinion, a secondary operation is almost a necessity for the improvement of both function and appearance of the digits. Thirty percent to 50% of replantation has problems related to bony healing. Nonunion rates range from 10% to 30% with K-wire fixation having the highest nonunion rates. Malunion rates are about 20% with screw fixation being associated with the highest rates of malunion. Intraosseous wires alone were found to have the lowest nonunion and complication rate. In cases of rotational deformity or nonunion, secondary revision with corrective osteotomy and internal fixation with or without bone graft are needed. To improve joint motion, artificial joint insertion or toe joint transfer is another option depending on the condition of the tissues surrounding the joint.

The indications for flexor tendon tenolysis of the replanted digits are almost the same as the general indications for tenolysis following isolated flexor tendon injury. These include significant discrepancy between passive and active flexion of the digital joints after a substantial period of more than 6 months. This allows sufficient time for wound healing and maximal rehabilitation therapy. The result of tenolysis after digital replantation is a useful and safe procedure to achieve an improvement in the active flexion of the digit. After tenolysis, secondary tendon rupture or subsequent bone fracture may happen due to aggressive rehabilitation. In extensor tenolysis, any hardware used in bone fixation should be removed at the same time. An intrinsic reconstruction and dorsal arthrolysis and capsulotomy are worthwhile when active and passive flexions are present. Certain procedures such as tenolysis, capsulotomy, and arthrolysis are performed together because all these procedures need no immobilization.

Soft tissue atrophy or cold intolerance of surviving replants is closely related with the type of injury and patency of microanastomosed arteries. Cold intolerance is present in most replanted digits and may or may not improve after 2 years. Normal thermoregulatory response returns as sensibility recovers.

PEARLS AND PITFALLS

- The only absolute contraindication for replantation is the case where the patient is medically unstable to tolerate the operation.
- Radical debridement of damaged soft tissue is a necessity for rapid wound healing.
- Bone shortening and rigid fixation shortens operation time and allows for more rapid rehabilitation.

- Tendon repair of both extensor and flexor should be performed with a four-strand repair. Periosteal repair provides a gliding surface for tendons.
- Meticulous repair of vessel guarantees survival of replantation and careful nerve repair ensures recovery of sensation.

RECOMMENDED READING

Backman C, Mystrom A, Backman C, et al. Arterial spasticity and cold intolerance in relation to time after digital replantation. *J Hand Surg Br.* 1993;18:551.

Barzin A, Hernandez-Boussard T, Lee GK, et al. Adverse events following digital replantation in the elderly. *J Hand Surg Am.* 2011;36:870.

Buncke GM, Buntic RF, Romeo O. Pediatric mutilating hand injuries. *Hand Clin.* 2003;19:121.

Chen ZW, Meyer VE, Kleinert HE, et al. Present indications and contra-indications for replantation. In: Watson HK, Weinzweig J, eds. *The Wrist.* Philadelphia, PA: Lippincott Williams & Wilkins; 2001:269–276.

Cheng GL, Pan DD, Zhang NP, et al. Digital replantation in children: a long-term follow-up study. *J Hand Surg Am.* 1998;23:635.

Chung KC, Alderman AK. Replantation of the upper extremity: indications and outcomes. *J Hand Surg Am.* 2002;2:78.

Faivre S, Lim A, Dautel G, et al. Adjacent and spontaneous neurotization after distal digital replantation in children. *Plast Reconstr Surg.* 2003;111:159.

Giladi AM, McGlinn EP, Shauver MJ, et al. Measuring outcomes and determining long-term disability after revision amputation for treatment of traumatic finger and thumb amputation injuries. *Plast Reconstr Surg.* 2014;134:746e.

Hanasono MM, Butler CE. Prevention and treatment of thrombosis in microvascular surgery. *J Reconstr Microsurg.* 2008;24:305.

Han SK, Lee BI, Kim WK. Topical and systemic anticoagulation in the treatment of absent or compromised venous outflow in replanted fingertips. *J Hand Surg Am.* 2000;25:659.

Hattori Y, Doi K, Ikeda K, et al. A retrospective study of functional outcomes after successful replantation versus amputation closure for single fingertip amputations. *J Hand Surg Am.* 2006;31:811.

Hattori Y, Doi K, Sakamoto S, et al. Fingertip replantation. *J Hand Surg Am.* 2007;32:548.

Hoffman R, Buck-Gramcko D. Osteosynthesis in digital replantation surgery. *Ann Chir Gynaecol.* 1982;71:14.

Ikeda K, Yamauchi S, Hashimoto F, et al. Digital replantation in children: a long-term follow-up study. *Microsurgery.* 1990;11:261.

Jones JM, Schenck RR, Chesney RB. Digital replantation and amputation: comparison of function. *J Hand Surg Am.* 1982;7:183.

Kay S, Werntz J, Wolff TW. Ring avulsion injuries: classification and prognosis. *J Hand Surg Am.* 1989;14:204.

Kim WK, Lee JM, Lim JH. Eight cases of nine-digit and ten-digit replantations. *Plast Reconstr Surg.* 1996;98:477.

Kleinert HE, Cash SL. Current guideline for flexor tendon repair within the fibro-osseous tunnel: Indication, timing and technique. In: Hunter JM, Schneider LH, Mackin EJ, eds. *Tendon Surgery in the Hand.* St. Louis, MO: CV Mosby; 1987:117–125.

Koshima I, Yamashita S, Sugiyama N, et al. Successful delayed venous drainage in 16 consecutive distal phalangeal replantations. *Plast Reconstr Surg.* 2005;115(1):149.

Kwon GD, Ahn BM, Lee JS, et al. Clinical outcomes of a simultaneous replantation technique for amputations of four or five digits. *Microsurgery.* 2016;36(3):225–229.

Lee CH, Han SK, Dhong ES, et al. The fate of microanastomosed digital arteries after successful replantation. *Plast Reconstr Surg.* 2005;116:805.

Lim BH, Tan BK, Peng YP. Digital replantations including fingertip and ring avulsion. *Hand Clin.* 2001;17:419.

Lineaweaver WC, Hill MK, Buncke GM, et al. *Aeromonas hydrophila* infections following use of medicinal leeches in replantation and flap surgery. *Ann Plast Surg.* 1992;29:238.

Meuli-Simmen C, Canova M, Bollinger A, et al. Long-term follow up after finger and upper limb replantation: clinical, angiologic, and lymphographic studies. *J Reconstr Microsurg.* 1998;14:131.

Morrison WA, O'Brien BM, MacLeod AM. Evaluation of digital replantation: a review of 100 cases. *Orthop Clin North Am.* 1977;8:295.

Nikolis A, Tahiri Y, St-Supery V, et al. Intravenous heparin use in digital replantation and revascularization: the Quebec provincial replantation program experience. *Microsurgery.* 2011;31:421.

Povlsen B, Nylander G, Nylander E. Cold-induced vasospasm after digital replantation does not improve with time: a 12-year prospective study. *J Hand Surg Br.* 1995;20:237.

Rawles RB, Deal DN. Treatment of the complete ring avulsion injury. *J Hand Surg Am.* 2013;38:1800.

Scott FA, Howar JW, Boswick JA Jr. Recovery of function following replantation and revascularization of amputated hand parts. *J Trauma.* 1981;21:204.

Sears ED, Chung KC. Replantation of finger avulsion injuries: a systematic review of survival and functional outcomes. *J Hand Surg Am.* 2011;36:686.

Sebastin SJ, Chung KC. A systematic review of the outcomes of replantation of distal digital amputation. *Plast Reconstr Surg.* 2011;128:723.

Shi D, Qi J, Li D, et al. Fingertip replantation at or beyond the nail base in children. *Microsurgery.* 2010;30:380.

Soucacos PN, Beris AE, Touliatos AS, et al. Current indications for single digit replantation. *Acta Orthop Scand Suppl.* 1995;264:12.

Urbaniak JR, Roth JH, Nunley JA, et al. The results of replantation after amputation of a single finger. *J Bone Joint Surg Am.* 1985;67:611.

VanderWilde RS, Wood MB, Zu ZG. Hand replantation after 54 hours of cold ischemia: a case report. *J Hand Surg Am.* 1992;17:217.

Waikakul S, Sakkarnkosol S, Vanadurongwan V, et al. Results of 1018 digital replantations in 552 patients. *Injury.* 2000;31:33.

Wei FC, Chang YL, Chen HC, et al. Three successful digital replantation in a patient after 84, 86, and 94 hours of cold ischemia time. *Plast Reconstr Surg.* 1988;82:346.

Weiland AJ, Villarreal-Rios A, Kleinert HE, et al. Replantation of digits and hands: analysis of surgical techniques and functional results in 71 patients with 86 replantations. *J Hand Surg Am.* 1977;2:1.

Whitney TM, Lineaweaver WC, Buncke HJ, et al. Clinical results of bony fixation methods in digital replantation. *J Hand Surg Am.* 1990;15:328.

Woo SH, Cheon HJ, Kim YW, et al. Delayed and suspended replantation for complete amputation of digits and hands. *J Hand Surg Am.* 2015;40:883.

Woo SH, Kim KC, Lee GJ, et al. A retrospective analysis of 154 arterialized venous flaps for hand reconstruction: an 11-year experience. *Plast Reconstr Surg.* 2007;119:1823.

Woo SH, Kim YW, Cheon HJ, et al. Management of complications relating to finger amputation and replantation. *Hand Clin.* 2001;31:319.

Xu JH, Gao ZJ, Yao JM, et al. Foster replantation of fingertip using neighbouring digital artery in a young child. *J Plast Reconstr Aesthet Surg.* 2010;63:e532.

Index

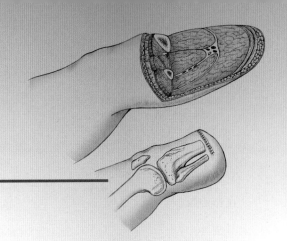

Note: Page numbers in *italics* indicate figures. Page numbers ending in *t* indicate tables.